Pediatric Neurocritical Care

Pediatric Neurocritical Care

Nicholas S. Abend, MD

Assistant Professor of Neurology and Pediatrics
Division of Neurology,
    The Children's Hospital of Philadelphia
Departments of Neurology and Pediatrics,
    Perelman School of Medicine at the
    University of Pennsylvania
Philadelphia, Pennsylvania

Mark A. Helfaer, MD

Professor Anesthesiology and Critical Care,
    Pediatrics, and Nursing,
Division of Critical Care Medicine,
    The Children's Hospital of Philadelphia
Department of Anesthesiology and Critical Care,
    Perelman School of Medicine at the
    University of Pennsylvania
Philadelphia, Pennsylvania

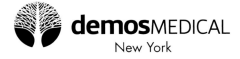
demosMEDICAL
New York

Visit our website at www.demosmedpub.com

ISBN: 978-1-936287-35-2
e-book ISBN: 9781617050695

Acquisitions Editor: Beth Barry
Compositor: The Manila Typesetting Company

Medicine is an ever-changing science. Research and clinical experience are continually expanding our knowledge, in particular our understanding of proper treatment and drug therapy. The authors, editors, and publisher have made every effort to ensure that all information in this book is in accordance with the state of knowledge at the time of production of the book. Nevertheless, the authors, editors, and publisher are not responsible for errors or omissions or for any consequences from application of the information in this book and make no warranty, express or implied, with respect to the contents of the publication. Every reader should examine carefully the package inserts accompanying each drug and should carefully check whether the dosage schedules mentioned therein or the contraindications stated by the manufacturer differ from the statements made in this book. Such examination is particularly important with drugs that are either rarely used or have been newly released on the market.

Library of Congress Cataloging-in-Publication Data

Abend, Nicholas S.
 Pediatric neurocritical care / Nicholas S. Abend, Mark A. Helfaer.
   p. ; cm.
 Includes bibliographical references and index.
 ISBN 978-1-936287-35-2 -- ISBN 978-1-61705-069-5 (e-book)
 I. Helfaer, Mark A. II. Title.
 [DNLM: 1. Child. 2. Trauma, Nervous System—therapy. 3. Critical Care—methods. WS 340]
 618.92'0028—dc23

                                                    2012035967

Special discounts on bulk quantities of Demos Medical Publishing books are available to corporations, professional associations, pharmaceutical companies, health care organizations, and other qualifying groups. For details, please contact:

Special Sales Department
Demos Medical Publishing, LLC
11 West 42nd Street, 15th Floor
New York, NY 10036
Phone: 800-532-8663 or 212-683-0072
Fax: 212-941-7842
E-mail: rsantana@demosmedpub.com

Made in the United States of America by Bang Printing.
12 13 14 15 / 5 4 3 2 1

I dedicate this book to my wife, Gayle. I could not have completed it without her daily encouragement and dedication to our family. Her professional efforts to improve the lives of children and their families continually inspire me. I am very appreciative of my parents' guidance and support. They have consistently demonstrated the value of working to help others while still making family a priority. I am very grateful for the support and encouragement of the many superb clinicians and neuroscientists with whom I have trained and worked. I particularly thank Harold Burton, Frances Jensen, Stephen Back, V. Leo Towle, Robert Clancy, Dennis Dlugos, Rebecca Ichord, Daniel Licht, Gihan Tennekoon, and Donald Younkin.

Nicholas S. Abend

I am grateful for a full and gratifying professional life focused on pediatric critical care and anesthesiology. The dovetail of this clinical focus has been in research in the area of neuropathophysiology. I am indebted to a host of trainees, collaborators, mentors, students, and teachers. I am also indebted to non-physicians including nurses, nurse practitioners, respiratory therapists, pharmacists, and so many others, without whom the entire enterprise would collapse, and of course to my family; especially Michele, Sam, and Jon, without whom life would not be nearly as much fun and certainly not as rewarding.

Mark A. Helfaer

Contents

Contributors

Nicholas S. Abend, MD
Assistant Professor of Neurology and Pediatrics
Division of Neurology, The Children's Hospital of
    Philadelphia
Departments of Neurology and Pediatrics, Perelman
    School of Medicine at the University of Pennsylvania
Philadelphia, PA
Approach to Acute Encephalopathy and Coma
Electroencephalography in Critically Ill Children
Hyperthermic Drug-Induced Disorders
Movement Disorders

Saba Ahmad, MD
Fellow in Child Neurology
Division of Neurology, The Children's Hospital of
    Philadelphia
Philadelphia, PA
Hyperthermic Drug-Induced Disorders
Movement Disorders

Stephen Ashwal, MD
Professor of Pediatrics
Department of Pediatrics, Loma Linda University
    School of Medicine
Loma Linda, CA
Brain Death

Lauren A. Beslow, MD, MSCE
Instructor of Child Neurology
Departments of Pediatrics and Neurology,
    Yale University School of Medicine
New Haven, CT
Nontraumatic Intracerebral Hemorrhage and
    Subarachnoid Hemorrhage
Neurologic Complications in Pediatric
    Cardiac Disease
Spinal Cord Disease and Injury
Cerebral Venous Sinus Thrombosis
Arterial Ischemic Stroke

Elena Cavazzoni, MD, PhD
Attending Intensivist and Clinical Lecturer
The Children's Hospital at Westmead
Discipline of Pediatrics & Child Health,
    University of Sydney
Sydney, Australia
Approach to Intracranial Pressure Management

Melissa G. Chung, MD
Former Chief Resident in Child Neurology
Division of Pediatric Neurology, Children's Memorial
    Hospital
Chicago, IL
Fellow in Pediatric Critical Care and Pediatric Stroke
Divisions of Critical Care and Neurology, Nationwide
    Children's Hospital
Columbus, OH
Status Epilepticus and Seizures

Basil T. Darras, MD
Joseph J. Volpe Professor of Neurology
Harvard Medical School
Division of Clinical Neurology, Neuromuscular
    Program, Boston Children's Hospital
Boston, MA
Neuromuscular Disorders

Dennis J. Dlugos, MD, MSCE
Associate Professor of Neurology and Pediatrics
Division of Neurology, The Children's Hospital of
    Philadelphia
Departments of Neurology and Pediatrics, Perelman
    School of Medicine at the University of Pennsylvania
Philadelphia, PA
Electroencephalography in Critically Ill Children

Tom Drake, MD
Adjunct Assistant Professor of Pediatrics
UMDNJ-Robert Wood Johnson Medical School at
    Camden

Pediatric Rehabilitation, Division of Neurology,
    Children's Regional Center at Cooper
Cooper University Hospital
Camden, NJ
Rehabilitation: Indications, Management, and Timing

Chris Feudtner, MD, PhD, MPH
Stephen D. Handler Endowed Chair of Medical Ethics
    and Associate Professor of Pediatrics
Department of Medical Ethics, The Children's Hospital
    of Philadelphia
Department of Pediatrics, Perelman School of Medicine
    at the University of Pennsylvania
Philadelphia, PA
Ethical Issues

Can Ficicioglu, MD, PhD
Associate Professor of Pediatrics
Section of Metabolism, The Children's Hospital of
    Philadelphia
Department of Pediatrics, Perelman School of Medicine
    at the University of Pennsylvania
Philadelphia, PA
Acute Metabolic Encephalopathy

Stuart H. Friess, MD
Assistant Professor of Anesthesiology, Critical Care
    Medicine, and Pediatrics
Division of Critical Care Medicine, The Children's
    Hospital of Philadelphia
Department of Anesthesiology and Critical Care,
    Perelman School of Medicine at the
    University of Pennsylvania
Philadelphia, PA
Mechanical Ventilation and Blood Pressure Management
Traumatic Brain Injury

Joshua L. Goldstein, MD
Assocciate Professor of Pediatrics
Division of Pediatric Neurology, Davee Pediatric
    Neurocritical Care Program, Anne and Robert H.
    Lurie Children's Hospital
Feinberg School of Medicine of Northwestern
    University
Chicago, IL
Status Epilepticus and Seizures

Abby M. Green, MD
Fellow in Infectious Diseases
Division of Infectious Diseases, The Children's Hospital
    of Philadelphia

Philadelphia, PA
Central Nervous System Infections

Fred Henretig, MD
Professor of Pediatrics and Emergency Medicine
Director, Section of Clinical Toxicology
Department of Pediatrics, The Children's Hospital of
    Philadelphia
Department of Pediatrics, Perelman School of Medicine
    at the University of Pennsylvania
Philadelphia, PA
Neurotoxicology

Gregory G. Heuer, MD, PhD
Assistant Professor of Neurosurgery
Division of Neurosurgery, The Children's Hospital of
    Philadelphia
Department of Neurosurgery, Perelman School of
    Medicine at the University of Pennsylvania
Philadelphia, PA
*Nontraumatic Intracerebral Hemorrhage and
    Subarachnoid Hemorrhage*

Jimmy Huh, MD
Assistant Professor of Anesthesiology, Critical Care
    Medicine, and Pediatrics
Division of Critical Care Medicine, The Children's
    Hospital of Philadelphia
Department of Anesthesiology and Critical Care,
    Perelman School of Medicine at the
    University of Pennsylvania
Philadelphia, PA
Traumatic Brain Injury

Robert Hurst, MD
Professor of Radiology
Department of Radiology, Perelman School of
    Medicine at the University of Pennsylvania
Philadelphia, PA
*Diagnosis and Endovascular Management of
    Cerebrovascular Malformations*

Rebecca N. Ichord, MD
Associate Professor of Neurology and Pediatrics
Division of Neurology, The Children's Hospital of
    Philadelphia
Department of Neurology and Pediatrics, Perelman
    School of Medicine at the University of Pennsylvania
Philadelphia, PA
Cerebral Venous Sinus Thrombosis

Stephen Jacobe, MD
Clinical Associate Professor and Attending Intensivist
The Children's Hospital at Westmead
Discipline of Pediatrics & Child Health University of Sydney
Sydney, Australia
Approach to Intracranial Pressure Management

Stacey J. Jacovini, M Arch
Research Assistant
Division of Neurosurgery, The Children's Hospital of Philadelphia
Department of Neurosurgery, Perelman School of Medicine at the University of Pennsylvania
Philadelphia, PA
Neurosurgical Postoperative Monitoring and Complications

H. Royden Jones, Jr., MD
Clinical Professor of Neurology
Harvard Medical School
Boston, MA
Jaime Ortiz-Patino Chair in Neurology
Lahey Clinic
Burlington, MA
Electromyography Laboratory, Boston Children's Hospital
Boston, MA
Neuromuscular Disorders

Lori C. Jordan, MD, PhD
Assistant Professor of Neurology and Pediatrics
Director, Pediatric Stroke Program
Division of Pediatric Neurology, Monroe Carell, Jr. Children's Hospital at Vanderbilt
Nashville, TN
Nontraumatic Intracerebral Hemorrhage and Subarachnoid Hemorrhage

Sudha Kilaru Kessler, MD
Assistant Professor of Neurology and Pediatrics
Division of Neurology, The Children's Hospital of Philadelphia
Departments of Neurology and Pediatrics, Perelman School of Medicine at the University of Pennsylvania
Philadelphia, PA
Approach to Acute Encephalopathy and Coma

Todd J. Kilbaugh, MD
Assistant Professor of Anesthesiology, Critical Care

Medicine, and Pediatrics
Division of Critical Care Medicine, The Children's Hospital of Philadelphia
Department of Anesthesiology and Critical Care, Perelman School of Medicine at the University of Pennsylvania
Philadelphia, PA
Mechanical Ventilation and Blood Pressure Management
Traumatic Brain Injury

Matthew P. Kirschen, MD, PhD
Fellow in Pediatric Critical Care and Child Neurology
Divisions of Critical Care Medicine and Neurology, The Children's Hospital of Philadelphia
Departments of Anesthesiology, Critical Care, and Neurology, Perelman School of Medicine at the University of Pennsylvania
Philadelphia, PA
Ethical Issues

Michael J. Kramarz, BSE
Kevin Heaney and Judi Marvel Research Fellow
Division of Neurosurgery, The Children's Hospital of Philadelphia
Department of Neurosurgery, Perelman School of Medicine at the University of Pennsylvania
Philadelphia, PA
Neurosurgical Postoperative Monitoring and Complications

Shih-Shan Lang, MD
Neurosurgery Resident
Department of Neurosurgery, Perelman School of Medicine at the University of Pennsylvania
Philadelphia, PA
Spinal Cord Disease and Injury

Daniel J. Licht, MD
Assistant Professor of Neurology and Pediatrics
Division of Neurology, The Children's Hospital of Philadelphia
Departments of Neurology and Pediatrics, Perelman School of Medicine at the University of Pennsylvania
Philadelphia, PA
Approach to Acute Encephalopathy and Coma
Neurologic Complications in Pediatric Cardiac Disease

Kimberly Y. Lin, MD
Assistant Professor of Pediatrics

Division of Cardiology, The Children's Hospital of
    Philadelphia
Department of Pediatrics, Perelman School of Medicine
    at the University of Pennsylvania
Philadelphia, PA
Neurologic Complications in Pediatric Cardiac Disease

Vanessa Madrigal, MD
Attending Physician
Division of Critical Care Medicine, The Children's
    Hospital of Philadelphia
Philadelphia, PA
End of Life Care

Mudit Mathur, MD, FAAP
Associate Professor of Pediatrics
Division of Pediatric Critical Care, Loma Linda
    University Children's Hospital
Loma Linda, CA
Brain Death

Jennifer L. McGuire, MD
Instructor of Neurology and Pediatrics
Division of Neurology, The Children's Hospital of
    Philadelphia
Department of Neurology, Perelman School of
    Medicine at the University of Pennsylvania
Philadelphia, PA
Central Nervous System Infections

Wynne Morrison, MD, MBE
Assistant Professor of Anesthesiology, Critical Care
    Medicine, and Pediatrics
Division of Critical Care Medicine, The Children's
    Hospital of Philadelphia
Department of Anesthesiology and Critical Care,
    Perelman School of Medicine at the
    University of Pennsylvania
Philadelphia, PA
End of Life Care

Sona Narula, MD
Fellow in Child Neurology
Division of Neurology, The Children's Hospital of
    Philadelphia
Philadelphia, PA
Approach to Acute Headache

Lewis S. Nelson, MD
Professor of Emergency Medicine
New York University School of Medicine

Director, Fellowship in Medical Toxicology
New York, NY
Neurotoxicology

Bryan Pukenas, MD
Assistant Professor of Radiology
Department of Radiology, Perelman School of
    Medicine at the University of Pennsylvania
Philadelphia, PA
*Diagnosis and Endovascular Management of
    Cerebrovascular Malformations*

Colleen M. Rivers, MD
Senior Fellow in Medical Toxicology
New York City Poison Control Center
Department of Emergency Medicine, New York
    University School of Medicine
New York, NY
Neurotoxicology

Paul M. Robins, PhD
Associate Professor of Clinical Psychology
Department of Child and Adolescent Psychiatry and
    Behavioral Sciences, The Children's Hospital of
    Philadelphia
Department of Psychiatry, Perelman School of
    Medicine at the University of Pennsylvania
Philadelphia, PA
Psychological Reactions to Critical Care Events

David Z. Rose, MD
Attending Neurologist
Department of Neurology (Stroke Division), The
    University of South Florida and Tampa General
    Hospital
Tampa, FL
Arterial Ischemic Stroke

Mary Rourke, PhD
Assistant Professor of Clinical Psychology
Institute of Graduate Clinical Psychology
Widener University
Chester, PA
Psychological Reactions to Critical Care Events

Michael J. Shumski, MD, MSE
Research Assistant
Division of Neurology, The Children's Hospital of
    Philadelphia
Philadelphia, PA
*Acquired Demyelinating Syndromes of the Central
    Nervous System*

Sabrina E. Smith, MD, PhD
Attending Neurologist
Department of Pediatrics, Division of Neurology
Kaiser Permanente Oakland Medical Center
Oakland, CA
Arterial Ischemic Stroke

Vijay Srinivasan, MD
Assistant Professor of Anesthesiology, Critical Care
    and Pediatrics
Perelman School of Medicine at the University of
    Pennsylvania
Attending Physician
Department of Anesthesiology and Critical Care
    Medicine, The Children's Hospital of Philadelphia
Philadelphia, PA
Nutrition and Glucose Management

Phillip B. Storm, MD
Associate Professor of Neurosurgery
Division of Neurosurgery, The Children's Hospital of
    Philadelphia
Department of Neurosurgery, Perelman School of
    Medicine at the University of Pennsylvania
Philadelphia, PA
*Neurosurgical Postoperative Monitoring and
    Complications*

Sally M. Sultan, MD
Post Doctorate Vascular Neurology/Childhood Stroke
Department of Neurology, Columbia University
    Medical Center
New York, NY
Cerebral Venous Sinus Thrombosis

Christina L. Szperka, MD
Attending Physician
Division of Neurology, The Children's Hospital of
    Philadelphia
Philadelphia, PA
Approach to Acute Headache

Gihan I. Tennekoon, MD
Professor of Neurology and Pediatrics
Division of Neurology, The Children's Hospital of
    Philadelphia
Departments of Neurology and Pediatrics, Perelman
    School of Medicine at the University of
    Pennsylvania
Philadelphia, PA
*Acquired Demyelinating Syndromes of the Central
    Nervous System*

Alexis A. Topjian, MD, MSCE
Assistant Professor of Anesthesiology and Critical Care
    Medicine
Division of Critical Care Medicine, The Children's
    Hospital of Philadelphia
Department of Anesthesiology and Critical Care
    Medicine, Perelman School of Medicine at the
    University of Pennsylvania
Philadelphia, PA
*Mechanical Ventilation and Blood Pressure
    Management*
*Temperature Management and Hypothermic
    Neuroprotection*

Amy T. Waldman, MD, MSCE
Assistant Professor of Neurology and Pediatrics
Division of Neurology, The Children's Hospital of
    Philadelphia
Departments of Neurology and Pediatrics,
    Perelman School of Medicine at the
    University of Pennsylvania
Philadelphia, PA
*Acquired Demyelinating Syndromes of the Central
    Nervous System*

Preface

The care of children with neurocritical illness often involves multi-specialty collaboration and is guided by a steadily expanding body of data. However, many clinicians treating these children are subspecialists and often only a portion of their time can be devoted to neurocritical care. This book provides up-to-date, concise, and clinically relevant guidance to clinicians providing acute care to children with neurologic disorders. The first set of chapters presents differential diagnosis and management approaches to common overarching problems. The second set of chapters discusses the evaluation and management of specific conditions. The final chapters address important associated psychological, social, and ethical issues.

Reflecting the spectrum of specialties involved in pediatric neurocritical care, this book is co-authored by an international group of experts from the fields of critical care medicine, anesthesia, neurology, neurosurgery, neuroradiology, rehabilitation medicine, psychology, and numerous pediatric specialties. We recognize that each author has spent countless hours crafting chapters which are detailed and clear, and we are exceedingly grateful for their time and effort. Guidance and encouragement from our publisher, Beth Barry, has been invaluable in bringing this text to fruition.

1 Approach to Acute Encephalopathy and Coma

SUDHA KILARU KESSLER, DANIEL J. LICHT, and NICHOLAS S. ABEND

■ INTRODUCTION

Acute encephalopathy is a recent alteration in mental status and refers to a range of altered states of attention and consciousness which can result from many different types of central nervous system (CNS) insults. The term is not a specific diagnosis unless the etiology is also stated. Coma is the most extreme of the altered states. It is relatively rare in children, but the consequences may be profound. The estimated incidence of nontraumatic coma is 30/100,000, with a higher incidence in children younger than 1 year of age (160 per 100,000) (1). The incidence of traumatic brain injury is dependent on age and mechanism but is about 10 to 30 per 100,000 (2–4). Morbidity and mortality are highly dependent on the etiology of coma (1,5).

A child with an acute alteration in consciousness requires immediate, detailed evaluation, general support, and specific treatment directed at the cause in order to avoid long term neurologic deficits. The history, physical examination, and tests should be directed at characterizing mental status in such a way that stability, improvement, and deterioration over time can be determined and the coma etiology can be identified, which will permit specific management. Tests and treatments should be tiered, initially targeting life threatening etiologies that are reversible and manageable. This chapter will describe the various types of acute encephalopathy, discuss pathophysiology, review etiologies, provide a strategy for evaluation, and discuss potential complications of encephalopathy.

It is important to recognize that all types of acute encephalopathy, ranging from mild confusion to greater loss of attention and intellect to coma, are serious disorders and involve largely the same differential diagnosis and approach to history, physical examination, testing, and treatment. The mildly confused patient can rapidly spiral down toward coma.

States of Altered Consciousness

Consciousness is defined by Plum and Posner (6) as *a state of wakefulness and awareness of self and surroundings*. This elegant definition is used in this chapter. Normal consciousness requires arousal (mediated by ascending projections from the pontine tegmentum, posterior hypothalamus, and thalamus) and awareness (mediated by cerebral and subcortical structures). Judging awareness may be difficult in neonates and young infants. Behaviors taken to indicate awareness include crying or being soothed in response to feeding and other external tactile, auditory, and visual stimuli. Conscious patients may have abnormal content of consciousness such as delirium, illusions, or hallucinations (see below). *Unconsciousness* is absence of wakefulness and complete unawareness of the self and environment.

Coma describes a state of altered consciousness involving sustained loss of wakefulness (arousal, vigilance) and apparent loss of awareness at least so far as can be determined with bedside testing. The patient has eyes closed and is completely unarousable and nonresponsive to all stimuli except for reflex responses. It differs from sleep in that the patient cannot be aroused by an appropriate stimulus. Sleep-wake cycles are absent. Coma may evolve toward normal consciousness, a minimally conscious state, a vegetative state, or brain death.

The spectrum of diminished consciousness extending from just below normal to coma has often been divided by convention into confusion, delirium, lethargy, obtundation, and stupor. These are all serious conditions that can become fixed deficits or spiral down along the spectrum if not promptly identified, diagnosed, and treated.

1. *Confusion* refers to inattention (eg, inability to give directed responses and distractibility), disorientation, and reduced awareness of surroundings. It can be very mild and not identified unless there is mental status testing and patient behavior and verbal responses are adequately judged.
2. *Delirium* is an acute confusional state characterized by a fluctuating course, changes in level of consciousness, impaired attention, disorientation, irritability, fear, and misperceptions such as illusions, delusions, and visual hallucinations. *Illusions* are misinterpretations of real stimuli (eg, altered size or form of a visual stimulus). *Hallucinations* are perceptions occurring in the absence of an apparent external stimulus. *Delusions* are incorrect thoughts or beliefs that persist when challenged by contradictory evidence or logic. Delirium occurs with toxic, metabolic, infectious, and seizure-related etiologies. It is particularly common when patients with preexisting cognitive abnormalities are in a new hospital environment and at night.

3. *Lethargy* refers to confusion with frequent appearance of mild sleepiness.
4. *Obtundation* refers to a reduction in alertness, delayed, slow, and brief conversational ability, and slower than usual reactivity to nonverbal stimuli. An obtunded patient can be aroused from sleep but appears drowsy or sleeps much of the time.
5. *Stupor* refers to a state in which the patient is unresponsive except that during a period of vigorous stimulation there is some degree of arousal, with eyes opening and perhaps a nonverbal vocalization or minimal verbal response. Stupor appears as deep sleep.

Except for coma, all of these terms are not uniformly defined or used by medical providers. Thus, especially in the acute setting when tracking changes in mental status is important, a detailed description of the patient's state and reactivity will convey more useful information than arbitrarily defined terms. For example, a patient can be described as appearing asleep and unresponsive to voice or light touch, but briefly arousable with painful stimuli.

Other chronic states of altered neurologic function must be differentiated from coma (Table 1.1). A patient in a *vegetative state* cycles through wakefulness and sleep and has complete or partial preservation of hypothalamic and brainstem autonomic processes, but is unaware of the self and environment. This is a clinical diagnosis that when present usually appears in the aftermath of coma, and, by convention, this state is not diagnosed until 1 month after onset of coma. Patients

■ **Table 1.1**	States of Severely Altered Consciousness					
State	Arousal	Awareness	State Changes (Sleep-Wake Cycling)	Motor Function	Respiratory Function	Pain and Suffering
Brain death	Absent	Absent	Absent	None or Spinal reflexes	Absent	No
Coma	Absent	Absent	Absent	Nonpurposeful	Variable	No
Vegetative State (unresponsive wakefulness syndrome)	Present	Absent	Present	Nonpurposeful	Present	No
Minimally conscious state	Present	Partial	Present	Intermittently purposeful or Absent but nonmotor evidence of responsiveness	Present	Yes
Akinetic mutism	Present	Partial	Present	Reduced	Present	Yes
Delirium	Present	Partial	Present	Normal	Present	Yes

are unconscious (no awareness of self or environment) but have alternating periods of wakefulness and sleep. The eyes may be open but there is no visual fixation or pursuit. Respiratory function is intact. There is no external evidence of pain or discomfort Patients may make sounds, facial expressions, and body movements but detailed testing does not demonstrate sustained, reproducible, or purposeful responses to visual, tactile, auditory, or noxious stimulation. The most common etiologies of a persistent vegetative state are: (1) acute brain injury which may be due to hypoxic-ischemic encephalopathy, traumatic brain injury, or CNS infection, (2) metabolic, chromosomal, and degenerative disorders, and (3) developmental malformations. One study of 847 patients in a vegetative state showed the following disease percentages: trauma (15%), nontraumatic (16%), infection (10%), perinatal (15%), chromosomal/developmental (13%), and other (28%) (7). The diagnosis is usually made clinically, but sometimes a responsiveness testing program involving detailed observation of potential responses to determine whether they are purposeful is required to distinguish between the vegetative and minimally conscious states. Patients in coma due to head trauma recover consciousness more often than those with nontraumatic etiologies. Thus the diagnosis of a persistent vegetative state may be made 3 months following nontraumatic brain injury, but not until 12 months following traumatic brain injury (8,9). Of children in the vegetative state 1 month following head injury, 1 year outcome was death (9%), persistent vegetative state (29%), and recovery of consciousness (62%). However, when the etiology was nontraumatic, outcome was worse, with death (22%), persistent vegetative state (65%), and recovery of consciousness in only 13%. Those who recovered consciousness generally retained severe cognitive disabilities (10). Children in a persistent vegetative state have a shortened life expectancy, with even shorter survival in younger children. Life expectancy is about 3 years in children younger than 1 year, 5 years in children aged 2 to 5 years, and 7 years in children aged 7 to 18 years (7,11).

A patient in a *minimally conscious state* has severely altered consciousness but has definite behavioral evidence of self or environmental awareness. A patient in this state may follow simple commands, make nonreflexive gestures or yes-no responses (regardless of response accuracy), or exhibit purposeful behaviors that are contingent on environmental stimuli. Examples include smiling or crying in response to appropriate stimuli but not neutral stimuli, vocalization or gestures in response to questions, reaching for objects, holding or touching objects in a manner dependent on the shape and size of the object, and pursuit eye movement or ocular fixation (12,13). Patients may evolve to the minimally conscious state following coma or the vegetative state. The most common causes of the minimally conscious state are acquired brain injury, neurodegenerative diseases, neurometabolic conditions, or congenital disorders (14). Survival is predicted more strongly by mobility than by the precise degree of awareness. Among 5073 children in the vegetative or minimally conscious states studied, 8 year survival was 65% for immobile minimally conscious patients, 81% for mobile minimally conscious patients, and 63% for patients in the vegetative state (15).

Recent studies have further blurred the distinction between the minimally conscious and vegetative states. Functional neuroimaging and electrophysiology studies have demonstrated that some patients considered to be in the vegetative state based on detailed examination and responsiveness testing actually demonstrate reproducible physiologic changes in response to tasks, indicating there may be some awareness despite the absence of behavioral signs of responsiveness (16–18). These findings have led to a recent shift toward the use of more neutral and descriptive terms (19,20). The vegetative state may be referred to as the *unresponsive wakefulness syndrome*. The minimally conscious state may be subdivided into the minimally conscious state plus (MCS+) if there are high-level behavioral responses, such as following commands or intelligible verbalizations, or the minimally conscious state negative (MCS–) if there are lower level behavioral responses, such as visual pursuit or contextually appropriate crying or smiling (19).

Akinetic mutism is an uncommon condition in which wakefulness and awareness are partially preserved, but there is extreme slowing or absence of bodily movement, reduced mental function, and loss of speech. This state may result from extensive bihemispheric disease and lesions involving the bilateral inferior frontal lobes, paramedian mesencephalic reticular formation, or the posterior diencephalon. Causes include tumors, bacterial and viral infections, and hydrocephalus. It may occur postoperatively following resection of posterior fossa tumors. Prognosis is dependent on etiology.

It is important to be aware of conditions with normal mental status that mimic coma since failure to recognize them will cause avoidable suffering. In these conditions, cognitive function is preserved and the electroencephalogram (EEG) is normal. The *locked-in syndrome* is a state of preserved consciousness and cognition with complete loss of voluntary motor functions (other than vertical eye movements and blinking). Cerebral cortical function is intact and EEG patterns are normal. The locked-in state is seen with lesions of the corticospinal and corticobulbar pathways at or below the pons (as in brainstem strokes). Vertical eye movements or blinking allow communication, such as answering yes/no questions. Some children with locked-in syndrome may show motor recovery (21). Similarly, *neuromuscular disorders* causing severe loss of cranial and limb movement may appear as coma but normal mental status can be demonstrated with careful testing. These include Miller-Fisher variant of Guillain-Barré syndrome, botulism, myasthenia gravis, and critical illness polyneuropathy. *Psychogenic unresponsiveness* may mimic coma.

Coma must also be distinguished from *brain death*, which is the permanent absence of all brain activity including brainstem function. The most recently published recommendations regarding brain death state that "determination of brain death in neonates, infants, and children relies on a clinical diagnosis that is based on the absence of neurologic function with a known irreversible cause of coma" (22). Patients must fulfill specific criteria, and many institutions have specific brain death protocols.

■ ANATOMY OF COMA

Wakefulness is maintained by the reticular activating system (RAS) while awareness is dependent on the cortex and subcortical connections. The RAS extends from the caudal medulla to the thalamus and basal forebrain. It receives input from all sensory pathways and projects to extensive areas of the cerebral cortex, thereby activating cortex and permitting feedback control to regulate incoming signals. The RAS may be partitioned into medial and lateral zones. The medial RAS zone has ascending axons emanating from the raphe nuclei, which regulate sleep cycles and utilize serotonin as their major neurotransmitter. Descending pathways regulate automatic motor functions including the automatic rhythms of breathing. The lateral RAS zone uses cholinergic and noradrenergic projections to the reticular nucleus of the thalamus to relay signals to the cortex, and this system is critical to maintaining wakefulness. A separate cholinergic pathway ascends through the hypothalamus and influences basal forebrain structures (including the limbic system) to influence conscious behavior, and lesions may result in akinetic mutism. A third noradrenergic pathway originates in the locus caeruleus and excites widespread areas of brain, mediating arousal and priming the brain to be activated by stimuli.

■ ENCEPHALOPATHY/COMA ETIOLOGIES

The causes of acute encephalopathy/coma in children are broad (Table 1.2). Multiple systems of categorization are possible. Etiology may be categorized as (1) traumatic or nontraumatic, (2) structural or toxic-metabolic, or (3) focal or diffuse. Nontraumatic subcategories include toxic-metabolic etiologies and structural abnormalities. Multiple interrelated etiologic factors may be present. For example, status epilepticus may occur in the setting of encephalitis, infection inducing a catabolic state may produce decompensation in a child with an inborn error of metabolism, and hyponatremia may accompany brain injury and contribute to cerebral dysfunction. Thus, identifying one etiology does not preclude consideration of other etiologies.

In a population-based study of 600,000 children experiencing 345 episodes of non-traumatic coma, the most common etiology was infection (38%), while intoxication, epilepsy, complications of congenital abnormalities, nontraumatic accidents (smoke inhalation, drowning), and metabolic causes each accounted for 6% to 10% of cases (1). Traumatic brain injury is the most common cause of coma in children, not only because trauma is common but also because it frequently leads to coma. Approximately 27% of patients with traumatic brain injury have an initial Glasgow Coma Score of less than 9 (4).

■ EVALUATION

The evaluation of the encephalopathic or comatose child must be rapid, systematic, and comprehensive. In those cases where the cause is reversible, the neurologic effects

■ **Table 1.2** Etiologies of Acute Encephalopathy

Traumatic Etiologies
Cerebral contusion
Intracranial hemorrhage
    Epidural hematoma
    Subdural hematoma
    Subarachnoid hemorrhage
    Intraparenchymal hematoma
Diffuse axonal injury
Nontraumatic Etiologies
Hypoxic-ischemic encephalopathy
    Shock
    Cardiopulomary arrest
    Cardiac or pulmonary failure
    Near drowning
    Carbon monoxide poisoning
    Cyanide poisoning
Vascular
    Intracranial hemorrhage (subdural, epidural,
        subarachnoid, parenchymal)
    Arterial ischemic infarct
    Venous sinus thromboses
    Vasculitis
    Carotid or vertebral artery dissection
        (cervical or intracranial)
Mass lesions
    Primary neoplasms
    Brain metastases
    Abscess
    Granuloma
Hydrocephalus
Infections
    Meningitis and encephalitis: bacterial, viral,
        rickettsial, fungal, protozoal
    Abscess
Inflammatory/autoimmune/postinfectious
    Acute disseminated encephalomyelitis
    Multiple sclerosis
    Sarcoidosis
    Sjögren disease
    Cerebritis (eg, systemic lupus erythematosus)
    Sepsis associated encephalopathy
Paroxysmal neurologic disorders
    Seizures, status epilepticus, nonconvulsive seizures,
        postictal state
    Acute confusional migraine

Hypertensive encephalopathy
Posterior reversible leukoencephalopathy
Systemic metabolic disorders
    Substrate deficiencies
        Hypoglycemia
        Cofactors: thiamine, niacin, pyridoxine,
            folate, B_{12}
    Electrolyte and acid-base imbalance: sodium,
        magnesium, calcium
    Hypoglycemia
    Diabetic ketoacidosis
    Endocrine
        Acute hypothyroidism
        Addison disease
        Acute panhypopituitarism
    Uremic encephalopathy
    Hepatic encephalopathy
    Reye Syndrome
    Sepsis associated encephalopathy
    Porphyria
    Inborn errors of metabolism
        Urea cycle disorders
        Aminoacidopathies
        Organic acidopathies
        Mitochondrial disorders
Toxins
    Medications: narcotics, sedatives,
        antiepileptics, antidepressants,
        analgesics, aspirin, valproic acid
        encephalopathy
    Environmental toxins:
        organophosphates, heavy metals,
        cyanide, mushroom poisoning
    Illicit substances: alcohol, heroine,
        amphetamines, cocaine, and
        many others
Drug induced
    Neuroleptic malignant syndrome
    Serotonin syndrome
    Malignant hyperthermia
Psychiatric
    Conversion disorder
    Catatonia
Other
    Hypothermia

may only be reversed if the cause is treated promptly. In the case of coma, systemic management including immediate life support must occur as etiology is being investigated to prevent development of secondary brain injury. An

algorithm for initial evaluation of acute encephalopathy/coma is outlined in Table 1.3. A recent guideline for the evaluation and management of a child with decreased consciousness by the Pediatric Accident and Emergency

■ Table 1.3   Initial Evaluation of Encephalopathy

- Airway, breathing, and circulation assessment and stabilization.
  - Ensure adequate ventilation and oxygenation.
  - Blood pressure management depends on considerations regarding underlying coma etiology. If hypertensive encephalopathy or intracranial hemorrhage then lower blood pressure. If perfusion dependent state such as some strokes or elevated intracranial pressure then reducing blood pressure may reduce cerebral perfusion.
  - Intubation for hypoxia, hypoventilation, or risk of aspiration. Intubation procedures must consider potential cervical spine injury and elevated intracranial pressure.
  - Establish intravenous access. Generally at least two intravenous access points are required.
- Draw blood for glucose, electrolytes, ammonia, arterial blood gas, liver and renal function tests, complete blood count, lactate, pyruvate, and toxicology screen.
- Focused history and examination.
- Neurologic assessment.
  - Glasgow Coma Score (or description of state).
  - Assess for evidence of raised intracranial pressure and herniation.
  - Assess for abnormalities suggesting focal neurologic disease.
  - Assess for history or signs of seizures.
- Administer glucose intravenously. In a young adult, consider thiamine first.
- Urgent head CT.
- If there is concern for infection and LP must be delayed then provide broad spectrum infection coverage (including bacterial, viral, and possibly fungal).
- Give specific antidotes if toxic exposures are known.
  - For opiate overdose administer naloxone.
  - For benzodiazepine overdose consider administering flumazenil.
  - For anticholinergic overdose consider administering physostigmine.
- Identify and treat critical elevations in intracranial pressure.
  - Neutral head position and elevated head by 20°–30°.
  - Sedation.
  - Hyperosmolar therapy with mannitol or hypertonic saline.
  - Hyperventilation as temporary measure.
  - Consider intracranial monitoring.
  - Consider neurosurgical intervention.
- Treat seizures with anticonvulsants. Consider prophylactic anticonvulsants.
- Investigate source of fever and use antipyretics and/or cooling devices to reduce cerebral metabolic demands.
- Consider: lumbar puncture, EEG or extended long term EEG monitoring, brain MRI, metabolic testing (amino acids, organic acids, acylcarnitine profile), autoimmune testing (ANA panel, antithyroid antibodies), thyroid testing (TSH, T3, T4).

Abbreviations: ANA, antinuclear antibody; CT, computed tomography; EEG, electroencephalogram; LP, lumbar puncture; MRI, magnetic resonance imaging; TSH, thyroid stimulating hormone.

Research Group of the Royal College of Paediatrics and Child Health and the British Association for Emergency Medicine (www.nottingham.ac.uk/paediatric-guideline) is based on extensive literature review and expert consensus and includes helpful flowcharts (23). Other reviews are also available (24–26).

History

Historical information may help identify the cause of encephalopathy and should include a detailed description of events leading up to the illness including timing of events, possible exposures, and initial symptoms (Table 1.4). Preceding somnolence or headache that progress suggests metabolic etiologies, toxin or medication exposures, infectious etiologies, hydrocephalus, or expanding mass lesions that may have been developing over time. In contrast, the sudden onset of illness without trauma suggests intracranial hemorrhage, seizure, cardiac arrhythmia producing hypoxic-ischemic encephalopathy, or ischemic stroke. A fluctuating course may occur with metabolic encephalopathy, seizures, or subdural hemorrhage. Head injury followed by a lucid period and then encephalopathy mandates a head computed tomography (CT) to evaluate for an epidural or expanding subdural hemorrhage. Focal symptoms

History	Etiology Considerations
Table 1.4 Clinical History in Patients With Encephalopathy	
Onset	
Abrupt	Seizure, ischemic stroke, intracranial hemorrhage, cardiac with hypoxic-ischemic encephalopathy
Gradual	Metabolic, toxic, infectious, tumor, venous thrombosis, hydrocephalus
Fluctuating	Seizure, metabolic, epidural or subdural hemorrhage
Prior similar episodes	Seizure, transient ischemic attack, inborn errors of metabolism, Munchausen syndrome by proxy
Altered behavior prior to coma	Toxic, metabolic, infectious, seizure
Focal symptoms prior to coma	Focal lesion
Potential toxin exposure	Toxin
Trauma	Epidural hemorrhage, subdural hemorrhage, subarachnoid hemorrhage, intraparenchymal hemorrhage
Dehydration	Metabolic, venous thrombosis
Recent illness or fever	Infectious
Neck stiffness	Infectious, carcinomatous, subarachnoid hemorrhage, herniation
Travel history or animal exposure	Infectious
Headache	Intracranial mass, hydrocephalus

followed by encephalopathy suggest a focal lesion that may have expanded, developed edema, or experienced intralesion hemorrhage.

Eliciting a history of trauma and the mechanism of injury can direct investigation. Base of the skull fractures may compromise blood flow in the carotid artery, as in carotid artery dissection, producing serious middle cerebral artery ischemia. Preceding headache with positional changes or Valsalva maneuver implies increased intracranial pressure secondary to hydrocephalus or a mass lesion. Headache with neck pain or stiffness suggests meningeal irritation from inflammation, infection, or hemorrhage. Fever suggests infection, but its absence does not rule it out, particularly in infants under 3 months of age or immunocompromised children. Recent fever or nonspecific illness can signal autoimmune or postinfectious processes such as acute disseminated encephalomyelitis. A survey of medications and poisons in the child's environment may suggest toxic ingestion. Travel history may explain exposure to infections prevalent in certain areas. Exposure to kittens in a patient with axillary or inguinal lymphadenopathy may be a clue to infection with *Bartonella henselae* induced cat scratch encephalopathy. Use of a heater or kerosene stove in an enclosed location may suggest carbon monoxide poisoning.

Past medical history may help elucidate etiology. Prior similar episodes can indicate transient ischemic attacks, recurrent ingestion, or Munchausen syndrome by proxy. Multiple episodes of encephalopathy or coma also raise a question about seizures or an inborn error of metabolism, especially if there is also history of developmental delay or other neurologic abnormalities. Cardiac disease raises the possibility of dysrhythmia or cardiac failure leading to hypoxic-ischemic encephalopathy, brain abscess, or stroke. A diagnosis of diabetes may suggest hypoglycemia or diabetic ketoacidosis. Weight changes, recent darkening of the skin, or other constitutional abnormalities may suggest endocrine dysfunction. Prior recurrent infections, known immunodeficiency, or use of immune suppressing medications may lead to consideration of infectious etiologies. A history of uncontrolled hypertension may suggest posterior reversible encephalopathy syndrome.

Physical Examination

The general physical examination should focus on identifying the etiology and complications that may produce secondary neurologic injury.

Encephalopathy, Coma, and Consciousness Rating Scales

A detailed description of the mental status, indicating what the child can and cannot do, is the ideal method for relaying detailed information to other providers and detecting changes over time. There is also value in including numerically scored rating scales of consciousness level, which provide objective description of a patient's consciousness and a tool for tracking the condition over time and conveying information quickly to other caregivers. The most widely used instrument is the Glasgow Coma Scale (GCS) which was initially developed to evaluate adults with head injury (27). Pediatric adaptations to the GCS, which are more developmentally appropriate for infants and children, include the Pediatric Coma Scale, the Children's Coma Scale, and the GCS Modified for Children (Table 1.5) (28–30). The GCS and the pediatric adaptations categorize the patient based on measures of verbal response, eye opening, and movement. The GCS Modified for Children yields a 3 to 15 score based on the best response of the 3 categories.

In response to limitations of the GCS, the FOUR score was recently developed for use in adults with coma (31). Each of 4 functional categories (eye response, motor response, brainstem reflexes, and respiration) receives a score of 0 (nonfunctioning) to 4 (normal functioning) (Table 1.6). Some differences from the GCS score include assessment of eye tracking in the eye response category, assessment of response to pain, ability to follow simple commands, the presence of generalized myoclonic status epilepticus in the motor response category, elimination of

verbal response from the scale, and addition of brainstem reflex and respiratory categories (31). The FOUR score has proven useful in adults in the medical intensive care unit (ICU) (32) and after resuscitation from cardiac arrest (33). One study has evaluated the interrater reliability and predictive value of the GCS Modified for Children and FOUR score in critically ill children. In a study of 60 children aged 2 to 18 years in an ICU with both traumatic and nontraumatic brain injury, the FOUR score had better interrater reliability than the GCS Modified for Children (excellent for FOUR score and good for GCS) and both predicted outcome similarly (34). While many coma scoring systems exist (35), further validation of these tools is needed in children.

Vital Signs

Hypertension may cause encephalopathy or result from another condition that is causing altered mental status. Primary or secondary hypertension may cause hypertensive encephalopathy. Primary hypertensive encephalopathy is suggested by a history of hypertension or renal disease, or by preceding headache, visual complaints, or seizures. Hypertension may occur with Cushing syndrome, thyrotoxicosis, pheochromocytoma, drug overdose (cocaine, amphetamine, phencyclidine), renal disease (such as acute glomerulonephritis or chronic renal

■ Table 1.5 Glasgow Coma Scale and Glasgow Coma Scale Modified for Children

Sign	Glasgow Coma Scale	Glasgow Coma Scale Modified for Children	Score
Eye opening	Spontaneous	Spontaneous	4
	To Command	To sound	3
	To pain	To pain	2
	None	None	1
Verbal response	Oriented	Age appropriate verbalization, orients to sound, fixes and follows, social smile	5
	Confused	Cries, but consolable	4
	Disoriented	Irritable, uncooperative, aware of environment	3
	Inappropriate words	Irritable, persistent cries, inconsistently consolable	
	Incomprehensible sounds	Inconsolable crying, unaware of environment or parents, restless, agitated	2
	None	None	1
Motor response	Obeys commands	Obeys commands, spontaneous movement	6
	Localizes pain	Localizes pain	5
	Withdraws	Withdraws	4
	Abnormal flexion to pain	Abnormal flexion to pain	3
	Abnormal extension	Abnormal extension	2
	None	None	1
Best total score			15

■ **Table 1.6** FOUR Score		
Eye response	4	Eyelids open or opened, tracking, or blinking to command
	3	Eyelids open but not tracking
	2	Eyelids closed but opens to loud voice
	1	Eyelids closed but opens to pain
	0	Eyelids remain closed with pain
Motor response	4	Thumbs up, fist, or peace sign to command
	3	Localizing to pain
	2	Flexion response to pain
	1	Extensor posturing
	0	No response to pain or generalized myoclonus status epilepticus
Brainstem reflexes	4	Pupil and corneal reflexes present
	3	One pupil wide and fixed
	2	Pupil or corneal reflexes absent
	1	Pupil and corneal reflexes absent
	0	Absent pupil, corneal, and cough reflex
Respiration	4	Not intubated, regular breathing pattern
	3	Not intubated, Cheyne-Stokes breathing pattern
	2	Not intubated, irregular breathing pattern
	1	Breathes above ventilator rate
	0	Breathes at ventilator rate or apnea

Wijdicks EF et al. Validation of a new coma scale: The FOUR score. *Ann Neurol.* 2005;58:585–93.

failure), medication exposure (such as immunomodulatory and chemotherapeutic drugs), and, rarely, essential hypertension. Importantly, in critically ill children, hypertension can be a physiologic response to elevated intracranial pressure that functions to maintain cerebral perfusion pressure. Differentiating between reactive/compensatory hypertension and a primary hypertensive encephalopathy may be difficult but is crucial in determining how to manage blood pressure. If hypertension is a response to elevated intracranial pressure, then acutely lowering blood pressure may worsen the neurologic injury by reducing cerebral perfusion. Hypertension, bradycardia, and irregular respiration (Cushing triad) is an ominous sign of elevated intracranial pressure and impending brain herniation. Management may require urgent measures to lower intracranial pressure such as hyperventilation, hyperosmolar therapy, and neurosurgical therapy.

Hypotension may cause encephalopathy or coma as a result of poor cerebral perfusion and associated diffuse or watershed hypoxic-ischemic injury. It may result in worse outcome in encephalopathy due to other causes. Hypotension may result from sepsis, cardiac dysfunction (which may be secondary to severe neurologic injury in neurogenic stunned myocardium), systemic hemorrhage, intracranial hemorrhage in neonate/infant, toxic ingestion, adrenal insufficiency, or hypothyroidism.

Tachycardia may occur with hypovolemic shock (due to dehydration or systemic hemorrhage), cardiogenic shock, sepsis, pain, toxin exposure (stimulants such as amphetamines, cocaine, nicotine, and caffeine), malignant hyperthermia, anemia, heart failure, hyperthyroidism, pheochromocytoma, or pulmonary embolism. Bradycardia may occur with intracranial hypertension, cardiac disease, hypothermia, toxin exposure (sedating drugs), uremic coma, or myxedema coma.

Abnormalities in respiratory rate and pattern of breathing may indicate pulmonary disease, acid-base derangement, or nervous system dysfunction. Tachypnea may occur with a primary abnormality of respiration (eg, asthma, pneumonia, or pulmonary embolism) or acidosis (eg, uremia or ketoacidosis). Cheyne-Stokes respiration describes a rhythmic and cyclic pattern of accelerating hyperpnea followed by decelerating respiratory rate and/or apnea. It is a nonspecific pattern seen with extensive bihemispheric cerebral dysfunction, diencephalic (thalamic and hypothalamic) dysfunction, or cardiac failure. Central neurogenic hyperventilation is characterized by rapid and deep hyperpnea and is caused by pontine or midbrain tegmental lesions. Apneustic breathing is characterized by prolonged inspiration, a few second pause, and then expiration. It is caused by damage to respiratory centers in the mid or lower pons. Apneusis also occurs with basilar artery occlusion (leading to pontine infarction), metabolic changes, or meningitis. Ataxic breathing is completely irregular in rate and tidal volume and occurs with damage to the reticular formation of the dorsomedial medulla. Kussmaul breathing refers to deep, rapid, and regular breaths and occurs with pontomesencephalic lesions or metabolic acidosis. Agonal gasps represent a terminal respiratory pattern and indicate damage to the bilateral lower brainstem (6). Respiratory patterns are summarized in Table 1.7.

Hyperthermia suggests an infectious etiology such as meningitis, encephalitis, or cerebral abscess or empyema. Systemic infection can cause sepsis encephalopathy. Fever may also occur with brain injury impacting temperature control mechanisms, heat stroke, or anticholinergic ingestion. The absence of fever does not rule out infection, especially in infants or children who are immunosuppressed. Hypothermia may also be due to intoxication, sepsis, hypothyroidism, adrenal insufficiency, chronic malnutrition, or environmental exposure.

General Examination

A complete general examination is important in identifying the cause of encephalopathy and associated conditions requiring management. Low weight may suggest pre-existing failure to thrive or neurodevelopmental conditions. Microcephaly may indicate a pre-existing neurodevelopmental disorder, while macrocephaly may indicate prior or new hydrocephalus. A full anterior fontanelle indicates elevated intracranial pressure while a sunken fontanelle may indicate dehydration.

Signs of meningeal inflammation/irritation include neck stiffness with resistance to passive flexion of the neck, involuntary hip flexion with passive flexion of the neck (Brudzinski sign), and resistance to knee extension with hips flexed (Kernig sign). These may occur with meningitis, subarachnoid hemorrhage, craniocervical pathology, or tonsillar herniation. They may take several hours to develop or remain minimal or absent, especially in immunocompromised patients.

Skin and mucosal examination are important. Bruises or lacerations, especially at the head, or cephalohematoma, suggest traumatic etiology. Bruising in the periorbital (raccoon eyes) or mastoid (Battle sign) regions strongly suggest fracture of the skull base. Telling skin abnormalities may include pallor due to hypotension, jaundice indicating hepatic encephalopathy, cherry red skin indicating carbon monoxide poisoning, gray-blue skin indicating hypoxia or methemoglobin intoxication, and hyperpigmentation indicating adrenal insufficiency or Addison disease. Petechiae and ecchymosis may occur with idiopathic or secondary thrombocytopenia, thrombotic thrombocytopenic purpura, disseminated intravascular coagulation, meningococcemia, Rocky Mountain spotted fever, vasculitis, or endocarditis. Erythema migrans is seen with Lyme disease. Splinter hemorrhages may occur with anemia, sepsis, endocarditis, or leukemia. Noting a neurocutaneous lesions may point to neurofibromatosis, tuberous sclerosis, or Sturge-Weber disease.

Nonaccidental trauma (inflicted trauma) is common in children younger than 2 years of age and is suggested by retinal hemorrhages, metaphyseal fractures, rib fractures, and subdural hemorrhages. About 10% have normal retinal examinations and skeletal surveys (36).

Clear fluid emanating from the nose or ears may indicate a cerebrospinal fluid (CSF) leak due to skull fracture. Cranial bruits may indicate a vascular

■ Table 1.7 Respiratory Patterns in Encephalopathy/Coma

Respiratory Pattern	Description	Localization/Etiology
Cheyne-Stokes	Alternating hyperpnea and apnea	Extensive bihemispheric dysfunction or diencephalic dysfunction
Central neurogenic hyperventilation	Rapid and deep hyperpnea	Pons or midbrain
Apneustic	Prolonged pause at end of inspiration	Pons
Ataxic	Irregular in rate and tidal volume	Medulla
Agonal gasps	Terminal pattern of intermittent, disorganized breaths	Lower brainstem
Kussmaul	Rapid, deep, regular breath	Pontomesencephalic, metabolic acidosis

malformation with turbulent blood flow. Organomegaly raises suspicion of metabolic, hematologic, hepatic diseases, or heart failure. Orthopedic injuries indicate unreported trauma or, rarely, injury caused by a seizure.

Neurologic Examination

The neurologic examination is directed at identifying the type of mental status disorder that is present, localizing brain dysfunction, identifying the cause of the encephalopathy, and determining early indicators of prognosis. If there is an initial impression of coma, this must be confirmed by demonstrating that there is no cranial nerve or motor or verbal response to verbal commands and other auditory stimuli, no response to visual stimuli such as visual threat, and no response to noxious stimuli such as nail-bed pressure, pinch, and sternal rub. Motor, brain stem, and reflex activity must be reviewed. Locked-in syndrome and psychogenic coma must be considered. If the child is not in coma, then mental status testing is used to determine the level of impairment, as reviewed above ("States of Altered Consciousness").

Fundoscopic examination yields information about the retina and optic nerves. Retinal hemorrhages may be seen in inflicted (nonaccidental) childhood trauma and in hypertensive encephalopathy. Flame-shaped hemorrhages and cotton-wool spots are seen in hypertensive encephalopathy. Papilledema or absence of venous pulsations may be seen with increased intracranial pressure. However, these may take hours or days to develop so the absence of these signs does not indicate that intracranial pressure is normal. If pharmacologic pupil dilation is needed for fundoscopic examination, the effects may last for 24 hours and may preclude evaluation of pupillary light response.

Pupil size and reactivity are controlled by the sympathetic (dilation) and parasympathetic (constriction) systems. Sympathetic control originates in the hypothalamus, descends to the lower cervical and upper thoracic spinal cord levels, exits the spinal cord, ascends in the cervical sympathetic chain to the superior cervical ganglion, and then travels in the wall of the internal carotid artery to the ophthalmic branch of the trigeminal nerve (cranial nerve V) to the pupil. Other sympathetic fibers follow this same course and innervate the eyelid smooth muscles and face sweat glands. Disruption of the sympathetic fibers results in unilateral pupil constriction (meiosis), anhidrosis, and ptosis (Horner syndrome). In traumatic encephalopathy, Horner syndrome might be due to carotid artery dissection. Parasympathetic fibers originate in the midbrain (Edinger-Westphal nucleus) and travel along the outer layers of the oculomotor nerve (cranial nerve III) to the pupil constrictors. Thus, mild extrinsic compression of the oculomotor nerve results in an abnormally dilated pupil. The interior of the oculomotor nerve contains extraocular motor fibers and thus more extensive compression results in parasympathetic dysfunction (pupil dilation) and also ptosis and ophthalmoparesis with the affected eye laterally and inferiorly deviated. One of the causes is uncal herniation.

Pupils are examined first by observing the size of both pupils in dim light and then by assessing reactivity to a bright light shined in each eye. Anisocoria (asymmetric pupils) is an important physical finding and differentiating whether a pupil is abnormally large or abnormally small is crucial to identifying underlying pathology. Pupil reactivity to light is mediated by an afferent limb (optic nerve, cranial nerve II) and an efferent limb (parasympathetic fibers traveling along the oculomotor nerve). Pupils that are more asymmetric in bright light indicate pathology with the larger pupil that is likely the result of oculomotor palsy. Investigations to rule out uncal herniation or an aneurysm of the posterior communicating artery may be indicated. Uncal herniation is a potentially treatable emergency so pupil asymmetry or lack of pupil reactivity requires immediate assessment and treatment. Pupils that are more asymmetric in the dark suggest pathology in the abnormally constricted pupil, that is, Horner syndrome (see above). Investigation of the carotid artery and the low cervical–high thoracic spinal cord or brachial plexus roots should be considered. Fixed and dilated pupils are concerning for herniation progressing to brain death, recent hypoxic-ischemic injury, or anticholinergic administration. Common pupil abnormalities are listed in Table 1.8.

Extraocular movements are controlled by three nerves with nuclei in the midbrain and pons: the oculomotor nerve (cranial nerve III), the trochlear nerve (cranial nerve IV), and the abducens nerve (cranial nerve VI). Supranuclear control originates in frontal (rapid, saccadic movements contralateral to the side stimulated) and parietal-occipital (smooth pursuit and tracking movements ipsilateral to the side stimulated) gaze centers. Conjugate gaze requires linking of these nuclei within the medial longitudinal fasciculus. Thus, abnormalities of eye position and motility may be signs of cortical, midbrain, or pontine dysfunction. Eye movement abnormalities are listed in Table 1.9.

■ Table 1.8 Pupil Abnormalities in Encephalopathy/Coma

Pupil Appearance	Etiology/Localization
Bilateral small and reactive	Metabolic encephalopathy Thalamic, hypothalamic, pontine lesions Intoxication (narcotics, benzodiazepines, organophosphates)
Bilateral dilated and unreactive	Midbrain lesion Severe hypoxic-ischemic encephalopathy Anticholinergic poisoning
Bilateral dilated and reactive	Seizure
Unilateral small	Ipsilateral sympathetic fiber tract (associated with Horner syndrome) including hypothalamus, cervical/thoracic cord, carotid artery, ophthalmic branch of cranial nerve V
Unilateral dilated and unreactive	Ipsilateral cranial nerve III dysfunction including related to herniation
Dilated and unreactive and hippus	Tectal lesion

Oculocephalic (doll's eyes) and oculovestibular (caloric) reflexes are useful for assessing the integrity of the midbrain and pons. Oculocephalic reflexes should not be tested if the patient has sustained cervical spine trauma or if the spine has not been cleared. Stimulus provoked testing should be performed in this case (see below). To test oculocephalic reflexes, the examiner holds the patient's eyelids open and quickly moves the head to one side. If the brainstem is intact, the eyes should move in the direction opposite the head motion. For example, if the head is moved to the right, the eyes should move conjugately to the left. After several seconds, the eyes may return to a neutral position. The head should be tested in both horizontal and vertical directions. Absence of the oculocephalic reflex may be seen with brainstem lesions (may be asymmetric loss) or toxic-metabolic encephalopathies (symmetric loss).

The oculovestibular reflex (cold calorics) tests the function above the pontomedullary junction. The child must have an open external auditory canal with an intact tympanic membrane (including the absence of pressure equalization tubes), so visual inspection of the canal is an important first step. With the head elevated at 30° (where possible), up to 120 ml of ice water is introduced in the ear canal with a small catheter. A conscious patient would experience nystagmus with slow deviation of the eyes toward the irrigated ear and a fast corrective movement away from the ear (the mnemonic COWS, *Cold Opposite, Warm Same,* applies to the fast phase). In a comatose patient, the fast correction mediated by the cortex is not seen. Instead, the eyes will deviate slowly toward the irrigated ear and remain fixed there. Testing should be performed in both ears, with a 5 minute delay between ears in order to allow for return of temperature equilibrium between the two ears. Vertical eye movements may be tested by simultaneously irrigating both auditory canals with cold water, producing downward deviation in the comatose patient. Warm water irrigation has the opposite effect and produces upgaze. Unilateral or asymmetric loss suggests a brainstem lesion while symmetric loss suggests a brainstem lesion or toxic-metabolic encephalopathy. If the brainstem vestibular nuclei on one side (pontomedullary junction) are impaired, then no response to stimulation from that side will be seen. Oculovestibular testing is also an important test for brain death determination.

■ Table 1.9 Eye Movements in Encephalopathy/Coma

Eye Movement	Etiology/Localization
Conjugate horizontal eye deviation	Lesions in ipsilateral cortex, pons Contralateral hemisphere seizure Contralateral thalamic lesion ("wrong way" eyes)
Downgaze	Dorsal midbrain
Ocular bobbing	Bilateral pons
Ocular dipping	Diffuse cortical injury
Eyes deviated down and in	Thalamic or upper midbrain
Eye deviated down and out	Oculomotor nerve (CN III) palsy
Eye deviated up	Trochlear nerve (CN IV) palsy
Eye(s) deviated in	Abducens nerve (CN VI) palsy, elevated intracranial pressure (thus considered "false localizing" sign)
Periodic alternating gaze (ping-pong gaze)	Extensive lesions of bilateral hemispheres, basal ganglia, thalamus, midbrain, intoxication with tricyclic antidepressants and monoamine oxidase inhibitors

Abbreviation: CN, cranial nerve.

The remaining brainstem reflexes provide information about the integrity of lower regions of the brainstem. The corneal reflex is tested by tactile stimulation of the cornea, which should elicit bilateral eyelid closure. The afferent (sensory) signal is carried by the trigeminal nerve (cranial nerve V), and the efferent (motor) pathway is carried by the facial nerve (cranial nerve VII). Completion of the reflex loop requires intact trigeminal and facial nerve nuclei in the mid and lower pons. The cough reflex, which may be seen with stimulation of the carina when a patient is intubated or undergoes suctioning, is mediated by medullary cough centers; sensory and motor signals are carried by the glossopharyngeal (cranial nerve IX) and vagus (cranial nerve X) nerves. When the soft palate is stimulated, the gag reflex is elicited, and the patient experiences the effects of pharyngeal contraction and elevation of the soft palate. As in the cough reflex, afferent and efferent signals are carried by the glossopharyngeal and vagus nerves, with processing in the medulla. Narcotics may suppress cough reflex, an important consideration for accurate assessment of brainstem function (37).

A comatose child may be flaccid or display an abnormal flexor or extensor posture. Flaccidity occurs with administration of paralytics, toxic-metabolic encephalopathy, or diffuse cortical-brainstem lesions (usually below the pontomedullary level). Asymmetric flaccidity suggests a cortical or subcortical lesion. Flaccidity may also occur with spinal cord injury and peripheral nervous system conditions, but coma will generally be absent. Decerebrate posturing is extension and internal rotation of arms and legs and may occur with toxic-metabolic encephalopathy and brainstem dysfunction. Decorticate posturing is flexion of the arms and extension of the leg and may occur with cortical or subcortical injury but with brainstem preservation.

Laboratory, Imaging, and Electrophysiologic Investigation

It is often appropriate for initial stabilization, basic management, and diagnostic testing to be carried out simultaneously with obtaining the history and performing the physical examination, as long as history and exam are not curtailed or seen as less important. Reference is again made to the excellent guideline with flowcharts for the care of a child with decreased consciousness (www.nottingham .ac.uk/paediatric-guideline) by the Pediatric Accident and Emergency Research Group of the Royal College of Paediatrics and Child Health and the British Association for Emergency Medicine (23).

All children should have a finger stick blood glucose measurement at the initial evaluation and, even if this is normal, laboratory glucose determination should be obtained. Hypoglycemia may cause altered mental status and seizures, and it may worsen outcome when associated with other etiologies. Hypoglycemia must be treated urgently with intravenous dextrose. Hyperglycemia may occur in diabetic ketoacidosis. All patients should have a blood gas testing. All patients should have electrolytes measured since abnormalities may cause encephalopathy or may occur secondary to intracranial abnormalities. A complete blood count with differential is indicated in all patients to detect infection, anemia, disseminated intravascular coagulopathy, lead encephalopathy, or sickle cell disease. Liver function tests including ammonia should be performed for possible hepatic encephalopathy and because liver injury can occur in the setting of systemic hypoxic-ischemic injury. If fever is present or infection is suspected, then blood, urine, stool, and, in some situations, CSF cultures should be obtained. Toxin screens should be performed in all children and should include acetaminophen, salicylate, and ethanol. Urine toxicology tests may be performed first, but are often supplemented with expanded blood testing. Specific tests for medications found in the home should be carried out as necessary. Lactate, pyruvate, and ammonia may be helpful in screening for inborn errors of metabolism. If abnormal or the history is suggestive of metabolic disease then measurement of organic acids, amino acids, very long chain fatty acids, and acylcarnitine profile may be indicated. Some patients may require endocrine testing including cortisol levels and thyroid function studies.

As soon as medically feasible, all children should have a head CT performed to evaluate for intracranial hemorrhage, space occupying lesions (such as tumor or abscess), edema, focal hypodensities (such as infarct, acute disseminated encephalitis, herpes simplex encephalitis), hydrocephalus, or brain tissue shifts (herniation). Contrast is rarely needed in the acute setting. A normal head CT does not rule out all structural intracranial processes. Thus, once the patient has been stabilized and if the etiology of coma remains unclear, then a brain MRI should be performed assuming there is no contraindication. MRI is superior to CT in assessing the subcortical structures, brainstem, and spinal cord and in detecting ischemic stroke and venous disease, early hypoxic-ischemic injury, hypertensive encephalopathy, demyelinating disease, toxic leukoenceph-alopathies, encephalitis, and diffuse axonal injury.

If the patient is febrile, infection is suspected, or no other etiology can be determined, then a lumbar puncture (LP) should be performed in order to test CSF for infection. The test can also be used to determine intracranial pressure and test for tumor cells and immune disorders. If there is clinical or radiologic contraindication for LP such as impending cerebellar herniation, then it should be deferred and treatment should be initiated for possible infections (bacterial, viral, and/or fungal). A normal CT does not rule out elevated intracranial pressure. The opening pressure should be obtained at the time of the LP, and, if it is elevated, then in some cases only a small amount of CSF should be removed to avoid decreasing pressure rapidly. Normal CSF glucose is usually about two-thirds of the serum level (the ratio can be different if the serum level is very high or very low), so serum glucose should be obtained as an aid in assessing the CSF glucose level. If the serum level is varying then it is best determined about 3 hours before the LP. CSF cell counts should be obtained on collection tubes 1 and 4 so that genuine abnormalities can be distinguished from the effects of a "traumatic tap." CSF testing should also include glucose, protein, gram stain, and other stains as indicated, bacterial cultures, viral cultures and PCRs, and additional cultures depending on clinical suspicion (eg, fungal or tuberculosis). Extra collection tubes may be needed in order obtain sufficient volume necessary for all the testing. Saving a tube of CSF may be useful when etiology is unknown in case later testing for metabolic and immune mediated conditions is required.

An EEG may be useful for several reasons. While most EEG findings are etiologically nonspecific, they may help distinguish between focal and diffuse etiologies. Focal abnormalities suggest focal dysfunction, such as with herpes simplex encephalitis or stroke associated periodic epileptiform discharges. An unexpectedly normal or only mildly abnormal EEG may raise concern for psychogenic, neuromuscular, or locked-in conditions. Additionally, an EEG may identify nonconvulsive seizures or nonconvulsive status epilepticus, which may cause encephalopathy and occur in response to other acute encephalopathies that are also contributing to producing altered mental status. Studies have indicated 10% to 40% of children with acute encephalopathy experience nonconvulsive seizures or status epilepticus (38–41). Continuous EEG monitoring has a much higher yield than a standard EEG when aiming to identify nonconvulsive seizures. Continuous

EEG monitoring or serial standard EEGs may be useful for following the evolution of encephalopathic states and identifying abrupt changes that could require evaluation and intervention. Tracking EEG features over time may help determine the depth of encephalopathy and can help establish whether brain dysfunction is improving, stable, or worsening. Finally, serial EEGs may help with prognostication, particularly if the coma etiology is known (42–44).

If the cause remains unknown, additional studies may be directed at uncommon causes of encephalopathy in pediatrics such as Hashimoto encephalitis (thyroid function tests and thyroid autoantibodies), cerebral vasculitis (erythrocyte sedimentation rate (ESR), antinuclear antibody (ANA) panel, and possibly angiography), or paraneoplastic disorders.

■ MANAGEMENT AND MONITORING

The clinical course in a comatose child depends largely on the underlying illness producing coma and timing of treatment. Because the child's systemic and neurologic function will evolve over time, continuous monitoring including frequent serial neurologic examinations are essential. Related chapters address the most common etiologies for neurocritical illness leading to encephalopathy and coma, and appropriate condition-specific management.

■ CONCLUSIONS

The various types of encephalopathy discussed in this chapter are all medical emergencies since, while many causes are reversible, the neurologic disorder may resolve only if the cause is identified and treated promptly. The history, examination, laboratory, imaging, and electrophysiologic evaluation may disclose the etiology of coma, allowing specific treatment.

■ REFERENCES

1. Wong CP et al. Incidence, aetiology, and outcome of non-traumatic coma: a population based study. *Arch Dis Child.* 2001;84:193–199.
2. Keenan HT et al. A population-based study of inflicted traumatic brain injury in young children. *JAMA.* 2003;290:621–626.

3. Langlois J, Rutland-Brown W, Thomas K. *Brain Injury in the United States: Emergency Department Visits, Hospitalizations, and Deaths.* Centers for Disease Control and Prevention, National Center for Injury Prevention and Control; 2004. http://www.cdc.gov/traumaticbraininjury/tbi_ed.html

4. Parslow RC et al. Epidemiology of traumatic brain injury in children receiving intensive care in the UK. *Arch Dis Child.* 2005;90:1182–1187.

5. Michaud LJ et al. Predictors of survival and severity of disability after severe brain injury in children. *Neurosurgery.* 1992;31:254–264.

6. Plum F, Posner JB. *The Diagnosis of Stupor and Coma.* 3rd ed. Philadelphia, PA: Oxford University Press; 1980.

7. Ashwal S, Eyman RK, Call TL. Life expectancy of children in a persistent vegetative state. *Pediatr Neurol.* 1994;10:27–33.

8. Ashwal S et al. The persistent vegetative state in children: report of the Child Neurology Society Ethics Committee. *Ann Neurol.* 1992;32:570–576.

9. Practice parameters: assessment and management of patients in the persistent vegetative state (summary statement). The Quality Standards Subcommittee of the American Academy of Neurology. *Neurology.* 1995;45:1015–1018.

10. Kriel RL, Krach LE, Jones-Saete C. Outcome of children with prolonged unconsciousness and vegetative states. *Pediatr Neurol.* 1993;9:362–368.

11. Ashwal S. Recovery of consciousness and life expectancy of children in a vegetative state. *Neuropsychol Rehabil.* 2005; 15:190–197.

12. Giacino JT et al. The minimally conscious state: definition and diagnostic criteria. *Neurology.* 2002;58:349–353.

13. Ashwal S, Cranford R. The minimally conscious state in children. *Semin Pediatr Neurol.* 2002;9:19–34.

14. Ashwal S. Medical aspects of the minimally conscious state in children. *Brain Dev.* 2003;25:535–545.

15. Strauss DJ et al. Life expectancy of children in vegetative and minimally conscious states. *Pediatr Neurol.* 2000;23:312–319.

16. Owen AM, Coleman MR. Detecting awareness in the vegetative state. *Ann N Y Acad Sci.* 2008;1129:130–138.

17. Owen AM, Schiff ND, Laureys S. A new era of coma and consciousness science. *Prog Brain Res.* 2009;177:399–411.

18. Landsness E et al. Electrophysiological correlates of behavioural changes in vigilance in vegetative state and minimally conscious state. *Brain.* 2011;134:2222–2232.

19. Bruno MA et al. From unresponsive wakefulness to minimally conscious PLUS and functional locked-in syndromes: recent advances in our understanding of disorders of consciousness. *J Neurol.* 2011;258:1373–1384.

20. Gosseries O et al. Disorders of consciousness: what's in a name? *NeuroRehabilitation.* 2011;28:3–14.

21. Bruno MA et al. Locked-in syndrome in children: report of five cases and review of the literature. *Pediatr Neurol.* 2009;41:237–246.

22. Nakagawa TA, Ashwal S, Mathur M. Guidelines for the determination of brain death in infants and children: An update of the 1987 task force recommendations. *Crit Care Med.* 2011;39(9):2139–2155.

23. The management of a child (aged 0–18 years) with a decreased conscious level. The Paediatric Accident and Emergency Research Group; 2006. http://www.nottingham.ac.uk/paediatric-guideline/.

24. Michelson DJ, Ashwal S. Evaluation of coma and brain death. *Semin Pediatr Neurol.* 2004;11:105–118.

25. Kirkham FJ. Non-traumatic coma in children. *Arch Dis Child.* 2001;85:303–312.

26. Seshia SS et al. Nontraumatic coma in children and adolescents: diagnosis and management. *Neurol Clin.* 2012;29:1007–1043.

27. Teasdale G, Jennett B. Assessment of coma and impaired consciousness. A practical scale. *Lancet.* 1974;2:81–84.

28. Reilly PL et al. Assessing the conscious level in infants and young children: a paediatric version of the Glasgow Coma Scale. *Childs Nerv Syst.* 1988;4:30–33.

29. Raimondi AJ, Hirschauer J. Head injury in the infant and toddler. Coma scoring and outcome scale. *Child's Brain.* 1984;11:12–35.

30. Hahn YS et al. Head injuries in children under 36 months of age. Demography and outcome. *Childs Nerv Syst.* 1988;4:34–40.

31. Wijdicks EF et al. Validation of a new coma scale: the FOUR score. *Ann Neurol.* 2005;58:585–593.

32. Iyer VN et al. Validity of the FOUR score coma scale in the medical intensive care unit. *Mayo Clin Proc.* 2009;84:694–701.

33. Fugate JE et al. The FOUR score predicts outcome in patients after cardiac arrest. *Neurocrit Care.* 2010;13:205–210.

34. Cohen J. Interrater reliability and predictive validity of the FOUR score coma scale in a pediatric population. *J Neurosci Nurs.* 2009;41:261–267; quiz 268–269.

35. Kornbluth J, Bhardwaj A. Evaluation of coma: a critical appraisal of popular scoring systems. *Neurocrit Care.* 2011;14:134–143.

36. Keenan HT et al. A population-based comparison of clinical and outcome characteristics of young children with serious inflicted and noninflicted traumatic brain injury. *Pediatrics.* 2004;114:633–639.

37. O'Connell F. Central pathways for cough in man—unanswered questions. *Pulm Pharmacol Ther.* 2002;15:295–301.

38. Abend NS et al. Nonconvulsive seizures are common in critically ill children. *Neurology.* 2011;76:1071–1077.

39. Williams K, Jarrar R, Buchhalter J. Continuous video-EEG monitoring in pediatric intensive care units. *Epilepsia.* 2011;52:1130–1136.

40. Jette N et al. Frequency and predictors of nonconvulsive seizures during continuous electroencephalographic monitoring in critically ill children. *Arch Neurol.* 2006;63:1750–1755.

41. Saengpattrachai M et al. Nonconvulsive seizures in the pediatric intensive care unit: etiology, EEG, and brain imaging findings. *Epilepsia.* 2006;47:1510–1518.

42. Kessler S et al. Short-term outcome prediction by electroencephalographic features in children treated with therapeutic hypothermia after cardiac arrest. *Neurocrit Care.* 2011;14:37–43.

43. Mandel R et al. Prediction of outcome after hypoxic-ischemic encephalopathy: a prospective clinical and electrophysiologic study. *J Pediatr.* 2002;141:45–50.

44. Mewasingh LD et al. Predictive value of electrophysiology in children with hypoxic coma. *Pediatr Neurol.* 2003;28:178–183.

2 | *Approach to Acute Headache*

CHRISTINA L. SZPERKA and SONA NARULA

■ INTRODUCTION

Nearly everyone experiences a headache at some time, but in rare cases these headaches can be so severe or the onset so sudden that there is concern for an ominous cause. Headaches are classified as "primary" when due to a headache disorder like migraine or tension-type headache, or "secondary," where headache is a symptom of an underlying problem.

The goal of this chapter is to review causes of headache that would present with such severe intensity or level of neurologic decompensation that the child would require care in the Intensive Care Unit. The first section will discuss features of the history and physical examination that are most important for determining the etiology of severe headaches. The second section organizes the differential diagnosis by "red flag" signs and symptoms. The third section discusses primary headache disorders that can mimic dangerous headaches.

■ HISTORY AND PHYSICAL EXAMINATION

Historical and physical examination features are important in differentiating dangerous secondary headaches from primary headache disorders. Table 2.1 lists key historical features that help distinguish between more and less worrisome headaches. Table 2.2 describes key elements of the physical examination.

1. Ask about the pain itself, including the severity, location, duration, and pattern. Did the pain start gradually or suddenly? What time of day does the headache occur? Has the pain changed over time? Has the patient had similar pain before? What things make the pain better? Do coughing, sneezing, lying down, or standing up make the pain worse?

2. Ask about associated features. Sensitivity to light and sound, nausea, vomiting, and neck pain all occur with migraine, but can also be signs of more serious conditions like meningitis. Unilateral rhinorrhea, tearing, and ptosis can be signs of primary headache disorders like cluster headache and paroxysmal hemicrania. If the patient describes pulsatile tinnitus or hearing the pulse in the ears it could be a sign of increased intracranial pressure (ICP).

3. Ask about changes in vision, sensation, and strength. Did these develop suddenly or over a few minutes? Has the patient had these problems before and if so what happened? Has the patient passed out or had seizures?

4. Ask about medications, including over-the-counter meds, and frequency of use. Were medications started or doses adjusted just prior to the onset of headache? Have analgesic medications been used excessively?

5. Collect the patient's past medical history and ask a thorough review of systems. Focus on general symptoms like fatigue, weight loss, and fever, signs of autoimmune disease like joint pain, bowel problems, and rashes, cardiovascular symptoms like dizziness and palpitations, and neurologic symptoms like tremor.

6. Ask about family history of headache, keeping in mind that family members may label their own headaches as "sinus headaches" when they actually

■ **Table 2.1** Headache Characteristics that Suggest a Serious Secondary Cause		
Feature	More Worrisome	Less Worrisome
General characteristics	New or different headache	Chronic or recurrent pain that feels similar with each episode
Pain intensity	Severe	Mild
Timing	Maximal at onset—"thunderclap" (suggests bleeding, vascular causes, or intermittent obstruction)	Pain that develops over minutes to hours
	Pain that awakens patient or always occurs upon awakening (suggests increased intracranial pressure [ICP] but could be primary headache)	Pain that comes consistently later in the day or sporadically
	Progressive pain (suggests structural cause)	Intermittent pain or constant pain that is spontaneously improving
Exacerbating factors	Position change: – Pain worse when lying down, often goes along with pain worse in the morning (suggests increased ICP) – Pain worse when upright (suggests cerebrospinal fluid (CSF) leak or orthostatic blood pressure problems) – Pain worse with cough, sneeze, or Valsalva maneuver (suggests Chiari malformation or increased ICP)	– Pain worse with any activity (not specific to position) can fit with migraine
Location	Occipital/neck pain (concerning for posterior fossa tumor or Chiari malformation, but could be primary headache)	Frontotemporal, periorbital pain
	Unilateral vs bilateral—not helpful. Migraine is classically one-sided in adults but often bilateral in children.	
Other symptoms	Vomiting, photophobia, phonophobia are nonspecific, can come from structural problems or from primary headaches	
	Symptoms or signs of serious systemic illness	Symptoms or signs of benign systemic illness (like upper respiratory infection)
	Constricted visual field, enlargement of blind spot, loss of vision, double vision (suggests increased ICP/papilledema or structural cause)	Blurry vision, flashing lights, spots in vision, scotoma suggestive of migraine, much less often caused by seizure
	Change in mental status, seizure, weakness	Sensory changes can occur with seizure or stroke but more likely fit with migraine
	Hearing problems: – Pulsatile tinnitus (suggests increased ICP or vascular malformation) – Muffled sound (suggests low pressure) or decreased hearing (suggests tumor)	– High pitched tinnitus during headache is nonspecific—can represent mass lesion or can be benign
	Baseline hearing abnormalities can also point to underlying mitochondrial disease.	
Age	Preschool age	School age/adolescence
Family history	No family history of primary headache disorder	Family history of primary headache disorder

■ **Table 2.2** Key Elements of Physical Examination

1. **General medical exam**

   a. Vital signs—Hypertension, bradycardia, and irregular respirations are the ominous triad suggesting increased ICP, but patients do not always have all three. Severe hypertension can cause headache, and low blood pressure can be a sign of pituitary dysfunction.

   b. Head—Look for signs of trauma (skull fracture, point tenderness, CSF rhinorrhea). Check head circumference, especially noting macrocephaly or dramatically increasing circumference.

   c. Neck—Look for meningismus. If there is no history of trauma examine for active range of motion.

   d. Cardiovascular—Occasionally brain or pituitary disease can cause cardiac dysfunction leading to poor perfusion. Listen for bruits over the carotid arteries, temporal arteries, and eyes.

   e. Abdominal—Examine for hepatosplenomegaly and masses. The finding of constipation is especially important in patients with shunts as increased abdominal pressure can lead to poor CSF drainage.

   f. Skin and mouth—Look for rash which can accompany infections and some inflammatory conditions. Birthmarks can signal neurocutaneous disorders.

2. **Neurologic exam**

   a. Mental status—Note change in level of consciousness, speech

   b. Cranial nerves—Look for ptosis, pupillary asymmetry, eye movement abnormalities. Make sure to examine fundus for papilledema even in young children—if needed, turn down the intensity of the light in the ophthalmoscope and keep looking. Check strength and sensation in the face.

   c. Motor—Asymmetric change from baseline is concerning. If the patient is not able to participate with full exam observe spontaneous movements and position of limbs. Check tone—acute brain lesions can cause decreased tone.

   d. Sensory—Asymmetric change from baseline is concerning. Check light touch/tickle on each limb and test more as needed.

   e. Cerebellar—Observe general coordination (is the patient able to sit up?) which reflects the medial cerebellum and test for dysmetria in finger-to-nose movements (have small children reach for a toy). Note that it is difficult to discern cerebellar function in a weak limb.

   f. Gait—Unless the patient is too ill, watch him or her walk in normal position, on heels, on toes, and in tandem. Look for asymmetry of leg and arm movements as well as coordination problems.

---

suffer from migraines. Also ask about family history of brain tumors, strokes, seizures, aneurysms, kidney disease, and autoimmune disease.

■ DIFFERENTIAL DIAGNOSIS OF HEADACHES BY PROMINENT HISTORICAL FEATURE

The red flags for serious headache conditions in children can be summarized by the mnemonic SNOOPY snoop4 (to remember the 4 Ps) secondary causes (1). The remainder of the chapter will be organized by this mnemonic. Some conditions fit into more than one category and are only listed once in the text. Table 2.3 provides a complete differential diagnosis.

Systemic disease signs or symptoms
Neurologic disease signs or symptoms

Onset sudden
Occipital location
Pattern: Progressive or new
          Parents—lack of family history
          Precipitated by Valsalva
          Positional
Years <3

Systemic Disease Signs and Symptoms

Infectious

Infectious causes of headache are very common in children; studies have shown an infectious etiology in 30% to 60% of children presenting to the emergency department with a chief complaint of headache (2,3).

Viral Infection

Viral infections such as influenza, adenovirus, Epstein-Barr virus (EBV) and cytomegalovirus, and bacterial pharyngitis

■ Table 2.3 Differential Diagnosis of Headaches Organized by SNOOPY Mnemonic

Systemic Disease Signs or Symptoms	Neurologic Disease Signs or Symptoms	Onset Sudden

Infectious
Viral infection
Sinusitis
Meningitis
Encephalitis
Intracranial abscess
Shunt infection
HIV infection
 	
Postinfectious
ADEM
 	
Metabolic
Hypoxia/hypercapnia
Hypothyroidism
Hypoglycemia/fasting
Hyperglycemia/DKA
Kidney disease/dialysis
Diabetes insipidus
 	
Rheumatologic disease
Systemic lupus erythematosus
Kawasaki
Rheumatoid arthritis
Behcet's
Sarcoidosis
Polyarteritis nodosa
CINCA syndrome
CNS vasculitis
 	
Other
Pregnancy
Drug-induced headache
Hypertension
	Focal symptoms or signs
	Seizure
	Ischemic stroke
	Intracranial hemorrhage
	Carotid or vertebral artery dissection
	Migraine with aura
	Hemiplegic migraine
	Basilar-type migraine
	Cluster headache
	Paroxysmal hemicrania
	SUNCT
	Ophthalmoplegic "migraine"
	Mitochondrial disease
	CADASIL
	PRES
	RCVS
	CNS vasculitis
	HaNDL
	Trauma
	Hypoglycemia
	ADEM
	Meningitis/encephalitis
	
	Symptoms of increased intracranial pressure
	Brain tumor
	Idiopathic intracranial hypertension
	Cerebral venous sinus thrombosis
	Pineal cyst/apoplexy
	Colloid cyst
	Pituitary apoplexy
	Arachnoid cyst
	Trauma with second impact syndrome
	
	Patients with prior CSF shunt
		Subarachnoid hemorrhage/aneurysm
		Cortical hemorrhage
		Cerebral sinus venous sinus
		  thrombosis
		Ischemic stroke
		Cervical artery dissection
		RCVS
		Pituitary apoplexy
		Colloid cyst
		Spontaneous intracranial
		  hypotension
		Sinusitis
		Meningitis/encephalitis
		
		Occipital Location
		Cervicogenic
		Arnold-Chiari malformation
		Brain tumor
		Vertebral artery dissection
		Trauma
		
		Pattern: Progressive or New
		Trauma
		Brain tumor
		IIH
		Cerebral sinus venous thrombosis
		Sinusitis
		Meningitis/encephalitis
		
		Pattern: Parents (Lack of Family History)
		Nonspecific
		
		Pattern: Precipitated by Valsalva
		Arnold-Chiari malformation
		All causes of increased CSF pressure
		  Spontaneous intracranial
		  hypotension
		
		Pattern: Positional
		Worse when upright
		Intracranial hypotension
		POTS
		Migraine
		Worse when lying down
		All causes of increased CSF pressure
		Worse with neck movements
		Trauma
		Cervicogenic
		
		Years <3
		Nonspecific
		Infectious causes

Conditions that fit into multiple categories are listed in all relevant places.
Abbreviations: ADEM, acute disseminated encephalomyelitis; CADASIL, cerebral autosomal dominant arteriopathy with subcortical infarcts and leukoencephalopathy; CINCA, chronic infantile neurologic, cutaneous, and articular; CNS, central nervous system; DKA, diabetic ketoacidosis ; HaNDL, headache and neurologic deficits with CSF lymphocytosis; IIH, idiopathic intracranial hypertension; POTS, postural orthostatic tachycardia syndrome; PRES, posterior reversible encephalopathy syndrome; RCVS, reversible cerebral vasoconstriction syndrome; SUNCT, short-lasting unilateral neuralgiform headache attacks with conjunctival injection and tearing.

and otitis media are some of the most common causes of acute headache in children. Fever and tachycardia frequently produce a pounding headache that abates when the child's temperature is lowered. Less common infections such as West Nile virus, Lyme disease, brucellosis, malaria, legionella, mumps, mycoplasma pneumonia, and tuberculosis of the central nervous system (CNS) may also cause headache (4–6). In these circumstances symptomatic treatment and antibiotics when indicated are usually all that are necessary. A type of chronic headache called New Daily Persistent Headache can start at the time of infections like EBV and the headache will persist for months to years, but this is rare (7). The presence of headache and seizure with fever is concerning, but does not always herald a severe condition, especially when the child has a history of febrile seizures and the seizure was generalized at onset.

Sinusitis

Sinusitis is another common cause of headache. It usually causes dull, periorbital pain and nasal congestion. However, when the symptoms are chronic or frequently recur, especially when the nasal congestion is mild, one should consider the diagnosis of migraine. Migraine frequently causes pain in the frontal and periorbital areas and involvement of the autonomic nervous system leads to nasal congestion (8). This overlap is further complicated because imaging studies done to evaluated headache often show incidental sinus disease, but treatment of the sinus disease does not affect the headache (9).

Acute isolated sphenoid sinusitis is seen in fewer than 3% of all cases of sinusitis. Although relatively rare, it is important to keep in mind as sphenoid sinusitis can present with subtle symptoms but can lead to multiple complications including intracranial spread (10). Headache is typically the most common presenting sign associated with sphenoid sinusitis and can present anywhere in the craniofacial region. The pain usually will increase over time and may interfere with sleep (11).

Meningitis, Encephalitis, Intracranial Abscess

Less common are intracranial infections like meningitis and encephalitis. These should be suspected when the child has a new severe headache with fever, nuchal rigidity, change in mental status, photophobia, phonophobia, nausea, pain with eye movements, rash, or abnormalities on neurologic examination. The headache may be anywhere on the head, but is usually holocranial, frontal, or occipital. The onset may be gradual or abrupt. Bacterial causes are the most dangerous, but viral and chemical causes are more common. Even rarer are intracranial abscesses which can arise in children with meningitis, otitis, mastoiditis or sinusitis, congenital heart disease, neurosurgical procedures, open head trauma, or immunocompromise. These may also cause focal neurologic signs or seizures. If intracranial infection is suspected, especially if there are any focal neurologic signs or symptoms, initial evaluation should include brain imaging prior to lumbar puncture (LP). Empiric antibiotic therapy should be started immediately (4,12,13).

HIV Infection

Headache can occur with HIV infection at almost any stage of the disease, from acute seroconversion to AIDS. Headache may be related to viral load, and especially in later stages of the disease, can be a sign of opportunistic infection (4).

Postinfectious

Acute Disseminated Encephalomyelitis

Acute disseminated encephalomyelitis (ADEM) is an inflammatory demyelinating disease generally thought to be provoked by infection or vaccination. ADEM is most commonly a monophasic illness and can present with a wide range of neurologic signs and includes some degree of encephalopathy. The diagnosis is confirmed with magnetic resonance imaging (MRI), which typically shows T2 hyperintense white matter lesions. While the presenting signs of ADEM may be varied and nonspecific, one case series reported headache to be one of the most common presenting signs. In this series, headaches were reported as part of the prodromal phase as well as part of the encephalopathy associated with an episode of ADEM (14).

Metabolic Derangements

Many metabolic derangements can cause headaches in children. If any of these disturbances are suspected based on a patient's history and exam, laboratory tests should be done to confirm the abnormality. Headaches should be temporally related to the metabolic disturbance in question and should improve as the abnormality is corrected.

Hypoxia/Hypercapnia

Headaches occur in conditions such as high altitude, diving, or sleep apnea. With high altitude, the headache is generally bilateral, frontal, and aggravated by exertion. It occurs above 2,500 meters within 24 hours of ascent and resolves within 8 hours of descent. Medical treatment of this disorder includes use of acetazolamide and possibly steroids (15). With sleep apnea, the typical headache is usually brief, bilateral, and occurs upon awakening. These children will often snore and have enlarged tonsils or signs of obesity on exam. If sleep apnea is suspected, a polysomnogram should be done (16).

Hypothyroidism

Hypothyroidism has been found to be a risk factor for daily headache, and about 30% of patients with hypothyroidism also have headaches. Headaches are typically described as bilateral and nonpulsatile, and occur within 2 months after the onset of hypothyroidism. The headaches should resolve within 3 months of adequate thyroid replacement therapy (15).

Hypoglycemia/Fasting

Hypoglycemia and fasting are 2 other common causes for headache in children. It is important to note that headaches that occur while fasting may be multifactorial as dehydration and possibly caffeine withdrawal may contribute to the pain (13).

Hyperglycemia/Diabetic Ketoacidosis

Cerebral edema occurs in 0.3% to 1% of children with diabetic ketoacidosis and can occur before or during treatment of diabetic ketoacidosis. Headache can be an early sign of cerebral edema and should be monitored with along with mentation and vital signs (17).

Kidney Dysfunction, Including Hemodialysis

Patients with severe underlying renal disease may complain of headaches, but it may be related to treatment with hemodialysis. In fact, 70% of patients getting hemodialysis complain of headache in more than half of their treatments (15). It has been reported that headaches resolve completely in these patients after successful transplantation and completion of hemodialysis treatments.

Diabetes Insipidus

Along with the characteristic symptoms of polyuria and polydipsia, headache can be a common complaint in children with diabetes insipidus. As sodium levels fluctuate in the setting of diabetes insipidus and its subsequent treatment, headaches can occur in the setting of initial hypernatremia or with aggressive treatment causing hyponatremia and cerebral edema.

Rheumatologic Disease

Headache is a frequent complaint in patients with rheumatologic disease. In fact, one study found that more than half of all systematic lupus erythematosus (SLE) patients reported either migraine or tension-type headache. There was no association found between type or severity of headache and SLE disease status, including whether the CNS was involved (18). Kawasaki disease is a disease that is characterized by persistent fever, conjunctivitis, rash, lymphadenopathy, and abnormalities in the lips and oral mucosa. The disease is characterized by vasculitis and headaches may occur. Patients with rheumatoid arthritis can have arthritic changes in their cervical vertebrae or atlantoaxial instability with associated headache. Headaches have also been reported in Behcet's disease with the etiology being aseptic meningitis or benign intracranial hypertension. Other rarer rheumatic disorders in children that have associated headaches are sarcoidosis, polyarteritis nodosa, and CINCA syndrome (chronic infantile neurologic, cutaneous, and articular syndrome). Secondary CNS vasculitis may cause headache in patients with rheumatologic disease (18).

Other Systemic Causes of Headache

Pregnancy

Headaches, both immediately before and after delivery, may be one of the most sensitive markers for severe complications such as eclampsia, sinus venous thrombosis (SVT), and posterior reversible encephalopathy syndrome (PRES). In order to determine the etiology of a headache, a careful history must be obtained.

Eclampsia occurs when a patient with preeclampsia (hypertension, proteinuria, and edema) develops generalized seizures. Though eclampsia typically occurs prior to delivery, it has also been reported in the postpartum period and can even occur more than 48 hours after delivery. One of the most sensitive presenting signs of eclampsia is headache, which has been reported in up to 87% of cases (19). Other associated symptoms may be nonspecific and include visual changes, nausea and vomiting, and abdominal pain.

Other serious causes of postpartum headaches include headaches secondary to PRES and cerebral sinus venous thrombosis. PRES is typically characterized by visual disturbance, seizure, encephalopathy, and hypertension in addition to headache. Patients with cerebral sinus venous thrombosis report that headache is the most common and earliest symptom (20). These headaches are typically gradual in onset. If associated with increased ICP, they are typically characterized as dull, severe, generalized pain that can worsen with Valsalva and lying down. To differentiate the above etiologies, brain MRI should be done. Vascular imaging may also be needed if a venous thrombosis is suspected.

Another cause of a postpartum headache is a low-pressure headache secondary to an inadvertent dural leak from epidural anesthesia during delivery. This type of headache should be differentiated based on history as these headaches are positional and worse when in an upright position (19).

Drug Induced Headache

Headaches can be associated with a variety of medications, with one of the most common being hormonal contraceptives. Other medications may cause headache due to aseptic meningitis which may be associated with meningismus. Examples of these medications include ibuprofen, intravenous immune globulin, penicillin, trimethoprim, and intrathecal agents. Evaluation of this type of headache may include removal of offending drug and subsequent observation. If meningismus is present, LP may be considered for further workup (16).

Alternately, medication overuse headache is a daily headache that occurs in the context of chronic analgesic use (greater than 3 times per week for at least 3 months), usually initiated for treatment of frequent migraine or tension-type headaches. Typically there are no other associated neurologic signs and the exam is normal. Evaluation includes withdrawal of offending agent with subsequent reevaluation (16).

Hypertension

Hypertensive crisis or encephalopathy may present with acute, severe headaches. While significant elevation of blood pressure may result in headache, typically mild to moderate hypertension does not cause severe headaches (21). See discussion of PRES below regarding hypertensive encephalopathy.

Neurologic Disease Signs and Symptoms

Headache With Focal Neurologic Symptoms or Signs

Seizure

The relationship between headache and epilepsy is complex, and they are comorbid more often that would be expected based on the prevalence of each condition. The pathophysiology of both conditions is related to brain hyperexcitability. There are many ways in which seizure and headache episodes can overlap, including postictal headache, preictal headache, headache that leads to seizure, and seizures with headache as a primary manifestation. Focal seizures can cause focal symptoms or abnormalities on exam, while primarily or secondarily generalized seizures cause loss of consciousness.

Surveys of patients with epilepsy have found that 12% to 52% experience postictal headache, which is defined as headache that starts within 3 hours of a seizure and resolves within 72 hours. It is usually moderate to severe in intensity, and can have features of migraine or tension-type headache. Patients with epilepsy who have migraine headache interictally and those with more severe and long-standing epilepsy are more likely to have postictal headache. Longer seizures and generalized tonic-clonic seizures are more likely to provoke postictal headache. Both analgesics and triptans have been used effectively to treat these headaches. It is not known if antiepileptic medications used for headache prevention (topiramate, valproic acid, etc) have any effect on postictal headache (22). Preictal headaches are less commonly reported (23).

Migralepsy, defined as an episode of migraine with aura progressing to an epileptic seizure, has been reported in about 50 cases. Other authors have criticized that those reports actually described occipital lobe seizures. There are some historical features that can distinguish migraine aura from ictal visual changes. Migraine visual aura usually starts as small flashes of lights or zigzag line which progress over 5 to 30 minutes, often followed by a scotoma. It is usually white or uncolored but can be colorful (24). The hallucinations of occipital lobe epilepsy are usually colorful and circular, develop within a few seconds, widen and multiply, and last a total of a few minutes (25).

There are two idiopathic focal epilepsy syndromes of childhood where headache is a major manifestation of the seizure itself. Idiopathic Childhood occipital epilepsy of Gastaut, also called late onset childhood occipital epilepsy, has been described in children aged 3 to 16 years who have brief visual hallucinations that may progress to other visual or ocular symptoms. Ictal or postictal headache may be orbital or migrainous. The electroencephalogram (EEG) shows paroxysms of spike-wave or sharp discharges in the occipital region with eye closure (26). Early onset benign childhood seizures with occipital spikes, also call Panayiotopoulos syndrome, is a syndrome of infrequent, usually lengthy, nocturnal seizures in children with nausea, retching, and vomiting. Other autonomic manifestations include pallor, pupillary changes, cardiorespiratory and thermoregulatory alterations, incontinence of urine or feces, and hypersalivation. Headache may be present, leading to the misdiagnosis as "atypical migraine." The seizure may secondarily generalize or progress to syncope. The EEG typically shows multifocal, high amplitude sharp and slow wave complexes. Children tend to have a small number of seizures over their lifetime and therefore may not need antiepileptic therapy (27,28).

Ischemic Stroke and Intracranial Hemorrhage

Headache, focal neurologic deficits, and altered mental status can be presenting signs of ischemic stroke or intracranial hemorrhage.

Cervical Artery Dissection

Dissection of the carotid or vertebral artery usually causes head and neck pain followed days to weeks later by symptoms of ischemia; ipsilateral Horner syndrome may accompany carotid dissection.

Primary Headache Disorders

These conditions will be discussed below in more detail.

Briefly, patients with migraine with aura can have focal abnormalities including visual, speech, and sensory disturbances. Patients with hemiplegic migraine have focal weakness associated with headache. Basilar-type migraines cause brainstem dysfunction including vertigo, visual disturbances, bilateral sensory symptoms, and ataxia. Rarely migraines are the presenting sign of progressive genetic or metabolic conditions.

Trigeminal autonomic cephalgias such as cluster headache, paroxysmal hemicrania, and SUNCT (short-lasting unilateral neuralgiform headache attacks with conjunctival injection and tearing) have prominent autonomic features including unilateral ptosis, conjunctival injection, lacrimation, and rhinorrhea. These conditions can be secondary to pituitary or vascular abnormalities, so children with these conditions require MRI to evaluate for a secondary cause.

Ophthalmoplegic "Migraine"

This migraine variant is defined as at least two episodes of headache accompanied or followed within 4 days by paresis of one or more of the third, fourth, and sixth cranial nerves. The most recent *International Classification of Headache Disorders* does not include this as a type of migraine, but recommends imaging to rule out parasellar, orbital fissure, and posterior fossa masses and to look for gadolinium-enhancement of the cranial nerves (21).

Mitochondrial Disease

Headaches and migraines are frequently seen in patients with known mitochondrial disease, but the pathophysiology is still unknown (29,30). As most patients with significant mitochondrial disease have notable neurologic dysfunction and effects on multiple organ systems, screening for mitochondrial disease in patients with isolated headache is not indicated (13). Headache is one of the most common complaints, and may be the presenting symptom, with mitochondrial encephalopathy lactic acidosis and strokelike episodes (MELAS) (31,32). MELAS is a multisystem disorder characterized by strokelike episodes, encephalopathy with seizures or dementia, and lactic acidosis. Other common features of MELAS include vomiting, short stature, hearing loss, and muscle weakness. MELAS is associated with mutations in mitochondrial DNA and is transmitted by maternal inheritance. It typically presents in childhood after a normal early development (33,34). Mutations in the POLG gene have also been associated with headache (35).

Cerebral Autosomal Dominant Arteriopathy With Subcortical Infarcts and Leukoencephalopathy

Cerebral autosomal dominant arteriopathy with subcortical infarcts and leukoencephalopathy (CADASIL) is an underrecognized condition caused by mutations in the Notch3 gene. While this entity is typically seen in adults, there have been case reports in children. Clinically, patients typically present with migraines first and then recurrent episodes of stroke or transient ischemic attacks (36). Other clinical features include the development of cognitive deficits and dementia in more than half of patients and neuropsychiatric symptoms such as mood disorders in 25% to 30% of patients (37). Apathy has been reported as one the most common neuropsychiatric problems associated with CADASIL and can occur independent of depression (38).

Since CADASIL is inherited in an autosomal dominant fashion, it should be suspected in patients with a strong family history of migraines and stroke at an early age in the absence of vascular risk factors. Although migraine with aura is most common, atypical patterns such as aura without headache, prolonged aura, and hemiplegic migraine may be seen (39). Brain MRI is helpful in diagnosis as T2 hyperintense lesions in the deep and periventricular white matter and anterior temporal poles are commonly seen. Definitive diagnosis can be made with genetic testing (screening of the Notch3 gene) or by skin biopsy as small vessel arteriopathy with granular osmiophilic material is diagnostic.

Posterior Reversible Encephalopathy Syndrome

PRES is also called reversible posterior leukoencephalopathy syndrome, and encompasses what was previously called hypertensive encephalopathy. Patients typically present with seizure, visual disturbances, headache, and altered mental status; a review of pediatric cases showed that 76% had 3 of those 4 symptoms (40). Seizures may be focal or generalized, and may lead to status epilepticus. Visual disturbances range from blurred vision to cortical blindness. Headaches are often severe. Mental status may wax and wane, and impairment may be so severe as to necessitate intubation. Nausea, vomiting, papilledema, and focal neurologic findings such as cranial nerve palsies may also be present (41). Stroke and hemorrhage are infrequent complications. There is substantial overlap with reversible cerebral vasoconstriction syndrome (RCVS) in that the same agents may provoke either, and many patients have evidence of both conditions (42).

PRES is associated with acute hypertension, preeclampsia and eclampsia, immunosuppressants (including tacrolimus, cyclosporine, and steroids), bone marrow or solid organ transplantation, chemotherapy, and autoimmune disease (41). Case series of children have also reported an association with transfusion, HIV infection (40), poststreptococcal glomerulonephritis (43),

hemolytic uremic syndrome, and intraabdominal neurogenic tumors (44).

The name of the syndrome refers to the typical pattern seen on imaging of edema in the parietal and occipital white matter. However, gray matter is often involved, and frontal cortex, basal ganglia, corpus callosum, brainstem, and cerebellum can be involved (44,45). While severe PRES can be detected on computed tomography (CT), MRI is more sensitive. Lesions are hypointense on T1-weighted images, hyperintense on T2-weighted and fluid-attenuated inversion recover (FLAIR) recovery images, isointense or bright on diffusion-weighted imaging (DWI), and bright on apparent diffusion coefficient (ADC) map images, consistent with vasogenic rather than cytotoxic edema (43,45). Sometimes the lesions enhance with gadolinium, but this is usually not a striking feature. A few cases reported in the literature have had repeated follow-up MRIs showing incomplete resolution less than 1 week after onset with normalization later (45). If PRES is diagnosed, magnetic resonance angiography (MRA) should also be performed to look for reversible cerebral vasoconstriction given the frequent clinical overlap, and the use of calcium channel blockers to treat the latter. LP is not needed for the diagnosis, but may show elevations in opening pressure up to 50 cm of water (40). Cerebrospinal fluid studies are usually normal, but a mild elevation in protein may be seen (41). EEG can be normal or show focal or diffuse slowing, focal epileptiform discharges, or seizures (43).

Treatment should be aimed at withdrawal of the causative agent when possible, aggressive management of hypertension, and symptomatic treatment of seizures. There has not been any report of how to treat the associated headache, but medications that could exacerbate hypertension should be avoided. While the name implies that the condition will resolve, permanent changes have been reported in up to one quarter of adult cases, and in a few pediatric cases. Recurrent PRES has also been described (45).

CNS Vasculitis

While secondary CNS vasculitis may be associated with systemic rheumatologic disease, primary CNS vasculitis is rare in the pediatric population and is generally accompanied by other signs of CNS inflammation or ischemia (13). Acute severe headache, focal neurologic deficits, and cranial nerve abnormalities are all common presenting features of primary CNS vasculitis in children. If CNS vasculitis is suspected, further evaluation with an LP may be pursued as studies in adults and children have shown the presence of either elevated protein or a pleocytosis in the cerebrospinal fluid of patients with vasculitis (18). Although MRA may be an additional diagnostic tool for detecting CNS vasculitis, brain biopsy is the gold standard for diagnosis. Serologic studies for evaluation of a possible systemic rheumatologic disorder may also be done as part of the workup if vasculitis is suspected.

Syndrome of Transient Headache and Neurologic Deficits With (CSF) Lymphocytosis (HaNDL)

Syndrome of transient headache and neurologic deficits with Cerebrospinal Fluid (CSF) lymphocytosis is characterized by recurrent episodes of neurologic deficits accompanied or followed by moderate to severe headache. The condition was previously called pseudomigraine with lymphocytic pleocytosis. Sensory symptoms are more common than aphasia, motor deficits, or visual changes, and usually last several hours. Patients usually have no history of headaches before these episodes start, but one-third have a viral prodrome. When performed, LP shows CSF lymphocytic pleocytosis (> 15 cells/μL), elevated CSF protein, and sometimes elevated opening pressure; cultures and microbiologic studies are usually normal, though there was one reported case with elevated human herpesvirus 6 (HHV-6) immunoglobulin M when symptoms developed after a viral prodrome (46). Nausea, vomiting, fever, and papilledema may be present. Routine imaging including MRI DWI is usually normal, but perfusion studies may show hypoperfusion in the affected area (47). EEG may show focal abnormalities consistent with symptoms. One case report describes resolution of symptoms with intravenous dexketoprofen (47). Patients are asymptomatic between episodes (21), and the recurrences usually cease within a few months. Multiple case series have been reported, including children as young as 7 years old (48).

Headache With Signs/Symptoms of Increased ICP

Signs of increased ICP include altered consciousness, vomiting, visual problems including blurred vision and diplopia, worsening of headache when supine, bending forward, or coughing, and pulsatile tinnitus.

Idiopathic Intracranial Hypertension

Idiopathic intracranial hypertension (IIH), also called pseudotumor cerebri, is elevated ICP without evidence of structural abnormality in the brain. The headache is usually dull and daily, sometimes accompanied by migrainous features, but can present more acutely. Historical features that suggest IIH includes transient obscurations of vision, blurred vision or diplopia, pulsatile tinnitus, and retro-orbital pain (49). Young children may also show neck stiffness, irritability, somnolence, and ataxia (13). Physical examination should be normal other than papilledema, though the absence of papilledema does not rule out IIH.

The pathophysiology of IIH is not well understood, but is believed to be related to an imbalance between CSF production and resorption. Obese adolescent girls and young women are most commonly affected, but in young children boys and girls are equally affected and there is no association with obesity. Vitamin A, retinoic acid, nitrofurantoin, withdrawal of steroids, thyroid replacement in children with hypothyroidism, and hyperparathyroidism have been associated with IIH. Previously found links with tetracycline, minocycline, oral contraceptives, and pregnancy have been called into question (49).

Particularly in young children the diagnosis is one of exclusion, and a thorough evaluation should include MRI to look for structural abnormalities and signs of infection, and magnetic resonance venography (MRV) to look for thrombosis of the cerebral veins. Magnetic resonance (MR) findings consistent with IIH include an empty sella, flattening of the globes, and stenosis of the cerebral veins. Patients should also have a thorough ophthalmologic evaluation, as decreased visual acuity and visual field loss are often not appreciated or reported by the patient (50).

Diagnosis is made by LP with measurement of opening pressure in the lateral decubitus position. However, the upper limit of normal CSF pressure is not well established in children. One prospective study proposed a value of 28 cm water, but the subjects included in that study all had LP performed due to clinical symptoms, including many with the primary complaint of headache (51). Other studies have shown that adult patients with chronic daily headache, some of whom had stenosis of the venous sinuses, can have significant fluctuation in CSF pressure even when the opening pressure is within the normal range (52,53). Abnormalities in the CSF analysis should prompt testing for chronic infections like Lyme and inflammatory conditions, and preclude the diagnosis of IIH.

Treatment involves several steps. The LP itself can be therapeutic. When the CSF opening pressure is greater than 20 cm water and the history suggests this diagnosis, CSF should be drained to bring the closing pressure to 10 to 20 cm water. Development of low pressure headache after LP does not exclude the diagnosis of IIH. If the headache returns after LP, medical therapy with acetazolamide or topiramate should be initiated. Both of these decrease CSF production by inhibiting the action of carbonic anhydrase. Carefully evaluating for worsening of vision is important and for severe cases where vision is threatened, intravenous steroids can be a temporizing measure, but surgical management with optic nerve sheath fenestration may be necessary. Lumboperitoneal or ventriculoperitoneal shunts are done for extreme cases, but are generally avoided due to a high incidence of shunt failure (50). In obese patients, weight loss is the best long term strategy.

Pineal Cysts/Apoplexy

Pineal cysts are very common, seen on up to 4% of MRIs and 20% to 40% of autopsies. Usually cysts are found incidentally, and are asymptomatic and benign, but rarely they enlarge and become symptomatic. This enlargement can cause obstruction of the third ventricle and hydrocephalus which in turn causes paroxysmal or chronic headache, papilledema, and altered mental status. Pressure on the midbrain causes eye movement abnormalities. An extremely rare complication of pineal cysts and tumors, pineal apoplexy involves sudden hemorrhage into the pineal gland with resultant acute hydrocephalus and abrupt worsening of headache and mental status. Patients may have been symptomatic for months or even years before the acute worsening. A few children have been reported. The youngest was 9 months old. Management options including treatment of the hydrocephalus with ventriculoperitoneal shunt and aspiration or excision of the lesion (54,55).

Arachnoid Cysts

Arachnoid cysts are collections of CSF within the arachnoidal membrane and subarachnoid space. These can occur in many locations, including along the cerebral fissures, in the sella, and at the cerebellopontine angle. They are relatively common, with a prevalence of about 0.7%, and are often found incidentally when head imaging is done after trauma. Bilateral cysts are unusual, and can be associated with glutaric aciduria type I. Arachnoid cysts are usually asymptomatic but can produce symptoms including headaches, seizures, weakness, and hydrocephalus. Long-term most of them remain stable, but they can acutely enlarge and cause symptoms (56) or reduce spontaneously (57). Infrequently after head trauma

the contents rupture, leading to subdural hygromas or intracranial hypertension (56). Most of the case series in the literature have been reported by neurosurgeons, and overall the majority of patients were reported to improve with surgery, especially when fenestration rather than shunting was performed (58). However, there is disagreement about whether all symptomatic patients should be referred for surgery (59).

Headache Associated With Intraventricular Shunts

Headache in a child with a CSF shunt is always worrisome because it can be a sign of shunt malfunction. Shunt malfunction occurs in as many as 50% within 2 years of placement. Patients usually present with nausea, vomiting, headache or irritability, and altered consciousness, but can also have seizures, weakness, cranial nerve abnormalities (especially VI), ataxic gait, and papilledema. Young children and infants can present with a bulging fontanel, splaying of the cranial sutures, or increasing head circumference. In most cases head imaging and a "shunt series," x-rays to image the shunt tubing throughout its course, should be performed. Due to its speed and availability in emergency situations, head CT is usually the study of choice, but MRI is more sensitive for detection of transependymal flow. Ideally, the scan should be compared to a prior image from a time when the child was well.

Causes of shunt malfunction include:

1. Infection—Most common cause of shunt failure in the immediate postoperative period. Typically presents in the days to weeks after surgery. Persistent infection can lead to multiple shunt revisions within a short period of time. Fever is usually present.
2. Shunt misplacement—Rare. Presents with signs of increased ICP in the immediate postoperative period.
3. Obstruction—Relatively common. Can present days to years after surgery. Obstruction can occur at the ventricular catheter, valve, or distal catheter (60).
4. Overdrainage—Refers to situations where the shunt is removing more fluid than desired. Rarely overdrainage leads to extraaxial fluid collections in the immediate postoperative period, but more commonly the excessive drainage leads to "slit ventricle syndrome" years later. Patients with slit ventricles often present with recurrent attacks of vomiting and headache which improve with lying down, whereas patients with obstruction typically experience acute or progressive symptoms that are worse when the

child is supine. Because patients with slit ventricle syndrome can have normal sized ventricles the diagnosis can be difficult; migraine medications or surgical revision of the shunt may be beneficial (61,62).

5. Loculation—Refers to noncommunicating fluid pockets within the ventricles. The shunt drains the fluid pocket to which it is connected, but the others can enlarge and create signs of hydrocephalus. Rarely patients can develop an enlarged, "trapped" fourth ventricle, and present with cranial nerve abnormalities from brainstem dysfunction (61).

6. Fracture, disconnection, or migration of the distal tubing—Typically presents with signs of local irritation around the tubing years after surgery. These patients may not have signs of increased ICP (60).

7. Abdominal complications—Ascites, pseudocyst, constipation, or perforation of an abdominal organ can all lead to hydrocephalus by preventing appropriate drainage from the shunt (61).

Patients with CSF shunts can also have primary headache disorders such as migraine headaches, but these must be diagnoses of exclusion. Given the high prevalence of primary headache disorders, these patients might have developed migraines even if they had never needed a shunt, or the hydrocephalus and shunting may have somehow lowered their threshold for migraine headaches (62). Once an ominous cause has been ruled out, the patient should be treated with migraine therapies (see below). Rarely, patients may complain of headache from allodynia at the shunt bubble or incision site on the scalp (S. Silberstein and W. Young, personal oral communication, 2010).

Onset Sudden

Headaches that are maximal intensity at onset, called thunderclap headache, raise concern for a serious underlying problem, especially a vascular cause like subarachnoid hemorrhage (42). Recurrent thunderclap headaches can be caused by repeated bleeds from aneurysm and by reversible cerebral vasoconstriction. When all other causes have been excluded the diagnosis Primary Thunderclap Headache has been described in adults, but there have been no reports of children with this condition.

Workup for Thunderclap Headache

The workup for Thunderclap Headache is much more aggressive than for other headaches, and should proceed

stepwise until an etiology is found. The timing of these tests will depend on the condition of the patient and availability of testing at your institution, but should proceed as rapidly as possible as most causes of thunderclap headache can cause significant morbidity and mortality. This list is based on the author's experience and review of the literature, but is not based on any formal recommendations.

1. Noncontrast head CT to evaluate for acute bleeding or early signs of ischemia.

2. LP to evaluate for bleeding or xanthochromia. Since it is difficult to differentiate a traumatic tap versus actual hemorrhage, make sure to check cell count in the first and last tubes collected. If the number of red blood cells is significantly elevated and relatively stable between the two tubes consider it positive for hemorrhage. Also measure the opening pressure. Opening pressure greater than 20 to 25 cm of water can be found with many conditions. Opening pressure less than 6 cm of water is diagnostic for intracranial hypotension (IH). If patient has focal neurologic deficits consider MRI before LP to evaluate for ischemia. If IH is suggested by history, the MRI should be done before LP, as LP may exacerbate the condition. If colloid cyst is suggested by history or found on imaging, LP should not be done.

3. MRI of the brain with diffusion-weighted sequences (looking for ischemia). If possible include both noncontrast and postcontrast sequences as IH is best detected with contrast. If the MRI shows ischemia, if reversible cerebral vasoconstriction is suspected, or if any of the above tests have shown hemorrhage, do an MRA of the head and neck. Some institutions may substitute computed tomography angiography (CTA) or other vascular imaging.

4. If the history is suspicious for arterial dissection *or if no other cause is found*, perform MRI of the neck with fat saturated images to best visualize the lumen of the artery.

5. If imaging or history point to SVT, and the imaging above has not been sufficient to visualize the veins, consider additional dedicated imaging with MR or CT venography or the venous phase of conventional angiography.

Vascular Causes

The most well-known causes of thunderclap headache are subarachnoid hemorrhage and unruptured intracranial aneurysm. However, if the patient has focal neurologic deficits the differential should include ischemic stroke, intraparenchymal hemorrhage, SVT, and cervical artery dissection. Blood near the circle of Willis points to hemorrhage from aneurysm whereas blood in the cortical convexities has been associated with SVT, reversible cerebral vasoconstriction, PRES, and cavernomas (42). Chapters 10, 11 and 12 discuss subarachnoid hemorrhage, aneurysm, intraparenchymal hemorrhage, ischemic stroke, arterial dissection, and SVT.

Reversible Cerebral Vasoconstriction Syndrome

The syndrome now called RCVS was previously given several other labels by different medical subspecialists including Call–Fleming syndrome, benign angiopathy of the CNS, and postpartum angiopathy. The current descriptive term highlights the major features of the condition—there is multifocal segmental constriction of intracranial vessels which must by definition resolve within 12 weeks. Vasoconstriction may not be demonstrated on initial imaging, so in patients with recurrent thunderclap headache repeated vascular imaging is recommended. The syndrome is more common in women, but the 4 reported pediatric cases have been in boys (64,65).

RCVS has been associated with the postpartum period and a number of drugs including cannabis, selective serotonin reuptake inhibitors, nasal decongestants, ecstasy 3,4-methylenedioxy-N-methamphetamine (MDMA), cocaine, amphetamines, alcohol, nicotine patches, ergot derivatives, triptans, tacrolimus, cyclophosphamide, erythropoietin, intravenous immune globulin, interferon-A (42), licorice (66), and oral contraceptive pills (67). There have been a few reported cases of RCVS in the setting of catecholamine-secreting tumors including pheochromocytoma, or triggered by orgasm or immersion in a hot bath (42). One of the pediatric cases occurred following a deep dive into a swimming pool (64).

Complications are quite serious and time-dependent. Cortical subarachnoid and intraparenchymal hemorrhage, PRES, and seizures tend to occur within 1 week of onset, while stroke and transient ischemic accidents tend to occur 1 to 2 weeks after the initial headache (68). Treatment involves removal of the inciting substance when possible. Calcium channel blockers, most commonly nimodipine, have been used to prevent vasospasm, and intravenous magnesium is often used in postpartum cases (42). The optimum duration of these treatments is unknown. Mild headache often persists, and depressed mood can be seen a few months later (68).

Pituitary Apoplexy

Pituitary apoplexy refers to the sudden onset of severe headache, vision loss, ophthalmoplegia, vomiting, pituitary failure, and sometimes altered consciousness or fever related to hemorrhage or infarction of a pituitary adenoma. Symptoms arise because sudden increase in the contents of the sella leads to compression and infarction of the pituitary gland, and puts pressure on the optic nerves/chiasm and cranial nerves of the cavernous sinus. Leakage of blood or necrotic tissue causes chemical meningitis and headache. While the injury almost always arises from an adenoma, the tumor can be nonsecreting, and in 60% of patients there is no preceding sign of illness. Trauma, hypotension or hypertension, history of radiation therapy, increased ICP, cardiac surgery, treatment with anticoagulation or dopamine agonists, and pituitary function testing have been reported as precipitants but usually the problem arises without clear provocation (69). Hemorrhage into or hemorrhagic infarction of a Rathke cleft cyst can present similarly, and can only be differentiated pathologically (70). Physical examination may reveal vital sign abnormalities indicating pituitary dysfunction, vision loss, eye movement abnormalities, and alteration in consciousness. CT and MRI will show a sellar mass, usually with hemorrhage. The differential diagnosis includes subarachnoid hemorrhage from ruptured anterior communicating artery aneurysm, and pituitary adenomas and cerebral aneurysms have a co-occurrence rate of ~7%, so vascular imaging may be needed. LP does not aid the diagnosis; CSF studies may be normal or may show hemorrhage or meningitis. Initial management should be focused on fluid and electrolyte balance and replacement of pituitary hormones. Many patients require surgical decompression of the adenoma (69,71). Rare cases in children as young as 6 years old have been reported (72).

Colloid Cyst

Colloid cysts are rare intracranial tumors, usually presenting in the fourth or fifth decade of life but have been found in children as young as 3 weeks of age. They are typically located in the anterior third ventricle, leading to obstruction of flow through the foramen of Monro and compression of the fornix. Bilateral frontal or diffuse headache is the most common presenting sign, caused by acute hydrocephalus. Typically the headache begins abruptly, lasts seconds to hours, and may improve with changing head position or lying down. Other symptoms include nausea, vomiting, alteration in personality, memory disturbance, blurred vision, leg weakness, ataxia, and problems with urination. An infrequent but diagnostic association is abrupt loss of consciousness at the peak of the headache. Sudden death has been reported in up to 10% of patients with colloid cyst, sometimes after a long period of symptoms (73). Airplane travel and head trauma have also been reported to precipitate sudden death (74). Overall, children with colloid cyst tend to have a more aggressive course, and present with signs or symptoms of increased ICP (75,76).

Physical exam may show papilledema, cerebellar abnormalities, nystagmus, and Babinski sign. Imaging is diagnostic. The cyst is usually hyperdense but can be hypodense or isodense on CT and may enhance with contrast. MR characteristics are similarly variable, but most frequently the lesion is hyperintense on T1-weighted images and hypointense on T2-weighted images. The differential diagnosis of a mass in the anterior third ventricle includes ependymoma, glioma, craniopharyngioma, choroid plexus papilloma, meningioma, pituitary adenoma, basilar artery aneurysm, or arteriovenous malformation. LP should be avoided if colloid cyst is suspected because it can provoke herniation. Because of the high rate of death, even in the absence of hydrocephalus at the time of imaging, all symptomatic colloid cysts should be removed surgically, and ventricular drainage may be necessary to relieve hydrocephalus. There is disagreement about whether incidentally found colloid cysts should be removed (73,74).

Occipital Location

This is a risk factor for serious secondary cause of headache (77).

Cervicogenic Headache

Cervicogenic headache refers to a head or facial pain that is referred from the neck. This type of headache should be considered in a patient with a history of neck trauma or surgery to the head, or if the headaches occur with movement or palpation of the neck. If this type of headache is suspected, consider imaging of the brain and cervical spine to exclude any acute fractures or injury to the cord. If no acute abnormality is found, physical therapy may be beneficial to the patient (13).

For patients with trisomy 21, the American Academy of Pediatrics recommends careful neurologic evaluation for signs and symptoms consistent with spinal cord injury, including loss of bowel or bladder control, neck pain, neck stiffness, as the most important clinical predictor of symptomatic atlantoaxial instability and dislocation (78). Patients with rheumatoid arthritis are also at risk for cervicogenic headache. It is important to remember that many of these patients may localize and actually describe their neck pain as headaches.

Pattern: Progressive or New

Headache Associated With Trauma

Mild head trauma is one of the most common causes of headache presenting to the pediatric emergency department (77). Posttraumatic headache is more common after mild injury and in patients with a prior history of a headache. By definition, the pain must start within 7 days of injury; it usually resolves within 4 weeks of injury, but can become chronic. The headache usually resembles tension-type headache or migraine without aura and may be accompanied by neuropsychological symptoms such as mood changes, reduced attention span, easy distractibility, decreased concentration, and sleep disorders. Whiplash injury can also cause headache (79).

Very rarely, trivial head trauma provokes episodes of hemiplegic migraine, diffuse brain edema, and early seizures. This has been linked to a mutation in the CACNA1A gene in 5 patients (80,81). Another rare effect is the "second impact syndrome," where repeated mild head trauma leads to diffuse brain edema (82). Worrisome problems like hemorrhage, carotid or vertebral artery dissection, brain edema, and seizures are more commonly the result of severe head trauma. Patients should be treated aggressively for these sequelae, and the headache should be managed symptomatically with analgesic medications. Acetaminophen and limited narcotics may be given acutely.

Nonsteroidal antiinflammatory drugs (NSAIDs) should be avoided for the first few days unless hemorrhage has been excluded. Chronic posttraumatic headache should be managed like the headache it resembles, focusing on a long-term strategy and avoiding overuse of analgesics.

Brain Tumor

When persistent headaches are present in children, families are often worried about the possibility of an underlying primary brain tumor. Characteristics that predict the presence of a space-occupying mass in children with recurrent headaches include headache lasting less than 1 month, the absence of a family history of migraine, an abnormal neurologic exam, gait abnormalities, and the occurrence of seizures. Other risk factors for brain tumor include sleep-related headache, vomiting, and confusion (83). Brain tumors should also be considered if a child has a history of exposure to ionizing radiation or an underlying syndrome such as tuberous sclerosis or neurofibromatosis (13).

If a patient is found to have a brain tumor, potential etiologies of headache include hydrocephalus, mass effect due to vasogenic edema, hemorrhage, and secondary metabolic disturbances, such as changes in serum sodium. For example, hypernatremia in the setting of diabetes insipidus can occur in the setting of both primary or secondary brain tumors as well as infiltrative diseases such as Langerhans cell histiocytosis (84). Alternatively, hyponatremia in the setting of cerebral salt wasting or syndrome of inappropriate antidiuretic hormone (SIADH) can also occur if a tumor is present.

While treating headaches associated with primary tumors can be challenging, choosing a treatment often depends on the underlying cause of the headache. For instance, if increased ICP is a leading cause, consider the use of acetazolamide. If the tumor is exerting mass effect, treatment with steroids may be helpful to reduce the edema. If awaiting definitive treatment with surgery, using narcotics as a bridge may be appropriate.

Pattern: Parents—Lack of Family History

This is a nonspecific risk factor for secondary cause of headache, including structural causes like brain tumor. Most patients with a primary headache disorder have a family history of headache. However, because primary headache disorders are so much more common than serious secondary causes of headache, most patients without a family history of headache will still have a primary headache disorder like migraine.

Pattern: Precipitated by Valsalva

Most headaches are briefly worsened by coughing, sneezing, and straining, so it is concerning only if the headache worsening is severe and/or sustained. Valsalva maneuvers can also lead to spontaneous CSF leak with resultant low pressure headache.

Chiari Malformation

Chiari malformation type I is defined as inferior displacement of the cerebellar tonsils at least 5 mm below the foramen magnum. It is detected on about 1% of MRIs in children, often incidentally when imaging is done for unrelated reasons. The only population-based study of children, extracted from the database of the Kaiser system, showed that 63% with this finding were symptomatic, including 55% with headache (85). Other associated symptoms include neck pain, syringomyelia (fluid in the center of the spinal cord), motor problems, scoliosis, dysphagia, ataxia, and rarely syncope. The headache can be nonspecific, but the classic presentation is short-lasting stabbing occipital pain precipitated by cough or Valsalva maneuvers like sneezing, laughing, straining, lifting, or bending over (86).

The relationship between the malformation and headache is not fully understood—since Chiari malformations are relatively common (1%) and headaches are very common, it is not always clear that the malformation is causing the headache. The question then arises whether these patients would benefit from surgery. Most of the information in the literature comes from case series of children who have had posterior fossa decompression surgery to relieve the symptoms. There is some disagreement among neurosurgeons about the appropriate criteria for surgery. In their series of 500 children who had surgery for Chiari I, Tubbs et al (87) described that > 80% of patients with Valsalva-induced headache/neck pain improved, but only 15% of those with non–Valsalva-induced headaches improved. Small case series of children under 6 years old have reported more favorable outcomes, with 76% to 100% improvement in headache, including Valsalva-induced and non–Valsalva-induced (88–90). McGirt et al (91) conducted a review of their 256 pediatric patients who had decompressive Chiari surgery to look at long-term outcomes and found that headache is more likely to recur after surgery than are other preoperative symptoms, and the risk is increased for frontal headaches and headaches of longer preoperative duration. Whereas all other studies were conducted from neurosurgical case series, the population-based Kaiser study reported that three of the 28 children who presented with headache had surgical decompression for intractable daily headache. All three improved postoperatively, but one had recurrence of the headache soon after surgery (85). Current research is using advanced imaging studies to look for factors that could predict who will benefit from surgery (92).

Pattern: Positional

When eliciting a history of headache worsened by change in position, it is imperative to clarify the conditions in which the headache is exacerbated.

Worse when upright: Migraine headaches worsen with movement, and therefore are usually worse when the patient is upright and better when the patient is lying down. However, this is different from the dramatic change expected with headache from IH soon after the CSF leak, where the headache should essentially disappear when the patient lies down for at least 15 minutes, and come back only when the patient gets up. This dramatic change can disappear over time, so ask about whether there was an effect of change in position early in the course of the headache. Postural orthostatic tachycardia syndrome (POTS) will also cause headache which is worse when upright and active.

Worse when lying down: This is a sign of increased CSF pressure. Patients will often report that they are more comfortable upright, or that they are awakened by headache in the middle of the night after lying down for several hours. While migraine and other primary headaches can come at night, this history should always raise concern for structural lesions that cause increased CSF pressure.

Worse with neck movements: Cervicogenic headaches and headaches related to trauma will worsen with neck movements. Many patients with migraine also complain of neck pain.

Intracranial Hypotension

Intracranial hypotension (IH) is a condition where the leak of CSF through the dura leads to low CSF volume and/or pressure. IH can develop spontaneously or from minor trauma, LP, epidural or spinal anesthesia, or surgery. All of these causes have been described in children (93,94).

Typically the presentation is insidious, with diffuse, dull pain which worsens when upright for 15 minutes, and improves when supine, but headache from spontaneous CSF leak can start with thunderclap onset. Over time the effect of position on the headache lessens. Muffled hearing, hyperacusis, tinnitus, blurred vision, nausea, neck pain, and stiffness often accompany the headache. When related to a procedure the pain usually starts within 24 to 48 hours, but can be as late as several weeks afterwards (95). The rate of post-LP headache in pediatric studies has varied between 4% and 50%, lower in children ≤ 12 years and with higher gauge (25 or 27) needles (94). Connective tissue diseases such as Ehlers-Danlos and Marfan syndrome have been associated with spontaneous leak. The presence of CSF rhinorrhea suggests leak at the cribriform plate, but most spontaneous leaks occur in the thoracic spine.

Brain MRI with gadolinium usually shows diffuse pachymeningeal enhancement, downward displacement of the brain (can mimic Chiari malformation), enlargement of the pituitary (can mimic pituitary tumors), and engorgement of the venous sinuses sometimes with subdural hygromas or hematomas. Rarely the brain MRI is normal and nuclear cisternogram or CT or MR myelogram must be pursued to document the leak.

Conservative treatment involves supine positioning, intravenous hydration, and intravenous caffeine. Often lumbar blood patch brings relief (96) (even if the leak is not in the lumbar area), but sometimes blood patch directed to the area of leak or even surgical repair are needed (42).

Postural Orthostatic Tachycardia Syndrome

POTS is a form of orthostatic intolerance that is thought to be secondary to autonomic dysfunction. While typically characterized by a constellation of symptoms including light-headedness, syncope, nausea, palpitations, and visual changes, headache is one of the most common symptoms. In terms of epidemiology, postpubescent adolescent females are generally most affected and its development has been commonly reported after an underlying trigger such as a prolonged illnesses or injury. Although diagnostic guidelines are not definitive, it has been suggested that an increase of more than 35 beats per minute with standing (without an obvious underlying cause) in the context of worsening clinical symptoms is consistent with this diagnosis (97). In terms of headache, patients typically report orthostatic headaches, ones that are worsened with standing and improved when recumbent and often occipital in location or affecting the nape of the neck. Additionally, migraines are often comorbid with POTS and it has been reported that up of 95% of patients affected with POTS have concurrent nonorthostatic headaches meeting the definition of migraine or probable migraine.

Years <3

This is a nonspecific risk factor for secondary headache, driven in part by the fact that it is difficult to get a full history and physical examination from a very young child. In their review of patients presenting to the emergency department for headache, Conicella et al (77) found age 2 to 5 years to be a risk factor for life-threatening secondary cause of headache. Because there is little data from which to derive a recommendation, the lower age cutoff of 3 years here is based on expert opinion (98; D. Lewis, A. Hershey, and M. Yonker, personal oral communication, April 14–15, 2011). While very young children can suffer from primary headache disorders like migraine, at initial presentation the clinician should look for signs and symptoms of secondary causes of headache like infection and tumor. In general for this age group, consider obtaining additional diagnostic tests like brain MRI.

■ PRIMARY HEADACHE DISORDERS THAT MIMIC DANGEROUS HEADACHES

In an emergent and critical care setting, it is important to be able to identify mimics of dangerous headaches. In fact, there are many primary headache disorders in children that have features that may resemble more serious neurologic conditions such as stroke, increased ICP, and shunt malfunctions. In addition, it also important to remember that a child may have more than one cause of headache. For instance, while children with shunts are at risk for headaches secondary to shunt malfunction and infection, they may also experience migraines. As a result, it is important to keep these primary headache disorders in the differential when a patient presents with headache and other paroxysmal neurologic signs or symptoms.

In one retrospective study that looked that the frequency and characteristics of headaches that presented to an emergency room in 1 year, 38% of patients presented with a headache secondary to a primary headache disorder. Migraine (especially migraine without aura) was most common followed by tension headache, chronic migraine, and cluster headache (77). Headaches attributed to a serious life-threatening intracranial disorder occurred in about 6% of patients; these etiologies included brain tumors, meningitis, ventriculoperitoneal shunt malfunction, IIH, and brain malformations (Dandy-Walker, Chiari malformations). In this study, all patients with primary headaches were able to describe the quality of their pain while the majority of patients with intracranial diseases were unable to do so. In addition, primary headaches represented about 70% of the unilateral headaches while those with headaches attributed to intracranial disease were either unable to locate their pain or described an occipital headache (77).

The need for additional diagnostic workup for a patient with headache depends on the quality, pattern, and associated symptoms that are identified. If a patient has recurrent paroxysmal headaches that are typical of migraines with a normal neurologic exam and a family history of migraine, typically no imaging or further workup is required (83). However, if a patient with a history of recurrent migraine with a previously normal exam presents with an atypical headache or is found to have an abnormal neurologic exam, additional testing should be considered to rule out other organic causes (99). Other elements in a patient's history that may prompt further diagnostic investigations include recent head or neck trauma, new onset acute headache, new symptoms of increased ICP, worsening severity, and systemic symptoms such as fever, weight loss, and nuchal rigidity (99,100).

Migraine can cause many different focal abnormalities. Migraine with aura, basilar-type migraine, and hemiplegic migraine may be mistaken for stroke at initial presentation. Migraine equivalents also include paroxysmal events without headache like cyclic vomiting, abdominal migraine, benign paroxysmal vertigo, and benign paroxysmal torticollis (101). Common migraine auras include visual, sensory, and speech disturbances. Patients with a history of migraine with aura who present with typical aura (defined as less than 60 minutes, but most important is that the timing be within the patient's typical range) do not require imaging, even if the aura is not followed by headache. Those with prolonged aura should be evaluated because these patients have an increased risk of ischemic stroke. Basilar-type migraine often presents with vertigo, visual disturbances, bilateral sensory symptoms, and ataxia. Should these symptoms present for the first time, a full workup must be done to exclude other disorders involving the posterior fossa.

Hemiplegic migraine is described as migrainous headache with an associated aura that produces fully reversible motor weakness. The weakness will often precede the headache, has been reported to persist even after resolution of the headache itself, and is more likely to affect the arm than the leg (102). Typically the headache is located contralateral to the focal deficit. Hemiplegic migraine is often familial, with at least 1 first- or second-degree relative being affected and 3 types have been described. Type 1 is an autosomal dominant disorder associated with mutation in the CACNA1A gene. Type 2 is associated with a mutation in the ATP1A2 gene (alpha2 subunit of the sodium potassium pump) and type 3 is associated with a mutation in the SCN1A gene. Sporadic hemiplegic migraine has also been described in patients with clinical episodes of hemiplegic migraine and no family history (103). Though no cases have been reported in children, a case series of adults described a condition called Migraine with Unilateral Motor Symptoms (MUMS) characterized by unilateral "give-way" weakness of arm and leg typically ipsilateral to the headache; the weakness could be prolonged, and was seen in patients with both episodic and chronic migraine (104). In terms of treatment, case reports have found verapamil and acetazolamide to be effective for hemiplegic migraine. Triptans are typically contraindicated (105).

Other primary headache disorders seen rarely in children include cluster headaches and paroxysmal hemicranias. Cluster headaches are severe stabbing headaches localized to the periorbital or temporal regions that are unilateral and associated with autonomic phenomenon such as rhinorrhea, lacrimation, and conjunctival injection. This headache syndrome is generally characterized by attacks of daily headaches lasting 15 minutes to 3 hours. These attacks can be ongoing for weeks and then remit for weeks to months at a time with the patient being headache free. Paroxysmal hemicrania is similar to cluster headaches in character though headaches are shorter (few minutes) and occur more frequently throughout the day during an attack than cluster headaches (21). Paroxysmal hemicrania is generally responsive to indomethacin while cluster headaches are not. If a patient presents with these particular headaches, it is important to get brain imaging as they can occur in the setting of pituitary or vascular abnormalities.

If other conditions have been ruled out by history or diagnostic tests and the diagnosis of migraine is most appropriate, acute treatment could include a wide variety of medications like NSAIDs, antidopaminergic medications, dihydroergotamine, and valproic acid (106,107). The best studied combination in children is prochlorperazine and ketorolac (108). Steroids and intravenous magnesium have not been studied in children but are also used. In critically ill patients, it is especially important to consider the side effects of many of the medications used. For example (this list is not exhaustive), NSAIDs and steroids can cause gastrointestinal upset and hypertension. Antidopaminergic medications like metoclopramide and prochlorperazine can cause restlessness or dystonic reaction. Dihydroergotamine is an alpha-adrenergic blocker and a weaker arterial vasoconstrictor; it is contraindicated in patients with hypertension, ischemic heart disease, and residual cardiac abnormalities from Kawasaki disease because it can cause sustained coronary artery constriction. Valproic acid is teratogenic, so a pregnancy test should be done on a patient before it is used. Acute migraine management has been reviewed recently (109).

CONCLUSIONS

Though headaches are very common, and a high proportion of children experience a severe headache at some time, there are many serious causes of headache. Headaches can be a symptom of a primary headache disorder like migraine, but even these can have unusual features. Headaches can also be secondary to another underlying problem. A thorough history and physical should guide the evaluation of headache to ensure that these serious causes are detected when present.

ACKNOWLEDGMENT

Special thanks to Dr William Young for discussion of the differential diagnosis of severe headaches.

REFERENCES

1. Dodick DW. Pearls: headache. *Semin Neurol.* 2010;30(1):74–81.
2. Burton LJ et al. Headache etiology in a pediatric emergency department. *Pediatr Emerg Care.* 1997;13(1):1–4.
3. Kan L, Nagelberg J, Maytal J. Headaches in a pediatric emergency department: etiology, imaging, and treatment. *Headache.* 2000;40(1):25–29.
4. Gladstone J, Bigal ME. Headaches attributable to infectious diseases. *Curr Pain Headache Rep.* 2010;14(4):299–308.
5. Hviid A, Rubin S, Muhlemann K. Mumps. *Lancet.* 2008;371(9616):932–944.

6. Farinha NJ et al. Tuberculosis of the central nervous system in children: a 20-year survey. *J Infect.* 2000;41(1):61–68.

7. Mack KJ. New daily persistent headache in children and adults. *Curr Pain Headache Rep.* 2009;13(1):47–51.

8. Levine HL et al. An otolaryngology, neurology, allergy, and primary care consensus on diagnosis and treatment of sinus headache. *Otolaryngol Head Neck Surg.* 2006;134(3): 516–523.

9. Senbil N et al. Sinusitis in children and adolescents with chronic or recurrent headache: a case-control study. *J Headache Pain.* 2008;9(1):33–36.

10. Tan HK, Ong YK. Acute isolated sphenoid sinusitis. *Ann Acad Med Singapore.* 2004;33(5):656–659.

11. Lahat E et al. Acute isolated sphenoid sinusitis in children. *Pediatr Infect Dis J.* 1997;16(12):1180–1182.

12. Rothner AD, Hershey A. Secondary headaches in children and adolescents. In: Winner P, Lewis D, Rothner AD, eds. *Headache in Children and Adolescents.* BC Decker Inc., Hamilton, Ontario, PMPHUSA; 2007.

13. Blume HK, Szperka CL. Secondary causes of headaches in children: when it isn't a migraine. *Pediatr Ann.* 2010;39(7): 431–439.

14. Gupte G et al. Acute disseminated encephalomyelitis: a review of 18 cases in childhood. *J Paediatr Child Health.* 2003;39(5):336–342.

15. Bigal ME, Gladstone J. The metabolic headaches. *Curr Pain Headache Rep.* 2008;12(4):292–295.

16. Szperka CL. Headache. In: Florin TA, Ludwig S, eds. *Netter Pediatrics.* Philadelphia, PA: Elsevier Saunders; 2011: 471–478.

17. Wolfsdorf J, Glaser N, Sperling MA. Diabetic ketoacidosis in infants, children, and adolescents: a consensus statement from the American Diabetes Association. *Diabetes Care.* 2006;29(5):1150–1159.

18. Duzova A, Bakkaloglu A. Central nervous system involvement in pediatric rheumatic diseases: current concepts in treatment. *Curr Pharm Des.* 2008;14(13):1295–1301.

19. Cantey JB, Tecklenburg FW, Titus MO. Late postpartum eclampsia in adolescents. *Pediatr Emerg Care.* 2007;23(6): 401–403.

20. Cumurciuc R et al. Headache as the only neurological sign of cerebral venous thrombosis: a series of 17 cases. *J Neurol Neurosurg Psychiatry.* 2005;76(8):1084–1087.

21. Headache Classification Subcommittee of the International Headache Society. *International Classification of Headache Disorders.* 2nd ed. Cephalgia. 2004; 24 Suppl 1:1–160

22. Ekstein D, Schachter SC. Postictal headache. *Epilepsy Behav.* 2010;19(2):151–155.

23. Forderreuther S et al. Headache associated with epileptic seizures: epidemiology and clinical characteristics. *Headache.* 2002;42(7):649–655.

24. Friedman DI. Characteristics of migraine visual aura. Paper presented at: American Headache Society 53rd Annual Scientific Meeting; 2011; Washington, DC.

25. Sances G et al. Migralepsy: a call for a revision of the definition. *Epilepsia.* 2009;50(11):2487–2496.

26. Panayiotopoulos CP. Late onset childhood occipital epilepsy. International League Against Epilepsy Web site. http://www. ilae-epilepsy.org/ctf/syn_frame.html. Updated October 3, 2003. Accessed March 4, 2011.

27. Panayiotopoulos CP. Early onset benign childhood seizures with occipital spikes (Panayiotopoulos syndrome). International League Against Epilepsy Web site. http://www.ilae-epilepsy. org/ctf/syn_frame.html. Updated August 20, 2003. Accessed March 4, 2011.

28. Covanis A. Panayiotopoulos syndrome: a benign childhood autonomic epilepsy frequently imitating encephalitis, syncope, migraine, sleep disorder, or gastroenteritis. *Pediatrics.* 2006;118(4):e1237–e1243.

29. Sparaco M et al. Mitochondrial dysfunction and migraine: evidence and hypotheses. *Cephalalgia.* 2006;26(4):361–372.

30. Zaki EA et al. Two common mitochondrial DNA polymorphisms are highly associated with migraine headache and cyclic vomiting syndrome. *Cephalalgia.* 2009;29(7): 719–728.

31. Chi CS et al. Clinical manifestations in children with mitochondrial diseases. *Pediatr Neurol.* 2010;43(3):183–189.

32. Rosen N. Headache and mitochondrial disorders. *Headache.* 2008;48(5):733–734.

33. DiMauro S, Hirano M. *Mitochondrial Encephalomyopathy, Lactic Acidosis, and Stroke-like Episodes (MELAS). GeneReviews.* Oct 2010. PMID: 20301411.

34. Ohno K, Isotani E, Hirakawa K. MELAS presenting as migraine complicated by stroke: case report. *Neuroradiology.* 1997;39(11):781–784.

35. Cohen BH, Chinnery PF, Copeland WC. *POLG-Related Disorders. GeneReviews.* March 2010. PMID: 20301791.

36. Granild-Jensen J et al. Cerebral autosomal dominant arteriopathy with subcortical infarcts and leukoencephalopathy resulting in stroke in an 11-year-old male. *Dev Med Child Neurol.* 2009;51(9):754–757.

37. Dichgans M et al. The phenotypic spectrum of CADASIL: clinical findings in 102 cases. *Ann Neurol.* 1998;44(5):731–739.

38. Reyes S et al. Apathy: a major symptom in CADASIL. *Neurology.* 2009;72(10):905–910.

39. Cleves C et al. Genetically confirmed CADASIL in a pediatric patient. *Pediatrics.* 2010;126(6):e1603–e1607.

40. Pavlakis SG, Frank Y, Chusid R. Hypertensive encephalopathy, reversible occipitoparietal encephalopathy, or reversible posterior leukoencephalopathy: three names for an old syndrome. *J Child Neurol.* 1999;14(5):277–281.

41. Staykov D, Schwab S. Posterior reversible encephalopathy. *J Intensive Care Med.* 2012 Feb;27(1):11–24.

42. Ju YE, Schwedt TJ. Abrupt-onset severe headaches. *Semin Neurol.* 2010;30(2):192–200.

43. Hu MH et al. Clinical experience of childhood hypertensive encephalopathy over an eight year period. *Chang Gung Med J.* 2008;31(2):153–158.

44. Kwon, S, Koo J., Lee S. Clinical spectrum of reversible posterior leukoencephalopathy syndrome. *Pediatr Neurol.* 2001;24(5):361–364.

45. Lee VH et al. Clinical spectrum of reversible posterior leukoencephalopathy syndrome. *Arch Neurol.* 2008;65(2):205–210.

46. Emond H et al. Syndrome of transient headache and neurological deficits with CSF lymphocytosis (HaNDL) associated with recent human herpesvirus-6 infection. *Cephalalgia.* 2009;29(4):487–491.

47. Segura T et al. Usefulness of multimodal MR imaging in the differential diagnosis of HaNDL and acute ischemic stroke. *BMC Neurol.* 2010;10:120.

48. Pascual J, Valle N. Pseudomigraine with lymphocytic pleocytosis. *Curr Pain Headache Rep.* 2003;7(3):224–228.

49. Wall M. Idiopathic intracranial hypertension (pseudotumor cerebri). *Curr Neurol Neurosci Rep.* 2008;8(2):87–93.

50. Wolf A, Hutcheson KA. Advances in evaluation and management of pediatric idiopathic intracranial hypertension. *Curr Opin Ophthalmol.* 2008;19(5):391–397.

51. Avery RA et al. Reference range for cerebrospinal fluid opening pressure in children. *N Engl J Med.* 2010;363(9):891–893.

52. Torbey MT et al. Utility of CSF pressure monitoring to identify idiopathic intracranial hypertension without papilledema in patients with chronic daily headache. *Cephalalgia.* 2004;24(6):495–502.

53. Bono F et al. Abnormal pressure waves in headache sufferers with bilateral transverse sinus stenosis. *Cephalalgia.* 2010;30(12):1419–1425.

54. Majeed K, Enam SA. Recurrent pineal apoplexy in a child. *Neurology.* 2007;69(1):112–114.

55. Patel AJ et al. Pineal cyst apoplexy: case report and review of the literature. *Neurosurgery.* 2005;57(5):E1066; discussion E1066.

56. Pradilla G, Jallo G. Arachnoid cysts: case series and review of the literature. *Neurosurg Focus.* 2007;22(2):E7.

57. Russo N et al. Spontaneous reduction of intracranial arachnoid cysts: a complete review. *Br J Neurosurg.* 2008;22(5):626–629.

58. Helland CA, Wester K. A population-based study of intracranial arachnoid cysts: clinical and neuroimaging outcomes following surgical cyst decompression in children. *J Neurosurg.* 2006;105(5 suppl):385–390.

59. Koch CA et al. Arachnoid cysts: does surgery improve epileptic seizures and headaches? *Neurosurg Rev.* 1995;18(3):173–181.

60. Browd SR et al. Failure of cerebrospinal fluid shunts: part I: Obstruction and mechanical failure. *Pediatr Neurol.* 2006;34(2):83–92.

61. Browd SR et al. Failure of cerebrospinal fluid shunts: part II: overdrainage, loculation, and abdominal complications. *Pediatr Neurol.* 2006;34(3):171–176.

62. Rekate HL. Shunt-related headaches: the slit ventricle syndromes. *Childs Nerv Syst.* 2008;24(4)423–430.

63. Silberstein, S. and W. Young, *Personal Communication.* 2010.

64. Kirton A et al. A pediatric case of reversible segmental cerebral vasoconstriction. *Can J Neurol Sci.* 2006;33(2):250–253.

65. Liu HY et al. Three paediatric patients with reversible cerebral vasoconstriction syndromes. *Cephalalgia.* 2010;30(3):354–359.

66. Chatterjee N et al. Licorice-associated reversible cerebral vasoconstriction with PRES. *Neurology.* 2010;75(21):1939–1941.

67. Soo Y et al. Reversible cerebral vasoconstriction syndrome with posterior leucoencephalopathy after oral contraceptive pills. *Cephalalgia.* 2010;30(1):42–45.

68. Ducros A et al. The clinical and radiological spectrum of reversible cerebral vasoconstriction syndrome. A prospective series of 67 patients. *Brain.* 2007;130(pt 12):3091–3101.

69. Nawar RN et al. Pituitary tumor apoplexy: a review. *J Intensive Care Med.* 2008;23(2):75-90.

70. Komatsu F et al. Clinicopathological characteristics in patients presenting with acute onset of symptoms caused by Rathke's cleft cysts. *Acta Neurochir (Wien).* 2010;152(10):1673–1678.

71. Turgut M. et al. Pituitary apoplexy: an overview of 186 cases published during the last century. *Acta Neurochir (Wien).* 2010;152(5):749–761.

72. Sakalas R et al. Pituitary apoplexy in a child. Case report. *J Neurosurg.* 1973;39(4):519–522.

73. Spears RC. Colloid cyst headache. *Curr Pain Headache Rep.* 2004;8(4):297–300.

74. Humphries RL, Stone CK, Bowers RC. Colloid cyst: a case report and literature review of a rare but deadly condition. *J Emerg Med.* 2011;40(1):e5–e9.

75. Kumar V et al. Pediatric colloid cysts of the third ventricle: management considerations. *Acta Neurochir (Wien).* 2010;152(3):451–461.

76. Alnaghmoosh N, Alkhani A. Colloid cysts in children, a clinical and radiological study. *Childs Nerv Syst.* 2006;22(5):514–516.

77. Conicella E et al. The child with headache in a pediatric emergency department. *Headache.* 2008;48(7):1005–1011.

78. Bull MJ. Health supervision for children with Down syndrome. *Pediatrics.* 2011;128(2):393–406.

79. Obermann M, Keidel M, Diener HC. Post-traumatic headache: is it for real? Crossfire debates on headache: pro. *Headache.* 2010;50(4):710–715.

80. Stam AH et al. Early seizures and cerebral oedema after trivial head trauma associated with the CACNA1A S218L mutation. *J Neurol Neurosurg Psychiatry.* 2009;80(10):1125–1129.

81. Kors EE et al. Delayed cerebral edema and fatal coma after minor head trauma: role of the CACNA1A calcium channel subunit gene and relationship with familial hemiplegic migraine. *Ann Neurol.* 2001;49(6):753–760.

82. Wetjen, NM, Pichelmann MA, Atkinson JL. Second impact syndrome: concussion and second injury brain complications. *J Am Coll Surg.* 2010;211(4):553–557.

83. Lewis DW et al. Practice parameter: evaluation of children and adolescents with recurrent headaches: report of the Quality Standards Subcommittee of the American Academy of Neurology and the Practice Committee of the Child Neurology Society. *Neurology.* 2002;59(4):490–498.

84. Grois N et al. Central nervous system disease in Langerhans cell histiocytosis. *J Pediatr.* 2010;156(6):873–881, 881 e1.

85. Aitken LA et al. Chiari type I malformation in a pediatric population. *Pediatr Neurol.* 2009;40(6):449–454.

86. Levin M. Teaching case: Chiari type I/ cerebellar ectopia headaches: complete resolution following posterior fossa decompressive surgery. *Headache.* 2008;48(7):1146–1149.

87. Tubbs RS et al. Institutional experience with 500 cases of surgically treated pediatric Chiari malformation Type I. *J Neurosurg Pediatr.* 2011;7(3):248–256.

88. Albert GW et al. Chiari malformation Type I in children younger than age 6 years: presentation and surgical outcome. *J Neurosurg Pediatr.* 2010;5(6):554–561.

89. Greenlee JD et al. Chiari I malformation in the very young child: the spectrum of presentations and experience in 31 children under age 6 years. *Pediatrics.* 2002;110(6):1212–1219.

90. Weinberg JS et al. Headache and Chiari I malformation in the pediatric population. *Pediatr Neurosurg.* 1998;29(1):14–18.

91. McGirt MJ et al. Symptom recurrence after suboccipital decompression for pediatric Chiari I malformation: analysis of 256 consecutive cases. *Childs Nerv Syst.* 2008;24(11):1333–1339.

92. McGirt MJ et al. Correlation of hindbrain CSF flow and outcome after surgical decompression for pediatric Chiari I malformation. *Childs Nerv Syst*. 2008;24(7):833–840.

93. Chan EK, Yan B, Ryan MM. Spontaneous intracranial hypotension in childhood: a case report and review of the literature. *J Child Neurol*. 2011;26(6):761–6.

94. Oliver A. Dural punctures in children: what should we do? *Paediatr Anaesth*. 2002;12(6):473–477.

95. Janssens E et al. Post-dural puncture headaches in children. A literature review. *Eur J Pediatr*. 2003;162(3):117-121.

96. Ylonen P, Kokki H. Management of postdural puncture headache with epidural blood patch in children. *Paediatr Anaesth*. 2002;12(6):526–529.

97. Celle ME, Carelli V, Fornarino S. Secondary headache in children. *Neurol Sci*. 2010;31(suppl 1):S81–S82.

98. Lewis, D., A. Hershey, and M. Yonker, *Personal Communication*. 2011.

99. Reuter D, Brownstein D. Common emergent pediatric neurologic problems. *Emerg Med Clin North Am*. 2002;20(1):155–176.

100. De Luca GC, Bartleson JD. When and how to investigate the patient with headache. *Semin Neurol*. 2010;30(2):131–144.

101. Ozge A et al. Overview of diagnosis and management of paediatric headache. Part I: diagnosis. *J Headache Pain*. 2011 Feb;12(1):13–23.

102. Thomsen LL et al. Evidence for a separate type of migraine with aura: sporadic hemiplegic migraine. *Neurology*. 2003;60(4)595–601.

103. Lewis DW. Pediatric migraine. *Neurol Clin*. 2009;27(2):481–501.

104. Young WB et al. Migraine with unilateral motor symptoms: a case-control study. *J Neurol Neurosurg Psychiatry*. 2007;78(6):600–604.

105. Gelfand, AA Fullerton HJ, Goadsby PJ. Child neurology: migraine with aura in children. *Neurology*. 2010;75(5): e16–e19.

106. Kabbouche MA, Linder SL. Management of migraine in children and adolescents in the emergency department and inpatient setting. *Curr Pain Headache Rep*. 2005;9(5): 363–367.

107. Walker DM, Teach SJ. Emergency department treatment of primary headaches in children and adolescents. *Curr Opin Pediatr*. 2008;20(3):248–254.

108. Brousseau DC et al. Treatment of pediatric migraine headaches: a randomized, double-blind trial of prochlorperazine versus ketorolac. *Ann Emerg Med*. 2004;43(2):256–262.

109. Kabbouche MA, Cleves C. Evaluation and management of children and adolescents presenting with an acute setting. *Semin Pediatr Neurol*. 2010;17(2):105–108.

3 Approach to Intracranial Pressure Management

ELENA CAVAZZONI and STEPHEN JACOBE

■ INTRODUCTION

Fusion of the cranial sutures at around 12 months of age results in a semirigid cranial vault with a fixed volume. The three main components constituting this volume are brain parenchyma, cerebrospinal fluid (CSF), and blood. Changes in the volume of one component directly impacts on the others, modifying the proportion each represents within the cranium, a principle referred to as the Monro-Kellie doctrine (1). The respective volumes of each of these 3 components are integral to the regulation of the pressure within the cranial vault, and the relationship between pressure and volume is known as elastance (2).

Intracranial pressure (ICP) usually lies between 5 and 15 mmHg in healthy children and adults (3). A number of compensatory mechanisms exist to minimize fluctuations in ICP, with CSF redistribution, changes in CSF flow, and increased absorption rate being the initial protective responses. If the ICP continues to rise unabated, cerebral blood flow (CBF) will eventually decrease, cerebral ischemia will occur, and finally brain tissue will herniate through the foramen magnum with catastrophic consequences.

This chapter is dedicated to discussing the physiologic and pathologic changes that occur with elevated ICP as well as reviewing current evidence-based treatments available to protect neural tissue.

CBF, Metabolism, Autoregulation, and Disruption of These Mechanisms

CBF in the healthy human brain is tightly regulated by a series of complex feedback systems. These can be classified as:

1. Metabolic: flow-metabolism coupling, in which flow is proportional to the partial pressure of carbon dioxide and oxygen
2. Myogenic: pressure autoregulation
3. Neurogenic: cerebral vascular innervation.

CBF can be expressed by the equation:

$$CBF = CPP/CVR$$

(CPP = cerebral perfusion pressure; CVR = cerebral vascular resistance), where CPP is the difference between the mean arterial blood pressure (MAP) and the ICP as seen in the equation below.

$$CPP = MAP - ICP$$

This pressure gradient ensures blood flow through the brain. Pathologic consequences occur if the CPP is either too low (ischemia) or too high (hyperoxia).

CBF and Metabolism

The gold standard for measurement of global CBF is the Kety-Schmidt technique (4). This relatively cumbersome technique requires cannulation of the jugular veins, and is not considered ideal for critically ill patients. Transcranial Doppler (TCD) sonography has been successfully used to measure blood flow velocities in the basal cerebral arteries. These measurements correlate well with changes in CBF (5,6) and the technique can be safely used at the bedside of critically ill patients.

CBF volume is significantly higher in children compared to adults. In the term neonate, blood flow volume averages ~70 mL/min (7), increasing 10-fold to ~700 mL/min by 3 years of age and peaking at ~900 mL by the age of 6.5 years before declining to ~700 mL at 15 years (8,9). The greatest increase occurs over the first 6 months of life (8). The increase in CBF volume occurs in parallel to increases in oxygen metabolic rate (10) and regional glucose metabolism (11) that reflect neuronal growth and maturation during infancy and early childhood (12). The coupling of blood flow to cerebral metabolism is an important concept, and has also been described during sleep (13) and general anesthesia (14).

Significant intracranial pathology often disrupts the mechanisms that regulate CBF, resulting in either excessive or insufficient blood flow to the brain. A recent study examining the relationship between CBF (by middle cerebral artery flow velocity, Vmca) and CPP in children following traumatic brain injury (TBI) found an inconsistent relationship between the two variables—79% of subjects with a CPP > 40 mmHg had a normal Vmca, while Vmca was decreased in 9% and increased in 12% (15).

Little data exists on the changes in metabolic rate or metabolism in the pediatric brain following trauma or other intracranial pathology; however, adult data suggests global cerebral metabolism is decreased following severe TBI (16). The association between hypotension, low CPP, and poor outcome in patients with severe TBI has been well documented (17,18). It has also been shown that CBF less than 10 to 12 mL/min/100 g causes irreversible global damage to neuronal tissue (19). Studies using microdialysis techniques to measure the metabolic requirements of injured versus noninjured tissue (20) demonstrate that injured brain may be more vulnerable to decreases in CBF and oxygen delivery (20).

Carbon Dioxide and Oxygen Vasoreactivity

Changes in the partial pressure of carbon dioxide rapidly alter CBF in a quasilinear fashion in the healthy adult. The vasodilatation associated with a 1 mmHg increase in $Paco_2$ results in a 2% to 4% increase in CBF (21). The reverse is also true—a decrease in $Paco_2$ causes marked vasoconstriction (22). These changes occur within seconds, making $Paco_2$ a potent cerebral vascular regulator (23). The effects are attenuated by hypotension (24), severe hypoxia (25), and barbiturates (26). Cerebral vasoreactivity is impaired during the initial acute phase following TBI (27,28), which predisposes the brain to either underperfusion or overperfusion.

Adverse outcomes are reported in adult patients hyperventilated following TBI (29), and poor vascular response to changes in $Paco_2$ have been associated with negative neurologic outcomes in children (30). The most recent evidence-based TBI guidelines recommend that prophylactic hyperventilation should be avoided in adult (31) and pediatric (32) patients.

The effect the partial pressure of oxygen has on the cerebral vasculature is less dramatic, with hypoxia-induced vasodilatation (33) and hyperoxia-induced vasoconstriction (34,35) taking several minutes to occur.

Pressure Autoregulation

In healthy adults cerebral autoregulation maintains CBF constant over a range of MAP between 60 and 160 mmHg. The cerebral vasculature responds to changes in pressure by constricting and dilating to avoid rapid changes in blood flow. The effect is achieved by regulating arteriolar diameter so that a decrease in blood pressure results in vasodilatation to maintain blood flow, and a rise in blood pressure leads to vasoconstriction to protect cerebral vascular beds. Beyond the autoregulatory limits, CBF passively increases with an increase in CPP and ICP. The inverse is true with hypotension with associated risk of neural tissue ischemia. The response that cerebral vasculature has to changes in blood pressure is believed to invoke a myogenic effect (36), with smooth muscle tone being altered by changes in transmural pressure.

The other mechanism of pressure autoregulation is neurogenically mediated. Cerebral vessels have both sympathetic and parasympathetic innervation. The former are believed to have a significant effect on vasoconstriction through noradrenaline and neuropeptide Y (37). This has been demonstrated with an increase in CBF with stellate ganglion block (38) and trigeminal ganglion stimulation (39). The sympathetic innervation seems to shift the upper limit of autoregulation to the right, protecting the brain from episodes of hypertension.

Following moderate to severe TBI, cerebral pressure autoregulation is disrupted in both adult (40) and pediatric patients (41). There is evidence that this disruption is greater in cases of nonaccidental versus accidental injury (42). The outcome of patients with impaired pressure autoregulation remains poor in children (42) and adults (43).

Microcirculatory Changes

First elaborated in 1896, the Starling equation essentially states that the net flux of fluid into or out of capillaries (J_v) in the tissues depends on the balance between the hydrostatic pressure within the capillary (P_c) and interstitium (P_i), the oncotic pressure within the capillary (π_c) and interstitium (π_i), the filtration coefficient of the capillary membrane (or how leaky the capillary membrane is to fluid) (K_f), and the reflection coefficient of the capillary membrane (how leaky it is—or is not—to particular molecules) (σ). This relationship can be expressed by the formula:

$$J_v = K_f([P_c - P_i] - \sigma[\pi_c - \pi_i])$$

This concept is relevant when discussing ICP management in a number of areas, in particular, hyperosmolar therapy as well as the basis of what has become known as "the Lund concept" of approaching ICP management (44) (discussed in more detail below).

■ INDICATIONS FOR ICP MONITORING

The clinical features of headache, nausea, or vomiting and decreased level of consciousness should alert the clinician to the possibility of intracranial hypertension. Pathologies that predispose to an increase in ICP can be divided into intracranial or extracranial (see Table 3.1). Fundoscopy and neuroimaging aid in the diagnosis, but elevated ICP may occur in the absence of either papilledema (45) or abnormal neuroimaging (46).

Indications for ICP monitoring in patients with TBI have been defined in adults (47) and—perhaps less clearly—children (48). Uncertainty persists regarding the value of ICP monitoring to positively influence outcome in other conditions such as hypoxic-ischemic injuries (49) and hepatic encephalopathy (50).

Evidence for ICP monitoring has been predominantly obtained from studies of adult patients; however, evidence-based pediatric guidelines were published by the Brain Trauma Foundation in 2003 (51) and these were updated in 2012 (48,52) (hereafter referred to as "the pediatric TBI management guidelines"). ICP monitoring is currently recommended for all children with "severe TBI," which is generally defined as a postresuscitation Glasgow Coma Score (GCS) of ≤ 8. Mild to moderate head injury does not routinely require ICP monitoring, but if the child is unable to be serially neurologically monitored, due to airway management, sedation, and analgesia concerns, then the treating physician may opt to monitor ICP invasively. The presence of an open fontanel and/or open sutures does not preclude the development of raised ICP.

A correlation between raised ICP and poor outcome has been demonstrated in both adult (53,54) and pediatric (55,56) studies of TBI. The purpose of monitoring ICP is to identify, and guide management of, raised ICP (generally defined as ICP ≥ 20 mmHg) (57).

In spite of published recommendations, variability in the implementation of ICP monitoring exists between centers. A prospective study examining ICP monitoring use in the United Kingdom found that overall only 59% of patients presenting to the emergency department with

■ **Table 3.1** Pathologies Associated With Raised Intracranial Pressure	
Intracranial	**Extracranial**
Neoplasm	Ventilation issues (high PEEP, hypercarbia, or hypoxia)
Traumatic head injury	Cardiovascular instability (hypertension or hypotension)
Nonaccidental head injury	Hyperthermia
Infections (meningitis/encephalitis)	Inadequate sedation or analgesia
Intracranial hemorrhage	Obstructed cerebral venous return
Ischemic stroke	Diabetic ketoacidosis
Hydrocephalus	Toxins and medication (lead, doxycycline, tetracycline, rofecoxib)
Status epilepticus	Hepatic failure
Postoperative complications (bleeding, edema, CSF drainage disruption)	

Abbreviations: CSF, cerebrospinal fluid; PEEP, positive end-expiratory pressure.

severe TBI (GCS ≤ 8) had ICP monitored, and the use in individual centers varied widely (7% to 100%) (58).

The adult literature is more specific with its recommendations (47), with level II evidence that ICP should be monitored in patients with severe TBI and a GCS between 3 and 8 following resuscitation and an abnormal computed tomographic (CT) scan of the head—defined as demonstrating either hematomas, swelling, contusions, herniation, or compression of the basal cisterns. There is level III evidence that ICP monitoring is indicated in patients with severe TBI and a normal head CT scan if two of the following three clinical features are noted on admission: age over 40 years, unilateral or bilateral posturing, or a systolic blood pressure < 90 mmHg.

Whether monitoring ICP has an impact on functional neurologic outcome remains uncertain. A retrospective study (59) of adult patients with blunt TBI treated in the United States from 1994 to 2001 actually found a 45% decrease in survival in those patients who had ICP monitoring as part of their treatment. This result needs to be interpreted with caution as treatment modalities subsequently shown to have a detrimental effect on outcome, such as hyperventilation and steroids, may have been used in response to intracranial hypertension. Many clinicians would be reluctant currently to enroll patients with severe TBI into a prospective trial which included randomization to a "no ICP monitoring" arm.

■ ICP MONITORING TECHNIQUES

ICP monitoring devices should be tailored to specific patient groups, but there are some generic characteristics that are favorable for all devices. These characteristics are accuracy, reliability, minimal patient morbidity, and cost effectiveness.

ICP may be measured by direct or indirect methods. Direct methods allow monitoring of true ICP, while indirect techniques allow only assessment of ICP trends.

Direct ICP Measurement

There are 3 types of invasive catheters currently available: (1) the external strain gauge, (2) microstrain gauge, and (3) fiberoptic catheter. Each type has advantages and disadvantages. Devices can be inserted in different locations within the injured central nervous system (CNS). The external strain gauge system relies on a fluid filled catheter in direct communication with the patient's intracranial cavity. The transducer must be calibrated in relation to a fixed point on the patient's head (usually the tragus) and adjusted each time the level of the head is moved. These devices have been shown to be reliable (60) and can be easily recalibrated, but air bubbles or obstruction to the catheter can cause inaccuracies. The microstrain gauge and fiberoptic technologies require calibration prior to surgical insertion and once in situ cannot be easily recalibrated. Catheters can be placed in a range of different locations within the neurologic system, and the commonly used sites and modalities are outlined below. Minimum standards for any ICP monitoring were established in the late 1980s by the Association for the Advancement of Medical Instrumentation, and include the ability to measure pressure in the range from 0 to 20 mmHg, accuracy to 2 mmHg within the stated range, and a maximum error of 10% in the range 20 to 100 mmHg.

1. Intraventricular Devices

    Lundberg in 1960 (60) published the first method to directly measure ICP using a fluid filled external strain gauge, and this remains the gold standard (61–64). A limitation of this catheter is that it can be difficult to insert when the ventricles are effaced. Ventricular catheters allow CSF to be drained if there is raised ICP, providing a therapeutic option not shared by other monitoring systems (65). Complications include hemorrhage, infection, and malposition. There is a paucity of studies looking at catheter complications in children, and the majority of the data is derived from adult studies. The rate of hemorrhagic complications in adults varies between 1% (62,66) to 5% (67) and varies according to the level of experience of the proceduralist. Around 0.5% of patients may require hematoma evacuation (62,66,67). The incidence of hemorrhagic complications in children has been reported to be much higher at up to 15% (68). The rate of infective complications has been reported to be up to 5% (69), and is affected by the number of times the catheter is accessed and by the number of days the device is in situ. Finally, the rate of malposition of intraventricular catheters in children has been reported to be as high as 9% (69).

    Microstrain gauge and fiberoptic catheters have been placed into the intraventricular space but these catheters do not have any therapeutic options. As a result, they have not been widely adopted as the sole monitors for ICP placed within the intraventricular space, unless the ventricles are effaced.

2. Parenchymal Devices

The intraparenchymal monitoring devices are available as microstrain gauge or fiberoptic catheters. They have been compared against the gold standard and both the micro strain gauge (63,64) and fiberoptic catheters (61) have been reported to be accurate. These catheters are calibrated prior to insertion into the parenchymal tissue and cannot be recalibrated once inserted. The deviation from the calibrated "zero" after a period of monitoring is called "drift" and has been assessed following removal of the catheter. Both microstrain gauge (64,70) and fiberoptic probes (62,71) show some drift over time, but both are considered clinically acceptable (72,73). The drift is an important factor to consider when aggressively treating ICPs in patients who have had these catheters in situ for over a week. Complication rates for the intraparenchymal catheter are relatively low. Hemorrhagic complications in children using fiberoptic catheters have been reported to be between 0% (74,75) and 6.5% (69). The clinical infection rate of these devices is also low at between 0% (69,74) and 2% (76). The microstrain gauge device has a very similar complication profile with very few hemorrhagic complications and infections reported (64,77). These types of catheters have increased in popularity in pediatric intensive care units due to the relatively low complication profile with clinically acceptable drift, but one of the major limitations is the lack of any therapeutic options. Whether it is optimal to monitor the noninjured parenchymal tissue, the penumbra area, or injured tissue with these devices remains uncertain.

3. Subdural and Epidural Devices

Epidural and subdural monitoring catheters are rarely used in pediatric patients although their risk profile is low. The subdural device requires anchoring the catheter probe to the skull, which makes it difficult to use in neonates and young infants. Cerebral edema increases the risk of probe malfunction due to brain tissue blocking the lumen of the catheter, and therapeutic CSF drainage is not possible with this device. The epidural device in practice has been found to frequently malfunction, become easily displaced, has significant baseline drift, and

provides no therapeutic option, and as a result has not been widely adopted.

Indirect ICP Measurement

Indirect techniques for measuring ICP are mainly used as screening tools and have not replaced invasive real-time assessment of ICP. In spite of being less invasive with a lower risk profile, the measurements obtained are merely surrogates for the ICP and the initiation of aggressive ICP treatment strategies without reliable monitoring of the actual ICP is usually considered inadequate. The majority of indirect methods only monitor ICP intermittently and continuous monitoring with early aggressive intervention aimed at minimizing episodes of raised ICP is still considered the best way to prevent long term neurologic morbidity.

1. Tonometry

The optic nerve sheath is in direct communication with the CNS so an increase in ICP directly impacts on the perioptic nerve space. This mode of measuring ICP has been used in the acute emergency setting as a screening tool to identify those patients who require more aggressive forms of ICP monitoring and treatment. Studies in adults (78,79) and children (80) have demonstrated a significant correlation between an increase in the optic nerve sheath diameter to 5 and 6 mm and elevated ICP. Ultrasonic assessment of intraocular pressure has also been reported to identify elevated ICP (81).

2. Visual Evoked Response

Visual evoke response (VER) was used in the early 1980s in an attempt to monitor changes in ICP (82). This method relies on an intact optic pathway and assesses a time latency of a specific wave called the N_2 wave following exposure to a visual flash. More recent studies in both children (83) and adults (84) have demonstrated a good correlation between VER and raised ICP. Although noninvasive with a low complication profile, this technique has not yet been adopted widely for patients with raised ICP.

3. Transcranial Doppler

TCD is used to assess the velocity of blood in blood vessels in the basal intracranial arteries. Studies in children (85) and adults (86) have demonstrated good correlation between changes in blood flow and a rise in ICP (87). This type of monitoring has been used as a screening tool to identify patients who might benefit from more invasive ICP monitoring and treatment. Uncertainty remains regarding the accuracy of this tool in predicting changes in ICP (88) and results appear to be highly operator dependent.

4. Jugular Bulb Oxygen Saturation Monitoring

This mode of indirect monitoring involves the retrograde insertion of an oximetry catheter into the jugular bulb to detect oxygen desaturation in the venous blood returning from the brain. This is based on the assumption that in the absence of any changes to the cerebral metabolic rate, any decrease in venous oxygen saturation will be secondary to a rise in ICP (89,90). Reports suggest that the use of this mode of monitoring, in conjunction with the use of brain tissue oxygenation monitoring (91), can aid in the early detection of low CPP and may prevent further secondary insult (92,93). As retrograde cannulation of the internal jugular vein is required, it has not been widely adopted in pediatric intensive care units, with a reported use in only 4% of children with suspected raised ICP in the United Kingdom in 2006 (58).

Newer Monitoring Techniques

1. Brain Tissue Oxygenation

Direct brain tissue oxygenation ($PbtO_2$) monitoring involves a specialized monitoring catheter placed into brain parenchyma measuring real-time partial pressure of oxygen. The majority of studies using this device have been performed in adults; however, there is increasing evidence that minimizing low tissue oxygen levels in the injured brain minimizes secondary damage and improves outcomes in patients with TBI (94–96). Results of pediatric studies are less conclusive about outcome improvements but have indicated that using $PbtO_2$ in conjunction with other modes of monitoring may aid in the treatment of children with TBI (97). Where direct brain tissue monitoring is used, it is recommended that $PbtO_2$ should be maintained ≥ 10 mmHg (98).

2. Near-Infrared Spectroscopy

Near-infrared spectroscopy (NIRS) is a noninvasive monitoring system that measures the percentage of oxygenated hemoglobin ($rScO_2$) in the interrogated tissue by passing a beam of near-infrared light and calculating the difference between oxygenated and deoxygenated blood. This noninvasive technique offers real-time information, and studies have shown an association between low $rScO_2$ and poor

outcome following brain injury (99,100). A limitation is that the relationship between raised ICP and $rScO_2$ may be influenced by the type of brain injury (101) and until a clearer understanding of this relationship is established, NIRS cannot be recommended as a standard ICP monitor.

■ ICP WAVEFORMS

In order to understand and interpret a measured ICP value, two aspects of ICP measurement must be considered.

First, the individual waveform has three peaks called P_1, P_2, and P_3 (Figure 3.1), and these provide varying information. These peaks are associated with the arterial and venous waveforms and changes in their morphology may indicate changes in the compliance within the cranial vault. The P_1 wave has a fairly sharp peak with

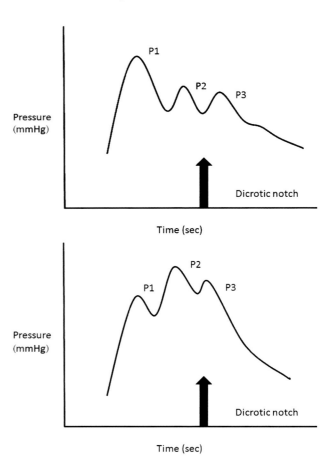

FIGURE 3.1 The intracranial pressure (ICP) waveform.

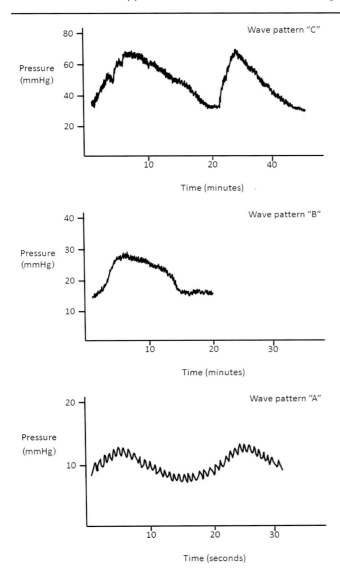

FIGURE 3.2 ICP wave patterns.

relatively constant amplitude; it is the tallest of the 3 waves and an increase in systolic blood pressure will increase the amplitude (102). The P_2 and P_3 waves end and follow the dicrotic notch. An increase in the amplitude of P_2 either indicates an increase in venous volume or a decrease in compliance within the cranial vault (102).

Second, ICP generates varying patterns over time. In the 1960s Lundberg et al (60,103,104) described three types of wave patterns which they labeled "A", "B," and "C" (Figure 3.2). The "C" wave is the result of normal variation in the cardiac cycle and is not considered pathologic. Wave "B" is characterized by a rise in ICP

to 30 to 50 mmHg for 5 to 10 minutes before returning to the baseline level. This wave pattern is considered pathologic if there more than three events in a 24 hour period. Wave "A" is a pathologic pattern characterized by a rise in ICP to above 50 mmHg for as long as 20 minutes and failing to return to the pre-event baseline.

■ MANAGEMENT OF RAISED ICP

Raised ICP has been consistently identified as an independent marker of a poor prognosis (18,54,105). As a consequence, ICP has long been used as a surrogate therapeutic target with management strategies largely focused on interventions to either prevent the development of raised ICP, or, when the ICP becomes elevated, to safely lower the ICP to a more "acceptable" (less harmful) range. Conclusive evidence that such strategies improve mortality and neurologic outcome are, however, lacking.

The underlying aim of ICP management is to prevent or minimize secondary ischemic insult to the brain by ensuring that oxygen delivery (DO_2) remains in excess of cerebral oxygen consumption ($CMRO_2$) at all times. This is best achieved by focusing on delivering good general intensive care, attending to the "airway, breathing, and circulation" ("ABC") of resuscitation, and optimizing CBF.

Patient management goals should be to (1) ensure adequate ventilation, oxygenation, and cardiac output, (2) optimize cerebral perfusion by either decreasing ICP or increasing the arterial blood pressure, (3) decrease cerebral metabolic requirements, and (4) ensure that adequate supplies of oxygen and glucose are available in the blood.

It follows from the Monro-Kellie doctrine referred to above that an ICP reduction may be achieved by either decreasing the volume of any of the intracranial contents (brain, CSF, blood, or pathologic space occupying mass), or increasing the size of the cranial compartment. Treatments to lower the ICP therefore might include: reducing the amount of interstitial fluid (edema) in the brain tissues (hyperosmolar therapy, manipulation of the microcirculation [eg, Lund approach]); decreasing the amount of intracerebral blood (hyperventilation, hyperosmolar therapy); decreasing the amount of CSF (drainage via a ventriculostomy); evacuating space-occupying masses/hematomas; and, finally, by increasing

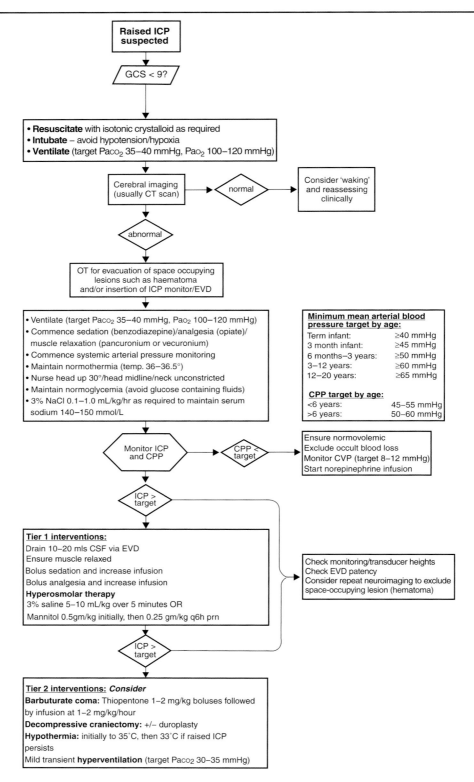

FIGURE 3.3 Suggested algorithm for the management of raised ICP.

the volume of the cranial compartment (decompressive craniectomy).

No single intervention is effective in all patients and given the lack of evidence for many of the available interventions, it is logical that interventions are introduced in a stepwise or "tiered" sequence such as that outlined in Figure 3.3. Tier 1 interventions are generally less invasive with fewer side effects, and are therefore implemented before those Tier 2 interventions that are often more invasive and carry increased risks of causing harm (106).

GENERAL MEDICAL MANAGEMENT

Initial Stabilization and Resuscitation

Patients with acute intracranial hypertension will often present with Cushing triad which is comprised of irregular respiration, hypertension, and bradycardia. Decreased level of consciousness and impaired airway protective reflexes are often present. Patients with TBI as a component of multisystem trauma may have hypotension due to associated hypovolemia or spinal cord injury. Many are also hypoxemic at presentation (107). A systematic ABC-style approach to resuscitation such as that taught in pediatric advanced life support courses requires focus on the rapid assessment and stabilization of the patient's airway (with cervical spine precautions), breathing, and circulation.

Induction and Intubation

All patients suspected of having raised ICP who are obtunded (GCS 8 or less) should be intubated to establish and maintain a secure airway. Secondary cerebral insults such as hypotension and hypoxia, as well as intracranial hypertension that may be seen during intubations—particularly in the partially conscious patient—must be avoided. Therefore induction and intubation in patients with raised ICP should be performed by the most experienced operator available.

Although the depolarizing muscle relaxant succinylcholine (suxamethonium) may cause a slight ICP elevation, this tends to be mild and transient, and the rapidity of onset which provides optimal intubating conditions generally outweighs any potential drawbacks. A defasciculating dose of a nondepolarizing neuromuscular blocker administered prior to succinylcholine prevents the rise in ICP; however, this is seldom used. An intubating dose of a nondepolarizing agent such as rocuronium (0.6–1.2 mg/kg) may be considered as an alternative to succinylcholine. Intravenous lignocaine (1.5 mg/kg) administered 3 minutes prior to intubation may also prevent the transient rise in ICP associated with intubation and may be considered as an adjunct to the procedure (108–110).

Induction agents such as thiopentone and propofol afford excellent cerebral protection during intubation but may cause transient hypotension, particularly in critically ill hypovolemic patients. Alternative agents such as ketamine and etomidate are less likely to cause hemodynamic instability. Etomidate has been associated with adrenal suppression and is best avoided in the patients who are likely to be unwell for some time. Ketamine has been considered contraindicated in patients with possibly raised ICP due to the widely held belief that it can elevate ICP further; however, this dogma has been recently challenged and appears to have little basis (111–113).

Mechanical Ventilation

Mechanical ventilation of the obtunded patient with raised ICP is essential to avoid hypoxemia, hypocarbia, and hypercarbia. Mechanical ventilation is not a benign intervention, however, and the sedation and muscle relaxation often used to facilitate it are associated with potential complications such as atelectasis and ventilator-associated pneumonia which must be recognized and prevented. Positive intrathoracic pressure can also impede venous return, including that from the head. Although the application of positive end-expiratory pressure (PEEP) may lead to an increase in ICP, this increase appears to be clinically insignificant even at levels as high as 15 cm H_2O, with preservation of CPP (114), and we recommend starting with PEEP of 4 to 6 cm H_2O. The patient's minute ventilation should be adjusted to maintain a $Paco_2$ 35 to 40 mmHg (4.7–5.6 kPa).

Chest physiotherapy should be provided as necessary to prevent atelectasis and ventilator-associated pneumonia. Although manual hyperinflation and endotracheal suctioning may increase ICP (115,116), particularly if treatment is begun when the ICP is > 15 mmHg (117,118), percussion can actually lower ICP (117,119). Pretreatment with analgesia, sedation, lignocaine (intravenous or endotracheal) (116), or neuromuscular blockade (118) can attenuate ICP rises and should be considered, and the treatment duration should be as brief as possible.

Volume Resuscitation

Even brief episodes of hypotension can be harmful in the setting of raised ICP and must be strenuously avoided. Patients with TBI may have suffered multitrauma and hypovolemia requiring fluid resuscitation. The choice of prehospital resuscitation fluid in patients with TBI has recently been studied in a randomized controlled trial, and no difference in outcome was identified between the patients resuscitated with hypertonic saline/dextran solution, hypertonic (7.5%) saline, and normal (0.9%) saline (120). These results are consistent with other studies (121), and therefore an isotonic crystalloid solution (normal saline or Hartmann solution) is recommended for prehospital fluid resuscitation.

In terms of in-hospital choice of resuscitation fluids, a recent post hoc subgroup analysis of the multicenter SAFE study (122,123) compared the administration of 4% albumin to crystalloid solution (0.9% saline) for volume resuscitation in adults with TBI. At 2 year follow-up, patients with severe TBI who received albumin had a relative risk of death of 1.88 (95% confidence interval 1.31–2.70, $P < .001$) compared to those who received normal saline. This finding strongly suggests that crystalloid fluids should be the preferred resuscitation fluid in adults with TBI and in the absence of contradictory evidence this should apply to pediatric practice as well.

Surgery

Once resuscitated and stabilized, any patient with suspected raised ICP should have a cerebral CT scan. A decision must be made regarding whether any significant space occupying lesions or other surgically remedial lesions are present that can be addressed, and whether ICP monitoring is indicated (see above). Although the value of surgical evacuation of significant extraaxial (subdural and extradural) hematomas is well established, a study is currently underway to examine whether evacuation of traumatic intracerebral hematomas is also beneficial (124).

Head Positioning and Posture

In patients with raised ICP, positioning with the head of the bed (trunk and head) elevated is thought to encourage CSF drainage and lower ICP, with a concomitant improvement in CPP. Overall, the empirical evidence supports elevation of the head of the bed by 15° to 30° to decrease ICP and improve CPP (125,126). Elevation of the head of the bed also minimizes the risk of pulmonary aspiration, particularly given that most of these patients will be muscle-relaxed. However, elevating the head places it higher than the heart, and this may decrease the MAP. This potential decrease is proportional to the height of the patient (decreased "pressure" [mmHg] at 30° = 0.5 × distance from the heart [fourth intercostal space in the midaxillary line] to the head [tragus][cm]/1.36). A recent study in children with TBI found that elevation of the head of the bed led to a lower ICP and MAP in most patients (127). The resultant CPP changes were negligible. Importantly, a paradoxical relationship between head elevation and ICP occurred in some patients, and the authors concluded that the optimal degree of elevation of the head of the bed should be established individually.

Venous outflow from the head must be unimpeded by ensuring that the head is in the midline, cervical collars are well fitted, and that any ties used to secure endotracheal tubes are not constricting.

Analgesia and Sedation

Patients with intracranial hypertension may suffer pain from a number of causes, particularly postoperative patients and those with traumatic injuries. Noxious stimuli may cause elevations in the ICP, and anxiety and pain can increase $CMRO_2$ consumption 2- to 3-fold. It is therefore important that all patients receive adequate sedation and analgesia.

A recent systematic review of randomized controlled trials comparing sedation agents for adults with severe TBI failed to find evidence that one drug is more efficacious than any other (128). The issue of analgesia is usually adequately addressed with an opiate infusion such as morphine (10–40 micrograms/kg/hour) or fentanyl (1–2 micrograms/kg/hour).

Adequate sedation is usually achieved with a benzodiazepine, and our usual practice is to commence a midazolam infusion at 1 to 2 micrograms/kg/minute. Intermittent boluses of diazepam or lorazepam may be given as an alternative. Diazepam has been shown to decrease $CMRO_2$ by up to 25% (129). Although propofol is often used in adult patients, long-term use as a sedative in intensive care children is contraindicated due to safety concerns raised by the United States Food and Drug Administration (130) as well as the United

Kingdom Committee on Medication Safety (131). Ketamine may be considered in certain situations, and may be helpful if there is hemodynamic instability with other sedatives (113).

Anticonvulsants

Seizures may occur in up to 22% of patients following moderate to severe TBI (132) as well as intracranial hemorrhages. Many of these seizures may be nonconvulsive and only detected by continuous electroencephalographic (EEG) monitoring. In addition, many patients with intracranial hypertension will be muscle-relaxed making seizure activity subtle or absent, and seizures may easily go unrecognized despite close clinical observation.

Benzodiazepines have the added advantage of having some anticonvulsant effects, although patients with either documented seizures or a high risk of seizures should receive prophylactic treatment with phenytoin. Phenobarbitone may be a reasonable alternative anticonvulsant in infants, and levetiracetam may be given intravenously in older children if phenytoin fails to adequately control seizures. A recent study by Vespa et al (133) found that despite therapeutic phenytoin levels, a significant number of adults with severe TBI experienced nonconvulsive seizures which were associated with elevated ICP as well as increased lactate to pyruvate ratios on microdialysis monitoring suggesting possible ischemia. Patients in this study with documented seizures also received levetiracetam; however, they uniformly required induction of burst suppression with midazolam, pentobarbital, or propofol before the seizures were adequately controlled.

The recent pediatric TBI management guidelines recommend that anticonvulsants be considered following severe TBI to reduce the incidence of posttraumatic seizures (134).

Sedation and Analgesia for Interventions

Bolus medications to blunt an anticipated rise in the ICP associated with planned interventions such as endotracheal suctioning and chest physiotherapy may be useful. Potentially useful agents may include narcotics, benzodiazepines, propofol, lignocaine (116), or even ketamine (113). Care must be exercised with bolus opiates as there is a risk these may increase ICP and decrease CPP (128).

For refractory intracranial hypertension, induced anesthesia with a thiopentone infusion will usually decrease ICP as well as decrease the cerebral metabolic rate of oxygen ($CMRO_2$). Such treatment is not without complications, however, and should be reserved for use as a Tier 2 intervention (see below). Monitoring with continuous or intermittent EEG is useful. Following prolonged infusion, plasma thiopentone levels can be monitored. Following prolonged infusions, thiopentone may accumulate in the body's fat stores and recovery may be delayed.

Neuromuscular Blockade

By producing relaxation of the chest wall and abdominal muscles, neuromuscular blockade decreases intrathoracic pressure, facilitates mechanical ventilation, and prevents patient-ventilator dyssynchrony and coughing, all of which may decrease ICP. The use of neuromuscular blockers is not without risk, however, and they should be discontinued as soon as possible.

Glucose and Nutritional Modifications

Following neurologic injury resting energy expenditure has been estimated to be markedly elevated (135). Several authors have addressed the timing of nutrition and a Cochrane Review concluded that early feeding is associated with a trend towards improved survival in adult patients with head injuries (136). The mode of nutrition is also important. Compared to parenteral nutrition, enteral nutrition may reduce complication rates and improve outcome in patients with neurologic injury (137). Children have significantly different metabolic requirements than adults and extrapolating conclusions from adult studies is inadequate. Further studies are needed to determine the optimal needs and timing of nutrition in children with neurologic injuries.

Although glutamine has been found to be beneficial in general trauma patients (138) it has not been specifically studied in either TBI patients or children. Supplements such as zinc (139) and vitamins C and E (140) also require further investigation to determine whether they have a role in improving neurologic outcome in children with neurologic injuries. The pediatric TBI management guidelines found no evidence to support the use of an immunomodulating diet in TBI patients (141).

Finally it remains unclear how hyperglycemia or hypoglycemia affects the injured brain. There are several studies demonstrating hypoglycemic episodes have a negative effect on neurologic outcome (142–144), as well as a substantial body of evidence that indicates that hyperglycemia is an independent risk factor for death in both adults (145–148) and children (148,149) with TBI. Studies in the pediatric population are few and, in view of the real risk of damage to the developing brain of an infant due to hypoglycemia, it is very important to determine if an upper glycemic threshold exists beyond which injury is caused to the brain.

Generally, normal saline (or Ringer lactate/ Hartmann solution) should be provided as maintenance fluids in the first instance, the patient's blood glucose should be monitored frequently to avoid episodes of hypoglycemia and hyperglycemia, and enteral nutrition should be commenced as soon as possible.

■ TREATMENT THRESHOLDS

Patients with a higher measured ICP have been demonstrated to have a worse outcome (death or neurologic morbidity) (18,54,105). Although it is recognized that intracranial hypertension in this setting may represent an epiphenomenon rather than be causally related to the poor outcome, the consistent association between elevated ICP and poor outcome has led to efforts to decrease ICP, and 20 mmHg has been broadly accepted as a threshold for treatment escalation in both adults (150) and children (151). Transient elevations may be tolerated, and many protocols stipulate a period of approximately 5 minutes before advising intervention. It is suspected that a lower ICP threshold should apply to younger children (152); however, the exact levels remain unclear and for the time being, at least, the consensus is that 20 mmHg be considered a reasonable threshold for treatment (151).

The focus on ICP is based on the understanding that an elevated ICP will impede cerebral perfusion. As discussed above, CPP is calculated as the difference between the MAP and mean ICP (CPP = MAP – ICP). The minimal level of "adequate" CPP in the adult population remains uncertain; however, an attempt to balance the risks of using aggressive measures to elevate MAP (such as acute respiratory distress syndrome) against the risks of cerebral hypoperfusion has led to a range of 50 to 70 mmHg being currently recommended (153).

For pediatric patients the ideal target CPP is even less clear, but the pediatric TBI management guidelines recommend that CPP should be maintained greater than 40 mmHg (154,155). It has been demonstrated that the secondary insults leading to adverse outcomes may be "dose responsive," that is, proportional to both the amount and duration the ICP is above or CPP is below the identified threshold (156).

Target the ICP or the CPP?

In the 1990s two somewhat divergent strategies emerged aimed at minimizing cerebral insults associated with raised ICP following TBI. The CPP-targeted strategy emphasized measures to maintain CPP above a target value of 70 mmHg based on the belief that a low CPP would lead to a decrease in CBF and cerebral hypoperfusion, which in turn results in a "spiral" involving reflex vasodilation, increased cerebral blood volume, raised ICP, and further decreased CPP (157). Therapy to stabilize the CPP included the use of vasopressor agents such as phenylephrine or norepinephrine to increase the systemic blood pressure, euvolemia or mild hypervolemia, and ICP-lowering measures such as CSF drainage and mannitol administration. Rosner et al (157) reported the initial results using this strategy on 158 adult patients following severe TBI. Over the first 10 days of treatment the mean ICP for the study population was 27 mmHg and mean CPP 83 mmHg. Overall mortality in the group treated was 29%, with a favorable outcome (Glasgow Outcome Score [GOS] = 4–5) in 59%. There was no control group in the study; however, when compared to matched patients from the Traumatic Coma Data Bank, both mortality and morbidity outcomes were significantly better in the CPP-targeted patients. The 40% of patients who received vasopressors in this study had a lower GCS and higher ICP at admission compared to those who did not, and the mortality rate was over twice as high (48% vs. 18%). Half the deaths were attributed to Acute Respiratory Distress Syndrome (ARDS), renal failure, sepsis, and pathologies other than neurologic.

The second approach—referred to as "Lund therapy" (158)—targeted a low ICP while accepting a CPP of 50 mmHg in adults (and 40 mmHg in children). This approach aims to decrease cerebral volume by encouraging the reabsorption of water across the transcapillary membrane by preserving the colloid oncotic pressure and decreasing the intracapillary hydrostatic pressure. The latter objective is achieved by decreasing the systemic blood pressure using a combination of a

β_1-antagonist (metoprolol) and an α_2-agonist (clonidine), and also producing moderate constriction of the precapillary resistance vessels using low-dose thiopental and dihydroergotamine. Dihydroergotamine also causes venous vasoconstriction which might also contribute to a decrease in ICP. The treatment protocol also includes furosemide administration as necessary to achieve a neutral or moderately negative fluid balance, and red blood cell transfusions and albumin as necessary to achieve a hemoglobin 125 to 140 g/L and serum albumin 40 g/L. Eker et al (159) reported their center's experience using Lund therapy [more recently referred to as the "Lund concept" (44)] in 53 adult patients with raised ICP (> 25 mmHg) following TBI. The results were excellent, with mortality rate of 8% and an overall favorable outcome (GOS 4–5) in 79% [compared to a mortality rate of 29% and "favorable outcome" of 59% in the series reported by Rosner et al (157)]. This also represented a significant improvement compared to a group of historical controls treated in the same unit (47% mortality and GOS 4–5 42%). Lund therapy has also been used in children following TBI, with similarly good outcomes (93% survival, and 80% survivors GOS 4–5) (160).

Robertson et al (161) randomized 189 adults with severe TBI to either an ICP-targeted or CBF-targeted management strategy. The CPP target was ≥ 50 mmHg in the ICP-target group, compared to ≥ 70 mmHg in the CBF-target group. Hyperventilation was permitted in the ICP-target group, but not in the CBF-target group. Measured outcomes included jugular venous desaturation ($sjvO_2$ < 50% for > 10 minutes), refractory intracranial hypertension, and functional outcome. After adjustment for potential confounding factors, the patients in the ICP-targeted group had a 2.4 times higher risk of having an episode of jugular venous desaturation than the CBF-targeted patients and the episodes were of longer duration. Despite these differences, there was no significant difference between the groups in terms of functional neurologic outcomes at 3 and 6 months. The incidence of refractory intracranial hypertension was also similar between the groups. Possibly as a result of therapy, the CBF-targeted group suffered a significantly increased incidence of ARDS (15% vs 3.3%, P = .007).

Despite the impressive outcomes reported from single centers, the implementation of Lund therapy has not become widespread, and CPP targeting remains the predominant strategy in the majority of units.

Norepinephrine produces a more reliable and predictable increase in blood pressure compared to dopamine (162) and is the preferred vasopressor.

■ TIER 1 INTERVENTIONS

CSF Drainage

Removal of CSF from within the cranial compartment, usually by way of an external ventricular catheter, is an efficient and rapid means of decreasing ICP.

In patients who have chronic "shunted" hydrocephalus and develop an acute shunt dysfunction with signs of herniation (apnea, anisocoria, bradycardia, and hypertension), rapid "decompression" may be achieved by "tapping the shunt" (or reservoir). Following sterile preparation of the area to be needled, a 25 gauge butterfly needle is introduced into the purpose-designed area of the shunt device or the Rickham reservoir and the CSF pressure is measured using a manometer. If elevated pressure is confirmed, then approximately 10 mL of CSF should be aspirated (163). More CSF can be aspirated if there is no clinical improvement, with intermittent checks of the CSF pressure.

Patients with TBI and potential raised ICP will often have an external ventricular drain (EVD) placed to permit both ICP monitoring as well as CSF drainage. The system must be "closed" to ensure sterility, and CSF may be drained either intermittently in response to elevated ICP, or the EVD may be set at a specific level above the tragus, a site that approximates the foramen of Munro. The conversion factor for mmHg to cm H_2O/CSF is approximately 1.36, so placing the drain at a level ~27 cm H_2O (CSF) above the tragus, for example, should result in drainage of CSF when the ICP rises above ~20 mmHg.

Complications include hyponatremia from excessive CSF drainage, catheter blockage, infection, and potential "overdrainage." CSF may not drain in the presence of profound cerebral edema with ventricular effacement. In addition, intermittent ICP assessment may lead to a delay in detection of significant ICP elevations, and a dual monitoring system should be considered if continuous CSF diversion is used (164).

CSF drainage via a lumbar drain may also be considered as an option if intracranial hypertension is refractory to medical management in the presence of a functioning ventricular drain, and appears to be safe

■ **Table 3.2** Sodium Content and Osmolality of Commonly Used Fluids

Solution	Sodium Content (mmol/L)	Osmolality (mOsm/L)
Saline 0.9%	154	308
Mannitol 20%	—	1098
Saline 3%	513	1026
Saline 7.5%	1283	2565
Saline 23.4%	4004	8008

Source: Modified from Qureshi AI, Suarez JI. Use of hypertonic saline solutions in treatment of cerebral edema and intracranial hypertension. *Crit Care Med.* 2000;28:3301–3313.

when there are open basal cisterns, and focal lesions with mass affect and shift have been excluded (165).

Hyperosmolar Therapy

In the healthy state, the blood-brain barrier is highly impermeable to even very small solutes. This unique property means that increases in plasma osmolality (and not merely colloid oncotic pressure) lead to an increase in the net flux of water into the capillaries in the cerebral circulation. This concept has resulted in a number of osmotically-active substances being used in an attempt to "dehydrate" the brain, thereby decreasing its volume and lowering the ICP (166,167). The "reflection coefficient" referred to earlier in this chapter in regard to Starling forces relates to how readily the molecule diffuses across a membrane and ranges from 0 (very easily) to 1 (none). Substances used therapeutically in the past have included urea (reflection coefficient 0.48), glycerol (reflection coefficient 0.59), mannitol (reflection coefficient 0.90), and sodium chloride (reflection coefficient 1.00) (168).

Mannitol 20% and varying (hypertonic) concentrations of saline are the osmotic agents most widely used currently (Table 3.2). The "dehydrating" properties of these agents were probably overemphasized previously, and more recent studies suggest their use is associated with a range of other potentially beneficial effects including an increase in intravascular volume and decrease in plasma viscosity. They may also reduce endothelial edema, increasing internal blood vessel diameter and thereby decreasing resistance. The accompanying increase in CBF, when autoregulation is intact, has been linked to reflex vasoconstriction (169), another mechanism for the decrease in ICP observed following their administration. Both agents are widely used to treat children with intracranial hypertension (170).

Mannitol

Mannitol has been the mainstay of hyperosmolar therapy for intracranial hypertension for many decades. It is usually available as a 20% solution (20 gm/100 mL), easy to administer, and the recommended initial dose is 0.5 to 1 gm/kg infused over 15 minutes. Further doses of 0.25 to 0.5 gm/kg can be given as long as serum osmolality remains < 320 mOsm/kg, or the osmole gap remains < 10 mOsm/kg. Plasma osmolality can be calculated using the formula (171):

$$(1.86 \times [Na + K]) + [urea] + [glucose] + 10 \text{ where all are expressed as mmol/L, or}$$

$$(1.86 \times [Na + K]) + [BUN] /2.8) + ([glucose]/18) + 10$$
where the glucose and blood urea nitrogen (BUN) concentrations are expressed as mg/dL.

The osmole gap can be calculated by subtracting the calculated osmolarity (mOsm/L) from the measured osmolality (normal range = 0–5) and reflects the quantity of unmeasured osmoles (mOsm/kg). While mannitol is being administered, the osmole gap correlates to some extent with the mannitol concentration, and although the correlation is far from precise, if the osmole gap is low, one can feel reassured that mannitol is being cleared and an additional dose can be safely administered (171).

Potential side effects of mannitol include hypovolemia (due to the induced osmotic diuresis), acute renal failure, hyperkalemia, hypotension, and rebound intracranial hypertension. Historically acute renal failure may have been due to acute tubular necrosis secondary to hypovolemia, and is rarely seen now that patients are generally maintained in a euvolemic state.

Hypertonic Saline

Hypertonic saline was one of the electrolyte solutions used by Weed and McKibben (166,167) in 1919 to demonstrate the potential for hypertonic solutions to decrease the ICP apparently by dehydrating the brain.

Hypertonic saline use has experienced a recent resurgence (172). Initially this was for minimal volume fluid resuscitation of hypervolemic patients, particularly following trauma; however, much research over the past decade has focused on its utility for the treatment of raised ICP. The reflection coefficient for sodium is higher than mannitol, and several studies have found hypertonic saline superior to mannitol (173) leading to suggestions that hypertonic saline should be considered the preferred hyperosmolar agent for the treatment of intracranial hypertension (173–175).

Reported systemic adverse effects include hyperosmolarity, hypernatremia, congestive cardiac failure, hypokalemia, hyperchloremic acidosis, coagulopathy, phlebitis, and renal failure (176). Adverse neurologic effects may include decreased level of consciousness, rebound intracranial hypertension, seizures, central pontine myelinolysis, and subdural and parenchymal hemorrhage (176).

Hypertonic saline is recommended in the recent pediatric TBI management guidelines for the treatment of severe TBI associated with intracranial hypertension (175). Three percent sodium chloride solution (3% NaCl) can be administered as either a slow bolus of 5 to 10 mL/kg, or as an infusion of 3% NaCl solution at a dose range of 0.1 to 1.0 mL/kg/hour. A continuous infusion may be associated with hypernatremia without additional ICP control, and intermittent bolus doses as required may be preferable (177). A recent retrospective study of ICU patients (178) found an association between hypernatremia and ICU mortality. A causal relationship was not proven, and the explanation for the finding may be that hypernatremia is a surrogate marker for disease severity or even reflects a possible increased incidence of diabetes insipidus. Until this becomes clear, it would appear prudent to aim to maintain sodium levels < 165 mEq/L and the serum osmolarity < 360 mOsm/L (179).

Hyperventilation

In the presence of preserved $Paco_2$ vasoreactivity, hyperventilation results in pH-dependent cerebral vasoconstriction with a decrease in ICP and corresponding increase in CPP. Despite a lack of evidence of improved outcomes, these observed positive effects led to hyperventilation being incorporated into ICP management protocols in the past.

However, more recent studies in patients following TBI involving imaging studies such as xenon-enhanced CT and positron emission tomography used to quantify global and regional CBF and brain tissue perfusion have demonstrated in both adult (180) and pediatric (181) TBI patients that any potential benefits of the decrease in ICP and increase in CPP produced by induced hypocarbia are outweighed by the decrease in CBF and resulting increase in regional brain tissue hypoperfusion/

ischemia. The $Paco_2$ threshold for the onset of significant increase in hypoperfused brain tissue appears to lie between 34 and 38 mmHg (4.5–5 kPa) (182). There was no relationship between CBF and ICP or CPP (181). Global indicators of brain perfusion such as $SjVO_2$ and Arteriojugular Venous Difference of Oxygen ($AVDO_2$) monitoring failed to provide a warning when significant regional hypoperfusion developed, and cannot be relied upon to provide an adequate safeguard when hyperventilation is used (180,182).

Based on these findings, routine ("prophylactic") hyperventilation should be avoided (32) and the use of hyperventilation should be limited to situations where clinical signs (such as the onset of bradycardia, systemic hypertension, and anisocoria) suggest that brain herniation due to refractory intracranial hypertension is imminent.

■ TIER 2 INTERVENTIONS

Therapies such as barbiturate coma, hypothermia, and decompressive craniectomy have been found to fairly consistently lower ICP, making these interventions attractive to treat intracranial hypertension. However, more recent studies looking at "patient-centric" outcomes such as morbidity and mortality have so far failed to demonstrate a beneficial effect. In spite of this lack of evidence of benefit on outcomes, it is understandable that many clinicians feel compelled to intervene to reduce severe intracranial hypertension that we know is associated with a poor prognosis. It is likely that these interventions may be useful in some instances and harmful in others, and it is hoped that further research may be able to identify the specific patients or circumstances where the likely benefits of these interventions outweigh the potential harms.

Barbiturate Coma

High-dose barbiturates such as thiopentone and pentobarbital decrease cerebral metabolism and oxygen consumption, leading to metabolism-regulated cerebral vasoconstriction resulting in decreased ICP. In addition, barbiturates have some free radical scavenging properties which may provide a degree of protection against ischemic damage. They are therefore attractive therapeutic options for patients with intracranial hypertension. Unfortunately, high-dose barbiturate therapy has numerous side effects which may outweigh these benefits, including hypotension due to systemic vasodilation and myocardial depression and pulmonary complications. Despite the fairly consistent effects on ICP, there has been no evidence that the use of high-dose barbiturates is associated with improved outcome in patients with raised ICP (183).

A laboratory-based animal study (26) found thiopentone (producing burst-suppression on EEG) produced a 16% decrease in mean blood pressure, 23% decrease in cardiac index, 45% increase in heart rate, no change in peripheral vascular resistance, and a 38% decrease in cerebral metabolic rate for oxygen. These changes remained constant over a range of $Paco_2$ levels between 20 and 60 mmHg. The degree of cerebral vasoconstriction induced by barbiturates was approximately equivalent to that seen with a drop in $PaCO_2$ from 40 to 20mmHg.

A number of reports describe unexpectedly good outcomes following the use of barbiturates. Sidi et al (184) described two patients with severe refractory ICP elevation who appeared to respond to thiopentone. Both patients made near-complete recoveries, and although the authors acknowledged this was anecdotal evidence, they recommended thiopentone be considered in patients with refractory ICP.

Pittman et al (185) reported on the use of pentobarbital for elevated ICP in 27 children with TBI. Fourteen patients (52%) had satisfactory control (ICP < 20 mmHg), 6 patients (22%) died within 48 hours, and 7 patients (26%) had extremely high ICP (ICP > 35 mmHg) and a sustained CPP of less than 50 mmHg despite pentobarbital treatment. Six of the 7 patients had a CPP of less than 30 mmHg for several hours. Hypotension was seen in all patients. All 7 patients survived: 3 with a good outcome, 2 moderately disabled, and 2 with vegetative outcomes, and the authors attributed the survival of these patients to beneficial effects of pentobarbital.

In an unpublished study by Bohn et al (186), patients with severe head injuries were randomized to receive either phenobarbitone or "standard therapy" (which at the time included routine steroids and hyperventilation to $Paco_2$ < 25 mmHg for episodes of raised ICP). There was no difference in terms of mortality, ICP control, or neurologic outcome between the groups at discharge or 6 month follow up.

Other studies have examined whether barbiturates administered prior to the onset of intracranial hypertension might somehow offer a degree of protection from ICP elevation and subsequent neurological injury. Ward et al (187) randomized patients older than 12 years with ICP monitoring following head injuries to receive either pentobarbital "prophylactically" to achieve burst suppression on EEG or no pentobarbital. There was no significant difference in hourly levels of ICP between the groups, incidence of patients with elevated ICP, duration of ICP elevation, or the response of ICP elevation to other treatments. This indicated there was no improvement in outcome when pentobarbital was used prophylactically.

Barbiturates should therefore be considered to treat intracranial hypertension refractory to maximal medical and surgical management (188). Thiopentone appears to be more effective at controlling the ICP than pentobarbital (189). The usual dose is 1 to 2 mg/kg as a slow bolus, observing for a decrease in the ICP (and blood pressure). Once ICP control is achieved, an infusion should be commenced at 1 to 5 mg/kg/hour via a central line—extravasation can cause tissue necrosis. EEG monitoring should be performed regularly aiming for a "burst-suppression" pattern. Blood levels can also be monitored. Systemic hypotension is common, and recalling that hypotension has been associated with poor outcomes, it is imperative that it is anticipated and treated promptly with fluid loading and an inotrope (eg, epinephrine) or vasopressor (eg, norepinephrine) infusion as necessary.

Induced Hypothermia

The potential of induced hypothermia to provide cerebral protection for patients with elevated ICP first appeared in the literature over 50 years ago (190–194), and support for its use in clinical practice has waxed and waned over the years since. Therapeutic hypothermia has been demonstrated to have numerous potentially beneficial neuroprotective effects in animal models of TBI (195,196), and has become the subject of many trials over the past decade following evidence of improved outcomes when used for neonates following hypoxic-ischemic injury (197) and adults following out-of-hospital cardiac arrest (198,199).

Following a number of small, single center studies with positive results, a large multicenter study (200) of adult TBI patients (GCS ≤ 8) failed to demonstrate a significant difference in outcomes between groups of patients randomized to hypothermia (initiated within 6 hours of injury, target 33°C) or normothermia, with similar mortality rates (28% and 27% in the hypothermia and normothermia groups respectively), and similar unfavorable neurologic outcomes (dead, vegetative, or severe disability: 57% in both groups). Recruitment was stopped early after 392 patients were randomized (out of a planned 500) due to futility. The investigators found a higher incidence of hypotension in the hypothermia group on days 3 and 4 during rewarming, with a higher mean CPP on day 1 but lower on days 3 and 4. Patients < 45 years of age who were both hypothermic at presentation and assigned to the hypothermia treatment arm had a better outcome than those who were hypothermic at presentation but subsequently rewarmed following assignment to the normothermic arm. This prompted the investigators and others (201) to speculate that the lack of demonstrated benefit may have been due to the hypothermia being instituted too late, and a further trial which aims to enroll patients with 2.5 hours and institute hypothermia within 4 hours of the injury, with strict avoidance of hypotension, has commenced (202).

A further study (Eurotherm3235Trial) is currently underway studying the effect of the rapid institution of hypothermia in patients following severe TBI for the treatment of intracranial hypertension refractory to other (Tier 1) ICP measures (196).

In a recent randomized controlled trial involving 17 centers in 3 countries over nearly 5 years, Hutchinson et al (203) randomized 225 children with severe TBI (GCS ≤ 8) to either the hypothermia (32.5 +/− 0.5°C) or normothermia (37 +/− 0.5°C) treatment group. The cooling had to be commenced within 8 hours of injury and rewarming commenced at 24 hours at a rate of 0.5°C every 2 hours. Somewhat unexpectedly, the hypothermia group had worse outcomes. The proportion of patients with an unfavorable neurologic outcome (the primary outcome) as assessed by the Pediatric Cerebral Performance Score at 6 months was higher in the hypothermia group (32 of 102, or 31%) compared to the normothermia group (23 of 103, or 22%). Mortality was also higher in the therapeutic hypothermia group (23% vs 14%); however, both results failed to reach statistical significance (*P* values .14 and .06 respectively). There was no difference between groups in other secondary outcomes including duration of ICP monitoring, mechanical ventilation, ICU length of stay, and hospital length of stay. The hypothermia group had a lower ICP (mean 14.7 vs 17.1 mmHg) and lower heart rate (81 vs 108 beats per minute) during the first 24 hours while cooled, and a lower blood pressure (77.7 vs 83.4 mmHg) and lower CPP (60.8 vs 66.0 mmHg) during

the rewarming phase (25–72 hours). Based on these findings, the authors concluded that the use of hypothermia following such a protocol is not warranted, but speculated that either earlier or more prolonged cooling might produce benefit. The potentially detrimental impact of hypotension and lower CPP was reinforced in a post hoc analysis of data from the study which confirmed more episodes of hypotension and low CPP in the hypothermia group compared with the normothermia group, and that hypotension and low CPP were associated with an unfavorable outcome in both groups (204).

The Hypothermia in Traumatic Brain Injury in Children (HiTBIC) Trial (ClinicalTrials.gov no. NCT00282269) randomized children with TBI (GCS ≤ 8 and abnormal cerebral CT scan) to be either cooled (32°C–33°C) for 72 hours and then rewarmed slowly (≤0.5°C every 2 hours) or maintained at normal temperature. The results are yet to be published.

The "CoolKids Trial" (ClinicalTrials.gov no. NCT00222742) aimed to examine the effect on mortality and functional outcome of pediatric patients following severe TBI (GCS ≤ 8) randomized to either cooling to 32° to 33°C commencing within 6 hours and lasting at least 48 hours, or the control arm. The rate of rewarming was 1°C every 12 to 24 hours. Recruitment for the study was halted for "futility" after an interim analysis found that continuing the trial was unlikely to provide an answer to the study hypothesis, and the final results and analysis are awaited.

A recent systematic review of evidence for the use of hypothermia in TBI (205) concluded that there was no evidence that hypothermia is beneficial. The pediatric TBI management guidelines also found no evidence to support a level 1 recommendation but suggested that moderate hypothermia (32°C–33°C) may be considered for refractory intracranial hypertension. Based on the Hutchinson trial, however, if cooling is instituted it should be continued for longer than 24 hours (and probably up to 48–72 hours), and the subsequent rate of rewarming should be slower than 0.5°C per hour, with careful monitoring for—and rapid reversal of—hypotension during this phase (206).

Decompressive Craniectomy

When intracranial hypertension is refractory to medical interventions, a decompressive craniectomy, with or without duroplasty, may be performed to enlarge the cranial compartment, thereby relieving ICP. This approach has been used for over a century, and is attractive based on first principles. Despite many case series and anecdotes reporting successful outcomes in both traumatic (207–213) and nontraumatic (214) causes of raised ICP, evidence for the efficacy of this approach is scant (215).

A range of surgical techniques for decompressive craniectomy are described in the literature, including unilateral or bilateral temporal, frontal, frontotemporoparietal, or posterior fossa craniectomies. While the dura mater is not always opened (216), a further significant decrease in ICP (217) as well as increase in $PbtO_2$ (218) following initial craniectomy have been observed following opening of the dura, and many consider dural opening and duroplasty to be a standard of care in this setting.

While the bone flap is usually removed and stored either in a bone bank at −80°C or in a fashioned subcutaneous abdominal pouch, a recent article reported a lower complication rate following a "hinge" craniectomy (219). In this procedure, the bone flap is secured to the surrounding skull by a Y-shaped plate immediately posterior to the coronal suture, with another 2 plates placed to prevent the bone flap subsequently "subsiding" following resolution of the swelling. In addition to fewer complications, this technique also obviates the need for a second procedure.

Complications of decompressive craniectomy may be seen early or late. The decrease in ICP and exposure of the brain to atmospheric pressure has been associated with hyperemia, herniation, venous engorgement with hemorrhagic contusions, and contralateral extraaxial hematomas. Late complications include infections, hydrocephalus, seizures, bone resorption, and CSF circulation abnormalities including CSF hygromas. In addition, a "syndrome of the trephined" has been described consisting of headache, dizziness, concentration difficulties, memory problems, and mood disturbances (220). A number of patients have also developed late onset reversible monoplegia usually affecting the contralateral upper limb (221).

Up until recently, the only published randomized controlled trial involved 27 pediatric patients with refractory raised ICP randomized to decompressive craniectomy or "routine medical management" which included 24 to 36 hours of induced hypothermia to 33°C (216). The decision to randomize was based on an ICP on day 1 of 20 to 24 mmHg for 30 minutes, 25 to 29 mmHg for 10 minutes, ≥ 30 mmHg for 1 minute, or clinical evidence of herniation. This study demonstrated both better ICP control following decompressive craniectomy as well as improved outcome—as assessed by the GOS (222) and Health State Utility Index at 6 month follow up.

A recently published study (223) known as the DECRA trial evaluated outcomes of 155 adults aged 15 to 59 years with diffuse TBI and refractory intracranial hypertension (defined as > 20 mmHg for > 15 minutes within a 1 hour period) randomized to either decompressive craniectomy or standard care. There was a significant decrease in ICP following craniectomy; however, patient outcomes at six months, assessed by the Extended GOS, were actually significantly worse in the decompressive craniectomy group compared to the patients who received standard care. There was no difference in mortality between groups (18% in decompressive craniectomy group vs 19% in standard care group). It should be noted that more patients in the decompressive craniectomy group had unreactive pupils prior to enrollment, and following adjustment for this factor, the differences in outcome failed to reach statistical significance. Also, the indication for decompressive craniectomy in the study of 15 minutes with ICP > 20 mmHg may not be widely accepted. Although it is important not to delay decompressive craniectomy in the setting of possible cerebral hypoperfusion/ischemia, many units would wait longer until proceeding to decompressive craniectomy. In fact, although the ICP in the "standard care" group remained significantly higher than the decompressive craniectomy group, it was generally less than the 20 mmHg threshold following randomization. These limitations have led some to question the generalizability of the study's findings (224,225).

The RESCUEicp Trial (International Standard Randomised Controlled Trial Number Register no. 66202560) is an ongoing multicenter international randomized controlled trial with 324 of a projected 400 subjects already recruited (226). The definition of "refractory raised ICP" for the purposes of randomization within this study is an ICP > 25 mmHg for > 1 to 12 hours despite optimal medical management (227). Recruitment is apparently proceeding well (228) and a result is expected in the next few years. Given the DECRA study was confined to patients 15 to 59 years of age, and RESCUEicp study looks at patients 10 to 65 years, it remains to be seen whether the results of these studies will be accepted as applicable to the pediatric population.

For now, it is reasonable to consider decompressive craniectomy for patients with raised ICP and signs of neurologic deterioration, including herniation, or intracranial hypertension refractory to other measures (229).

■ FUTURE DIRECTIONS

Although neurologic injury is the leading cause of morbidity in the pediatric population the impact that has been made on long term neurologic outcome has not been encouraging and therefore clinicians are striving to improve treatment strategies. Below, a number of new therapeutic concepts are outlined that either remain in the experimental realm or have been adopted in centers but have not become standard of care.

Newer Pharmacologic Interventions

Progesterone

Progesterone is a hormone that has been demonstrated to have neurosteroidal and neuroactive properties in the CNS. There has been significant interest in the role progesterone has in modifying cerebral edema in the setting of TBI. Several different animal models have been used to investigate this and consistently have shown that there is a reduction in ICP and improvement of neurologic scores (230–232). There is little data on humans with only 3 randomized controlled studies in adults subjects with TBI treated with progesterone. Results are so far encouraging with improved neurologic outcomes at 1 month (233) and 6 months (234) and decreased mortality. Patient numbers are small, however, and a Cochrane Review (235) concluded that larger randomized controlled trials are needed before progesterone can be recommended as a neuroprotective treatment. Furthermore the safety and efficacy of using progesterone in prepubertal children needs to be established before this therapy can be considered in children.

Aquaporin-Channel Modifying Agents

Aquaporins (AQPs) are a relatively recently described family of water channel proteins that appear to regulate water transport in and out of cells. To date, 13 AQPs (236) have been described in mammals but one—AQP4—is considered to be the principal water channel of the cells in the brain. AQP4 is expressed mainly on astrocyte foot process, in particular the cell surface of the blood-brain and CSF-brain barrier (237).

The role that this water channel has in the formation of cerebral edema has been investigated using several animal models. The pathophysiologic mechanisms leading to cerebral edema can be classified broadly into three processes: cytotoxic, vasogenic, and hydrocephalic. The role of AQP4 in the development of cerebral edema has been studied in AQP4 channel deficient (knockout) mice. The cerebral injury model used in these mice differentiated between a vasogenic process (hemorrhagic stroke) and cytotoxic process (ischemic stroke). While a lack of AQP4 expression was found to be beneficial following a cytotoxic injury, resulting in decreased brain water content, infarct size, and lower ICP with improved survival (238), AQP4 deficiency was detrimental in the vasogenic model and associated with increased brain water content, increased ICP, and worse neurologic outcome (239). In pathologies driven mainly by cytotoxic injury, such as hypoxic-ischemic injury, TBI, meningitis, and metabolic derangements, administration of a specific therapeutic agent to inhibit the action of AQP4 might therefore represent a novel way to limit and possibly reduce cerebral edema.

Arginine-vasopressin has been identified as a possible AQP4 modulator. At this stage, studies of an arginine-vasopressin (V1a) receptor inhibitor in both TBI (240) and hemorrhagic brain injury (241) have been limited to animal models; however, the results of these studies show a reduction in cerebral water content and improved neurologic outcomes. Although these early results are encouraging, further studies are needed before AQP-targeted interventions can be trialed in human subjects.

Erythropoietin

Human recombinant erythropoietin has been shown to have neuroprotective properties but the dose required to exert this effect overstimulates the bone marrow (242). To overcome these side effects carbamylated erythropoietin was used in animal studies with a reduction of cerebral edema and improved functional outcomes reported in both ischemic brain injury (243) and TBI (244) models. There has only been one human study in which 16 patients with TBI were randomized to receive erythropoietin or a control. The results of this study showed no difference in outcome (245), but the study was significantly underpowered and much larger multicenterd randomized controlled trials need to be performed to establish the efficacy of this therapy for cerebral edema.

■ CONCLUSIONS

Many questions regarding intracranial hypertension and its management remain unanswered, and it is important that we acknowledge these areas of uncertainty. A number of robust studies have identified various factors and practices that are associated with poor outcomes, and these must be carefully avoided. These include: hypotension (particularly early), early resuscitation with albumin, hyperthermia, hypocarbia, hyperglycemia and hypoglycemia, hypoxemia, raised ICP, and decreased CPP. Whether an ICP-targeted approach to management is superior to one directed at CPP remains uncertain. The role of so-called Tier 2 treatments such as barbiturate coma, decompressive craniectomy, and hypothermia also remains unclear, for although these interventions have been demonstrated to decrease ICP, recent studies looking at longer-term patient-centric outcomes suggest that they may, in fact, cause harm. These findings remind us that we must not focus merely on surrogate markers or endpoints (246,247), and it is too simplistic to assume that an intervention that produces a decrease in ICP or an increase in CPP will necessarily benefit our patient. As with all clinical interventions, we are obliged to "first, do no harm," and must therefore ensure that we administer those therapies—and only those therapies—that we believe, based on all the available evidence, are likely to provide more benefits than harms to our patients.

■ REFERENCES

1. Mokri B. The Monro-Kellie hypothesis: applications in CSF volume depletion. *Neurology.* 2001;56(12):1746–1748.
2. Lanier WL, Warner DO. Intracranial elastance versus intracranial compliance: terminology should agree with that of other disciplines. *Anesthesiology.* 1992;77(2):403.
3. Meyer MJ et al. Acute management of acquired brain injury: an evidence-based review of pharmacological interventions. *Brain Inj.* 2010;24(5):706–721.
4. Kety SS, Schmidt CF. The nitrous oxide method for the quantitative determination of cerebral blood flow in man: theory, procedure and normal values. *J Clin Invest.*1948;27(4):476–483.
5. Bishop CC et al. Transcranial Doppler measurement of middle cerebral artery blood flow velocity: a validation study. *Stroke.* 1986;17(5):913–915.
6. Totaro R et al. Reproducibility of transcranial Doppler sonography: a validation study. *Ultrasound Med Biol.* 1992;18(2):173–177.
7. Kehrer M et al. The development of cerebral perfusion in healthy preterm and term neonates. *Neuropediatrics.* 2003;34(6):281–286.
8. Kehrer M, Schoning M. A longitudinal study of cerebral blood flow over the first 30 months. *Pediatr Res.* 2009;66(5):560–564.
9. Schoning M, Hartig B. Age dependence of total cerebral blood flow volume from childhood to adulthood. *J Cereb Blood Flow Metab.* 1996;16(5):827–833.
10. Vavilala MS, Lee LA, Lam AM. Cerebral blood flow and vascular physiology. *Anesthesiol Clin North Am.* 2002;20(2):247–264, v.
11. Chugani HT. Positron emission tomography: principles and applications in pediatrics. *Mead Johnson Symp Perinat Dev Med.* 1987(25):15–18.
12. Huttenlocher PR. Morphometric study of human cerebral cortex development. *Neuropsychologia.* 1990;28(6):517–527.
13. Zoccoli G et al. The cerebral circulation during sleep: regulation mechanisms and functional implications. *Sleep Med Rev.* 2002;6(6):443–455.
14. Smith AL, Wollman H. Cerebral blood flow and metabolism: effects of anesthetic drugs and techniques. *Anesthesiology.* 1972;36(4):378–400.
15. Philip S et al. Variation in cerebral blood flow velocity with cerebral perfusion pressure > 40 mmHg in 42 children with severe traumatic brain injury. *Crit Care Med.* 2009;37(11):2973–2978.
16. Steiner LA et al. Assessment of cerebrovascular autoregulation in head-injured patients: a validation study. *Stroke.* 2003;34(10):2404–2409.
17. Chesnut RM et al. The role of secondary brain injury in determining outcome from severe head injury. *J Trauma.* 1993;34(2):216–222.
18. Chambers IR et al. Age-related differences in intracranial pressure and cerebral perfusion pressure in the first 6 hours of monitoring after children's head injury: association with outcome. *Childs Nerv Syst.* 2005;21(3):195–199.
19. Harris RJ et al. Changes in extracellular calcium activity in cerebral ischaemia. *J Cereb Blood Flow Metab.* 1981;1(2):203–209.
20. Nordstrom CH et al. Assessment of the lower limit for cerebral perfusion pressure in severe head injuries by bedside monitoring of regional energy metabolism. *Anesthesiology.* 2003;98(4):809–814.
21. Kety SS, Schmidt CF. The effects of altered arterial tensions of carbon dioxide and oxygen on cerebral blood flow and cerebral oxygen consumption of normal young men. *J Clin Invest.* 1948;27(4):484–492.
22. Wasserman AJ, Patterson JL Jr. The cerebral vascular response to reduction in arterial carbon dioxide tension. *J Clin Invest.* 1961;40:1297–1303.
23. Severinghaus JW, Lassen N. Step hypocapnia to separate arterial from tissue Pco_2 in the regulation of cerebral blood flow. *Circ Res.* 1967;20(2):272–278.
24. Harper AM, Glass HI. Effect of alterations in the arterial carbon dioxide tension on the blood flow through the cerebral cortex at normal and low arterial blood pressures. *J Neurol Neurosurg Psychiatry.* 1965;28(5):449–452.
25. Quint SR et al. Enhancement of cerebrovascular effect of CO_2 by hypoxia. *Stroke.* 1980;11(3):286–289.
26. Kassell NF et al. Influence of changes in arterial pCO_2 on cerebral blood flow and metabolism during high-dose barbiturate therapy in dogs. *J Neurosurg.* 1981;54(5):615–619.
27. Cold GE, Jensen FT, Malmros R. The effects of $Paco_2$ reduction on regional cerebral blood flow in the acute phase of brain injury. *Acta Anaesthesiol Scand.* 1977;21(5):359–367.
28. Marmarou A et al. Measurement of vascular reactivity in head injured patients. *Acta Neurochir Suppl (Wien).* 1993;59:18–21.

29. Muizelaar JP et al. Adverse effects of prolonged hyperventilation in patients with severe head injury: a randomized clinical trial. *J Neurosurg.* 1991;75(5):731–739.

30. Adelson PD et al. Cerebrovascular response in infants and young children following severe traumatic brain injury: a preliminary report. *Pediatr Neurosurg.* 1997;26(4):200–207.

31. Bratton SL et al. Guidelines for the management of severe traumatic brain injury: hyperventilation. *J Neurotrauma.* 2007;24(suppl 1):S87–S90.

32. Kochanek PM et al. Guidelines for the acute medical management of severe traumatic brain injury in infants, children, and adolescents (2nd edition): hyperventilation. *Pediatr Crit Care Med.* 2012;13:S58–S60.

33. Liu Y, Harder DR, Lombard JH. Interaction of myogenic mechanisms and hypoxic dilation in rat middle cerebral arteries. *Am J Physiol Heart Circ Physiol.* 2002;283(6):H2276–H2281.

34. Omae T et al. Effects of high atmospheric pressure and oxygen on middle cerebral blood flow velocity in humans measured by transcranial Doppler. *Stroke.* 1998;29(1):94–97.

35. Floyd TF et al. Independent cerebral vasoconstrictive effects of hyperoxia and accompanying arterial hypocapnia at 1 ATA. *J Appl Physiol.* 2003;95(6):2453–2461.

36. Folkow B. Description of the myogenic hypothesis. *Circ Res.* 1964;15(suppl):279–287.

37. Gulbenkian S, Uddman R, Edvinsson L. Neuronal messengers in the human cerebral circulation. *Peptides.* 2001;22(6):995–1007.

38. Umeyama T et al. Changes in cerebral blood flow estimated after stellate ganglion block by single photon emission computed tomography. *J Auton Nerv Syst.* 1995;50(3):339–346.

39. Visocchi M et al. Cerebral blood flow velocities and trigeminal ganglion stimulation. A transcranial Doppler study. *Stereotact Funct Neurosurg.* 1996;66(4):184–192.

40. Sahuquillo J et al. Evaluation of cerebrovascular CO_2-reactivity and autoregulation in patients with post-traumatic diffuse brain swelling (diffuse injury III). *Acta Neurochir Suppl.* 1998;71:233–236.

41. Vavilala MS et al. Cerebral autoregulation in pediatric traumatic brain injury. *Pediatr Crit Care Med.* 2004;5(3):257–263.

42. Vavilala MS et al. Neurointensive care; impaired cerebral autoregulation in infants and young children early after inflicted traumatic brain injury: a preliminary report. *J Neurotrauma.* 2007;24(1):87–96.

43. Myburgh JA. Quantifying cerebral autoregulation in health and disease. *Crit Care Resuscitation.* 2004;6(1):59–67.

44. Grände PO. The "Lund concept" for the treatment of severe head trauma–physiological principles and clinical application. *Intensive Care Med.* 2006;32(10):1475–1484.

45. Selhorst JB et al. Papilledema after acute head injury. *Neurosurgery.* 1985;16(3):357–363.

46. Marshall LF et al. The diagnosis of head injury requires a classification based on computed axial tomography. *J Neurotrauma.* 1992;9(suppl 1):S287–S292.

47. Bratton SL et al. Guidelines for the management of severe traumatic brain injury: Indications for intracranial pressure monitoring. *J Neurotrauma.* 2007;24(suppl 1):S37–S44.

48. Kochanek PM et al. Guidelines for the acute medical management of severe traumatic brain injury in infants, children, and adolescents (2nd edition): indications for intracranial pressure monitoring. *Pediatr Crit Care Med.* 2012;13:S11–S17.

49. Tasker RC et al. Intracranial pressure monitoring following hypoxic-ischaemic cerebral insults. *Childs Nerv Syst.* 1989;5:280.

50. Wendon JA, Larsen FS. Intracranial pressure monitoring in acute liver failure. A procedure with clear indications. *Hepatology.* 2006;44(2):504–506.

51. Adelson PD et al. Guidelines for the acute medical management of severe traumatic brain injury in infants, children and adolescents. *Pediatr Crit Care Med.* 2003;4(3):S1–S74.

52. Kochanek PM et al. Guidelines for the acute medical management of severe traumatic brain injury in infants, children, and adolescents (2nd edition). *Pediatr Crit Care Med.* 2012;13(1)(suppl):S1–S82.

53. Narayan RK et al. Improved confidence of outcome prediction in severe head injury. A comparative analysis of the clinical examination, multimodality evoked potentials, CT scanning, and intracranial pressure. *J Neurosurg.* 1981;54(6):751–762.

54. Marmarou A et al. Impact of ICP instability and hypotension on outcome in patients with severe head trauma. *Special Supplements.* 1991;75(1s):S59–S66.

55. Pfenninger J et al. Treatment and outcome of the severely head injured child. *Intensive Care Med.* 1983;9(1):13–16.

56. Esparza J et al. Outcome in children with severe head injuries. *Childs Nerv Sys.* 1985;1(2):109–114.

57. Adelson PD et al. Guidelines for the acute medical management of severe traumatic brain injury in infants, children, and adolescents: threshold for treatment of intracranial hypertension. *Pediatr Crit Care Med.* 2003;4(3 suppl):S25–S27.

58. Morris KP et al. Intracranial pressure complicating severe traumatic brain injury in children: monitoring and management. *Intensive Care Med.* 2006;32(10):1606–1612.

59. Shafi S et al. Intracranial pressure monitoring in brain-injured patients is associated with worsening of survival. *J Trauma.* 2008;64(2):335–340.

60. Lundberg N. Continuous recording and control of ventricular fluid pressure in neurosurgical practice. *Acta Psychiatr Scand Suppl.* 1960;36(149):1–193.

61. Shapiro S et al. The fiberoptic intraparenchymal cerebral pressure monitor in 244 patients. *Surg Neurol.* 1996;45(3):278–282.

62. Munch E et al. The Camino intracranial pressure device in clinical practice: reliability, handling characteristics and complications. *Acta Neurochir.* 1998;140(11):1113–1119; discussion 1119–1120.

63. Signorini DF et al. A clinical evaluation of the Codman MicroSensor for intracranial pressure monitoring. *Br J Neurosurg.* Jun 1998;12(3):223–227.

64. Koskinen LO, Olivecrona M. Clinical experience with the intraparenchymal intracranial pressure monitoring Codman MicroSensor system. *Neurosurgery.* 2005;56(4):693–698; discussion 693–698.

65. Aschoff A et al. The scientific history of hydrocephalus and its treatment. *Neurosurg Rev.* 1999;22(2–3):67–93; discussion 94–65.

66. Guyot LL et al. Cerebral monitoring devices: analysis of complications. *Acta Neurochir Suppl.* 1998;71:47–49.

67. Kakarla UK et al. Safety and accuracy of bedside external ventricular drain placement. *Neurosurgery.* 2008;63(1)(suppl 1):ONS162–166; discussion ONS166–167.

68. Miller MT et al. Initial head computed tomographic scan characteristics have a linear relationship with initial intracranial pressure after trauma. *J Trauma.* 2004;56(5):967–972; discussion 972–963.

69. Anderson RC et al. Complications of intracranial pressure monitoring in children with head trauma. *J Neurosurg.* 2004;101(1 suppl):53–58.

70. Al-Tamimi YZ et al. Assessment of zero drift in the Codman intracranial pressure monitor: a study from 2 neurointensive care units. *Neurosurgery.* J2009;64(1):94–98; discussion 98–99.

71. Poca MA et al. Fiberoptic intraparenchymal brain pressure monitoring with the Camino V420 monitor: reflections on our experience in 163 severely head-injured patients. *J Neurotrauma.* Apr 2002;19(4):439–448.

72. Luerssen TG. Intracranial pressure: current status in monitoring and management. *Semin Pediatr Neurol.* 1997;4(3):146–155.

73. Gelabert-Gonzalez M et al. The Camino intracranial pressure device in clinical practice. Assessment in a 1000 cases. *Acta Neurochir.* 2006;148(4):435–441.

74. Jensen RL, Hahn YS, Ciro E. Risk factors of intracranial pressure monitoring in children with fiberoptic devices: a critical review. *Surg Neurol.* 1997;47(1):16–22.

75. Blaha M et al. Hemorrhagic complications of intracranial pressure monitors in children. *Pediatr Neurosurg.* 2003;39(1):27–31.

76. Pople IK et al. Results and complications of intracranial pressure monitoring in 303 children. *Pediatr Neurosurg.* 1995;23(2):64–67.

77. Gray WP et al. A clinical study of parenchymal and subdural miniature strain-gauge transducers for monitoring intracranial pressure. *Neurosurgery.* 1996;39(5):927–931; discussion 931–922.

78. Geeraerts T et al. Non-invasive assessment of intracranial pressure using ocular sonography in neurocritical care patients. *Intensive Care Med.* 2008;34(11):2062–2067.

79. Major R, Girling S, Boyle A. Ultrasound measurement of optic nerve sheath diameter in patients with a clinical suspicion of raised intracranial pressure. *Emerg Med J.* 2011;28(8):679–681.

80. Newman WD et al. Measurement of optic nerve sheath diameter by ultrasound: a means of detecting acute raised intracranial pressure in hydrocephalus. *Br J Ophthalmol.* 2002;86(10):1109–1113.

81. Spentzas T et al. Correlation of intraocular pressure with intracranial pressure in children with severe head injuries. *Pediatr Crit Care Med.* 2010;11(5):593–598.

82. York D et al. Further studies with a noninvasive method of intracranial pressure estimation. *Neurosurgery.* 1984;14(4):456–461.

83. Desch LW. Longitudinal stability of visual evoked potentials in children and adolescents with hydrocephalus. *Dev Med Child Neurol.* 2001;43(2):113–117.

84. Zhao YL, Zhou JY, Zhu GH. Clinical experience with the noninvasive ICP monitoring system. *Acta Neurochir Suppl.* 2005;95:351–355.

85. Melo JR et al. Transcranial Doppler can predict intracranial hypertension in children with severe traumatic brain injuries. *Childs Nerv Syst.* 2011;27(6):979–984.

86. Prunet B et al. Noninvasive detection of elevated intracranial pressure using a portable ultrasound system. *Am J Emerg Med.* 2012;30(6):936–941.

87. Hassler W, Steinmetz H, Gawlowski J. Transcranial Doppler ultrasonography in raised intracranial pressure and in intracranial circulatory arrest. *J Neurosurg.* 1988;68(5):745–751.

88. Behrens A et al. Transcranial Doppler pulsatility index: not an accurate method to assess intracranial pressure. *Neurosurgery.* 2010;66(6):1050–1057.

89. Lewis SB, Myburgh JA, Reilly PL. Detection of cerebral venous desaturation by continuous jugular bulb oximetry following acute neurotrauma. *Anaesth Intensive Care.* 1995;23(3):307–314.

90. Steiner LA, Andrews PJ. Monitoring the injured brain: ICP and CBF. *Br J Anaesth.* 2006;97(1):26–38.

91. Stevens WJ. Multimodal monitoring: head injury management using SjvO$_2$ and LICOX. *J Neurosci Nurs.* 2004;36(6):332–339.

92. Vigue B et al. Early SjvO$_2$ monitoring in patients with severe brain trauma. *Intensive Care Med.* 1999;25(5):445–451.

93. Schoon P et al. Incidence of intracranial hypertension related to jugular bulb oxygen saturation disturbances in severe traumatic brain injury patients. *Acta Neurochir Suppl.* 2002;81:285–287.

94. Meixensberger J et al. Brain tissue oxygen guided treatment supplementing ICP/CPP therapy after traumatic brain injury. *J Neurol Neurosurg Psychiatry.* 2003;74(6):760–764.

95. Stiefel MF et al. Reduced mortality rate in patients with severe traumatic brain injury treated with brain tissue oxygen monitoring. *J Neurosurg.* 2005;103(5):805–811.

96. Narotam PK, Morrison JF, Nathoo N. Brain tissue oxygen monitoring in traumatic brain injury and major trauma: outcome analysis of a brain tissue oxygen-directed therapy. *J Neurosurg.* 2009;111(4):672–682.

97. Figaji AA et al. Brain tissue oxygen tension monitoring in pediatric severe traumatic brain injury. Part 2: Relationship with clinical, physiological, and treatment factors. *Childs Nerv Syst.* 2009;25(10):1335–1343.

98. Kochanek PM et al. Guidelines for the acute medical management of severe traumatic brain injury in infants, children, and adolescents (2nd edition): advanced neuromonitoring. *Pediatr Crit Care Med.* 2012;13:S30-S32.

99. Dunham CM et al. Cerebral hypoxia in severely brain-injured patients is associated with admission Glasgow Coma Scale score, computed tomographic severity, cerebral perfusion pressure, and survival. *J Trauma.* 2004;56(3):482–489; discussion 489–491.

100. Highton D, Elwell C, Smith M. Noninvasive cerebral oximetry: is there light at the end of the tunnel? *Curr Opin Anaesthesiol.* 2010;23(5):576–581.

101. Zuluaga MT et al. Diagnosis influences response of cerebral near infrared spectroscopy to intracranial hypertension in children. *Pediatr Crit Care Med.* 2010;11(4):514–522.

102. Kirkness CJ et al. Intracranial pressure waveform analysis: clinical and research implications. *J Neurosci Nurs.* 2000;32(5):271–277.

103. Lundberg N, West KA. Leakage as a source of error in measurement of the cerebrospinal fluid pressure by lumbar puncture. *Acta Neurol Scand Suppl.* 1965;13(pt 1):115–121.

104. Lundberg N, Troupp H, Lorin H. Continuous recording of the ventricular-fluid pressure in patients with severe acute

traumatic brain injury. A preliminary report. *J Neurosurg.* 1965;22(6):581–590.

105. Carter BG, Butt W, Taylor A. ICP and CPP: excellent predictors of long term outcome in severely brain injured children. *Childs Nerv Syst.* 2008;24(2):245–251.

106. Robertson CS. Management of cerebral perfusion pressure after traumatic brain injury. *Anesthesiology.* 2001;95(6):1513–1517.

107. Adelson PD et al. Guidelines for the acute medical management of severe traumatic brain injury in infants, children, and adolescents: prehospital airway management. *Pediatr Crit Care Med.* 2003;4(3 suppl):S9–S11.

108. Tam S, Chung F, Campbell M. Intravenous lidocaine: optimal time of injection before tracheal intubation. *Anesth Analg.* 1987;66(10):1036–1038.

109. Murphy D et al. Intravenous lignocaine pretreatment to prevent intraocular pressure rise following suxamethonium and tracheal intubation. *Br J Ophthalmol.* 1986;70(8):596–598.

110. Robinson N, Clancy M. In patients with head injury undergoing rapid sequence intubation, does pretreatment with intravenous lignocaine/lidocaine lead to an improved neurological outcome? A review of the literature. *Emerg Med J.* 2001;18(6):453.

111. Sehdev RS, Symmons DA, Kindl K. Ketamine for rapid sequence induction in patients with head injury in the emergency department. *Emerg Med Australas.* 2006;18(1):37–44.

112. Filanovsky Y, Miller P, Kao J. Myth: ketamine should not be used as an induction agent for intubation in patients with head injury. *Can J Emerg Med.* 2010;12(2):154–157.

113. Bar-Joseph G et al. Effectiveness of ketamine in decreasing intracranial pressure in children with intracranial hypertension. *J Neurosurg: Pediatr.* 2009;4(1):40–46.

114. McGuire G et al. Effects of varying levels of positive end-expiratory pressure on intracranial pressure and cerebral perfusion pressure. *Crit Care Med.* 1997;25(6):1059–1062.

115. Tume LN, Baines PB, Lisboa PJG. The effect of nursing interventions on the intracranial pressure in paediatric traumatic brain injury. *Nurs Crit Care.* 2011;16(2):77–84.

116. Donegan MF, Bedford RF. Intravenously administered lidocaine prevents intracranial hypertension: during endotracheal suctioning. *Anesthesiology.* 1980;52(6):516–518.

117. Paratz J, Burns Y. The effect of respiratory physiotherapy on intracranial pressure, mean arterial pressure, cerebral perfusion pressure and end tidal carbon dioxide in ventilated neurosurgical patients. *Physiother Theory Pract.* 1993;9(1):3–11.

118. Garradd J, Bullock M. The effect of respiratory therapy on intracranial pressure in ventilated neurosurgical patients. *Aust J Physiother.* 1986;32:107–111.

119. Olson DWM et al. Changes in intracranial pressure associated with chest physiotherapy. *Neurocrit Care.* 2007;6(2):100–103.

120. Bulger EM et al. Out-of-hospital hypertonic resuscitation following severe traumatic brain injury: a randomized controlled trial. *JAMA.* 2010;304(13):1455–1464.

121. Tan PG et al. Prehospital fluid management in traumatic brain injury. *Emerg Med Australas.* 2011;23(6):665–676.

122. Investigators TSS. Saline or albumin for fluid resuscitation in patients with traumatic brain injury. *N Engl J Med.* 2007;357:874–884.

123. Myburgh J et al. Saline or albumin for fluid resuscitation in patients with traumatic brain injury. *N Engl J Med.* 2007;357(9):874–884.

124. Investigators ST. Surgical Trial in Traumatic intraCerebral Haemorrhage STITCH (trauma). http://research.ncl.ac.uk/trauma.stitch/. Accessed June 12, 2011.

125. Meyer MJ et al. Acute management of acquired brain injury: an evidence-based review of non-pharmacological interventions. *Brain Inj.* 2010;24(5):694–705.

126. Feldman Z et al. Effect of head elevation on intracranial pressure, cerebral perfusion pressure, and cerebral blood flow in head-injured patients. *J Neurosurg.* 1992;76(2):207–211.

127. Agbeko RS et al. Intracranial pressure and cerebral perfusion pressure responses to head elevation changes in pediatric traumatic brain injury. *Pediatr Crit Care Med.* 2012;13(1):e39–e47.

128. Roberts DJ et al. Sedation for critically ill adults with severe traumatic brain injury: a systematic review of randomized controlled trials. *Crit Care Med.* 2011;39(12):2743.

129. Cotev S, Shalit MN. Effects on diazepam on cerebral blood flow and oxygen uptake after head injury. *Anesthesiology.* 1975;43(1):117–122.

130. FDA. FDA advisory against using propofol for prolonged sedation in the PICU. Food and Drug Administration Web site. http://www.fda.gov/Safety/MedWatch/SafetyInformation/SafetyAlertsforHumanMedicalProducts/ucm172351.htm. Accessed December 6, 2011.

131. MCA/CSM. Propofol (Diprivan) infusion: sedation in children aged 16 years or younger contraindicated. *Curr Probl Pharmacovigilance.* 2001;27:10.

132. Vespa PM et al. Increased incidence and impact of nonconvulsive and convulsive seizures after traumatic brain injury as detected by continuous electroencephalographic monitoring. *J Neurosurg.* 1999;91(5):750–760.

133. Vespa PM et al. Nonconvulsive electrographic seizures after traumatic brain injury result in a delayed, prolonged increase in intracranial pressure and metabolic crisis. *Crit Care Med.* 2007;35(12):2830.

134. Kochanek PM et al. Guidelines for the acute medical management of severe traumatic brain injury in infants, children, and adolescents (2nd edition): antiseizure prophylaxis. *Pediatric Crit Care Med.* 2012;13:S72–S75.

135. Anonymous. Guidelines for the management of severe traumatic brain injury: nutrition. *J Neurotrauma.* 2000;17(6–7):539–547.

136. Perel P et al. Nutritional support for head-injured patients. *Cochrane Database Syst Rev.* 2006(4):CD001530.

137. Koc D et al. Percutaneous endoscopic gastrostomy in the neurosurgical intensive care unit: complications and outcome. *J Parenter Enteral Nutr.* 2007;31(6):517–520.

138. McClave SA et al. Guidelines for the provision and assessment of nutrition support therapy in the adult critically ill patient. *J Parenter Enteral Nutr.* 2009;33(3):277–316.

139. Young B et al. Zinc supplementation is associated with improved neurologic recovery rate and visceral protein levels of patients with severe closed head injury. *J Neurotrauma.* Jan 1996;13(1):25–34.

140. Wilson RF, Tyburski JG. Metabolic responses and nutritional therapy in patients with severe head injuries. *J Head Trauma Rehabil.* 1998;13(1):11–27.

141. Kochanek PM et al. Guidelines for the acute medical management of severe traumatic brain injury in infants, children,

and adolescents (2nd edition): glucose and nutrition. *Pediatr Crit Care Med*. 2012;13:S68–S71.

142. Vespa PM et al. Persistently low extracellular glucose correlates with poor outcome 6 months after human traumatic brain injury despite a lack of increased lactate: a microdialysis study. *J Cereb Blood Flow Metab*. 2003;23(7):865–877.

143. McMullin J et al. Lowering of glucose in critical care: a randomized pilot trial. *J Crit Care*. 2007;22(2):112–118; discussion 118–119.

144. Meier R et al. Differential temporal profile of lowered blood glucose levels (3.5 to 6.5 mmol/l versus 5 to 8 mmol/l) in patients with severe traumatic brain injury. *Crit Care*. 2008;12(4):R98.

145. Griesdale DE et al. Glucose control and mortality in patients with severe traumatic brain injury. *Neurocrit Care*. 2009;11(3):311–316.

146. Liu-DeRyke X et al. Clinical impact of early hyperglycemia during acute phase of traumatic brain injury. *Neurocrit Care*. 2009;11(2):151–157.

147. Salim A et al. Persistent hyperglycemia in severe traumatic brain injury: an independent predictor of outcome. *Am Surg*. 2009;75(1):25–29.

148. Smith RL et al. Relationship between hyperglycemia and outcome in children with severe traumatic brain injury. *Pediatr Crit Care Med*. 2012;13(1):85–91.

149. Cochran A et al. Hyperglycemia and outcomes from pediatric traumatic brain injury. *J Trauma*. 2003;55(6):1035–1038.

150. Bratton SL et al. Guidelines for the management of severe traumatic brain injury: Intracranial pressure thresholds. *J Neurotrauma*. 2007;24(suppl 1):S55–S58.

151. Kochanek PM et al. Guidelines for the Acute medical management of severe traumatic brain injury in infants, children, and adolescents (2nd edition): threshold for treatment of intracranial hypertension. *Pediatr Crit Care Med*. 2012;13:S18–S23.

152. Chambers I et al. Age-related differences in intracranial pressure and cerebral perfusion pressure in the first 6 hours of monitoring after children's head injury: association with outcome. *Childs Nerv Syst*. 2005;21(3):195–199.

153. Bratton SL et al. Guidelines for the management of severe traumatic brain injury: cerebral perfusion thresholds. *J Neurotrauma*. 2007;24(suppl 1):S59–S64.

154. Adelson PD et al. Guidelines for the acute medical management of severe traumatic brain injury in infants, children, and adolescents: cerebral perfusion pressure. *Pediatr Crit Care Med*. 2003;4(3 suppl):S31–S33.

155. Kochanek PM et al. Guidelines for the acute medical management of severe traumatic brain injury in infants, children, and adolescents (2nd edition): cerebral perfusion pressure thresholds. *Pediatr Crit Care Med*. 2012;13:S24–S29.

156. Chambers IR et al. Critical thresholds of intracranial pressure and cerebral perfusion pressure related to age in paediatric head injury. *J Neurol Neurosurg Psychiatry*. 2006;77(2):234.

157. Rosner MJ, Rosner SD, Johnson AH. Cerebral perfusion pressure: management protocol and clinical results. *J Neurosurg*. 1995;83(6):949–962.

158. Eker C et al. Improved outcome after severe head injury with a new therapy based on principles for brain volume regulation and preserved microcirculation. *Crit Care Med*. 1998;26(11):1881–1886.

159. Eker C et al. Improved outcome after severe head injury with a new therapy based on principles for brain volume

regulation and preserved microcirculation. *Crit Care Med*. 1998;26(11):1881–1886.

160. Wahlström MR et al. Severe traumatic brain injury in pediatric patients: treatment and outcome using an intracranial pressure targeted therapy—the Lund concept. *Intensive Care Med*. 2005;31(6):832–839.

161. Robertson CS et al. Prevention of secondary ischemic insults after severe head injury. *Crit Care Med*. 1999;27(10):2086–2095.

162. Steiner LA et al. Direct comparison of cerebrovascular effects of norepinephrine and dopamine in head-injured patients. *Crit Care Med*. 2004;32(4):1049–1054.

163. Greenberg MS. *Handbook of Neurosurgery*. 6th ed. Thieme Medical Publishers; New York, USA. 2006.

164. Exo J et al. Intracranial pressure-monitoring systems in children with traumatic brain injury: combining therapeutic and diagnostic tools. *Pediatr Crit Care Med*. 2011;12(5):560.

165. Levy DI et al. Controlled lumbar drainage in pediatric head injury. *J Neurosurg*. 1995;83(3):453–460.

166. Weed LH, McKibben PS. Experimental alteration of brain bulk. *Am J Physiol*. 1919;48(4):531–564.

167. Weed LH, McKibben PS. Pressure changes in the cerebrospinal fluid following intravenous injection of solutions of various concentrations. *Am J Physiol*. 1919;48(4):512–530.

168. Qureshi AI, Suarez JI. Use of hypertonic saline solutions in treatment of cerebral edema and intracranial hypertension. *Crit Care Med*. 2000;28:3301–3313.

169. Muizelaar JP, Lutz HA III, Becker DP. Effect of mannitol on ICP and CBF and correlation with pressure autoregulation in severely head-injured patients. *J Neurosurg*. 1984;61(4):700–706.

170. Bennett TD et al. Osmolar therapy in pediatric traumatic brain injury. *Crit Care Med*. 2012;40(1):208–215.

171. García-Morales, EJ et al. Osmole gap in neurologic-neurosurgical intensive care unit: its normal value, calculation, and relationship with mannitol serum concentrations. *Crit Care Med*. 2004;32(4):986–991.

172. Strandvik GF. Hypertonic saline in critical care: a review of the literature and guidelines for use in hypotensive states and raised intracranial pressure. *Anaesthesia*. 2009;64(9):990–1003.

173. Kamel H et al. Hypertonic saline versus mannitol for the treatment of elevated intracranial pressure: a meta-analysis of randomized clinical trials. *Crit Care Med*. 2011;39(3):554–559.

174. Marko NF. Hypertonic saline, not mannitol, should be considered gold-standard medical therapy for intracranial hypertension. *Crit Care*. 2012;16:113.

175. Kochanek PM et al. Guidelines for the acute medical management of severe traumatic brain injury in infants, children, and adolescents (2nd edition): hyperosmolar therapy. *Pediatr Crit Care Med*. 2012;13:S36–S41.

176. Froelich M et al. Continuous hypertonic saline therapy and the occurrence of complications in neurocritically ill patients. *Crit Care Med*. 2009;37(4):1433–1441.

177. Muizelaar JP, Shahlaie K. Hypertonic saline in neurocritical care: Is continuous infusion appropriate? *Crit Care Med*. 2009;37(4):1521–1523.

178. Maggiore U et al. The relation between the incidence of hypernatremia and mortality in patients with severe traumatic brain injury. *Crit Care*. 2009;13(4):R110.

179. Zygun DA. Sodium and brain injury: do we know what we are doing? *Crit Care*. 2009;13(5):184.
180. Coles JP et al. Hyperventilation following head injury: effect on ischemic burden and cerebral oxidative metabolism. *Crit Care Med*. 2007;35(2):568.
181. Skippen P et al. Effect of hyperventilation on regional cerebral blood flow in head-injured children. *Crit Care Med*. 1997;25(8):1402.
182. Coles JP et al. Effect of hyperventilation on cerebral blood flow in traumatic head injury: Clinical relevance and monitoring correlates. *Crit Care Med*. 2002;30(9):1950.
183. Roberts I, Sydenham E. Barbiturates for acute traumatic brain injury. *Cochrane Database Syst Rev*. 1999;3.
184. Sidi A et al. Long-term barbiturate infusion to reduce intracranial pressure. *Crit Care Med*. 1983;11(6):478–481.
185. Pittman T, Bucholz R, Williams D. Efficacy of barbiturates in the treatment of resistant intracranial hypertension in severely head-injured children. *Pediatr Neurosci*. 1989;15(1):13–17.
186. Bohn DJ et al. High-dose barbiturate therapy in the management of severe pediatric head trauma: a randomised controlled trial. *Crit Care Med*. 1989;17:S118.
187. Ward JD et al. Failure of prophylactic barbiturate coma in the treatment of severe head injury. *J Neurosurg*. 1985;62(3):383–388.
188. Kochanek PM et al. Guidelines for the acute medical management of severe traumatic brain injury in infants, children, and adolescents (2nd edition): barbiturates. *Pediatr Crit Care Med*. 2012;13:S49–S52.
189. Pérez-Bárcena J et al. Pentobarbital versus thiopental in the treatment of refractory intracranial hypertension in patients with traumatic brain injury: a randomized controlled trial. *Crit Care*. 2008;12(4):R112.
190. Sedzimir C. Therapeutic hypothermia in cases of head injury. *J Neurosurg*. 1959;16(4):407.
191. Lazorthes G, Campan L. Hypothermia in the treatment of craniocerebral traumatism. *J Neurosurg*. 1958;15(2):162.
192. Hendrick EB. The use of hypothermia in severe head injuries in childhood. *Arch Sur*. 1959;79(3):362.
193. Drake C, Jory T. Hypothermia in the treatment of critical head injury. *CMAJ*. 1962;87(17):887.
194. Harley HRS. The use of hypothermia and dehydration in the treatment of severe cerebral hypoxia. *Br J Anaesth*. 1964;36:581–590.
195. Rosomoff H et al. Experimental brain injury and delayed hypothermia. *Surg Gynecol Obstet*. 1960;110:27.
196. Sinclair HL, Andrews PJD. Bench-to-bedside review: hypothermia in traumatic brain injury. *Crit Care*. 2010;14(1):204.
197. Jacobs S et al. Cooling for newborns with hypoxic ischaemic encephalopathy. *Cochrane Database Syst Rev*. 2007;4(4).
198. Bernard SA et al. Treatment of comatose survivors of out-of-hospital cardiac arrest with induced hypothermia. *N Engl J Med*. 2002;346(8):557–563.
199. Mild therapeutic hypothermia to improve the neurologic outcome after cardiac arrest. *N Engl J Med*. 2002;346(8):549–556.
200. Clifton GL et al. Lack of effect of induction of hypothermia after acute brain injury. *N Engl J Med*. 2001;344(8):556–563.
201. Sakas DE et al. Lack of effect of induction of hypothermia after acute brain injury. *N Engl J Med*. 2001;345(1):66.
202. Clifton GL et al. Multicenter trial of early hypothermia in severe brain injury. *J Neurotrauma*. 2009;26(3):393–397.
203. Hutchison JS et al. Hypothermia therapy after traumatic brain injury in children. *N Engl J Med*. 2008;358(23):2447–2456.
204. Hutchison JS et al. Impact of hypotension and low cerebral perfusion pressure on outcomes in children treated with hypothermia therapy following severe traumatic brain injury: a post hoc analysis of the Hypothermia Pediatric Head Injury Trial. *Dev Neurosci*. 2010;32(5–6):406–412.
205. Sydenham E, Roberts I, Alderson P. Hypothermia for traumatic head injury. *Cochrane Database Syst Rev*. 2009;2.
206. Kochanek PM et al. Guidelines for the acute medical management of severe traumatic brain injury in infants, children, and adolescents (2nd edition): temperature control. *Pediatric Crit Care Med*. 2012;13:S42–S45.
207. Adamo MA, Drazin D, Waldman JB. Decompressive craniectomy and postoperative complication management in infants and toddlers with severe traumatic brain injuries. *J Neurosurg Pediatr*. 2009;3(4):334–339.
208. Jagannathan J et al. Outcome following decompressive craniectomy in children with severe traumatic brain injury: a 10-year single-center experience with long-term follow up. *J Neurosurg Pediatr*. 2007;106(4):268–275.
209. Josan VA, Sgouros S. Early decompressive craniectomy may be effective in the treatment of refractory intracranial hypertension after traumatic brain injury. *Childs Nerv Syst*. 2006;22(10):1268–1274.
210. Rutigliano D et al. Decompressive craniectomy in pediatric patients with traumatic brain injury with intractable elevated intracranial pressure. *J Pediatr Surg*. 2006;41(1):83–87; discussion 83–87.
211. Dickerman RD, Morgan JT, Mittler MA. Decompressive craniectomy for traumatic brain injury: when is it too late? *Childs Nerv Syst*. 2005;21(12):1014–1015.
212. Thomale UW et al. Severe traumatic brain injury in children—a single center experience regarding therapy and long-term outcome. *Childs Nerv Syst*. 2010;26(11):1563–1573.
213. Ruf B et al. Early decompressive craniectomy and duraplasty for refractory intracranial hypertension in children: results of a pilot study. *Crit Care*. 2003;7(6):R133–R138.
214. Aghakhani N et al. Decompressive craniectomy in children with nontraumatic refractory high intracranial pressure. *J Neurosurg Pediatr*. 2009;3(1):66–69.
215. Sahuquillo J. Decompressive craniectomy for the treatment of refractory high intracranial pressure in traumatic brain injury. *Cochrane Database Syst Rev*. 2009(1):CD003983.
216. Taylor A et al. A randomized trial of very early decompressive craniectomy in children with traumatic brain injury and sustained intracranial hypertension. *Childs Nerv Syst*. 2001;17(3):154–162.
217. Yoo DS et al. Ventricular pressure monitoring during bilateral decompression with dural expansion. *J Neurosurg*. 1999;91(6):953–959.
218. Figaji AA et al. Intracranial pressure and cerebral oxygenation changes after decompressive craniectomy in a child with traumatic brain swelling. *Childs Nerv Syst*. 2007;23(11):1331–1335.
219. Kenning TJ, Gandhi RH, German JW. A comparison of hinge craniotomy and decompressive craniectomy for the treatment of malignant intracranial hypertension: early clinical and radiographic analysis. *Neurosurg Focus*. 2009;26(6):E6.

220. Li LM et al. The surgical approach to the management of increased intracranial pressure after traumatic brain injury. *Anesth Analg.* 2010;111(3):736–748.

221. Stiver SI, Wintermark M, Manley GT. Reversible monoparesis following decompressive hemicraniectomy for traumatic brain injury. *J Neurosurg.* 2008;109(2):245–254.

222. Jennett B, Bond M. Assessment of outcome after severe brain damage: a practical scale. *Lancet.* 1975;305(7905):480–484.

223. Cooper DJ et al. Decompressive Craniectomy in Diffuse Traumatic Brain Injury. *N Engl J Med.* 2011; 364:1493-1502.

224. Servadei F. Clinical value of decompressive craniectomy. *N Engl J Med.* 2011;364(16):1558–1559.

225. Ma J et al. Is decompressive craniectomy useless in severe traumatic brain injury? *Crit Care.* 2011;15(5):193.

226. RESCUEicp Study 2011. http://www.rescueicp.com. Accessed November 28, 2011.

227. Hutchinson P et al. Decompressive craniectomy in traumatic brain injury: the randomized multicenter RESCUEicp study (www.RESCUEicp.com). *Brain Edema XIII.* 2006:17–20.

228. Hutchinson PJ et al. Update on the RESCUEicp decompressive craniectomy trial. *Crit Care.* 2011;15(suppl 1):312.

229. Kochanek PM et al. Guidelines for the acute medical management of severe traumatic brain injury in infants, children, and adolescents (2nd edition): decompressive craniectomy for the treatment of intracranial hypertension. *Pediatr Crit Care Med.* 2012;13:S53–S57.

230. Roof RL, Hall ED. Gender differences in acute CNS trauma and stroke: neuroprotective effects of estrogen and progesterone. *J Neurotrauma.* 2000;17(5):367–388.

231. Djebaili M et al. The neurosteroids progesterone and allopregnanolone reduce cell death, gliosis, and functional deficits after traumatic brain injury in rats. *J Neurotrauma.* 2005;22(1):106–118.

232. Shahrokhi N et al. Effect of sex steroid hormones on brain edema, intracranial pressure, and neurologic outcomes after traumatic brain injury. *Can J Physiol Pharmacol.* 2010;88(4):414–421.

233. Wright DW et al. ProTECT: a randomized clinical trial of progesterone for acute traumatic brain injury. *Ann Emerg Med.* 2007;49(4):391–402, 402 e391–e392.

234. Xiao G et al. Improved outcomes from the administration of progesterone for patients with acute severe traumatic brain injury: a randomized controlled trial. *Crit Care.* 2008;12(2):R61.

235. Junpeng M, Huang S, Qin S. Progesterone for acute traumatic brain injury. *Cochrane Database Syst Rev.* 2011(1): CD008409.

236. Verkman AS. Aquaporins: translating bench research to human disease. *J Exp Biol.* 2009;212(pt 11):1707–1715.

237. Nielsen S et al. Specialized membrane domains for water transport in glial cells: high-resolution immunogold cytochemistry of aquaporin-4 in rat brain. *J Neurosci.* 1997;17(1): 171–180.

238. Manley GT et al. Aquaporin-4 deletion in mice reduces brain edema after acute water intoxication and ischemic stroke. *Nat Med.* 2000;6(2):159–163.

239. Papadopoulos MC et al. Aquaporin-4 facilitates reabsorption of excess fluid in vasogenic brain edema. *FASEB J.* 2004;18(11):1291–1293.

240. Taya K et al. Modulation of AQP4 expression by the selective V1a receptor antagonist, SR49059, decreases trauma-induced brain edema. *Acta Neurochir Suppl.* 2008;102:425–429.

241. Manaenko A et al. Arginine-vasopressin V1a receptor inhibition improves neurologic outcomes following an intracerebral hemorrhagic brain injury. *Neurochem Int.* 2011;58(4):542–548.

242. Brines M, Cerami A. Emerging biological roles for erythropoietin in the nervous system. *Nat Rev Neurosci.* 2005;6(6):484–494.

243. Villa P et al. Reduced functional deficits, neuroinflammation, and secondary tissue damage after treatment of stroke by nonerythropoietic erythropoietin derivatives. *J Cereb Blood Flow Metab.* 2007;27(3):552–563.

244. Bouzat P et al. Reduced brain edema and functional deficits after treatment of diffuse traumatic brain injury by carbamylated erythropoietin derivative. *Crit Care Med.* 2011;39(9):2099–2105.

245. Nirula R et al. Safety and efficacy of erythropoietin in traumatic brain injury patients: a pilot randomized trial. *Crit Care Res Pract.* 2010;2010.

246. Yudkin JS, Lipska KJ, Montori VM. The idolatry of the surrogate. *Br Med J.* 2011;343.

247. Kochanek PM et al. Guidelines for the acute medical management of severe traumatic brain injury in infants, children, and adolescents (2nd edition): methods. *Pediatr Crit Care Med.* 2012;13:S7–S10.

4 | *Mechanical Ventilation and Blood Pressure Management*

TODD J. KILBAUGH, ALEXIS A. TOPJIAN, and STUART H. FRIESS

■ INTRODUCTION

Traumatic brain injury (TBI) is the most common cause of death in childhood (1). Despite advances in resuscitation care, morbidity following pediatric TBI remains high. TBI is composed of two components: (1) an initial primary injury due to direct mechanical deformation of brain parenchyma and (2) a subsequent secondary injury that may develop over hours to days. Secondary injury may be the result of multiple mechanisms including ischemia, excitotoxicity, metabolic failure and eventual apoptosis, cerebral swelling, axonal injury and inflammation, and regeneration (2). For improvements in outcome to be achieved in the pediatric critical care setting, secondary brain injury must be prevented or minimized.

Conventional wisdom about TBI has dictated that ischemia plays a major role in secondary brain injury. While reversal of ischemia is crucial, simply delivering oxygen to injured areas of the brain does not abate the onslaught of secondary injury cascades destroying vulnerable areas of potentially viable brain following TBI. Recent evidence suggests that secondary injury persists despite adequate oxygen delivery to brain tissue due to persistent metabolic crisis (3,4). Furthermore, hyperoxia is not effective in completely reversing metabolic crisis and may lead to persistent secondary injury due to superoxide and free radical generation. There is widespread metabolic heterogeneity following TBI such that some regions have increased glucose and oxygen utilization (likely due in part to electrical instability) while in other regions oxidative metabolism is reduced to a critical threshold with critically low cerebral metabolic rates

of oxygen ($CMRO_2$) (5). Low $CMRO_2$ coupled with ongoing low cerebral blood flow (CBF) following TBI places viable brain tissue at risk (5,6). Understanding how the neurovascular bundle regulates CBF to brain regions in metabolic crisis and how to manipulate CBF in this context remain important areas of investigation.

■ CEREBRAL PERFUSION PRESSURE AND CBF

In children, developing effective treatments for TBI is complicated by the rapid changing responses of the immature brain to each type of brain injury during development (7,8). Therefore, evaluation of therapies for children with brain injury must utilize immature animal models as a translational pathway to human trials in children. Much of the research that drives clinical guidelines and recommendations is derived from adult clinical studies and adult aged small animal research. Translating this data to the child provides some direction, but should catalyze further research focusing on the immature brain. This is especially true when the practitioner must indirectly target metabolic delivery in the face of secondary brain injury by attempting to modulate CBF and predict regulation or lack of regulation in the neurovascular bundle. Even in the healthy brain, CBF regulation is complex and poorly understood (9–11). Additionally, CBF is likely heterogeneous following brain injury and is dependent on the injury mechanism, age, and even gender. Optimal global CBF is an elusive clinical target, with a lower inflection point associated with ischemic injury and an upper inflection point associated with hyperemia increasing CBF and intracranial pressure (ICP). In early post-TBI, cerebral hypoperfusion may greatly contribute to secondary brain injury ultimately increasing morbidity and mortality (6,12). In adults, areas of contusions have low CBF similar to the ischemic penumbral zones surrounding areas of acute ischemic stroke (13,14). Low CBF states have been demonstrated in children by xenon computed tomographic (CT) scans following TBI within 24 hours of the initial injury, but by 48 hours these patients had normal or supernormal blood flows (12). Furthermore, using CBF as a neuroresuscitation target is a theoretical point of manipulation due to limited options of continuous measurement in the clinical setting. Therefore, cerebral perfusion pressure (CPP) is a commonly used surrogate. CPP is defined as mean arterial blood pressure (MAP) minus ICP.

When cerebral autoregulation is impaired, CBF and the metabolic needs of the injured brain may depend on maintaining adequate CPP. The difficulty comes in identifying the term *adequate*. Currently, pediatric CPP thresholds (40–60 mm Hg) have been mostly extrapolated from adult experimental and clinical TBI as well as limited stroke studies (13,15). However, recently it has been reported in adults that ischemia following TBI may occur at much higher levels of CBF compared to stroke (13). Chambers et al (16–18) have published much needed age-specific pediatric thresholds for critical CPP, below which cerebral ischemia occurs with unfavorable neurologic outcomes and increased mortality. These studies identified inadequate CPP levels but did not identify an "optimal treatment" CPP, and therefore assumed that these CPP levels were equivalent to brain injury insult thresholds.

From these studies it is not clear if a CPP of 40 mmHg is a minimal threshold and/or that an optimal CPP to prevent brain injury may be higher (19). Using currently accepted pediatric CPP guidelines (CPP > 40 mmHg) may not ensure adequate oxygen delivery to brain tissue (20,21). This raises the question: is a CPP > 40 mmHg in the pediatric TBI patient high enough? Mild induced hypertension after ischemic stroke has shown promise in animal models but remains controversial in the clinical setting (22,23). Adult TBI studies have observed an increased risk of adult respiratory distress syndrome (RDS) associated with targeting a CPP > 70 mmHg, but it is unclear how applicable this is to pediatric neurocritical

care (24,25). A retrospective study of 146 pediatric TBI patients observed a strong association of poor outcome at discharge with hypotension within the first 6 hours of injury (26). The window for treatment of hypoperfusion appears to be early after pediatric TBI, and may be of relatively short duration in children. We believe that early aggressive intervention of blood pressure support especially during early critical periods, such as initial resuscitation of a multitrauma patient, intubation, and placement of support lines and neuromonitoring devices, is critical to neuroresuscitation. *Guidelines released in 2012, based on Class III evidence for pediatric TBI, suggest that a minimum CPP of 40 mmHg should be maintained and that a CPP of 50 mmHg may be required in older children (27).*

Targeting CPP often requires vasopressor support. While central venous access should not delay administration of vasopressor support, it is important to understand the risks of extravasation of these infusions and have qualified individuals place central venous access as soon as possible to mitigate these risks. Initial stabilization of the pediatric TBI patient may occur in limited resource environments where complex invasive intracranial monitoring may not be available. Early stabilization of cerebrovascular hemodynamics with phenylephrine and targeting a higher MAP or CPP may reduce brain injury and improve long-term outcomes. A common first line vasopressor to improve MAP in pediatric brain injury is phenylephrine. Phenylephrine is an alpha-adrenergic agonist that may have little or no effect on cerebral vasculature resistance (28–31). Another vasoactive medication gaining favor is norepinephrine. Norepinephrine primarily targets alpha-receptors for peripheral vasoconstriction, but has additional effects on beta-receptors increasing inotropy. There are several published reports now in adults that show the rising use of norepinephrine as a preferred vasoactive medication, and that it may provide more predictable CPP augmentation when compared to dopamine (32–34). Further research is critical to determine which vasopressor should be considered a first line agent in pediatric brain injury; this should be determined by local experience and comfort of use.

In summary, to date there are no pharmacologic therapies for the brain injured child. Therefore the tenets of neuroresuscitation for pediatric TBI focus on preventing secondary injury by limiting ischemia. In this chapter we will focus on oxygen delivery to the injured brain by manipulating mechanical ventilation and cerebral perfusion. We believe that the next generation of treatments will build upon the tenets of ischemic neuroresuscitation and combine early directed metabolic neuroresuscitation.

Often the care of a critically ill child is fraught with competing physiology. Limiting ischemia in a child with brain injury is no exception to this observation. For example, attempts to optimize CPP by increasing MAP with the delivery of crystalloids and vasopressor therapy may be accompanied by an associated pulmonary capillary leak and acute RDS (ARDS).

■ RESPIRATORY MANAGEMENT

Airway Management

The comatose and brain injured patient is at severe risk for respiratory failure due to loss of airway protective reflexes and impaired central regulation of respiratory function. In addition, progression of acute lung injury (ALI) and ARDS can be exacerbated by concomitant injuries (pulmonary contusions, aspiration, left ventricular dysfunction or failure, and systemic inflammation due to trauma or infection) and treatments to improve cerebral perfusion (crystalloid administration, hyperchloremic metabolic acidosis, hypernatremia, and vasopressor therapy). It is critical that the physician caring for these patients have a neuroprotective plan in place for induction and intubation, as well as adequate training and skill to obtain an artificial airway. In addition, the physician needs to be adept at ongoing neuroresuscitation in the face of progressive lung disease and hemodynamic instability from systemic inflammatory response syndrome and rising pulmonary mean airway pressures (mP_{AW}) increasing intra-thoracic pressure and thus impeding cardiac preload.

The initial step in treating the head-injured pediatric patient is always to promote adequate oxygenation and ventilation, and to prevent or treat hypotension thereby limiting ischemia. Criteria for tracheal intubation include hypoxemia not resolved with supplemental oxygen, apnea, hypercarbia ($Paco_2 > 45$ mmHg), Glasgow Coma Scale (GCS) ≤ 8, an incremental decrease in GCS > 3 independent of the initial GCS (combined with clinical correlation, anisocoria > 1 mm, cervical spine injury compromising ventilation, loss of pharyngeal reflex, and any clinical evidence of a herniation pattern or Cushing triad) (35).

Induction and Intubation

Patients with neurologic injury are at a high risk for aspiration during induction of anesthesia due to loss of airway protective reflexes. In addition, there is a heightened risk of cervical spine injury due to trauma and most patients will be in a cervical collar requiring manual in-line stabilization. The goal of intubation in the neurologically impaired patients should be (1) rapid sequence from induction to placement of an endotracheal tube to reduce the risk of pulmonary aspiration, (2) blunt nociceptive reflexes that may further elevate ICP or cerebral hypertension that may exacerbate intracranial hemorrhage or facilitate herniation, (3) maintain adequate, age-appropriate CPP, and (4) limit ischemia by maximizing adequate oxygen delivery and maintaining $Paco_2$ in a normal range to ensure appropriate CBF (36). It should be assumed that all patients are at risk for a full stomach and cervical spine injury, so intubation should be performed utilizing a neuroprotective, rapid-sequence induction whenever possible. Supplemental oxygen (100%) should be delivered by face-mask to allow nitrogen washout from the patient's functional residual capacity (FRC) to allow sufficient oxygenation prior to tracheal intubation attempts. To avoid risk of aspiration, bag-valve-mask (BVM) ventilation should not be done unless the patient has signs and symptoms of impending herniation or life threatening desaturation events. Outside of impending herniation, if BVM ventilation is conducted it is imperative to not overventilate the patient, decreasing $Paco_2$, and thereby increasing cerebral vascular resistance, resulting in decreased CBF and metabolic delivery in a brain-injured patient. A separate health care professional's sole responsibility is to maintain the child's neck in a neutral position by mild axial traction during airway maneuvers to prevent or perpetuate cervical spinal injury. Cricoid pressure should be done by a third individual only if the individual is appropriately trained in the technique and it should be abandoned if it hinders a rapid intubation attempt. Orotracheal intubation by direct laryngoscopy should be performed, and nasotracheal intubation should be avoided due to potential for direct intracranial damage in a patient with a basilar skull fracture.

Because tracheal intubation is a noxious stimulus and can increase ICP, appropriate sedative and analgesic medications should be administered during rapid-sequence induction. The hemodynamic and neurologic status of the patient dictates the choice of agents.

Patients usually receive lidocaine (1–1.5 mg/kg) intravenously (IV) before intubation to help blunt the rise in ICP that occurs during direct laryngoscopy (43). For the hemodynamically unstable patient, the combination of lidocaine, etomidate (0.2–0.6 mg/kg), and neuromuscular blockade with rocuronium (1 mg/kg) or succinylcholine (1 mg/kg) IV is a popular choice. The authors believe that succinylcholine may still be an option for rapid sequence intubation (RSI) in children who may have a difficult airway due to its rapid recovery, as opposed to the nondepolarizing intermediate neuromuscular blockade of rocuronium. There are several choices for induction agents in the critically ill child with acute brain injury. In the following sections we will discuss the pros and cons of each induction agent.

Etomidate

Etomidate is a short acting IV drug that produces sedation, anxiolysis, and amnesia. Side effects include respiratory depression, hypotension, myoclonus, and adrenal suppression. Thus, etomidate should not be used in children with suspected adrenal insufficiency and sepsis (37). Etomidate has the benefits of decreasing ICP by reductions in CBF and $CMRO_2$ and has the advantage of producing less cardiovascular depression than barbiturates or propofol, preserving CPP (38,39). These neuroprotective qualities are counterbalanced by its ability to increase cerebral vascular resistance by a greater magnitude than its reduction of $CMRO_2$ resulting in an increased metabolic deficit (40,41). The increased metabolic deficit has the potential to expand the ischemic core and penumbra in brain injured tissue. This increase in cerebrovascular tone is thought to be attributed to etomidate's inhibition of nitric oxide (NO) synthase (42). Particular attention should also be paid to the rapid recovery of etomidate; once the airway is secured etomidate's effects on consciousness dissipates quickly, principally due to the redistribution of the drug from the brain to inactive tissue sites. Recovery of consciousness can occur in 5 to 15 minutes. Since rocuronium may lead to 45 minutes of paralysis, if it is used in combination with etomidate for RSI, then the patient will need ongoing sedation while paralyzed. The addition of a short-acting opioid such as fentanyl may be necessary especially if the patient has concomitant injuries, such as bone fractures.

An alternative is the combination of lidocaine, fentanyl (1–4 micrograms/kg), and rocuronium. The short-acting narcotic fentanyl, when used with lidocaine, can decrease the catecholamine release associated with direct laryngoscopy (43). In the hemodynamically stable patient, either of the above combinations should utilize the fast-acting benzodiazepine midazolam (0.05–0.2 mg/kg) as an adjuvant amnestic.

Ketamine

Ketamine is a phenylcyclidine derivative typically formulated as a mixture of two enantiomers in a hydrochloride salt form. It has a low pH of around 4, which can produce pain at the injection site when administered intramuscularly or IV. Ketamine is a N-methyl-D-aspartate antagonist, which produces increases in CBF and $CMRO_2$ (44,45). Early studies in patients with obstructed cerebrospinal fluid pathways reported ketamine administration increased ICP with reductions in CPP (46,47). More recent studies in adult patients with severe head injury have demonstrated improvements in CPP and minimal increases in ICP with ketamine (48–50). One recent report of 30 intubated pediatric head injury patients observed that single doses of ketamine lowered ICP without producing decreases in blood pressure or CPP (51). It is still unclear what ketamine's effect is on neurologic outcome in these patients or in patients where ventilation is not being tightly controlled. However, we believe that ketamine can be used in the brain injured patient, especially in multitrauma patients and if etomidate is not indicated.

Propofol

Propofol is a short-acting sedative-hypnotic IV agent that can be used to provide moderate or deep sedation. Propofol can induce a deep state of sedation rapidly, provide a short duration of effect, and have a pleasant recovery phase. Propofol is a very popular agent for sedating pediatric patients with neurologic conditions for noninvasive diagnostic imaging, such as a CT or magnetic resonance (MR) imaging. Due to the fast onset and recovery following administration, repeated neurologic examinations can be assessed. Propofol also has anticonvulsant properties and reduces ICP, which can be advantageous in sedating a patient with seizures or a patient with concerns for obstructive hydrocephalus due to a malfunctioning ventriculoperitoneal shunt to obtain diagnostic neuroradiologic imaging (52). While there have been cases of propofol providing adequate sedation and successfully treating intracranial hypertension

(52,53), several pediatric TBI case reports have reported metabolic acidosis and death in patients on prolonged (>24 hours) continuous infusion of propofol (54–58). Furthermore, a rare but potentially fatal "propofol infusion syndrome" associated with lactic acidosis, hyperlipidemia, and multiorgan system failure was first described in pediatric patients who received prolonged (>24 hours) continuous infusion and at higher dosages (> 4.5 mg/kg/h) (59). Current guidelines suggest that in the care of pediatric TBI patients, "continuous infusion of propofol is not recommended" (60).

Adverse effects of propofol include pain at the injection site, apnea or respiratory depression, hypotension, and bradycardia, which can be detrimental in a patient at risk for brain ischemia. If used, particular attention should be paid to the decrease in MAP with the administration of propofol. Crystalloid bolus and vasopressor usage will likely be needed to counteract the effects of propofol to maintain proper CPP and avoid ischemic insult. Propofol is a profound hypnotic but it does not provide any analgesia.

Dexmedetomidine

Dexmedetomidine, a centrally acting α_2-adrenergic agonist, is a recently approved agent by the Food and Drug Administration (FDA) for short-term (< 24 hours) continuous IV sedation of adults who are tracheally intubated (61). Like propofol, it has a rapid onset and a relatively rapid elimination half-life and is administered as a loading dose followed by continuous IV infusion. Advantageously, it provides sedation with a lower risk of respiratory depression than many other sedative medications. There is increased interest with this agent as a sedative during noninvasive neuroradiologic imaging studies in children who are not intubated. In one study, dexmedetomidine was compared to propofol in children undergoing MR imaging (62). While the onset of sedation and recovery time were significantly shorter in the children who received propofol, hypotension, respiratory depression, and desaturation were more common compared to the children receiving dexmedetomidine (62).

There is increased interest in the use of dexmedetomidine as a sedative and potential neuroprotective agent in both adults and children, as animal studies revealed neuroprotection from hypoxia-ischemia and decreased apoptosis and adult human studies in healthy volunteers demonstrated parallel decrease in $CMRO_2$ and CBF, which may potentially be helpful in briefly sedating patients who are at risk for intracranial hypertension such as head trauma, brain tumor, and obstructive hydrocephalus (63). In pediatric TBI case reports, no detrimental effects on ICP were observed. However, systemic hypertension was observed in 1 child who was receiving dexmedetomidine with other sedatives, while bradycardia was observed in 2 other children who were receiving dexmedetomidine, other sedatives, and therapeutic hypothermia (64,65). Further studies are warranted on the potential use of this agent in children at risk for intracranial hypertension.

The most common adverse side effects of dexmedetomidine appear to be cardiovascular. Bradycardia with rare reports of sinus pause or cardiac arrest has been reported. Hypotension has been reported as well as hypertension, the latter thought to be due to peripheral α_{2B} agonism with peripheral vasoconstriction. There are conflicting reports on the effects of ventilatory function, with some studies suggesting mild respiratory depression, while others show no effect. While ICP does not appear to increase, CPP and CBF have been shown to decrease. The effects on seizure threshold appear to be mixed (66). The authors do not recommend dexmedetomidine as an induction agent; however, it may be a useful agent for patients with brain injury and ongoing sedation needs; however, further study in pediatric patients is needed.

Postintubation Management

After successful tracheal intubation, oxygen saturation of 100%, normocarbia (35–39 mmHg confirmed by arterial blood gas and trended with an end-tidal CO_2), and a chest x-ray showing the tracheal tube in good position above the carina (right mainstem tracheal intubation is common in pediatrics) should be confirmed. Unless the patient has signs or symptoms of herniation, prophylactic hyperventilation ($Paco_2$ < 35 mm Hg) should be avoided. Hyperventilation causes cerebral vasoconstriction, which decreases CBF and subsequent cerebral blood volume. While this will lower ICP, it may lead to ischemia (67). However, in the presence of signs and symptoms of herniation, such as Cushing triad (irregular respirations, bradycardia, systemic hypertension), pupillary dysfunction, lateralizing extremity weakness, or extensor posturing, hyperventilation with 100% oxygen can be a lifesaving maneuver. Hyperoxia is to be avoided and Fio_2 should be titrated to maintain Sao_2 greater than 90%. Elevating the head to 30° (with C-spine precautions) increases venous drainage and lowers ICP (68,69). Furthermore, the head should be midline to prevent obstruction of venous return from the brain. If these maneuvers do not relieve the signs and symptoms of herniation, additional sedative and analgesic agents, can be administered as long as hypotension is avoided.

Supraglottic Airway Devices

While supraglottic airways are not considered a permanent airway in critically ill patients, competency in placement is critical for all individuals participating in resuscitation of a brain-injured child. Supraglottic airway devices such as a laryngeal mask airway (LMA) device can be life saving and in a situation where there is difficulty with direct laryngoscopy and inadequate bag-mask ventilation, an LMA should be placed to limit hypoxia and control ventilation until a physician with advanced airway skills can arrive to place an endotracheal tube.

■ VENTILATORY STRATEGIES FOR CHILDREN WITH ACUTE BRAIN INJURY

Definitions of Lung Injury

ALI develops initially in response to a variety of pulmonary and extrapulmonary disease processes, ultimately resulting in widespread alveolar-capillary leak with extravasation of protein rich, noncardiogenic pulmonary edema (Table 4.1). This acute phase leads to atelectasis, consolidation, surfactant degradation, and

ultimately decreased lung compliance with progressive hypoxemia. Further progression of the disease process leads to a chronic stage, also known as the fibroproliferative stage, characterized by improvement in compliance despite continued poor lung function, due to fibrous scarring and thickening of the lung interstitium. If the patient survives, the acute and fibroproliferative (chronic) stages, his or her lung function can vary from complete recovery to substantial long-lasting pulmonary functional deficits.

Clinical features of lung injury can vary from mild, self-limiting dyspnea to rapidly progressive and fatal respiratory failure. The clinical course of ALI can be generalized in 4 phases; however, not every patient passes through all these phases and the condition may resolve at any stage (Table 4.1). Extensive research continues to try to develop predictive biomarkers and genomic arrays for severity and resolution of lung injury; however, to date there are no useful clinical biomarkers or genomic readouts for prediction or goal directed therapy.

Consensus clinical definitions have been constructed to define lung injury and give a common vernacular among clinicians based on the pathophysiologic response to lung injury (Table 4.2). The definitions for ALI and ARDS are similar and include: a diffuse, bilateral disease process; pulmonary edema due to capillary leak (not hydrostatic edema from cardiogenic failure represented by a pulmonary capillary wedge pressure [PCWP] less than 18 cm H_2O); and hypoxemia. The PCWP is rarely measured and is often inferred by exam or ECHO. ALI and ARDS only *differ* by the degree of hypoxemia (measured by a decrease in arterial oxygen tension: Pao_2) and rising oxygen requirements (measured by an increase in the inspired fraction of oxygen: Fio_2). This ratio is numerically expressed as the $Pao_2/$

■ Table 4.1 Four Phases in the Clinical Development of Lung Injury

1. Dyspnea and tachypnea with no other abnormalities on chest radiograph.
2. Hypoxemia with normal or subnormal $Paco_2$. Minor abnormalities on CXR, lasts 24–48 hours.
3. Diagnostic criteria of ALI established, severe arterial hypoxemia. Decreased pulmonary compliance with characteristic bilateral diffuse infiltrates on CXR.
4. Massive bilateral consolidation with unremitting hypoxemia. Increased deadspace, and rising $Paco_2$. This phase is often terminal.

Abbreviations: ALI, acute lung injury; CXR, chest radiograph.

■ Table 4.2 ALI vs. ARDS

ALI[a]	ARDS[a]
• Bilateral infiltrates on CXR	• Bilateral infiltrates on CXR
• PCWP < 18 cm H_2O	• PCWP < 18 cm H_2O
• Hypoxemia	• Hypoxemia
• Pao_2/Fio_2 ratio > 200 and < 300	• Pao_2/Fio_2 ratio < 200

Abbreviations: ARDS, acute respiratory distress syndrome; PCWP, pulmonary capillary wedge pressure.
[a]Requires 4 criteria.

FiO_2 ratio (P/F ratio). The P/F ratio acts as a surrogate, quantitative data point to define worsening lung injury. A patient with a P/F ratio between 300 and 200, bilateral infiltrates on chest radiograph (CXR), and a PCWP less than 18 cm H_2O by definition has *ALI*. As the P/F ratio falls below 200, a patient's lung injury can be defined as *ARDS*. Unfortunately, the P/F ratio can be misleading in a mechanically ventilated patient, because it does not factor the level of mechanical support necessary for a patient to maintain an adequate PaO_2 for a given FiO_2. Therefore, physicians often discuss the degree of lung injury and progressive mechanical support in terms of oxygenation index (OI), which factors in the mean airway pressure (mP_{AW}), the amount of supplemental inspired oxygen, and the resulting PaO_2 (Figure 4.1). As with P/F ratios, the OI is a numerical representation attempting to quantify the degree of mechanical support and thus the degree of lung injury. OI, like P/F ratios, can be used to trend disease progression.

If lung injury can result from a varied group of disease processes, how can we use a broad, common set of definitions, such as ALI and ARDS, to define/discuss lung injury? In response to this question, Gattinoni and others have proposed that patients with ALI/ARDS should be considered as two separate groups (70) (Table 4.3). *Pulmonary lung injury* results from clinical conditions that cause direct lung injury (ie, pneumonia) whereas *extrapulmonary lung injury* follows an indirect mechanism of injury via systemic mediators of inflammation (ie, sepsis). In fact, despite meeting the same criteria for ARDS, the two subgroups of lung injury may differ with respect to pathologic mechanisms, appearances on CT, respiratory mechanics, and response to ventilatory strategies. However, despite diverse etiologies, the ultimate histologic appearances of lung injury are remarkably consistent. This ultimate, consistent histologic appearance, despite varied direct or indirect injury, allows ARDS to be considered a discrete clinical entity and this definition of ARDS has been used to study incidence and mortality.

■ Table 4.3 Direct and Indirect Lung Injury

Direct Lung Injury	Indirect Lung Injury
Common	Common
• Pneumonia	• Sepsis
• Aspiration	• Severe nonthoracic trauma
• Pulmonary embolism	• TRALI
Less common	Less common
• Pulmonary contusion	• Acute pancreatitis
• Near drowning	• Cardiopulmonary bypass
• Inhalational injury	• Burns
• Fat/amniotic fluid embolism	
• Reperfusion edema	

Abbreviation: TRALI, transfusion associated acute lung injury.

Principles of Lung Protective Strategies: Limiting Ventilator Associated Lung Injury

As lung injury progresses, in response to pulmonary or extrapulmonary injury, the lungs can be divided into three hypothetical regions: (1) Areas with severe collapse and alveolar flooding referred to as "dependent areas," (2) recruitable areas with alveolar atelectasis referred to as "intermediate areas," (3) normal lung referred to as "nondependent areas." (Figure 4.2) The goal of mechanical ventilation is to recruit intermediate areas allowing improved gas exchange, spare normal areas of lung from ventilator associated lung injury (VALI), and give dependent collapsed regions of lung with alveolar flooding time to recover from the primary process (ie, pneumonia, sepsis). Lung recruitment of intermediate

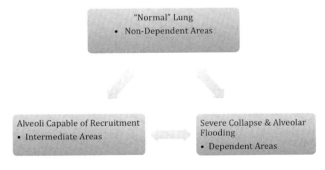

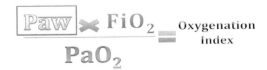

FIGURE 4.1 Formula to determine oxygenation index.

FIGURE 4.2 ALI/ARDS hypothetical lung sections.

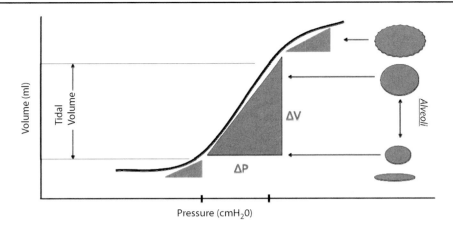

FIGURE 4.3   Volume-pressure curve.

areas and prevention of VALI is accomplished by using peak end expiratory pressure (PEEP) and limiting tidal volume and plateau pressures. This can be a complicated task. Figure 4.3 provides a theoretical pressure-volume curve of the lung. As alveolar airway pressure increases there is an opening pressure (Pflex) required to overcome airway resistance and alveolar compliance (Compliance = DV/DP). Pressures below Pflex will lead to alveolar collapse, termed atelectasis. If airway pressure cycles above and below Pflex, alveoli will continually open and collapse, leading to wall shear stress and eventual damage referred to as atelectrauma. Following the hysteresis curve to the upper extent of the inspiratory limb, as pressure increases, there comes a point, termed Pmax, whereby the alveoli start to become overdistended. Above Pmax, shear stress again leads to alveolar damage referred to as volutrauma. Therefore, in theory, we attempt to keep tidal volumes on the most compliant part of the volume-pressure curve which is located above Pflex and below Pmax. This strategy is referred to as "open lung ventilation." Triggered by the ARDSnet's initial study, the use of low tidal volumes (6–8 mL/kg) with the addition of PEEP (open lung strategy) may reduce morbidity and mortality in patients with ARDS (Figure 4.4) (71). However, as lung injury to the normal and intermediate areas of the lungs progresses, the volume-pressure curve moves to the right as the compliance of the lungs decreases, leaving a smaller therapeutic window requiring an increase in PEEP, resulting in higher MAP to maintain recruitment of areas of normal and recruitable lung (Figure 4.5).

Lung protective strategy attempts to decrease VALI by inhibiting: volutrauma, barotrauma, atelectrauma, oxygen toxicity, and biotrauma (Figure 4.6).

Low tidal volume: Despite using usual control groups in the ARDSnet original study, employing a low tidal volume approach of 6–8 mL/kg has become a standard of care.

PEEP: The advantages of PEEP as a distending pressure include increase in FRC, improvement of respiratory compliance, improvement of ventilation/perfusion mismatch, and redistribution of lung water/edema. PEEP ultimately improves arterial oxygenation. The use of low tidal volumes has been consistent across multiple recent trials, but the selection of PEEP in these trials has been highly variable. Animal models have shown that setting PEEP just above Pflex minimizes lung injury and inflammation (72). It can be difficult to determine the critical opening pressure of alveoli clinically. Therefore,

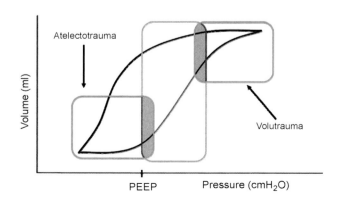

FIGURE 4.4   Lung protective ventilation.

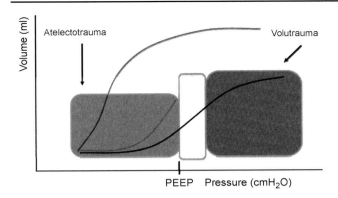

FIGURE 4.5 Lung protective ventilation.

most clinicians initially use a minimal distention strategy by setting PEEP between 5 and 9 cm H_2O; as lung injury progresses and hypoxemia worsens, PEEP may be increased to increase mean plateau pressures (keep < 30–35 cm H_2O) and aid in recruitment. These strategies have yet to show a decrease in mortality but have shown improvement in secondary outcomes (73). More precise methods of determining optimal PEEP in patients with ARDS include titration using dynamic compliance or static pressure-volume loops to identify the critical opening pressure. It is important to remember that as PEEP is increased and lung is recruited, intrathoracic pressure is also increased and may inhibit cardiac output by reducing venous return. Therefore, despite an improvement in oxygenation, oxygen delivery to vital organs may be compromised.

Plateau airway pressures: Sustained plateau airway pressures > 35 cm H_2O can lead to barotraumas producing pneumothorax, pneumomediastinum, and subcutaneous emphysema. In an attempt to limit barotrauma, $Paco_2$ is allowed to increase in the face of inadequate minute

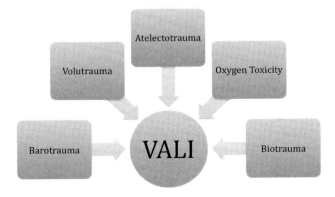

FIGURE 4.6 Factors leading to ventilator associated lung injury.

ventilation. This permissible hypercapnea can be employed as long as the patient tolerates the acidosis and is able to buffer with the renal retention of HCO_3 and there are no contraindications from coexisting disease.

Partial ventilatory support: By avoiding neuromuscular blockade and paralysis of the muscles of the diaphragm, spontaneous ventilation can occur during mechanical ventilation. Partial ventilatory support can lead to improved alveolar recruitment and ventilation/perfusion (VQ) mismatch, improved venous return and cardiac output, and enhanced weaning from mechanical ventilation. Avoidance of neuromuscular blockade may also lead to decreased need for sedation.

■ BASIC MODES OF MECHANICAL VENTILATION

The most basic mode of mechanical ventilation is controlled mandatory ventilation (CMV) which delivers a set tidal volume at a set respiratory rate, thereby ensuring a constant minute-ventilation (Minute Ventilation = Tidal Volume · Respiratory Rate). CMV delivers a preset tidal volume at a preset rate regardless of the patient's effort. Unlike CMV, intermittent mandatory ventilation (IMV) allows the patient to breath spontaneously between mandatory ventilator breaths. The most common type of IMV is synchronized IMV (SIMV), where mandatory ventilator breaths are synchronized via a timing window with the patient's spontaneous breaths. SIMV has an assist window which is a period of time measured in seconds that is dependent on the set mandatory breaths. For example, if the set ventilator rate is 10 breaths per minute then the assist window is 6 seconds. During the assist window, if the ventilator does not sense a spontaneous breath from the patient, the ventilator will deliver a mandatory breath. SIMV is commonly combined with pressure support (PS): SIMV + PS. When a ventilator is placed into SIMV + PS, the machine senses the patient initiating a breath and a preset positive pressure is delivered during the patient's breath in an attempt to support an adequate tidal volume and, thus, minute ventilation. PS is often set between 5 and 20 cm H_2O. SIMV + PS is advantageous because it allows for partial ventilatory support which improves cardiopulmonary mechanics and improves a patient's ability to wean from mechanical support. The disadvantage of SIMV + PS is that it does not assure minute ventilation as the mechanical breaths are decreased and the patient becomes less dependent on mandatory breaths to maintain minute ventilation. If the patient is not ready for decreased support the work of breathing may increase and ventilation will be impaired.

Once the mode of ventilation is set (CMV, IMV, SIMV, SIMV + PS) the clinician must determine the type of ventilator breath delivered to the patient. The most common types of breaths delivered are either pressure controlled (PC) or volume controlled (VC) and are referred to as SIMV-PC + PS or SIMV-VC + PS, respectively.

Pressure-controlled ventilation: PC ventilation delivers a pressure limited breath at a preset respiratory rate and inspiratory time (Ti). Tidal volume is a dependent variable during PC ventilation, and is determined by the preset pressure limit and the compliance and resistance of the respiratory system. If the respiratory systems compliance decreases or airway resistance increases, the preset pressure limit may not be adequate to maintain a tidal volume necessary to support a patient's minute ventilation. The flow waveform during PC ventilation is a decelerating pattern that follows a pressure gradient between the pressure delivered and alveolar pressure. Gas flows into airways along this pressure gradient, and as the alveolar volume increases and the pressure gradient between delivered breath and alveolar pressure narrows, gas flow will slow. When the clinician sets the Ti, gas flow maintains a decelerating pattern and even after the gas flow has stopped, MAP is maintained for the length of the set Ti. This combination of a high initial flow with a decelerating flow pattern and maintained set airway pressure over set Ti, may improve aeration by recruiting stiff, noncompliant sections of lung in ALI and ARDS. PC may also be useful in patients with air leak, either via a fistula or around the endotracheal tube, by maintaining gas flow until the set pressure is obtained and tidal volume achieved.

Volume-controlled ventilation: VC ventilation delivers a preset tidal volume breath during a preset Ti and at a preset respiratory rate. By setting volume control, alveolar overdistention may be avoided, limiting ventilator induced lung injury (volutrauma). During VC ventilation, airway and alveolar pressures are dependent variables, and as lung injury worsens mandatory tidal volumes may be maintained despite rising high peak inspiratory pressures to guarantee minute ventilation. These rising peak airway pressures may also lead to ventilator induced lung injury. Gas flow is constant during Ti. VC may be advantageous in patients with changing airway compliance, that is, intraoperative chest or abdominal surgery, so tidal volume may be consistent.

■ ADVANCED MODES OF MECHANICAL VENTILATION

Conventional mechanical ventilation fails due to inadequate CO_2 clearance (despite permissive hypercapnea, usually with persistent acidosis), poor oxygen delivery, exacerbation of lung injury beyond limits of protective ventilation, and inhibition of cardiovascular function due to increasing intrathoracic pressure. Traditionally, high frequency oscillatory ventilation (HFOV) and airway pressure release ventilation (APRV) have evolved as alternatives to failed conventional ventilation; however, APRV and HFOV may be used as a primary mode of ventilation in certain situations such as with air leak syndrome or postpneumonectomy. Both modes have the advantage of ventilating patients at full lung volumes on the expiratory limb of the pressure-volume curve while attempting to avoid phasic changes.

High frequency oscillatory ventilation: HFOV has become the mainstay of mechanical ventilation in pediatric patients with evolving ALI that is unresponse to conventional modes of ventilation. In fact, some authors have suggested that early institution of HFOV during ALI may improve survival by providing open lung ventilation without overdistention and further VALI (74). Therefore, HFOV allows for optimal alveolar recruitment with lower airway pressures, while minimizing atelectrauma associated with phasic alveolar opening and closing. A piston/diaphragm creates gas flow through by three methods: bulk axial flow, interregional gas mixing (pendelluft), and molecular diffusion. Tidal volumes are *dependent* on the patient's compliance, endotracheal tube size, device frequency, and device amplitude. Tidal volume is *inversely* related to cyclic frequency: $V_{CO_2} >$ Frequency $\times VT^2$. Transitioning from conventional modes of ventilation to HFOV, the initial power setting (ΔP/amplitude) is adjusted to visible chest "wiggle" from the clavicles to the abdomen or pelvis. Mean airway pressures (mP_{AW}) is initially set approximately 5 cm H_2O greater than the last mP_{AW} on conventional ventilation just prior to the initiation of HFOV. Traditionally, tidal volumes in HFOV are considered to be just above FRC; however, it is difficult to measure actual tidal volumes and provide precise "optimal" lung volume strategy. Clinically, mean airway pressure (mP_{AW}) is titrated by upward by 1 to 2 cm H_2O till oxygenation improves and inspired oxygen concentrations can be weaned to less toxic levels (below 0.60). While titrating mP_{AW} it is important to assess for overdistention by following chest radiographs. Overdistention/hyperinflation is determined by greater than 9 posterior ribs or flattened hemidiaphragms on chest x-ray. Table 4.4 lists initial frequency settings.

■ **Table 4.4** HFOV: Initial Frequency Settings

Patient Weight	Initial Frequency Setting
< 2 kg	15 Hz
2–15 kg	10 Hz
16–20 kg	8 Hz
21–30 kg	7 Hz
31–50 kg	6 Hz
> 50 kg	5 Hz

HFOV is the only mode of ventilation with active expiration. If hypercarbia, despite allowances for permissible hypercapnea, leads to profound respiratory acidosis and patient instability, then minute ventilation can be improved by several means during HFOV. First, one of the drawbacks of HFOV is the lack of spontaneous ventilation and adequate airway clearance, therefore inline suction (without breaking into the circuit causing derecruitment) should be used to ensure adequate airway and endotracheal tube patency and lung recruitment. Second, ΔP should be increased to maximize lung recruitment and increase minute ventilation. Third, frequency (Hz) can be slowly decreased to enhance lung recruitment and increase minute ventilation. Finally, the endotracheal tube cuff should be deflated to allow additional escape of CO_2 around the endotracheal tube.

Disadvantages of HFOV include lack of partial ventilatory support leading to increased sedation and paralysis requirements, cardiopulmonary interactions due to higher mP_{AW} and decreased venous return, and loss of alveolar recruitment if circuit detached for suctioning or manual ventilation.

Airway pressure release ventilation: APRV is essentially continuous positive airway pressure (CPAP) with brief, intermittent release coupled with spontaneous ventilation. The high CPAP level (Phigh) maintains alveolar recruitment and aids in oxygenation over a period of time (Thigh), and the timed release to a low pressure (Plow) minimizes resistance to expiratory flow and carbon dioxide removal. In addition, the patient is able to spontaneous breath during all phases, Phigh and Plow, potentially allowing for improved pulmonary mechanics and gas exchange. APRV differs from other modes of ventilation because it relies on an intermittent decrease in airway pressure, instead of an increase in airway pressure to maintain an open lung strategy for ventilation. Therefore, the release time (Tlow) should be set long enough to allow for an adequate tidal volume (6–8 mL/kg), but short enough to avoid alveolar collapse and atelectrauma.

In summary, the operator-controlled parameters in APRV are: Phigh, Thigh, Plow, Tlow, and FiO_2. Recommendations for implementing APRV are limited in pediatrics, and thus extrapolated from adult recommendations (75). Plow is initially set a zero. Phigh can be set by several methods such as plateau pressures or 75% of peak inspiratory pressure; however, when transitioning from conventional modes of ventilation Phigh is often determined by mP_{AW} pressure formula (see Table 4.5) where the mP_{AW} is set 2 to 3 cm H_2O above conventional mP_{AW}. To determine Thigh and Tlow, first determine the total cycle time according to a normal respiratory rate range for the patient's age (ie, a respiratory rate of 20 yields a total cycle time of 3 seconds). Thigh will be the total cycle time minus a Tlow of 0.2 to 0.6 seconds, initially starting at 0.4 seconds (ie, Total cycle time of 3 seconds yields a Thigh of 2.6 seconds and Tlow of 0.4 seconds). Transitioning to APRV, like transitioning to HFOV, will take time for optimal lung recruitment. After several hours if patient continues to have severe hypoxemia, Thigh can be increased to aid in oxygenation. Once established, Plow and Tlow usually do not require further changes; however, as lung compliance improves, Phigh and Thigh can be decreased and increased respectively to wean a patient toward a target of a continual CPAP of 5 to 6 cm H_2O in preparation for extubation.

APRV may be advantageous to other modes of advanced mechanical ventilation because of the patient's ability to breath spontaneously throughout the entire ventilatory cycle. This improves respiratory mechanics and reduces the need for sedation and neuromuscular blockade.

■ PRINCIPLES OF LUNG PROTECTIVE STRATEGIES FOR PATIENTS WITH ACUTE BRAIN INJURY

While there are clear tenets on how to treat ALI and ARDS (Figure 4.7), some of these strategies may conflict with usual neuroprotective strategies. For example, avoiding oxygen toxicity and permitting hypercapnea may be protective to the lungs, but may impact brain ischemia and ICP.

■ **Table 4.5** APRV Formulas

mP_{AW} formula: (Phigh · Thigh) + (Plow · Tlow)/Thigh + Tlow
Number of cycles (respiratory rate) = 60 seconds/Thigh + Tlow

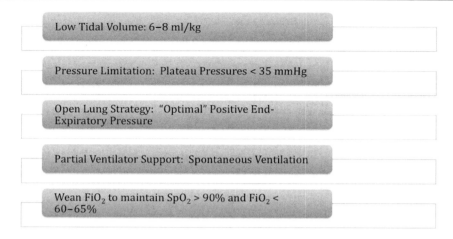

FIGURE 4.7 *Evolution of protective ventilation strategy.*

Oxygenation

There are no clear recommendations for baseline Pao_2 levels in pediatric brain injured patients. Guidelines released in 2012 suggest that a practitioner should consider maintaining a $Pbto_2$ greater than 10 mmHg measured by a parenchymal oxygen electrode in pediatric patients with severe TBI (27). There is very little evidence on the thresholds of arterial hypoxemia in the brain injured child; however, it is clear that arterial hypoxemia results in decreased cerebral oxygen delivery, resulting in cerebral vasodilation with intact autoregulation and thus an increase in ICP and a reduction in CPP. Where the inflection point for arterial hypoxemia results in cerebral vasodilation is a matter of debate in children (although classically taught as 50 mmHg). The Brain Trauma Foundation guidelines recommend avoidance of hypoxia (Pao_2 < 60 mm Hg) (76). We suggest that Pao_2 greater than 60 mm Hg be maintained in patients with brain injury and that an arterial Pao_2 between 70 and 80 mmHg may be necessary in a patient whose $Pbto_2$ measured by a parenchymal oxygen electrode is interpreted as low, or other evidence of ischemia is exhibited from advanced neuromonitoring, such as cerebral microdialysis or neuroimaging. The use of PEEP to maintain open lung strategies of mechanical ventilation and improve oxygenation in patients with ARDS can be implemented in patients with severe brain injury, provided that MAP is maintained and ICP is monitored to maintain an age appropriate CPP (77).

Minute Ventilation and $Paco_2$

Permissive hypercapnea has become a tenet of mechanical ventilation in patients with ARDS in an effort to limit ventilator induced lung injury (78). In pediatric patients with ARDS *without* brain injury, $Paco_2$ well above normal range is tolerated as long as the patient has a pH greater than 7.2 and is hemodynamically stable. Unfortunately, this becomes much more difficult in patients who have ARDS combined with a brain injury. Current pediatric level III recommendations suggest that practitioners should avoid prophylactic hyperventilation ($Paco_2$ < 30 mm Hg) in the first 48 hours, and if therapeutic hypoventilation is used for refractory intracranial hypertension then advanced neuromonitoring to evaluate ischemia should be considered (27). Additionally, most practitioners adjust minute ventilation in patients with severe brain injury and concern for intracranial hypertension to maintain normocapnea (approximately 35 mmHg). Balancing the need to minimize ventilator induced lung injury by adjusting tidal volumes and limiting minute ventilation can be in direct conflict with the need to limit $Paco_2$ in patients with severe TBI. Although advanced monitoring measuring partial pressures of cerebral oxygen, CBF, or cerebral metabolism are rarely used in pediatric, pediatric patients with brain injury and ARDS may necessitate placement, advanced neuromonitoring or neuroimaging that will allow the practitioner to direct neuroresuscitation in a complex critically ill child.

Adjuvant Therapies: Prone Positioning, NO, Surfactant Therapy

Prone Positioning

Prone positioning can improve oxygenation in patients with ARDS, and has been safely applied in pediatric patients. Prone positioning improves lung recruitment in select patients. Patient selection and duration of prone positioning is unclear; however, it is likely that a subgroup of patients respond to prone positioning early after lung injury, and immediate responders may benefit from prolonged prone positioning (79). While prone positioning improves oxygenation, this improvement has not been shown to improve mortality; however, in pediatric patients with brain injury and worsening hypoxemia, prone positioning may be attempted with careful monitoring of ICP (80,81).

Surfactant Therapy

Exogenous surfactant therapy is standard of care in neonates suffering from respiratory distress syndrome (RDS); however, the utility of surfactant therapy in the treatment of ALI and ARDS is uncertain and continues to be researched. In pediatric patients, recent studies have shown immediate improvement in oxygenation and a trend toward improved survival with the exogenous surfactant therapy, calfactant. Research is ongoing to determine patient selection, timing, and combination with other therapies for treatment of ALI and ARDS, and how this may be applied to the brain injured patient.

Nitric Oxide

Inhaled NO (iNO) acts as a selective pulmonary vasodilator to improve V/Q mismatch, decrease pulmonary hypertension, and reduce right ventricular cardiac work. NO upregulates cyclic guanosine monophosphate (cGMP), ultimately resulting in smooth muscle relaxation and pulmonary arteriolar vasodilatation. iNO is delivered directly to ventilated lung units and improves perfusion in these areas of lung without significant effects on the rest of the pulmonary vascular bed and systemic vasculature, thereby improving V/Q mismatch and oxygenation in patients with ARDS. Much like prone positioning and surfactant therapy, iNO can result in transient improvements in oxygenation. iNO may have antiinflammatory properties that may benefit patients with TBI and may improve CBF; however, these mechanisms are likely complex and further research is needed (82,83). We feel that in pediatric patients with brain injury and TBI with worsening hypoxemia, iNO should be used as an adjuvant therapy pending further research in the immature brain.

Extracorporeal Membrane Oxygenation

Extracorporeal membrane oxygenation (ECMO) remains a rescue strategy for pediatric patients with ARDS that fails to respond to advanced modes of mechanical ventilation. There are case reports of the use of ECMO with (84) and without (85) systemic heparinization in patients with TBI that have resulted in good neurologic outcomes. It is unclear whether ECMO improves outcomes in pediatric patients with ARDS; however, with the increasing use of bicaval dual lumen venovenous cannulas there may be a role for institution of ECMO in patients with coexisting ARDS and brain injury to maintain adequate oxygen delivery to the brain and limit ischemic injury.

■ CONCLUSIONS

In conclusion, there is a great deal of work that needs to be done to define goal directed neuroresuscitation for children with brain injury. However, maintaining a minimal CPP and optimizing oxygenation in patients with lung injury may improve outcomes in brain injured children by improving oxygen delivery and limiting ischemia. While this may only be a piece of the puzzle to decreasing secondary brain injury, the tenets of pediatric neurocritical care will provide the skeleton of future research and treatment algorithms, combined with neuroprotective agents, that will likely change the future of goal directed neuroresuscitation.

■ REFERENCES

1. Hamilton BE et al. Annual summary of vital statistics: 2005. *Pediatrics.* 2007;119:345–360.
2. Kochanek PM et al. Biochemical, cellular, and molecular mechanisms in the evolution of secondary damage after severe traumatic brain injury in infants and children: Lessons learned from the bedside. *Pediatr Crit Care Med.* 2000;1:4–19.

3. Hillered L, Vespa PM, Hovda DA. Translational neurochemical research in acute human brain injury: the current status and potential future for cerebral microdialysis. *J Neurotrauma.* 2005;22:3–41.

4. Marcoux J et al. Persistent metabolic crisis as measured by elevated cerebral microdialysis lactate-pyruvate ratio predicts chronic frontal lobe brain atrophy after traumatic brain injury. *Crit Care Med.* 2008;36:2871–2877.

5. Glenn TC et al. Energy dysfunction as a predictor of outcome after moderate or severe head injury: indices of oxygen, glucose, and lactate metabolism. *J Cereb Blood Flow Metab.* 2003;23:1239–2350.

6. Kilbaugh TJ et al. Cyclosporin A preserves mitochondrial function after traumatic brain injury in the immature rat and piglet. *J Neurotrauma.* 2011;28:763–774.

7. Raghupathi R, Margulies SS. Traumatic axonal injury after closed head injury in the neonatal pig. *J Neurotrauma.* 2002;19:843–53.

8. Duhaime AC et al. Maturation-dependent response of the piglet brain to scaled cortical impact. *J Neurosurg.* 2000;93:455–462.

9. Udomphorn Y, Armstead WM, Vavilala MS. Cerebral blood flow and autoregulation after pediatric traumatic brain injury. *Pediatr Neurol.* 2008;38:225–234.

10. Wintermark M et al. Brain perfusion in children: evolution with age assessed by quantitative perfusion computed tomography. *Pediatrics.* 2004;113:1642–1652.

11. Vavilala MS et al. Gender differences in cerebral blood flow velocity and autoregulation between the anterior and posterior circulations in healthy children. *Pediatr Res.* 2005; 58:574–578.

12. Adelson PD et al. Cerebrovascular response in infants and young children following severe traumatic brain injury: a preliminary report. *Pediatr Neurosurg.* 1997;26: 200–207.

13. Cunningham AS et al. Physiological thresholds for irreversible tissue damage in contusional regions following traumatic brain injury. *Brain.* 2005;128:1931–1942.

14. von Oettingen G et al. Blood flow and ischemia within traumatic cerebral contusions. *Neurosurgery.* 2002;50:781–790.

15. Jackson S, Piper IR. A study of the effects of using different cerebral perfusion pressure (CPP) thresholds to quantify CPP "secondary insults" in children. *Acta Neurochir Suppl.* 2000;76:453–456.

16. Chambers IR et al. Critical thresholds of intracranial pressure and cerebral perfusion pressure related to age in paediatric head injury. *J Neurol Neurosurg Psychiatry.* 2006;77:234–240.

17. Chambers IR et al. Age-related differences in intracranial pressure and cerebral perfusion pressure in the first 6 hours of monitoring after children's head injury: association with outcome. *Childs Nerv Syst.* 2005;21:195–199.

18. Chambers IR, Kirkham FJ. What is the optimal cerebral perfusion pressure in children suffering from traumatic coma? *Neurosurg Focus.* 2003;15:E3.

19. Adelson PD et al. Guidelines for the acute medical management of severe traumatic brain injury in infants, children, and adolescents. *Pediatr Crit Care Med.* 2003;4:S1–S75.

20. Stiefel MF et al. Reduced mortality rate in patients with severe traumatic brain injury treated with brain tissue oxygen monitoring. *J Neurosurg.* 2005;103:805–811.

21. Stiefel MF et al. Brain tissue oxygen monitoring in pediatric patients with severe traumatic brain injury. *J Neurosurg.* 2006;105:281–286.

22. Llinas RH. Ischemic stroke and ICU care. *Semin Neurol.* 2008;28:645–656.

23. Broderick JP, Hacke W. Treatment of acute ischemic stroke: part II: neuroprotection and medical management. *Circulation.* 2002;106:1736–1740.

24. Robertson CS et al. Prevention of secondary ischemic insults after severe head injury. *Crit Care Med.* 1999;27:2086–2095.

25. Contant CF et al. Adult respiratory distress syndrome: a complication of induced hypertension after severe head injury. *J Neurosurg.* 2001;95:560–568.

26. Samant UBT et al. Time of hypotension and discharge outcome in children with severe traumatic brain injury. *J Neurotrauma.* 2008;25:495–502.

27. Kochanek PM et al. Guidelines for the acute medical management of severe traumatic brain injury in infants, children, and adolescents—second edition. *Pediatr Crit Care Med.* 2012;13(suppl 1):S1–S82.

28. Johnston WE et al. Phenylephrine does not reduce cerebral perfusion during canine cardiopulmonary bypass. *Anesth Analg.* 1994;79:14–18.

29. Duebener LF et al. Effects of hemodilution and phenylephrine on cerebral blood flow and metabolism during cardiopulmonary bypass. *J Cardiothorac Vasc Anesth.* 2004;18:423–428.

30. Strebel SP et al. The impact of systemic vasoconstrictors on the cerebral circulation of anesthetized patients. *Anesthesiology.* 1998;89:67–72.

31. Cherian L et al. Cerebral hemodynamic effects of phenylephrine and L-arginine after cortical impact injury. *Crit Care Med.* 1999;27:2512–2517.

32. Di Gennaro JL et al. Use and effect of vasopressors after pediatric traumatic brain injury. *Dev Neurosci.* 2010;32:420–430.

33. Pfister D, Strebel SP, Steiner LA. Effects of catecholamines on cerebral blood vessels in patients with traumatic brain injury. *Eur J Anaesthesiol Suppl.* 2008;42:98–103.

34. Steiner LA et al. Direct comparison of cerebrovascular effects of norepinephrine and dopamine in head-injured patients. *Crit Care Med.* 2004;32:1049–1054.

35. Kochanek PK, Forbes ML, Ruppel R. Severe head injury in the infants and children. In: Furman BP, Zimmerman JJ, eds. *Pediatric Critical Care.* Philadelphia PA: Mosby; 2006:1595–1617.

36. Kilbaugh TJ et al. Sedation and analgesia in children with developmental disabilities and neurologic disorders. *Int J Pediatr.* 2010;2010.

37. Bergen JM, Smith DC. A review of etomidate for rapid sequence intubation in the emergency department. *J Emerg Med.* 1997;15:221–230.

38. Moss E et al. Effect of etomidate on intracranial pressure and cerebral perfusion pressure. *Br J Anaesth.* 1979;51: 347–352.

39. Renou AM et al. Cerebral blood flow and metabolism during etomidate anaesthesia in man. *Br J Anaesth.* 1978;50:1047–1051.

40. Drummond JC et al. Focal cerebral ischemia during anesthesia with etomidate, isoflurane, or thiopental: a comparison of the extent of cerebral injury. *Neurosurgery.* 1995;37:742–748; discussion 8–9.

41. Edelman GJ, Hoffman WE, Charbel FT. Cerebral hypoxia after etomidate administration and temporary cerebral artery occlusion. *Anesth Analg.* 1997;85:821–825.
42. Drummond JC et al. The role of nitric oxide synthase inhibition in the adverse effects of etomidate in the setting of focal cerebral ischemia in rats. *Anesth Analg.* 2005;100:841–846, table of contents.
43. Lev R, Rosen P. Prophylactic lidocaine use preintubation: a review. *J Emerg Med.* 1994;12:499–506.
44. Langsjo JW et al. Effects of subanesthetic doses of ketamine on regional cerebral blood flow, oxygen consumption, and blood volume in humans. *Anesthesiology.* 2003;99:614–623.
45. Langsjo JW et al. S-ketamine anesthesia increases cerebral blood flow in excess of the metabolic needs in humans. *Anesthesiology.* 2005;103:258–268.
46. Gibbs JM. The effect of intravenous ketamine on cerebrospinal fluid pressure. *Br J Anaesth.* 1972;44:1298–1302.
47. Wyte SR et al. Ketamine-induced intracranial hypertension. *Anesthesiology.* 1972;36:174–176.
48. Albanese J et al. Ketamine decreases intracranial pressure and electroencephalographic activity in traumatic brain injury patients during propofol sedation. *Anesthesiology.* 1997;87:1328–1334.
49. Bourgoin A et al. Safety of sedation with ketamine in severe head injury patients: comparison with sufentanil. *Crit Care Med.* 2003;31:711–717.
50. Kolenda H et al. Ketamine for analgosedative therapy in intensive care treatment of head-injured patients. *Acta Neurochir (Wien)* 1996;138:1193–1199.
51. Bar-Joseph G et al. Effectiveness of ketamine in decreasing intracranial pressure in children with intracranial hypertension. *J Neurosurg Pediatr.* 2009;4:40–46.
52. Spitzfaden AC, Jimenez DF, Tobias JD. Propofol for sedation and control of intracranial pressure in children. *Pediatr Neurosurg.* 1999;31:194–200.
53. Farling PA, Johnston JR, Coppel DL. Propofol infusion for sedation of patients with head injury in intensive care. A preliminary report. *Anaesthesia.* 1989;44:222–226.
54. Bray RJ. Propofol infusion syndrome in children. *Paediatr Anaesth.* 1998;8:491–499.
55. Cray SH, Robinson BH, Cox PN. Lactic acidemia and brady-arrhythmia in a child sedated with propofol. *Crit Care Med.* 1998;26:2087–2092.
56. Parke TJ et al. Metabolic acidosis and fatal myocardial failure after propofol infusion in children: five case reports. *BMJ.* 1992;305:613–616.
57. Canivet JL et al. Massive ketonuria during sedation with propofol in a 12 year old girl with severe head trauma. *Acta Anaesthesiol Belg.* 1994;45:19–22.
58. Veldhoen ES, Hartman BJ, van Gestel JP. Monitoring biochemical parameters as an early sign of propofol infusion syndrome: false feeling of security. *Pediatr Crit Care Med.* 2009;10:e19–e21.
59. Cray SH, Robinson BH, Cox PN. Lactic acidemia and brady-arrhythmia in a child sedated with propofol. *Crit Care Med.* 1998;26:2087–2092.
60. Adelson PD et al. Guidelines for the acute medical management of severe traumatic brain injury in infants, children, and adolescents. Chapter 19. The role of anti-seizure prophylaxis following severe pediatric traumatic brain injury. *Pediatr Crit Care Med.* 2003;4:S72–S75.
61. Phan H, Nahata MC. Clinical uses of dexmedetomidine in pediatric patients. *Paediatr Drugs.* 2008;10:49–69.
62. Mason KP et al. Dexmedetomidine for pediatric sedation for computed tomography imaging studies. *Anesthesia and Analgesia.* 2006;103:57–62, table of contents.
63. Tobias JD. Dexmedetomidine: applications in pediatric critical care and pediatric anesthesiology. *Pediatr Crit Care Med.* 2007;8:115–131.
64. Tobias JD. Bradycardia during dexmedetomidine and therapeutic hypothermia. *J Intensive Care Med.* 2008;23:403–408.
65. Erkonen G, Lamb F, Tobias JD. High-dose dexmedetomidine–induced hypertension in a child with traumatic brain injury. *Neurocrit Care.* 2008;9:366–369.
66. Ray T, Tobias JD. Dexmedetomidine for sedation during electroencephalographic analysis in children with autism, pervasive developmental disorders, and seizure disorders. *J Clin Anesth.* 2008;20:364–368.
67. Skippen P et al. Effect of hyperventilation on regional cerebral blood flow in head-injured children. *Crit Care Med.* 1997;25:1402–1409.
68. Feldman Z et al. Effect of head elevation on intracranial pressure, cerebral perfusion pressure, and cerebral blood flow in head-injured patients. *J Neurosurg.* 1992;76:207–211.
69. Huh JW, Raghupathi R. New concepts in treatment of pediatric traumatic brain injury. *Anesthesiol Clin.* 2009;27:213–240.
70. Pelosi, P et al. Pulmonary and extrapulmonary acute respiratory distress syndrome are different. Eur Respir J. 2003;42;48s–56s.
71. Ventilation with lower tidal volumes as compared with traditional tidal volumes for acute lung injury and the acute respiratory distress syndrome. The Acute Respiratory Distress Syndrome Network. *N Engl J Med.* 2000;342:1301–1308.
72. Villar J et al. A high positive end-expiratory pressure, low tidal volume ventilatory strategy improves outcome in persistent acute respiratory distress syndrome: a randomized, controlled trial. *Crit Care Med.* 2006;34:1311–1318.
73. Mercat A et al. Positive end-expiratory pressure setting in adults with acute lung injury and acute respiratory distress syndrome: a randomized controlled trial. *JAMA.* 2008;299:646–655.
74. Bollen CW, Uiterwaal CS, van Vught AJ. Systematic review of determinants of mortality in high frequency oscillatory ventilation in acute respiratory distress syndrome. *Crit Care.* 2006;10:R34.
75. Daoud EG, Farag HL, Chatburn RL. Airway pressure release ventilation: what do we know? *Respir Care.* 2012;57:282–292.
76. Foundation TBT. Guidelines for the management of severe traumatic brain injury. Introduction. *J Neurotrauma.* 2007;24(suppl 1):S1–S106.
77. McGuire G et al. Effects of varying levels of positive end-expiratory pressure on intracranial pressure and cerebral perfusion pressure. *Crit Care Med.* 1997;25:1059–1062.
78. Network TARDS. Ventilation with lower tidal volumes as compared with traditional tidal volumes for acute lung injury. *N Engl J Med.* 2000;342:1301–1308.
79. Mancebo J et al. A multicenter trial of prolonged prone ventilation in severe acute respiratory distress syndrome. *Am J Respir Crit Care Med.* 2006;173:1233–1239.
80. Thelandersson A, Cider A, Nellgard B. Prone position in mechanically ventilated patients with reduced

intracranial compliance. *Acta Anaesthesiol Scand.* 2006;50: 937–941.

81. Beuret P et al. Prone position as prevention of lung injury in comatose patients: a prospective, randomized, controlled study. *Intensive Care Med.* 2002;28:564–569.

82. Papadimos TJ. The beneficial effects of inhaled nitric oxide in patients with severe traumatic brain injury complicated by acute respiratory distress syndrome: a hypothesis. *J Trauma Manage Outcomes.* 2008;2:1.

83. Sinz EH et al. Inducible nitric oxide synthase is an endogenous neuroprotectant after traumatic brain injury in rats and mice. *J Clin Invest.* 1999;104:647–656.

84. Friesenecker BE et al. Craniotomy during ECMO in a severely traumatized patient. *Acta Neurochir (Wien).* 2005;147:993–996; discussion 6.

85. Yen TS et al. Extracorporeal membrane oxygenation resuscitation for traumatic brain injury after decompressive craniotomy. *Clin Neurol Neurosurg.* 2008;110:295–297.

5 | *Nutrition and Glucose Management*

VIJAY SRINIVASAN

■ INTRODUCTION

Optimizing nutrition is essential to good outcomes in pediatric neurocritical care. Children requiring neurocritical care are often malnourished at admission, especially if they have preexisting comorbidities. Lack of careful attention to nutrition support while administering "more intensive therapies" can result in further deficiencies (or excesses) developing during the course of illness. The changing metabolic milieu of the critically ill state coupled with difficulties in the nutritional assessment of children pose hurdles to the successful provision of nutrition during pediatric neurocritical illness, leading to both underfeeding and overfeeding. The lack of nutrition research and paucity of evidence-based guidelines for nutrition support in this population also constitute major barriers to good outcomes. In particular, abnormalities in blood glucose (BG) concentrations (both hyperglycemia and hypoglycemia) often occur during critical illness and pose threats to the vulnerable pediatric brain. Recent research suggests that strategies to carefully manage BG concentrations might improve clinical outcomes in pediatric neurocritical care. This chapter will review: (1) key concepts of cerebral metabolism during health, as well as changes in metabolism during critical illness that impact the brain, and (2) the importance of nutrition support and BG management in commonly seen conditions in pediatric neurocritical care.

■ CEREBRAL METABOLISM DURING HEALTH

The developing healthy brain almost exclusively uses glucose as a metabolic fuel for energy needs and biosynthesis (1). Since the brain has limited glycogen stores (chiefly in the astrocyte), normal brain function depends on a continuous supply of glucose via the bloodstream. Glucose transport into the brain occurs via members of the family of glucose transport proteins (GLUT) (2). Glucose travels from the blood into the brain across the blood-brain barrier (BBB) in conjunction with GLUT-1 (located in the endothelium of the BBB). After crossing the BBB, glucose is available to both neurons and astrocytes. A little over half of the glucose that crosses the BBB enters neurons via GLUT-3, while astrocytes utilize the rest via GLUT-1. During the resting state, "coupling" of oxygen delivery and glucose metabolism occurs by changes in cerebral blood flow (CBF) to match regional demand. Most of the glucose that enters the brain undergoes aerobic metabolism, with only a small amount converted to lactate under resting conditions (3). During periods of activity, cerebral oxygen consumption increases much less than CBF and glucose utilization. Correspondingly, there is an increase in nonoxidative glucose metabolism through glycolysis to generate pyruvate and lactate in neurons and astrocytes to meet the increased metabolic demands of activated neurons (4). Monocarboxylate transport proteins (MCT) transport lactate and pyruvate into and out of neural cells: MCT-1 in the BBB and astrocytes and MCT-2 in neurons. While the earlier astrocyte-neuron lactate shuttle hypothesis postulated that the astrocyte was the primary source of lactate production, recent studies have challenged this assertion and suggest that the neuron is likely the major source of lactate in the brain (2). Additionally, the developing brain also uses ketone bodies, free fatty acids, and amino acids as alternative fuels, especially when glucose supplies are limited. MCT-1 protein in the BBB mediates transport of ketones which may also play a role in biosynthetic precursors for developmental membrane and myelin formation.

Cerebral metabolism undergoes substantial alterations during growth and development with respect to energy utilization, metabolic rate, and distribution of activity. The fetal brain relies primarily on an uninterrupted supply of maternal glucose for its energy needs. Towards the end of gestation, brain expression of ketone metabolizing enzymes increases. Immediately after birth following interruption of maternal supplies of glucose, the fetus largely depends on its own stores of glycogen to provide glucose. The neonatal brain also metabolizes lactate during this period. As the neonate commences breast-feeding, ketone metabolism rapidly increases and remains high while the infant continues to breast-feed during infancy, along with a corresponding increase in the MCT-1 protein in the BBB to facilitate transport of ketones into the brain (5). When the infant stops breast-feeding, ketone metabolism declines sharply. During the early postnatal period, cerebral glucose metabolic rate is highest in the sensory and motor cortices, thalamus, and brain stem (6). Over the next few years, cerebral glucose metabolic rate continues to gradually increase in the cortex and thalamus, peaking by 4 years of age. Between 4 and 9 years of age, both CBF and cerebral glucose metabolic rate remain high in the cortex, corresponding to the period of rapid cognitive development. Subsequently, both CBF and cerebral glucose metabolic rate decline to adult values by 18 to 20 years of age (7).

■ METABOLIC ALTERATIONS DURING CRITICAL ILLNESS

During critical illness, a number of changes occur in multiple metabolic pathways including carbohydrate, protein, and lipid metabolism. Abnormalities in carbohydrate metabolism typically alter BG homeostasis during critical illness. Various factors such as hypoxia, oxidative stress, systemic inflammation, and changes in blood flow disrupt pathways of glucose metabolism during critical illness. Additionally, various therapeutic interventions used in the intensive care unit (ICU) have the potential to cause abnormalities in BG concentrations. Low BG concentrations (hypoglycemia) can result in neuroglycopenia with consequent neurologic injury, particularly in vulnerable younger age groups. Elevated BG concentrations (hyperglycemia) may affect pathways involved in the immune-inflammatory response to critical illness and result in poor outcomes. Changes in protein metabolism include greater protein turnover and loss, principally from skeletal muscle. This results in negative nitrogen balance and predisposes to the wasting syndrome of critical illness. Lipid metabolism undergoes several changes during critical illness, including decreases in total and high-density lipoprotein cholesterol levels. Critical illness predisposes to lipolysis resulting in elevated free fatty acids and glycerol. While free fatty acids contribute to insulin resistance seen commonly during critical illness, glycerol serves as a substrate for gluconeogenesis and predisposes to hyperglycemia.

Hypoglycemia During Critical Illness

Critical illness disrupts homeostatic mechanisms that regulate glucose metabolism (Figure 5.1), frequently resulting in hypoglycemia. Hypoxia can increase peripheral glucose utilization due to the inherent inefficiency of anaerobic glycolysis. Temperature instability and cold stress can increase metabolic demands and glucose utilization due to stimulation of the sympathetic nervous system and thyroid hormones. Critical illness is often associated with inadequate nutrient delivery and deficiencies of counterregulatory hormones (growth hormone or cortisol), which in turn lead to inadequate hepatic glucose production. Sepsis and multiple-organ failure frequently result in liver and renal dysfunction with resulting impairment in gluconeogenesis. Infants and children with preexisting disorders of fatty acid oxidation or carbohydrate metabolism, disorders of amino acid or organic acid metabolism, and deficiencies of growth hormone, thyroid hormone, or adrenal hormones are also at risk of hypoglycemia during critical illness due to inhibition of gluconeogenesis. Additionally, the practice of using intravenous insulin infusions to control

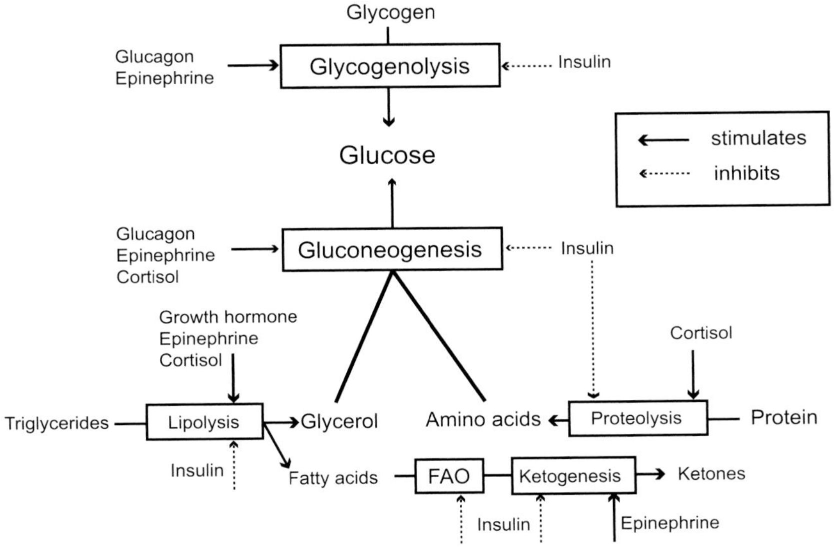

FIGURE 5.1 Glucose homeostasis. Abbreviation: FAO, fatty acid oxidation.

hyperglycemia is a major risk factor for hypoglycemia during critical illness. Often, therapies in the ICU such as mechanical ventilation, vasoactive infusions, nutrition support, and sedation and neuromuscular blockade can mask the symptoms of hypoglycemia, so that the practitioner is unaware of this occurrence. The catabolic state of critical illness together with numerous therapies that interfere with glucose metabolism disrupts the normal mechanisms that prevent hypoglycemia.

Impact on Cerebral Metabolism

The brain exhibits age-specific differences in its response to hypoglycemia. While the mature brain is quite vulnerable to the effects of hypoglycemia, the immature brain appears to resist the deleterious effects of low BG concentrations under normal conditions. Physiologic mechanisms that facilitate this in the immature brain include the ability to use alternate fuels such as lactate and ketones as well as increases in CBF and extraction of glucose from blood into brain (7). However, even in the immature brain, symptomatic, prolonged, or recurrent severe hypoglycemia can result in neurologic injury, especially in the setting of hypoxia and ischemia. Insulin-induced hypoglycemia might be more dangerous to the immature neonatal and pediatric brain than spontaneous hypoglycemia due to the lack of available alternative fuels such as ketones and fatty acids in the former state. The resulting energy failure mediates neuronal

damage via glutamate induced excitotoxicity, accumulation of oxygen free radicals, and activation of cellular apoptosis. Long-term sequelae of severe prolonged hypoglycemia in the neonatal period include mental retardation, seizures, or both. Recurrent episodes of severe hypoglycemia may be associated with mild neurocognitive dysfunction, memory deficits, and subtle changes in personality. Pathologic changes corresponding to severe prolonged hypoglycemia include cerebral atrophy, decrease in myelination of cerebral white matter, and gyral atrophy, with parietal and occipital lobes being the most severely affected (8). It is unclear at this time how hypoglycemia affects the brain in older children during critical illness. Preliminary studies suggest that hypoglycemia in older children with critical illness may be associated with higher mortality, worsening of organ failure, and greater ICU lengths of stay. The short-term and long-term consequences of critical illness hypoglycemia (spontaneous or insulin-induced) on the pediatric brain are unknown (9).

Hyperglycemia During Critical Illness

In the setting of critical illness, hyperglycemia develops principally through a combination of: (1) an increase in gluconeogenesis (relative to glucose clearance), and (2) insulin resistance affecting cellular uptake of glucose. Figure 5.2 depicts the pathogenesis of hyperglycemia during critical illness. The principal mechanisms appear

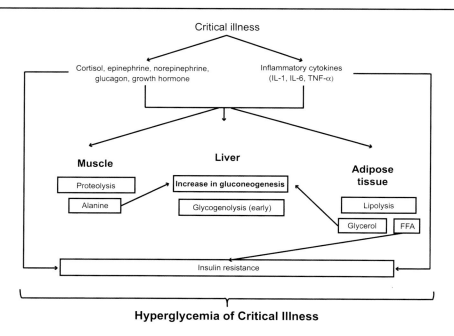

FIGURE 5.2 Pathogenesis of hyperglycemia of critical illness. Abbreviations: FFA, free fatty acids; IL-1, interleukin 1; IL-6, interleukin 6; TNF-α, tumor necrosis factor alpha.

to involve counterregulatory hormones (epinephrine, norepinephrine, glucagon, cortisol, growth hormone) and proinflammatory cytokines (tumor necrosis factor alpha, interleukin 1, interleukin 6). Additionally, proinflammatory cytokines may directly inhibit insulin secretion. The overall effect of hyperglycemia in critical illness is to increase BG concentrations and provide a ready source of fuel for vital organs in the body at a time of increased metabolic demand (10). Although hyperglycemia may represent an adaptive response by the body during the acute phase of illness to improve the likelihood of survival, persistence of hyperglycemia during chronic illness may be harmful. Under normal conditions, elevated BG concentrations stimulate the secretion of insulin by the pancreas, which in turn blocks hepatic glucose production and stimulates glucose uptake by the liver, muscle, and adipose tissue. The GLUT family of proteins regulate peripheral glucose uptake via facilitated diffusion. Typically, acute elevations in BG concentrations downregulate insulin-independent GLUT-1, GLUT-2, and GLUT-3 to prevent cellular glucose overload (11). Critical illness causes an overexpression of these transporters, leading to glucose overload and toxicity in organ systems that express these transporters. The upregulation of these insulin-independent GLUTs occurs in the central and peripheral nervous

systems as well as in renal tubules, gastrointestinal mucosa, and endothelial, hepatic, and immune cells.

Impact on Cerebral Metabolism

Glucose overload results in excessive glycolysis and oxidative phosphorylation with increased production of reactive oxygen species such as peroxynitrite and superoxide in the brain. These highly reactive species cause mitochondrial dysfunction and direct neuronal damage via lipid peroxidation, protein carbonylation, and DNA damage (12). Neutralization of nitric oxide by superoxide may also impair vasodilation at the endothelial level, thus compromising microcirculatory perfusion. These alterations in energy metabolism lead to increased apoptosis and, consequently, neuronal failure in critically ill patients. Insufficient cellular autophagy exacerbated by hyperglycemia may worsen cellular damage and delay recovery from critical illness. Hyperglycemia may exacerbate preexisting acidosis and increase availability of glutamate to the ischemic brain. This effect may promote N-methyl-D-aspartate (NMDA) mediated excitotoxicity and lead to additional mitochondrial damage from calcium overload (13). Hyperglycemia in critical illness also impairs macrophage and neutrophil activity and alters complement fixation. Hyperglycemia can worsen the inflammatory state by increasing binding of nuclear factor kappa B, leading to increases in transcription of proinflammatory cytokines. Hyperglycemia may contribute to other abnormalities commonly seen during critical illness, such as endothelial dysfunction, alterations in vascular smooth muscle tone, and abnormalities in coagulation that further worsen the cerebral milieu (11).

Alterations in Protein and Lipid Metabolism

Critical illness predisposes to a state of hypercatabolism with increases in protein turnover and losses, principally from skeletal muscle. Albumin levels often decline during the state of hypercatabolism. In the acute phases of critical illness, there is a net transfer of alanine from muscle to liver to support gluconeogenesis. In critical illness, especially sepsis, the skeletal muscle, lung, and kidney release glutamine for uptake by the liver. The liver utilizes glutamine for gluconeogenesis, ureagenesis, and synthesis of proteins and glutathione. Glutamine stores decline to a greater extent than other amino acids in critical illness. Arginine is another amino acid that decreases during critical illness, especially with burn injury. As the acute phase gives way to the chronic phase, persistence of these changes result in negative nitrogen balance and predisposes to the wasting syndrome of critical illness (14).

Lipid metabolism exhibits numerous alterations during critical illness. Inflammation results in increases in free fatty acids and triglycerides, while levels of high-density lipoprotein cholesterol decline. The increases in catecholamines and cytokines inhibit lipoprotein lipase and reduce extracellular lipolysis by endothelial cells. Simultaneously, upregulation of hormone sensitive lipase enhances lipolysis in adipose tissue to an extent that far exceeds demands. Elevated levels of free fatty acids mediate insulin resistance by affecting phosphorylation. This prevents translocation of GLUT-4 to the cell surface and in turn affects uptake of glucose. During critical illness, the liver is unable to secrete enough very low density lipoprotein to match production of triglycerides. The resulting hypertriglyceridemia can cause lipotoxicity, affect endothelial cell function, and exacerbate the state of inflammation by activating toll-like receptor 4. Increases in inflammatory cytokines coupled with limited intake of cholesterol reduce levels of high-density lipoprotein cholesterol during critical illness which predispose to adrenal insufficiency (15).

Impact on Cerebral Metabolism

Critical illness can impair neuronal energetics and predispose to glutamate excitotoxicity even when glutamate is present in physiologic concentrations. Additionally, high levels of nitric oxide generated during the glutamate-glutamine cycle can also cause toxicity and energy failure (16). Hypertriglyceridemia increases oxidative stress and impairs NMDA mediated hippocampal long-term synaptic potentiation. Hypertriglyceridemia affects the ability of leptin to cross the BBB. Since leptin enhances cognition, this could result in cognitive impairments. Additionally, elevated triglyceride levels also modify the release of feeding peptides, many of which affect cognition, via nitric oxide dependent pathways. Collectively, these changes in lipid metabolism predispose to memory loss and cognitive deficits (17).

■ NUTRITION SUPPORT AND GLUCOSE MANAGEMENT

Nutrition support with particular attention to glucose management forms an important aspect of pediatric neurocritical care. This section will cover common conditions in pediatric neurocritical care such as traumatic brain injury (TBI), stroke, hypoxic-ischemic encephalopathy, neuromuscular disorders, and spinal cord injury (SCI). Early provision of enteral nutrition with adequate calories and protein is associated with improved outcomes in adults and children with neurocritical illness. Glucose management to avoid hyperglycemia and hypoglycemia is also very important to improve clinical outcomes. It is less clear at this time if tight glucose control with intensive insulin therapy results in improved outcomes in pediatric neurocritical care.

General Principles

The hypermetabolic stress response in these children places enormous and often variable demands on energy. The body responds to this state with glucose intolerance, dyslipidemia, and protein losses, resulting in negative nitrogen balance and wasting with loss of lean body mass. Supply of protein and glucose during the hypermetabolic state does not necessarily reduce protein breakdown and nitrogen loss. However, net protein balance may improve with protein synthesis. Various nutritional deficiencies can develop during this phase and result in further worsening of critical illness. An anabolic phase follows the hypermetabolic state of critical illness in children who recover. Nutrition support is essential during this recovery phase to improve outcomes.

Assessment of Nutritional Status

Estimates suggest that 1 in 4 children is malnourished at the time of admission to the ICU. Nutritional status of the child with neurocritical illness requires careful assessment at admission and at regular intervals during the course of the ICU duration. Anthropometry is often challenging to perform and difficult to interpret in these critically ill children. Measures of body composition may be more useful, but are difficult to obtain in this population with the possible exception of bioelectrical impedance assessment. Biochemical assessment of visceral protein (albumin, prealbumin, and retinol binding protein) and acute-phase protein (C-reactive protein) pools, nitrogen loss, and energy expenditure are perhaps the most practical to follow in the ICU, but are subject to confounding by a number of variables. Failure to accurately estimate energy needs in children with neurocritical illness can result in both underfeeding and overfeeding, with undesirable consequences. Methods such as indirect calorimetry perform better than predictive clinical energy equations to measure energy expenditure and prescribe appropriate nutrition support in this population (18).

Nutrition Support

The energy burden imposed by the stress of critical illness is often difficult to estimate accurately and varies depending on the phase of illness. Nutrition support, therefore, requires an individualized prescription with frequent monitoring to avoid both overfeeding and underfeeding. Overfeeding critically ill children is associated with lipogenesis, hepatic steatosis, and liver dysfunction. Additionally, increase in carbon dioxide production results in difficulties with weaning from ventilator support (19). While hypocaloric diets in critically ill adults may be beneficial via protein sparing, the evidence of benefit of permissively underfeeding critically ill children is unclear, especially in the face of preexisting malnutrition.

The provision of dietary protein sufficient to optimize protein synthesis and preserve skeletal muscle protein mass is the most important nutrition intervention in critically ill children. A supply of adequate proteins and

energy intake improves protein balance by increasing protein synthesis without affecting protein breakdown due to catabolism. The amount of protein required to maintain a positive nitrogen balance may vary according to the severity of illness. The ideal amount and proportion of amino acids required during critical illness are unknown (18). Carbohydrates and fat should ideally make up nonprotein calories in a ratio of 1.2 to 1.8. Essential fatty acid deficiency may develop during critical illness in the absence of adequate lipid supplementation in the diet (20). Lipids typically constitute about 30% to 40% of the total calories. The practitioner should commence administering lipids at 1 g/kg/day, and gradually increase the dose to 2 to 4 g/kg/day, depending on the observed triglyceride levels. Micronutrients including vitamins and trace elements may also play important roles in critical illness and subsequent recovery. Table 5.1 summarizes protein and energy requirements in critically ill children (18).

Traumatic Brain Injury

Following TBI in children, mean energy expenditure increases significantly (up to 130%–173% from predicted energy expenditure) and variably between individuals (21,22). Seizures and elevated temperatures are common derangements that occur following TBI and may result in the increased mean energy expenditure observed. Additionally, muscle tone may account for a significant component of this increase in energy expenditure (23). Control of these factors with antiepileptic medications, antipyretic therapies, and sedation with neuromuscular blockade can significantly reduce mean energy expenditure. Most victims of TBI lose weight and attain

■ Table 5.1 Protein and Energy Requirements in Critically Ill Children

	Age (y)	Protein (g/kg/d)	Energy (kcal/kg/d)
Infants	0–1	2.0–2.2	105–115
Toddlers	1–3	1.8	100
School age children	4–10	1.2–1.5	85
Adolescents			
Males	11–14	1.0	60
	15–18	0.8	42
Females	11–14	1.0	48
	15–18	0.8	38

nitrogen balance only after 4 to 14 days, suggesting the importance of careful nutrition support in enhancing an earlier recovery.

The benefits of commencing early nutrition (whether enteral or parenteral) to reach full nutritional replacement by 7 days following injury appear to be associated with better outcomes in adults with TBI (24). A similar approach may be beneficial in children with TBI, but data are lacking. In those children with TBI who have a functioning gastrointestinal tract, enteral nutrition is preferable to parenteral nutrition for ease of administration, lower cost, and safer profile. However, postpyloric tube feedings and continuous feedings may be necessary to reach energy goals and optimize nutritional status. The use of immune-enhancing diets containing glutamine, arginine, omega-3 fatty acids, and antioxidants is not associated with better outcomes from pediatric TBI (25).

Stroke

Limited data from adult stroke survivors suggest that there is a slight increase in energy expenditure compared to predicted values, but this increase is not sustained (26). Decrease in physical activity and reduction in muscle tone may contribute to these findings. Extensive stroke may be associated with elevated intracranial pressure (ICP) with resulting gastric atony and feeding intolerance. In such circumstances, nasojejunal tube feeding may be necessary to reach caloric goals. Subsequently, after ICP normalizes, it may be possible to switch to nasogastric tube feedings and eventually an oral diet. Dysphagia following stroke may be a major impediment to successful nutrition. In such circumstances, nasogastric or nasojejunal tube feedings are important to optimize nutrition and deliver goal calories. If dysphagia persists, a percutaneous or surgical gastrostomy or jejunostomy tube may be required for continued nutrition support. The risk of reflux of gastrointestinal contents with aspiration remains high if the swallowing mechanism is impaired following stroke. Weaning from tube feedings requires close involvement of speech-language therapists with calorie counts to determine the exact amount of nutrition intake (27).

Hypoxic-ischemic Encephalopathy

Patients with hypoxic-ischemic encephalopathy may have lower energy expenditure. However, intercurrent seizures and autonomic dysreflexia can result in episodic hypermetabolism profound enough to cause severe weight loss and protein breakdown (28). Indirect calorimetry may be invaluable in such circumstances to accurately study energy requirements and prescribe appropriate nutrition therapy. Due to significant neurologic impairments, tube feedings are often required to deliver target calories. Constipation and gastroesophageal reflux are major impediments to successful nutrition in this population. Additionally, overfeeding is a common problem in this group of children.

Neuromuscular Disorders

Children with spinal muscular atrophy often have impaired swallowing mechanisms with limited mouth opening and difficulties chewing due to bulbar dysfunction (29). Critical illness and death is often due to aspiration pneumonia and respiratory failure. While growth failure is common in those with more severe disease, overfeeding and excessive weight gain is common in those with milder forms of the disease. Gastroesophageal reflux, delays in gastric emptying, and constipation commonly complicate the picture further in this group. While nasogastric or nasojejunal tube feedings may overcome some of the problems, percutaneous or surgical gastrostomy or jejunostomy tubes may be superior to consistently deliver nutrition without compromising the delicate respiratory status in these children. During acute illness, these children are more prone to hypoglycemia due to severe muscle wasting (30). Additionally, disorders of fatty acid oxidation may coexist in this group of children rendering them more vulnerable to fasting states (31). Prompt provision of calories and avoidance of prolonged fasting states can prevent muscle breakdown in these children during critical illness.

Guillain-Barré syndrome (GBS) is another entity in the ICU that poses tremendous challenges to nutrition support. Although the patient with GBS is immobile and appears to have reduced energy expenditure, hypermetabolism is common in GBS (32). In addition, patients are often malnourished at admission as bulbar weakness precludes adequate oral intake (33). If nutritional demands are not promptly met, patients rapidly become undernourished and have an increased incidence of pressure sores and infections. Patients with GBS should receive a high calorie (40–45 nonprotein calories/day) and high-protein (2–2.5 g/kg) enteral formula for optimal nutrition. Continuous enteral nutrition is preferable to intermittent or bolus feeding in these patients who also frequently experience delayed gastric emptying with gastroesophageal reflux, constipation, and erosive gastritis.

Spinal Cord Injury

Data from adults experiencing SCI suggest that energy expenditure is reduced acutely (34). Although these patients exhibit a negative nitrogen balance, this negative balance is obligatory, and attempts to correct it by increasing caloric intake may result in overfeeding with its attendant consequences. Indirect calorimetry may provide a more accurate reflection of the patient's caloric requirements, and could prevent overfeeding by allowing adjustments of intake based on measured energy expenditure rather than predicted energy expenditure. Enteral feeding is preferable to the parenteral route, as it produces a lower incidence of infectious complications and hyperglycemia. Nasogastric or nasojejunal tube feedings may be necessary if swallowing mechanisms are impaired. Percutaneous or surgical feeding tubes are preferable for long-term nutritional support in these patients.

Glucose Management

Hyperglycemia in pediatric critical illness is very common, with an estimated 49% to 72% of children experiencing BG concentrations greater than 150 mg/dL (35–38). Notably, 20% to 35% of critically ill children experience BG concentrations greater than 200 mg/dL. BG concentrations in critically ill children can often peak as high as 283 ± 115 mg/dL. Sustained hyperglycemia is also common over a prolonged period of ICU admission and may persist for up to half the duration of ICU stay. In the last decade, several studies have demonstrated the association of hyperglycemia in critically ill children with mortality (35–38). Specifically, peak BG concentrations and sustained elevation of BG concentrations appear to be associated with mortality. This association of hyperglycemia with mortality consistently appears across different pediatric conditions, including septic shock, burns, TBI, postcardiac surgery, and trauma. Hyperglycemia is also associated with longer periods of ICU and hospital stay as well as more frequent organ failure and nosocomial infections in critically ill children (35–38).

Studies of tight glucose control in critically ill adults have had mixed results with some observing worse outcomes from tight glucose control (39–41). Notably, all studies of tight glucose control in critically ill adults observed significant increases in hypoglycemia. Consequently, the initial rush to embrace this therapy has justifiably given way to a more cautious approach in the critical care community. It is worrying that studies suggest that hypoglycemia is also associated with mortality and worsening organ failure in critically ill children (42). Multicenter studies of tight glucose control in critically ill children are currently underway to answer this important question of whether tight glucose control can improve outcomes in critically ill children experiencing hyperglycemia (43).

Traumatic Brain Injury

Studies in children experiencing TBI have shown that admission hyperglycemia is associated with mortality and poor neurologic outcomes following injury (44,45). Persistent hyperglycemia, especially beyond 48 hours, is also associated with poor neurologic outcomes in children with TBI (46,47). Most studies of tight glucose control in adults with TBI have not observed any benefits, with some observing worse outcomes (48,49). Additionally, there is increasing concern about hypoglycemia and its risks to the injured brain. Studies employing microdialysis in adults with severe TBI have demonstrated increased metabolic stress in the cerebral milieu with tight glucose control compared with less rigorous BG targets (50). The practice of tight glucose control may reduce levels of lactate and ketones, which are likely to be the preferred fuels in the injured brain. The optimal BG target concentration following pediatric TBI remains unknown. It is, therefore, prudent to avoid extremes of hyperglycemia and hypoglycemia in pediatric survivors of TBI.

Stroke

Data from adults experiencing stroke observe that hyperglycemia is associated with worse outcomes (51). However, studies of tight glucose control in adult victims of stroke have not demonstrated any benefits, most likely due to increases in hypoglycemia that might negate any advantages of tight glucose control (52). Extrapolating from adult stroke guidelines, it would be reasonable to target BG concentrations in a more "moderate" range, taking care to avoid extremes of hyperglycemia and hypoglycemia.

Hypoxic-ischemic Encephalopathy

Hyperglycemia is common after cardiac arrest due to the upregulated metabolic state of the post cardiac arrest syndrome and may be associated with poor outcomes (53). However, studies have observed that tight glucose control may not be necessary to improve outcomes, with a more moderate BG target up to 150 mg/dL being clinically comparable (54,55). It is extremely important to avoid hypoglycemia at all costs to prevent further neuronal damage in this state.

Spinal Cord Injury

There is no pediatric data on the association of hyperglycemia with SCI and outcomes. Extrapolating from TBI, it would be reasonable to avoid tight glucose control in this group and target a modest BG range, taking care to avoid hypoglycemia.

■ CONCLUSION

Nutrition support with attention to BG management forms an important aspect of pediatric neurocritical care. Early provision of enteral nutrition with adequate calories and protein is important in children with neurocritical illness. Protocols to ensure adequate nutrition support may improve outcomes in neurocritical care by minimizing energy deficits or excesses. Techniques such as indirect calorimetry, if available, are helpful to provide targeted nutrition support. BG management to avoid hyperglycemia and hypoglycemia is also very important to improve clinical outcomes. Studies are underway to determine if tight glucose control with intensive insulin therapy results in improved outcomes in critically ill children. The results from these studies will help inform practice in pediatric neurocritical care.

■ REFERENCES

1. Sokoloff L et al. The [14C] deoxyglucose method for the measurement of local cerebral glucose utilization: theory, procedure, and normal values in the conscious and anesthetized albino rat. *J Neurochem.* 1977;28:897–916.
2. Simpson IA, Carruthers A, Vannucci SJ. Supply and demand in cerebral energy metabolism: the role of nutrient transporters. *J Cereb Blood Flow Metab.* 2007;27:1766–1791.
3. Clarke DD, Sokoloff L. Circulation and energy metabolism. In: Siegel GJ et al, eds. *Basic Neurochemistry: Molecular, Cellular, and Clinical Aspects.* 6th ed. New York, NY: Raven Press; 1999;637–669.
4. Fox PT et al. Nonoxidative glucose consumption during focal physiologic neural activity. *Science.* 1988;241:462–464.
5. Vannucci RC, Vannucci SJ. Glucose metabolism in the developing brain. *Semin Perinatol.* 2000;24:107–115.
6. Kinnala A et al. Cerebral metabolic rate for glucose during the first six months of life: an FDG positron emission tomography study. *Arch Dis Child Fetal Neonatal Ed.* 1996;74:F153–F157.
7. Vannucci RC, Vannucci SJ. Hypoglycemic brain injury. *Semin Perinatol.* 2001;6:147–155.
8. Sperling MA. Hypoglycemia. In: Kliegman RM et al, eds. *Nelson Textbook of Pediatrics.* 19th ed. Philadelphia, PA: Elsevier Saunders; 2011:517–531.
9. Faustino EV, Hirshberg EL, Bogue CW. Hypoglycemia in critically ill children. *J Diabetes Sci Technol.* 2012;6:48–57.
10. Srinivasan V. Stress hyperglycemia in pediatric critical illness: the intensive care unit adds to the stress! *J Diabetes Sci Technol.* 2012;6:37–47.
11. Van den Berghe G. How does blood glucose control with insulin save lives in intensive care? *J Clin Invest.* 2004;114:1187–1195.
12. Tomlinson DR, Gardiner NJ. Glucose neurotoxicity. *Nat Rev Neurosci.* 2008;9:36–45.
13. Li PA et al. Hyperglycemia enhances extracellular glutamate accumulation in rats subjected to forebrain ischemia. *Stroke.* 2000;31:183–192.
14. Latifi R. Nutritional therapy in critically ill and injured patients. *Surg Clin N Am.* 2011;91:579–593.
15. Dhar A, Castillo L. Insulin resistance in critical illness. *Curr Opin Pediatr.* 2011;23:269–274.
16. Bittigau P, Ikonomidou C. Glutamate in neurologic diseases. *J Child Neurol.* 1997;12:471–485.
17. Farr SA et al. Obesity and hypertriglyceridemia produce cognitive impairment. *Endocrinology.* 2008;149:2628–2636.
18. Mehta NM. Nutrient metabolism and nutrition therapy during critical illness. In: Fuhrman BP, Zimmerman JJ, eds. *Pediatric Critical Care.* 4th ed. Philadelphia, PA: Elsevier Saunders; 2011:1073–1088.
19. Garcia-de-Lorenzo A et al. Parenteral administration of different amounts of branch-chain amino acids in septic patients: clinical and metabolic aspects. *Crit Care Med.* 1997;25:418–424.
20. Goode HF, Cowley HC, Walker BE. Decreased antioxidant status and increased lipid peroxidation in patients with septic shock and secondary organ dysfunction. *Crit Care Med.* 1995;23:646–651.
21. Phillips R et al. Nutritional support and measured energy expenditure of the child and adolescent with head injury. *J Neurosurg.* 1987;67:846–851.
22. Moore R, Najarian MP, Konvolinka CW. Measured energy expenditure in severe head trauma. *J Trauma.* 1989;29:1633–1636.
23. Goran MI, Kaskoun M, Johnson R. Determinants of resting energy expenditure in young children. *J Pediatr.* 1994;125:362–367.
24. Bratton SL et al. Guidelines for the management of severe traumatic brain injury. XII. Nutrition. *J Neurotrauma.* 2007;24(suppl 1):S77–S82.

25. Briassoulis G et al. Temporal nutritional and inflammatory changes in children with severe head injury fed a regular or an immune-enhancing diet: a randomized, controlled trial. *Pediatr Crit Care Med.* 2006;7:56–62.

26. Finestone HM et al. Measuring longitudinally the metabolic demands of stroke patients, resting energy expenditure is not elevated. *Stroke.* 2003;34:502–507.

27. Corrigan ML et al. Nutrition in the stroke patient. *Nutr Clin Pract.* 2011;26:242–252.

28. Mehta NM et al. Severe weight loss and hypermetabolic paroxysmal dysautonomia following hypoxic ischemic brain injury: the role of indirect calorimetry in the intensive care unit. *JPEN J Parenter Enteral Nutr.* 2008;32:281–284.

29. Wang CH et al. Consensus statement for standard of care in spinal muscular atrophy. *J Child Neurol.* 2007;22:1027–1049.

30. Bruce AK et al. Hypoglycaemia in spinal muscular atrophy. *Lancet.* 1995;346:609–610.

31. Crawford TO et al. Abnormal fatty acid metabolism in childhood spinal muscular atrophy. *Ann Neurol.* 1999;45:337–343.

32. Roubenoff RA, Borel CO, Hanley DF. Hypermetabolism and hypercatabolism in Guillain-Barré syndrome. *JPEN J Parenter Enteral Nutr.* 1992;16:464–472.

33. Fulgham JR, Wijdicks EFM. Guillain-Barré syndrome. In: Diringer M, ed. *Critical Care Clinics: Update on Neurologic Critical Care.* Philadelphia, PA: WB Saunders; 1997:1–15.

34. Thibault-Halman G et al. Acute management of nutritional demands after spinal cord injury. *J Neurotrauma.* 2011;28:1497–1507.

35. Srinivasan V et al. Association of timing, duration, and intensity of hyperglycemia with intensive care unit mortality in critically ill children. *Pediatr Crit Care Med.* 2004;5:329–336.

36. Faustino EV, Apkon M. Persistent hyperglycemia in critically ill children. *J Pediatr.* 2005;146:30–34.

37. Yung M et al. Paediatric Study Group; Australian and New Zealand Intensive Care Society. Glucose control, organ failure, and mortality in pediatric intensive care. *Pediatr Crit Care Med.* 2008;9:147–152.

38. Hirshberg E, Larsen G, Van Duker H. Alterations in glucose homeostasis in the pediatric intensive care unit: hyperglycemia and glucose variability are associated with increased mortality and morbidity. *Pediatr Crit Care Med.* 2008;9:361–366.

39. van den Berghe G et al. Intensive insulin therapy in the critically ill patients. *N Engl J Med.* 2001;345:1359–1367.

40. Van den Berghe G et al. Intensive insulin therapy in the medical ICU. *N Engl J Med.* 2006;354:449–461.

41. NICE-SUGAR Study Investigators, Finfer S, Chittock DR, et al. Intensive versus conventional glucose control in critically ill patients. *N Engl J Med.* 2009;360:1283–1297.

42. Faustino EV, Bogue CW. Relationship between hypoglycemia and mortality in critically ill children. *Pediatr Crit Care Med.* 2010;11:690–698.

43. Srinivasan V. Stress hyperglycemia in pediatric critical illness: the intensive care unit adds to the stress! *J Diabetes Sci Technol.* 2012;6:37–47.

44. Michaud LJ et al. Elevated initial blood glucose levels and poor outcome following severe brain injuries in children. *J Trauma.* 1991;31:1356–1362.

45. Cochran A et al. Hyperglycemia and outcomes from pediatric traumatic brain injury. *J Trauma.* 2003;55:1035–1038.

46. Chiaretti A et al. Prognostic factors and outcome of children with severe head injury: an 8-year experience. *Childs Nerv Syst.* 2002;18:129–136.

47. Smith RL et al. Relationship between hyperglycemia and outcome in children with severe traumatic brain injury. *Pediatr Crit Care Med.* 2012;13:85–91.

48. Green DM et al. Intensive versus conventional insulin therapy in critically ill neurologic patients. *Neurocrit Care.* 2010;13:299–306.

49. Graffagnino C et al. Intensive insulin therapy in the neurocritical care setting is associated with poor clinical outcomes. *Neurocrit Care.* 2010;13:307–312.

50. Vespa P et al. Intensive insulin therapy reduces microdialysis glucose values without altering glucose utilization or improving the lactate/pyruvate ratio after traumatic brain injury. *Crit Care Med.* 2006;34:850–856.

51. Capes SE et al. Stress hyperglycemia and prognosis of stroke in nondiabetic and diabetic patients: a systematic overview. *Stroke.* 2001;32:2426–2432.

52. Bellolio MF, Gilmore RM, Stead LG. Insulin for glycaemic control in acute ischaemic stroke. *Cochrane Database Syst Rev.* 2011;(9):CD005346.

53. Calle PA, Buylaert WA, Vanhaute OA. Glycemia in the post-resuscitation period. The Cerebral Resuscitation Study Group. *Resuscitation.* 1989;17(suppl):S181–S188.

54. Oksanen T et al. Strict versus moderate glucose control after resuscitation from ventricular fibrillation. *Intensive Care Med.* 2007;33:2093–2100.

55. Losert H et al. Strict normoglycaemic blood glucose levels in the therapeutic management of patients within 12h after cardiac arrest might not be necessary. *Resuscitation.* 2008;76:214–220.

6 Temperature Management and Hypothermic Neuroprotection

ALEXIS A. TOPJIAN

■ INTRODUCTION

Over the last hundred years no other therapy has been as widely lauded for the treatment of neurologic injury as induced hypothermia. Hypothermia has been evaluated, utilized, and reevaluated over the years with proven benefit in several populations. Therapeutic temperature control for neuroprotection describes using temperature as a treatment. While monitoring temperature as a vital sign is routine, it is a paradigm shift for the clinician to use temperature as a therapeutic intervention. Temperature management includes both controlled normothermia, which is keeping a patient's temperature in the normothermic range, and induced hypothermia, maintaining a patient's temperature in the hypothermic range (Table 6.1).

The impact of hyperthermia prevention and induced hypothermia to minimize neurologic injury has been evaluated in both animal models and clinical trials across multiple types of brain injury. Both spontaneous hyperthermia and spontaneous hypothermia are associated with worse outcomes following brain injury (1). Therapeutic temperature management has been evaluated in neonates, children, and adults and in multiple etiologies of neurologic injury including: hypoxia ischemia, traumatic brain injury (TBI), cardiac arrest, and stroke. However, to date, the only pediatric population that may benefit from induced hypothermia is neonates following asphyxia.

To safely utilize therapeutic temperature control, whether aiming to achieve controlled normothermia or induced hypothermia, the clinician must understand the pathophysiology of the specific brain injury and the risks and benefits of therapeutic temperature control. It is paramount to consider the etiology of the underlying brain injury, the goal temperature range and duration, and the means by which to achieve the goal temperature and minimize side effects.

■ HISTORY

Some of the first descriptions of the benefits of hypothermia go back to the Baron Larrey (2) who described that during the Napoleonic wars wounded soldiers who were put close to a campfire died earlier than those who were not rewarmed. In the 1950s hypothermia was used in conjunction with anesthesia for neuroprotection during cardiac surgery. Patients were placed in large tubs of ice to reduce the body temperature and metabolic rate. In the early 1960s hypothermia was frequently used following resuscitation from cardiac arrest. At low temperature levels (28°C–32°C), multiple complications were observed including arrhythmia, bleeding, and infection. For comatose pediatric drowning victims, HYPER therapy, which consisted of multiple therapeutic modalities including induced hypothermia to 30 +/– 1°C, was utilized to minimize brain edema (3). Systematic evaluation of this therapy in the late 1970s to early 1980s showed HYPER therapy to be deleterious with worse mortality in those who were cooled (4). Induced hypothermia for treatment of pediatric brain injury fell out of favor due to concerns that it might be harmful.

■ Table 6.1 Temperature Ranges	
Hyperthermia	
Severe	Core temperature ≥ 39°C
Moderate	Core temperature 38.1°C–38.9°C
Mild	Core temperature 37.5°C–38.0°C
Normothermia	Core temperature 36°C–37.4°C
Hypothermia	
Mild	Core temperature 34°C–35.9°C
Moderate	Core temperature 32°C–33.9°C
Deep	Core temperature < 31.9°C

Adapted from Polderman CCM 2009 (79).

By the mid 1980s mild induced hypothermia was "rediscovered." Peter Safar (5–7) and his trainees evaluated multiple animal models of induced hypothermia and repeatedly found functional and histologic benefits in the cooled group (32–34°C). These studies are the foundation for the recent clinical trials evaluating temperature control for the treatment of brain injury.

■ CELLULAR PATHOPHYSIOLOGY

To understand the impact of temperature management on the brain injured patient it is important to understand the cellular pathophysiology of primary brain injury and the impact of secondary brain injury. While TBI, stroke, and global hypoxic-ischemic injury are mechanistically different, the resultant injuries culminate in cellular necrosis and apoptosis. Therapeutic temperature management attempts to minimize these pathologic processes.

Global Hypoxic Ischemic

Global hypoxic-ischemic injury is defined by a period of primary injury when the brain has inadequate oxygen and blood flow. Secondary injury occurs following a period of reperfusion when blood flow and oxygen delivery are restored. Reperfusion injury may be as severe as or even worse than the initial ischemic injury. Clinically, during the initial ischemic injury, there is loss of consciousness and electroencephalography rapidly becomes flat. On the cellular level, intracellular calcium increases, interstitial potassium increases, intracellular adenosine triphosphate (ATP) decreases, cellular pH decreases, and there is an influx of water and calcium into cells (8–9). With reinstitution of blood flow there is initial cerebral hyperemia and then subsequent cerebral hypoperfusion.

Intracellular and extracellular electrolytes are rapidly restored. However, ATP is not as readily repleted. Cellular death is potentiated by caspases, which lead to ongoing apoptosis, and calpains, which lead to neuronal necrosis.

Traumatic Brain Injury

TBI consists of primary injury during which the brain parenchyma is directly damaged. While this injury can be prevented through safety measures, it cannot be reversed. Secondary brain injury occurs in the time period following primary injury and may be reversible and preventable. Secondary injury is caused by low cerebral blood flow, excitotoxic injury including glutamate release and calcium influx, oxidative stress, and inflammation causing cytotoxic edema resulting in cellular necrosis and apoptosis (10). Physiologic abnormalities in patients following brain injury such as high or low levels of partial pressure of arterial oxygen or carbon dioxide, hypotension, and temperature derangements may exacerbate and potentiate secondary injuries.

Impact of Temperature on the Injured Brain

Fever following brain injury has been shown to potentiate secondary brain injury. Fever increases metabolic rate, neuronal excitotoxicity, proinflammatory cytokines, glutamate levels, intracellular acidosis, free radical production, and apoptosis (11–15). These processes can increase damage in ischemic tissue leading to infarction (16). Animal models of induced hyperthermia following either focal ischemia or global asphyxial injury resulted in worse outcomes (16–18). In contrast, prevention of fever by maintaining normothermia can decrease the severity of these processes (19–22).

Induced hypothermia may decrease brain injury by ameliorating the cascade of events that are ongoing during secondary injury. Induced hypothermia decreases cerebral metabolism by 6% to 10% for each 1°C decrease in body temperature (23). Following ischemia and reperfusion injury, hypothermia decreases glutamate release and neuronal injury (24), minimizes free radical production and decreases inflammation and apoptosis (25).

Hyperthermia further exacerbates reperfusion injury from stroke and hypoxia ischemia and secondary injury following TBI. Maintaining normothermia to prevent fever can minimize the ongoing processes that result in apoptosis and necrosis. Inducing hypothermia, even prior to restoration of blood flow following cardiac arrest, may substantially decrease reperfusion injury. Delayed initiation of hypothermia, even up to 20 minutes after achievement of return of spontaneous circulation in an animal model of cardiac arrest, was associated with worse outcomes (6,26).

■ CLINICAL IMPACT OF TEMPERATURE

Hyperthermia's Ill Effects

Fever is common following brain injury and may occur spontaneously or when trying to warm the hypothermic patient. Up to 70% of neurologically injured patients have fever in the days following the primary injury, but only half of these patients have an infectious cause (27,28). Fever is common following TBI, intracerebral hemorrhage, focal stroke, and subarachnoid hemorrhage and may be due to thermoregulatory centers damage, inflammation, or blood within the intraventricular and cerebral spinal fluid containing spaces (29–30).

Following pediatric cardiac arrest, hyperthermia is common (1,31). The 2010 American Heart Association cardiopulmonary resuscitation (CPR) and emergency cardiovascular (ECC) guidelines recommend that "providers should closely monitor patient core temperature after return of spontaneous circulation and actively intervene to avoid hyperthermia" (32). In one study, following in-hospital cardiac arrest, almost half of children had one temperature $> 38°C$ in the first 24 hours following return of spontaneous circulation (1). Fever was associated with unfavorable outcome in these patients. Following resuscitation from adult cardiac arrest, patients with hyperthermia were more likely to progress to brain death, and in those who survived, neurologic outcome was worse (33–37). Following neonatal asphyxia injury, for every 1°C increase in temperature above normothermia, infants had a 3.6 to 4 times increase in disability and mortality (38).

Following TBI, fever worsens intracranial pressure, prolongs intensive care unit hospitalization, and is associated with worse outcomes (39–42). Following pediatric TBI, early hyperthermia is associated with worse discharge neurologic outcomes (43).

To date, the most extensively studied impact of fever and fever prevention on neurologic outcome has been in the ischemic stroke population. Following focal ischemic stroke in adults, fever within the first 24 hours of injury is associated with worse neurologic outcome and larger cerebral infarcts (44). Two meta-analyses of ischemic stroke patients found that fever significantly increased morbidity and mortality (42,45). Similar findings have been reported in patients with subarachnoid hemorrhage and other forms of intracranial hemorrhage (42,46).

The high incidence of fever following neurologic injury and its association with morbidity and mortality have lead to the conclusion that fever should be treated and preferably prevented. Despite these conclusions, patients often become febrile following injury as clinicians are often more reactive than proactive. Steps to prevent fever and maintain normothermia should be taken. Because hyperthermia is detrimental to potential cerebral recovery, hypothermia to mitigate ongoing injury has been clinically evaluated in certain populations.

Induced Hypothermia's Potential Benefits

Induced hypothermia to improve neurologic outcome and prevent secondary injury has been evaluated following cardiac arrest, perinatal asphyxia, TBI, and ischemic stroke. Adult and pediatric populations have been evaluated separately because the etiology of events and age-dependent physiology differ. We will review the clinical investigations performed for these disease processes and how they have impacted current clinical care.

Adult Cardiac Arrest

In 2010 the American Heart Association, following the International Liaison Committee on Resuscitation's evidence evaluation process, recommended cooling all unconscious adults following successful resuscitation from an out-of-hospital ventricular fibrillatory (VF) cardiac arrest (47). These guidelines were formed based on two landmark papers published in 2002 evaluating the use of induced hypothermia following witnessed adult out-of-hospital VF arrest. Bernard et al (48) randomized 77 patients to either normothermia or hypothermia (33°C for 12 hours). Forty-nine percent (21/43) of patients in the hypothermia group had a good outcome (discharge to home or a rehab facility) as compared to 26% (9/34) patients in the control group (odds ratio [OR], 5.25; 95% confidence interval [CI], 1.47–18.76; $P = .046$). The hypothermia after cardiac arrest (HACA) study randomized 273 patients to hypothermia (32°C–34°C) for 24 hours or normothermia (49). Good neurologic outcome was defined as a 6 month Cerebral Performance Category of 1 or 2 (normal or mild dysfunction). Fifty-three percent (75/136) of subjects in the hypothermic arm had a good outcome as compared to 36% (54/137) of subjects in the control group (OR, 1.4; 95% CI, 1.08–1.81; P = .009). Of note, approximately 25% of subjects in the normothermic arm had bladder temperatures above 38°C. Some experts have questioned whether this was a testament to the benefits of hypothermia or harms of hyperthermia. Despite these studies' shortcomings, induced hypothermia following adult VF arrest is now considered standard of care (47).

Induced hypothermia for treatment of adult cardiac arrest due to nonshockable rhythms has not been as rigorously evaluated and results from retrospective evaluations are equivocal. One large retrospective evaluation of out-of-hospital cardiac arrest patients treated with induced hypothermia showed improvement in neurologic outcomes in those with an initial shockable rhythm, but no benefit in those with initial asystole/pulseless electrical activity (PEA) (50) Another retrospective study of induced hypothermia to treat adults following asystole/PEA concluded that hypothermia improved neurologic outcome and mortality (51). One small prospective randomized controlled trial evaluating induced hypothermia following adult asystole/PEA showed an outcome benefit, however, it was underpowered and not designed to evaluate an outcome difference (52). A Cochrane Review of induced hypothermia following adult cardiac arrest concluded the hypothermia was beneficial for adult VF/VT arrest. Due to small numbers, no recommendations could be made regarding in-hospital arrest, nonshockable rhythms, and cardiac arrest of noncardiac origin (53).

Pediatric Cardiac Arrest

To date, there are no published randomized controlled trials evaluating the efficacy of induced hypothermia following pediatric cardiac arrest. Current published evaluations are limited and show no benefit of induced hypothermia following pediatric cardiac arrest. The American Heart Associations' 2010 recommendation is: "Therapeutic hypothermia (32°C–34°C) may be considered for children who remain comatose after resuscitation from cardiac arrest. It is reasonable for adolescents resuscitated from sudden, witnessed, out-of-hospital VF cardiac arrest" (54). This statement is in part extrapolated from the adult data presented above.

Two recent retrospective studies compared induced hypothermia and normothermia in children successfully resuscitated from pediatric cardiac arrest (55,56). Both studies showed that there was no benefit to treating

patients with induced hypothermia once controlling for potential confounders. Doherty et al (56) performed a multicenter retrospective cohort study across five centers, of which only three utilized hypothermia. Eighty-eight percent of the study population was children with underlying heart disease and 94% of the arrests were in-hospital. There was variability in the temperature patients were cooled to (33.7 +/– 1.3°C) and the duration they were maintained at that temperature (20.8 +/– 11.9 hours). Despite baseline differences between the hypothermia and normothermia groups, there were no was difference in outcome after controlling for multiple variables. Fink et al (57) evaluated a single center's retrospective experience with induced hypothermia for primarily asphyxia-associated cardiac arrests. Only 8% of patients had underlying heart disease and only 9% suffered in-hospital arrests. There was no standard protocol for induction, maintenance, or rewarming. While they observed no significant difference in outcome between the normothermic and hypothermic groups, it was evident that patients treated with hypothermia had suffered more severe injury, as reflected in their longer durations of cardiac arrest and more epinephrine doses required to obtain return of spontaneous circulation. Both of these studies provide important initial assessments of induced hypothermia following pediatric cardiac arrest, but are limited by their retrospective approach and lack of explicit protocols.

A third study systematically evaluated the feasibility of a standard algorithm for induction and maintenance of induced hypothermia following pediatric cardiac arrest using a surface cooling protocol (58). Following resuscitation from cardiac arrest children were cooled to 32°C to 34°C using a standardized surface protocol and achievement of goal temperatures, and side effects were observed. Rectal temperature of ≤ 34°C was achieved in 1.5 hours from cooling initiation. Approximately 80% of the time patients were maintained between 32°C and 34°C. Overshoot hypothermia (< 32°C) was observed in 15% of measurements, a finding that was common in an adult study as well (58,59). Other expected and observed side effects of hypothermia were hypokalemia (67%) and bradycardia (< second percentile for age in 58%). However, there were no episodes of bleeding or ventricular tachyarrhythmia that required treatment. Six of 12 (50%) patients survived to discharge (58). This study was small and was not designed to evaluate the efficacy of induced hypothermia to improve neurologic outcome after cardiac arrest.

Despite protocols to induce and maintain hypothermia in children following cardiac arrest, to date, it has not been shown to be an efficacious therapy to prevent neurologic morbidity and mortality. A multicenter randomized clinical trial (Therapeutic Hypothermia After Pediatric Cardiac Arrest, www.thapca.org) is underway comparing induced hypothermia (32°C–34°C) to controlled normothermia (36°C–37.5°C).

Perinatal Asphyxia

Induced hypothermia has been most rigorously studied in the neonatal population following birth asphyxia. Shankaran et al randomized moderately or severely encephalopathic neonates to induced hypothermia (33.5°C esophageal) versus usual care for 72 hours. Forty-four percent (45/102) of subjects treated with hypothermia had a poor outcome (death or disability at 18–22 months) compared to 62% (64/106) of patients in the control group (relative risk (RR), 0.72; 95% CI, 0.54–0.95, P = .01). When death was evaluated as an isolated outcome there was no difference between the hypothermic and control groups (P = .08).

A second study evaluated the selective head cooling of neonates with moderate and severe encephalopathy. Severity of brain injury was stratified based on amplitude electroencephalogram (EEG) recordings within 5.5 hours of birth. Neonates were randomized to receive head cooling to a target rectal temperature of 34°C to 35°C for 72 hours or usual care. Fifty-five percent (59/108) of neonates treated with hypothermia had a poor outcome (death or disability at 18 months) compared to 66% (73/110) treated with usual care (P = .1) (61). Interestingly, a subanalysis evaluating only patient's with moderately abnormal amplitude integrated EEG background patterns showed a decrease in poor outcome for those treated with hypothermia vs usual care (48% vs 66% [OR, 0.47; 95% CI, 0.22–0.8; P =.009]).

Most recently, a third trial of induced hypothermia following neonatal asphyxia randomized 325 infants to hypothermia or usual care. There was no difference in the primary outcome of severe disability or death (62). Despite these mixed findings, induced hypothermia for the treatment of perinatal hypoxic-ischemic encephalopathy is standard of care.

Traumatic Brain Injury

TBI is the leading cause of mortality and severe morbidity in children. According to the Centers for Disease Control and Prevention, approximately 475,000 children under the age of 14 sustain TBI annually (63). Induced hypothermia has been systematically evaluated in the adult TBI population and while initially found to be beneficial in a small single institution study, a large systematic review of induced hypothermia showed no benefit (64,65). For pediatric TBI, three early phase clinical trials showed the implementation of induced hypothermia to be feasible (66) and safe (67,68), but were not powered for efficacy. Subsequently, a randomized controlled trial of induced hypothermia (32°C–33°C) for 24 hours following severe pediatric TBI found hypothermia to be no more effective than normothermia. Subjects were randomly assigned to hypothermia or normothermia within 8 hours of brain injury, cooled for 24 hours and rewarmed by 0.5°C every 2 hours back to normothermia. There was a trend for higher mortality in the cooled group and there was no difference in neurologic outcomes between the normothermia and hypothermia groups. Subjects in the hypothermia group had more hypotension in the rewarming period which may be independently associated with worse outcome following TBI (69). Criticisms of this study were that cooling was initiated too late after initial injury and not maintained through the period of peak swelling (approximately 48 hours), and hypotension was not adequately controlled during the rewarming period.

Adult Stroke

Induced hypothermia for the treatment of adult stroke has been evaluated in multiple small pilot studies and several small randomized controlled trials that were not powered to determine the impact on neurologic mortality and morbidity (70). These trials evaluated the safety and feasibility of inducing and maintaining hypothermia in stroke patients utilizing either an endovascular cooling catheter or external cooling devices (71–74). The cooling for acute ischemic brain damage (COOL AID) trials evaluated the feasibility of induced hypothermia for the treatment of adult ischemic stroke, and while they were able to cool patients safely, there was no significant difference in outcomes between groups (75). Prospective evaluation of hypothermia to minimize neurologic morbidity and mortality after adult ischemic stroke is underway. To date there is no pediatric data evaluating the efficacy of this therapy.

■ CLINICAL IMPLEMENTATION OF TEMPERATURE CONTROL

Implementation of temperature control, whether it be controlled normothermia (goal 36°C–37.8°C) or induced hypothermia (32°C–34°C) requires appropriate equipment, monitoring, trained personnel, and expertise to minimize the side effects of controlled normothermia and induced hypothermia. Both pharmacologic and nonpharmacologic methods of temperature control have been evaluated. Pharmacologic interventions may be effective at preventing fever but have not been effective for inducing hypothermia (30). In children, nonpharmacologic temperature control is most commonly performed with an external cooling blanket (55). Other potential, but less commonly used techniques are bladder irrigation, cold intravenous fluid administration, and gastric lavage. Below we will describe the equipment needed, the available protocols, and the common side effects that must be considered to safely maintain normothermia, induce and maintain hypothermia, and rewarm patients back to normothermia.

Pharmacologic Intervention

Both fever treatment and fever prevention are performed utilizing antipyretic agents such as acetaminophen and nonsteroidal antiinflammatory medications such as ibuprofen. While these drugs have standardly been used for fever prevention and treatment they are not always effective at achieving normothermia following brain injury. Acetaminophen for adults following ischemic stroke may be effective for fever prevention (76). A randomized controlled trial of high dose acetaminophen vs low dose acetaminophen vs placebo following adult ischemic stroke resulted in a 0.4°C decrease in rectal temperature in the high dose group but no difference in the low dose and placebo groups (77). When ibuprofen was compared to these groups, there was no difference in temperature reduction between ibuprofen and placebo (78). Therefore, when temperature control is desired, external devices should be utilized independently or in conjunction with antipyretics.

Nonpharmacologic Intervention

Equipment and Monitoring

To control a patient's temperature it is necessary to have (1) two core temperature probes and (2) a cooling device (such as an external cooling blanket and machine) (Table 6.2). Core temperature probes are most commonly placed in the rectum, esophagus, or bladder. The esophageal probe is placed directly behind the left atrium in the distal esophagus and measures changes in temperature more rapidly than bladder and rectal probes. One temperature probe, preferably the esophageal probe, should be connected to the cooling machine (primary probe). A second temperature probe should continuously monitor temperature. The two temperature probes should have temperature measurements that are within 1°C of each other. It is important to have two temperature probes to ensure that the measured temperatures are reliable.

Core temperature can be measured in variable locations: rectum, bladder, pulmonary artery, esophagus, tympanic membrane of nasopharynx. When using therapeutic temperature control, these monitoring sites are surrogates for brain temperature as it is rare to have a direct brain temperature probe in place. While these temperatures are highly accurate, the difference between brain temperature and these core temperatures can range from 0°C to 2°C. Pulmonary artery temperature is the most accurate and reflects immediate temperature changes. Esophageal, bladder, nasopharyngeal, and rectal temperatures are highly accurate; however, during induction of hypothermia and rewarming, bladder and rectal temperatures may lag behind the true core temperature (79).

External cooling devices can be used to maintain controlled normothermia or to induce and maintain hypothermia and then rewarm patients. Cooling blankets are placed against the patient's skin and cool the body by direct transference of heat. This can be done via conduction (circulating cold water) or convection (circulating cold air) blankets. Many devices are able to servo-control temperature, controlling the patient's temperature via an

■ Table 6.2 Temperature Monitoring Sites

Core	
Tympanic	Moderately accurate
Rectum	Highly accurate
Bladder	Highly accurate
Esophagus	Highly accurate
Nasopharynx	Highly accurate
Pulmonary artery	Highly accurate
Peripheral	
Skin/axillary	Inaccurate

internal device algorithm with a patient temperature input into the machine and the machine controlling the blanket temperature in response. The clinician sets a goal temperature in an automatic mode, the patient's temperature probe is connected to the machine, and the machine adjusts the blanket's temperature to maintain the patient's temperature at the set goal. Many devices can administer temperatures ranging from 4°C to 42°C.

■ SIDE EFFECTS OF INDUCED HYPOTHERMIA AND THERAPEUTIC TEMPERATURE CONTROL

Utilizing a cooling device to induce normothermic or hypothermic temperatures is associated with side effects. To safely implement temperature control it is important to understand the effects of actively controlling temperature as well as the effects of inducing and maintaining hypothermia and rewarming the body. When therapeutic temperature control is utilized it is often in a brain injured patient with the goal of minimizing the risk of secondary injury. Therefore, closely monitoring patients can help prevent side effects from becoming complications.

The clinician should closely monitor the patient and understand how the patient's exam and physiology will be impacted by actively titrating temperature. All patients should have continuous electrocardiogram (EKG), pulse oximetry, and respiratory monitoring. Patients treated with induced hypothermia should have central venous pressure monitoring and continuous arterial blood pressure monitoring. Peripheral vasoconstriction occurs with hypothermia and placement of these catheters is more easily achieved prior to inducing hypothermia.

Side Effects of Therapeutic Temperature Control

The act of controlling temperature can be uncomfortable for the patient as the blanket temperature decreases to cool the patient. This happens when maintaining normothermia for fever prevention or inducing hypothermia. It is also common for patients to become more agitated and tachycardic as they have colder temperatures against their skin. The cooling blanket itself can cause skin injury and therefore the skin must be assessed regularly to evaluate for local trauma. Sedation with narcotics and benzodiazepines can treat this discomfort and continuous sedating infusion should be considered during the duration of temperature control.

Side Effects of Hypothermia

Cardiovascular Effects

During the induction of hypothermia, normal physiology is disrupted. As the body temperature is initially decreased toward 35.5°C, patients initially become mildly tachycardic and then subsequently bradycardic (79). The bradycardia does not usually require treatment, but resolves with rewarming or chronotropic support. Atropine is usually ineffective. Other EKG changes associated with hypothermia are prolonged PR interval, mildly widened QRS, and prolonged QT interval. At 32°C patients have a decrease in cardiac output, mostly due to the decrease in heart rate. Systemic vascular resistance increases and there may be an associated increase in blood pressure. As long as the temperature is maintained above 32°C there is no increased risk of life-threatening arrhythmias. Below 30°C the risk of ventricular arrhythmias is substantially higher. If there are concerns for inadequate cardiac output based on clinical exam, a central venous oxygen saturation and lactate level can be evaluated to confirm that patients have adequate oxygen supply to meet their metabolic demand.

As systemic vascular resistance is increase, there is an increase in central venous pressure and blood return to the right side of the heart. This leads to an increase in atrial natriuretic peptide and a "cold diuresis." The cold diuresis occurs during induction of hypothermia and usually resolves once hypothermia is achieved and stabilized. If hypotension occurs during this period, a lower central venous pressure may be noted and intravenous fluid should be administered in conjunction with vasopressors.

Electrolyte Abnormalities

During induction of hypothermia multiple electrolyte shifts occur. Patients become transiently insulin resistant and have associated hyperglycemia. Although the ideal blood glucose range for prevention of mortality and morbidity has yet to be determined, treatment of hyperglycemia with insulin can prevent osmotic diuresis. Hypokalemia, hypophosphatemia, hypomagnesemia, and hypocalcemia also occur during induction. These changes are due to renal wasting as well as intracellular shifts which can be further potentiated by brisk diuresis and insulin administration. They should be aggressively managed to decrease the risk of arrhythmia. Frequent laboratory examination to monitor these levels is important.

Shivering

Shivering is commonly seen when the patient's body temperature decreases below their internal set-point and is the body's attempt to normalize temperature. Shivering increases the patient's metabolic rate and therefore should be prevented to both decrease the risk of brain injury as well as to facilitate cooling. Treatment of shivering can be achieved by administering sedation and/or paralysis, magnesium, or dexmedetomidine (Table 6.3). Multiple classes of agents have been evaluated to treat hypothermia induced shivering with mixed efficacy and side effect profiles (79). Benzodiazepines and narcotics are the most commonly used in children in conjunction with paralysis. Once the body temperature is below 34°C shivering improves, although it does not always completely resolve. In the already brain injured patient, seizures can be confused for shivering and therefore when in doubt EEG monitoring may help differentiate shivering and other nonepileptic events from seizures.

Drug Metabolism

Drug metabolism is impacted by hypothermia. Various agents may have slowed metabolism due to decrease in hepatic enzymatic processes and drug metabolism. Opiates and benzodiazepines are likely decreased which can lead to increased circulating levels of these medications. Fentanyl, morphine, barbiturates, and midazolam levels may be higher in the patient treated

■ **Table 6.3** Medications to Treat Shivering

Focal warming of the skin, hands and face	
Propofol	General anesthetic
Meperidine	Opioid
Fentanyl	Opioid
Midazolam	Benzodiazepines
Magnesium	
Clonidine	Alpha 2 agonist
Dexmedetomidine	Alpha 2 agonist
Paralytic	Neuromuscular blocking agent
Buspirone	Serotonin

with induced hypothermia (79). Lower doses of these medications may be needed to achieve the same effect as in the normothermic patient, and therefore it is important to assess sedation scores and titrate medication appropriately. Following treatment with hypothermia and sedatives, neurologic examination be impacted by delayed medication clearance. Clinicians should be careful not to underestimate the impact of sedating medications administered to the patient during hypothermia, event after they have returned to normothermic temperatures.

Hematologic Effects

Hypothermia impacts clinical laboratory parameters of the clotting cascade and has an associated increased risk of bleeding. Hypothermia causes decreased platelet counts and platelet function and a mild increase in bleeding time. Despite these effects, there has been no significant increase in bleeding in patients treated with hypothermia (49). In fact, in several studies patients have received heparin or thrombolysis and have had no more bleeding complications than their normothermic counterparts (49). The immunosuppression associated with cooling may be in part due to the antiinflammatory effects of hypothermia. A decrease in white blood cell count can be seen. At low temperatures for prolonged durations, the risk of infection can increase. Because patients being treated with controlled normothermia or induced hypothermia are actively having their temperature controlled they may not be able to mount a fever and clinicians should consider screening cultures to evaluate for the presence of infection.

Laboratory Changes

During hypothermia, laboratory measurements may be mildly abnormal, but usually do not reflect ongoing pathology. Blood lactate levels, serum amylase, and liver enzymes may be increased. Patients may have a mild acidosis and ketosis. Severe derangements in these parameters are usually not due to hypothermia but are due to underlying pathology.

Blood Gas Measurement

Blood gas measurements during hypothermia are affected by temperature's impact on gas solubility in blood. Cold blood dissolves less gas and therefore Pao_2 and $Paco_2$ levels are lower in patients who are hypothermic.

Blood gases are routinely analyzed at 37°C. When the blood gas is analyzed at 37°C not accounting for the patients' body temperature it is called *alpha-stat* measurement. When the blood gas is analyzed accounting for the patient's temperature it is called *pH-stat*. Blood gas analysis temperature is important because $Paco_2$ affects cerebral vasoconstriction and pH. If $Paco_2$ is underestimated and therefore higher than the clinician expects there may be excessive cerebral vasodilation. If $Paco_2$ is overestimated (thought to be higher than it is) cerebral vasoconstriction in the already ischemic brain may occur. It is unclear whether the method of blood gas analysis impacts care and outcomes in the cardiac arrest patient being treated with therapeutic hypothermia. Regardless, clinicians should utilize one method of blood gas analysis to minimize the variability of results attributable to analysis technique.

Side Effects of Rewarming

Rewarming is a period when patients with neurologic injury are at an increased risk for complications due to hypotension, seizures, and electrolyte abnormalities.

Hemodynamic Effects

During body rewarming, systemic vascular resistance decreases and patients may appear relatively volume deplete. They may become tachycardic, hypotensive, and have decreased urine output. Hypotension is common and may require treatment with intravenous fluids and vasopressor support. Vasopressor support alone may not be adequate to treat hypotension as adequate circulating blood volume needs to be restored. Inadequate treatment of hypotension may negate the potential benefits of induced hypothermia (69). Slower rates of rewarming may minimize the incidence of hypotension.

Seizures

Seizures, which are common following brain injury, may have increased occurrence during rewarming. As the metabolic activity of the brain increases new seizures may occur. It is important to be aware that repetitive or paroxysmal movements may be seizure activity and are common following cardiac arrest (80). Some seizures are not clinically identifiable and can only be diagnosed on electroencephalography. Therefore, if clinicians have the ability to monitor

for seizures, especially during rewarming, they should consider doing so.

Electrolyte Abnormalities

During rewarming intracellular shifts of potassium occur from within the cell to the intravascular space and patients are at increased risk for hyperkalemia. Clinicians should be aware of the amount of exogenous supplemental potassium patients are receiving and should frequently monitor electrolytes.

Skin Injury

Patients should be directly placed on the cooling blankets to control temperature. Blanket temperature can fluctuate between 4°C and 42°C and therefore skin should be frequently assessed for signs of redness, burns, and cold injury.

Protocols

The only pediatric population that has benefited from induced hypothermia are neonates following perinatal asphyxia. The neonatal cooling protocols attempt to implement therapeutic hypothermia to approximately 33.5°C within 6 hours of birth and cool for 72 hours often with passive rewarming (81,82). Following adult cardiac arrest, patients are often cooled for up to 12 to 24 hours before rewarming. Depth of temperature and location of monitoring has varied across investigations and rewarming has ranged from increasing 1°C every 2 to 6 hours. To safely treat patients with controlled normothermia or induced hypothermia it is important that physicians and nurses collaborate and that explicit temperature monitoring parameters and blanket titration orders are communicated. Electrolytes should be monitored at least every 6 hours during large temperature changes, including induction from hyperthermia to normothermia, to identify and manage electrolyte abnormalities. Invasive blood pressure monitoring and central venous pressure monitoring also aid in managing patients with altered perfusion and physiology. Screening laboratories for infection and clotting dysfunction should be considered.

While several protocols have been described in the literature, induced hypothermia has not been proven beneficial in children following cardiac arrest and may in fact be harmful in children following TBI (69). Therefore, it is important to weigh the risks and benefits before applying this therapy. Clinicians should make sure they have skilled resources to assist in implementation of this therapy if they choose to do so.

■ SUMMARY

Temperature control as a therapeutic intervention has been evaluated and reevaluated for brain injury over the better part of a century. Hyperthermia is detrimental to the damaged brain and worsens brain injury. Controlled normothermia to prevent fever is underutilized but may be efficacious to minimize secondary brain injury. To date, adult out-of-hospital VF arrest and perinatal asphyxia are the only neurologic injuries that have been shown to benefit from induced hypothermia. Evaluation of hypothermia for prevention of secondary brain injury following stroke, TBI, and pediatric cardiac arrest are ongoing. To safely study and treat subjects with therapeutic temperature control it is important to understand the impact of temperature on physiology. In the future, temperature control may be individualized for patients to minimize secondary brain injury and improve survival and neurologic recovery.

■ REFERENCES

1. Bembea MM et al. Temperature patterns in the early postresuscitation period after pediatric inhospital cardiac arrest. *Pediatr Crit Care Med.* 2010;11:723–730.
2. Larrey D. *Memoirs of Military Surgery and Campaigns of the French Armies.* Baltimore, MD: Joseph Cushing/University Press of Sergeant Hall. 1987.
3. Conn AW, Edmonds JF, Barker GA. Cerebral resuscitation in near-drowning. *Pediatr Clin North Am.* 1979;26:691–701.
4. Bohn DJ et al. Influence of hypothermia, barbiturate therapy, and intracranial pressure monitoring on morbidity and mortality after near-drowning. *Crit Care Med.* 1986;14:529–534.
5. Sterz F et al. Mild hypothermic cardiopulmonary resuscitation improves outcome after prolonged cardiac arrest in dogs. *Crit Care Med.* 1991;19:379–389.
6. Kuboyama K et al. Delay in cooling negates the beneficial effect of mild resuscitative cerebral hypothermia after cardiac arrest in dogs: a prospective, randomized study. *Crit Care Med.* 1993;21:1348–1358.
7. Weinrauch V et al. Beneficial effect of mild hypothermia and detrimental effect of deep hypothermia after cardiac arrest in dogs. *Stroke.* 1992;23:1454–1462.
8. Small DL, Morley P, Buchan AM. Biology of ischemic cerebral cell death. *Prog Cardiovasc Dis.* 1999;42:185–207.
9. Uematsu D et al. In vivo fluorometric measurement of changes in cytosolic free calcium from the cat cortex during anoxia. *J Cereb Blood Flow Metab.* 1988;8:367–374.
10. Bayir H, Kochanek PM, Clark RS. Traumatic brain injury in infants and children: mechanisms of secondary damage and treatment in the intensive care unit. *Crit Care Clin.* 2003;19:529–549.
11. Busija DW, Leffler CW, Pourcyrous M. Hyperthermia increases cerebral metabolic rate and blood flow in neonatal pigs. *Am J Physiol.* 1988;255:H343–H346.
12. Takagi K et al. Effect of hyperthermia on glutamate release in ischemic penumbra after middle cerebral artery occlusion in rats. *Am J Physiol.* 1994;267:H1770–H1776.
13. Huang T et al. Traumatic injury activates MAP kinases in astrocytes: mechanisms of hypothermia and hyperthermia. *J Neurotrauma.* 2009;26:1535–1545.
14. Mitani A, Kataoka K. Critical levels of extracellular glutamate mediating gerbil hippocampal delayed neuronal death during hypothermia: brain microdialysis study. *Neuroscience.* 1991;42:661–670.
15. Kil HY, Zhang J, Piantadosi CA. Brain temperature alters hydroxyl radical production during cerebral ischemia/reperfusion in rats. *J Cereb Blood Flow Metab.* 1996;16:100–106.
16. Hickey RW et al. Induced hyperthermia exacerbates neurologic neuronal histologic damage after asphyxial cardiac arrest in rats. *Crit Care Med.* 2003;31:531–535.
17. Baena RC et al. Hyperthermia delayed by 24 hours aggravates neuronal damage in rat hippocampus following global ischemia. *Neurology.* 1997;48:768–773.
18. Kim Y et al. Delayed postischemic hyperthermia in awake rats worsens the histopathological outcome of transient focal cerebral ischemia. *Stroke.* 1996;27:2274–2280; discussion 2281.
19. Coimbra C et al. Diminished neuronal damage in the rat brain by late treatment with the antipyretic drug dipyrone or cooling following cerebral ischemia. *Acta Neuropathol.* 1996;92:447–453.
20. Shibata M. Hyperthermia in brain hemorrhage. *Med Hypotheses.* 1998;50:185–190.
21. Busto R et al. Small differences in intraischemic brain temperature critically determine the extent of ischemic neuronal injury. *J Cereb Blood Flow Metab.* 1987;7:729–738.
22. Dietrich WD et al. Delayed posttraumatic brain hyperthermia worsens outcome after fluid percussion brain injury: a light and electron microscopic study in rats. *Neurosurgery.* 1996;38:533–541; discussion 541.
23. Otis AB, Jude J. Effect of body temperature on pulmonary gas exchange. *Am J Physiol.* 1957;188:355–359.
24. Takata K et al. Effects of hypothermia for a short period on histologic outcome and extracellular glutamate concentration during and after cardiac arrest in rats. *Crit Care Med.* 2005;33:1340–1345.
25. Novack TA, Dillon MC, Jackson WT. Neurochemical mechanisms in brain injury and treatment: a review. *J Clin Exp Neuropsychol.* 1996;18:685–706.
26. Abella BS et al. Intra-arrest cooling improves outcomes in a murine cardiac arrest model. *Circulation.* 2004;109:2786–2791.
27. Diringer MN et al. Elevated body temperature independently contributes to increased length of stay in neurologic intensive care unit patients. *Crit Care Med.* 2004;32:1489–1495.
28. Kilpatrick MM et al. Hyperthermia in the neurosurgical intensive care unit. *Neurosurgery.* 2000;47:850–855; discussion 855–856.

29. Axelrod YK, Diringer MN. Temperature management in acute neurologic disorders. *Neurol Clin.* 2008;26:585–603, xi.
30. Badjatia N. Hyperthermia and fever control in brain injury. *Crit Care Med.* 2009;37:S250–S257.
31. Hickey RW et al. Hypothermia and hyperthermia in children after resuscitation from cardiac arrest. *Pediatrics.* 2000;106:118–122.
32. Peberdy MA et al. Part 9: post-cardiac arrest care: 2010 American Heart Association Guidelines for Cardiopulmonary Resuscitation and Emergency Cardiovascular Care. *Circulation.* 2010;122:S768–S786.
33. Takasu A et al. Hyperthermia: is it an ominous sign after cardiac arrest? *Resuscitation.* 2001;49:273–277.
34. Zeiner A et al. Hyperthermia after cardiac arrest is associated with an unfavorable neurologic outcome. *Arch Intern Med.* 2001;161:2007–2012.
35. Takino M, Okada Y. Hyperthermia following cardiopulmonary resuscitation. *Intensive Care Med.* 1991;17:419–420.
36. Langhelle A et al. In-hospital factors associated with improved outcome after out-of-hospital cardiac arrest. A comparison between four regions in Norway. *Resuscitation.* 2003;56:247–263.
37. Suffoletto B et al. Body temperature changes are associated with outcomes following in-hospital cardiac arrest and return of spontaneous circulation. *Resuscitation.* 2009;80:1365–1370.
38. Laptook A et al. Elevated temperature after hypoxic-ischemic encephalopathy: risk factor for adverse outcomes. *Pediatrics.* 2008;122:491–499.
39. Stocchetti N et al. Pyrexia in head-injured patients admitted to intensive care. *Intensive Care Med.* 2002;28:1555–1562.
40. Jones PA et al. Measuring the burden of secondary insults in head-injured patients during intensive care. *J Neurosurg Anesthesiol.* 1994;6:4–14.
41. Jiang JY et al. Early indicators of prognosis in 846 cases of severe traumatic brain injury. *J Neurotrauma.* 2002;19:869–874.
42. Greer DM et al. Impact of fever on outcome in patients with stroke and neurologic injury: a comprehensive meta-analysis. *Stroke.* 2008;39:3029–3035.
43. Natale JE et al. Early hyperthermia after traumatic brain injury in children: risk factors, influence on length of stay, and effect on short-term neurologic status. *Crit Care Med.* 2000;28:2608–2615.
44. Castillo J et al. Timing for fever-related brain damage in acute ischemic stroke. *Stroke.* 1998;29:2455–2460.
45. Hajat C, Hajat S, Sharma P. Effects of poststroke pyrexia on stroke outcome: a meta-analysis of studies in patients. *Stroke.* 2000;31:410–414.
46. Oliveira-Filho J et al. Fever in subarachnoid hemorrhage: relationship to vasospasm and outcome. *Neurology.* 2001;56:1299–1304.
47. Neumar RW et al. Part 8: adult advanced cardiovascular life support: 2010 American Heart Association Guidelines for Cardiopulmonary Resuscitation and Emergency Cardiovascular Care. *Circulation.* 2010;122:S729–S767.
48. Bernard SA et al. Treatment of comatose survivors of out-of-hospital cardiac arrest with induced hypothermia. *N Engl J Med.* 2002;346:557–563.
49. HACA. Mild therapeutic hypothermia to improve the neurologic outcome after cardiac arrest. *N Engl J Med.* 2002;346:549–556.
50. Dumas F et al. Is hypothermia after cardiac arrest effective in both shockable and nonshockable patients? Insights from a large registry. *Circulation.* 2011;123:877–886.
51. Testori C et al. Mild therapeutic hypothermia is associated with favourable outcome in patients after cardiac arrest with non-shockable rhythms. *Resuscitation.* 2011;82:1162–1167.
52. Hachimi-Idrissi S et al. Mild hypothermia induced by a helmet device: a clinical feasibility study. *Resuscitation.* 2001;51:275–281.
53. Arrich J et al. Cochrane corner: hypothermia for neuroprotection in adults after cardiopulmonary resuscitation. *Anesth Analg.* 2010;110:1239.
54. Kleinman ME et al. Part 14: pediatric advanced life support: 2010 American Heart Association Guidelines for Cardiopulmonary Resuscitation and Emergency Cardiovascular Care. *Circulation.* 2010;122:S876–S908.
55. Fink EL et al. A tertiary care center's experience with therapeutic hypothermia after pediatric cardiac arrest. *Pediatr Crit Care Med.* 2009;11:66–74.
56. Doherty DR et al. Hypothermia therapy after pediatric cardiac arrest. *Circulation.* 2009;119:1492–1500.
57. Fink EL et al. A tertiary care center's experience with therapeutic hypothermia after pediatric cardiac arrest. *Pediatr Crit Care Med.* 2009;11(1):66–74.
58. Topjian A et al. Induction and maintenance of therapeutic hypothermia after pediatric cardiac arrest: efficacy of a surface cooling protocol. *Pediatr Crit Care Med.* 2010;12(3):e127–35.
59. Merchant RM et al. Therapeutic hypothermia after cardiac arrest: unintentional overcooling is common using ice packs and conventional cooling blankets. *Crit Care Med.* 2006;34:S490–S494.
60. Shankaran S et al. Whole-body hypothermia for neonates with hypoxic-ischemic encephalopathy. *N Engl J Med.* 2005;353:1574–1584.
61. Gluckman PD et al. Selective head cooling with mild systemic hypothermia after neonatal encephalopathy: multicentre randomised trial. *Lancet.* 2005;365:663–670.
62. Azzopardi DV et al. Moderate hypothermia to treat perinatal asphyxial encephalopathy. *N Engl J Med.* 2009;361:1349–1358.
63. Langlois JA, Rutland-Brown W, Thomas KE. Traumatic Brain Injury in the United States: Emergency Department Visits, Hospitalizations, and Deaths. Atlanta (GA): Centers for Disease Control and Prevention, National Center for Injury Prevention and Control; 2004.
64. Marion DW et al. Treatment of traumatic brain injury with moderate hypothermia. *N Engl J Med.* 1997;336:540–546.
65. Alderson P, Gadkary C, Signorini DF. Therapeutic hypothermia for head injury. *Cochrane Database Syst Rev.* 2004:CD001048.
66. Hutchison J et al. Hypothermia pediatric head injury trial: the value of a pretrial clinical evaluation phase. *Dev Neurosci.* 2006;28:291–301.
67. Adelson PD et al. Phase II clinical trial of moderate hypothermia after severe traumatic brain injury in children. *Neurosurgery.* 2005;56:740–754; discussion 754.
68. Biswas AK et al. Treatment of acute traumatic brain injury in children with moderate hypothermia improves intracranial hypertension. *Crit Care Med.* 2002;30:2742–2751.
69. Hutchison JS et al. Hypothermia therapy after traumatic brain injury in children. *N Engl J Med.* 2008;358:2447–2456.

70. Froehler MT, Ovbiagele B. Therapeutic hypothermia for acute ischemic stroke. *Expert Rev Cardiovasc Ther*. 2010;8: 593–603.

71. Martin-Schild S et al. Combined neuroprotective modalities coupled with thrombolysis in acute ischemic stroke: a pilot study of caffeinol and mild hypothermia. *J Stroke Cerebrovasc Dis*. 2009;18:86–96.

72. Lyden PD et al. Intravascular Cooling in the Treatment of Stroke (ICTuS): early clinical experience. *J Stroke Cerebrovasc Dis*. 2005;14:107–114.

73. Els T et al. Safety and therapeutical benefit of hemicraniectomy combined with mild hypothermia in comparison with hemicraniectomy alone in patients with malignant ischemic stroke. *Cerebrovasc Dis*. 2006;21:79–85.

74. Schwab S et al. Feasibility and safety of moderate hypothermia after massive hemispheric infarction. *Stroke*. 2001;32:2033–2035.

75. Krieger DW et al. Cooling for acute ischemic brain damage (cool aid): an open pilot study of induced hypothermia in acute ischemic stroke. *Stroke*. 2001;32:1847–1854.

76. Koennecke HC, Leistner S. Prophylactic antipyretic treatment with acetaminophen in acute ischemic stroke: a pilot study. *Neurology*. 2001;57:2301–2303.

77. Dippel DW et al. Effect of paracetamol (acetaminophen) on body temperature in acute ischemic stroke: a double-blind, randomized phase II clinical trial. *Stroke*. 2001;32: 1607–1612.

78. Dippel DW et al. Effect of paracetamol (acetaminophen) and ibuprofen on body temperature in acute ischemic stroke PISA, a phase II double-blind, randomized, placebo-controlled trial [ISRCTN98608690]. *BMC Cardiovasc Disord*. 2003; 3:2.

79. Polderman KH, Herold I. Therapeutic hypothermia and controlled normothermia in the intensive care unit: practical considerations, side effects, and cooling methods. *Crit Care Med*. 2009;37:1101–1120.

80. Abend NS et al. Electroencephalographic monitoring during hypothermia after pediatric cardiac arrest. *Neurology*. 2009;72:1931–1940.

81. Shankaran S et al. Whole-body hypothermia for neonatal encephalopathy: animal observations as a basis for a randomized, controlled pilot study in term infants. *Pediatrics*. 2002;110:377–385.

82. Azzopardi D et al. The TOBY Study. Whole body hypothermia for the treatment of perinatal asphyxial encephalopathy: a randomised controlled trial. *BMC Pediatr*. 2008;8:17.

7 Traumatic Brain Injury

STUART H. FRIESS, TODD J. KILBAUGH, and JIMMY HUH

■ INTRODUCTION

Traumatic brain injury (TBI) is the leading cause of mortality and severe morbidity in children. The primary goal in the acute management of the severely head-injured pediatric patient is to prevent or ameliorate factors that promote secondary brain injury, such as hypoxemia, hypotension, intracranial hypertension, hypercarbia, hyperglycemia or hypoglycemia, electrolyte abnormalities, enlarging hematomas, coagulopathy, seizures, and hyperthermia. It is integral to recognize the signs and symptoms of severe pediatric TBI, initiate appropriate interventions, and activate the necessary specialty services in a timely manner. Unfortunately, there is a paucity of randomized clinical trials in pediatric TBI, and the majority of recommendations have been based on consensus or adult data (1). With that in mind, this chapter focuses on a practical approach to the management of the pediatric patient with severe TBI in the critical care setting.

■ EPIDEMIOLOGY

Approximately 475,000 children under the age of 14 sustain TBI annually (2). Rates of hospitalization and mechanisms of injury vary by age secondary to developmental milestones (3). In infants (age less than 1 year), inflicted or nonaccidental TBI must always be considered. The median age for inflicted TBI is 2 to 4 months and intensive care hospitalization rates have been estimated at approximately 30 per 100,000 children yearly

(2,4). Estimating the accurate incidence of inflicted TBI is challenging due to the fact that many children may not present for treatment or may have an extended interval between injury and presentation for medical care. Motor vehicle crashes and falls from parents' arms are the main causes of TBI in this age group with intensive care admission rates of 20 per 100,000 children annually.

Toddler-aged children have developed the motor capabilities to encounter more hazards but lack the cognitive ability for avoidance. TBI requiring hospitalization is much less common in this age group (4 per 100,000 annually) for inflicted TBI and for noninflicted TBI (10 per 100,000 annually) (4). In school-aged children, falls requiring hospitalization decrease with age, while there is a rise in injuries associated with bicycle crashes. By adolescence, there is a dramatic rise in TBI-related death rates, with violence being an unfortunate common cause (24.3 per 100,000).

■ PATHOPHYSIOLOGY

TBI can be classified into primary and secondary injury. Primary brain injury results directly from the initial forces generated by impact following trauma. Contact linear forces are generated when the head is struck by a moving object and generally result in focal injuries (skull fracture, hematomas, and contusions) that are localized to the impact site or immediately opposite, known as contrecoup lesions. Severe inertial, angular forces produced by acceleration-deceleration can produce immediate physical shearing or tearing of axons termed "primary" axotomy. Following primary brain injury, a cascade of cellular, molecular, and biochemical events occurs in the minutes to weeks after the primary brain injury that lead to ongoing or "secondary" traumatic axonal injury (TAI) and neuronal cell damage (secondary brain injury) and, ultimately, neuronal cell death (5–7). Some of these important cellular mechanisms are discussed below.

Cerebrovascular Dysregulation

Following TBI, injury to cerebral blood vessels and alterations in cerebral blood flow (CBF) and cerebral metabolism are thought to contribute to secondary brain injury. Decreased CBF (< 20 mL/100 g/min) in the initial 24-hour period following TBI has been associated with poor outcome in infants and young children (8). Mechanisms that may underlie posttraumatic hypoperfusion include reduced cerebral perfusion pressure (CPP), reduced levels of vasodilators (including nitric oxide, cyclic guanosine 3',5'-monophosphate, cyclic adenosine 3',5'-monophosphate, and prostaglandins) (9–11), and increased levels of vasoconstrictors (such as endothelin 1) (12).

Excitotoxicity and Apoptosis

After TBI, the release of excessive amounts of the excitatory amino acid glutamate is thought to occur (excitotoxicity), which can lead to neuronal injury in two phases. The first phase is characterized by sodium-dependent neuronal swelling, which is then followed by delayed, calcium-dependent neuronal degeneration (13). Increased intracellular calcium initiates numerous processes, including activation of proteases, lipases, and endonucleases which can lead to neuronal degeneration and necrotic cell death. In contrast to necrotic cell death which is marked by neuronal cell swelling and dissolution of cell membranes, apoptotic cell death is marked by internucleosomal DNA fragmentation and the formation of apoptotic cell bodies associated with nuclear condensation and neuronal cell shrinkage. Apoptosis requires a cascade of intracellular events for completion of "programmed cell death," and is initiated by intracellular (intrinsic) or extracellular (extrinsic) signals.

Cerebral Swelling

Diffuse cerebral swelling following pediatric TBI may lead to intracranial hypertension, resulting in further ischemia and herniation. Swelling may result from blood-brain barrier disruption (vasogenic edema), osmolar changes, and edema at the cellular level (cytotoxic or cellular edema). Episodes of hypoxia and hypoperfusion are thought to worsen cerebral swelling. Osmolar shifts occur primarily in areas of necrosis where the osmolar load increases with the degradation of neurons. As reperfusion and recovery occurs, water is drawn into the area secondary to the high osmolar load, and the surrounding neurons become edematous. Cellular swelling independent of osmolar load primarily occurs in astrocyte foot processes and is thought to be brought on by excitotoxicity and uptake of glutamate. Glutamate uptake is coupled to sodium-potassium adenosine triphosphatase, with sodium and water being accumulated in astrocytes (14). Emerging literature suggests that cellular edema, rather than hyperemia or vasogenic edema, may be the primary contributor to cerebral swelling (15).

Traumatic Axonal Injury

A common pathology observed in infants and young children, in both accidental and in nonaccidental or inflicted closed-head injuries, is TAI or diffuse axonal injury. TAI involves widespread damage to axons in the white matter of the brain. While immediate or primary axotomy or immediate physical tearing of the axon can occur following injury, TAI is thought to primarily occur by a delayed process called "secondary" axotomy. Hypoxic-ischemic injury, calcium and ionic flux dysregulation, and mitochondrial and cytoskeletal dysfunction may play important roles in axonal damage (16). TAI most commonly occurs in the corpus callosum, basal ganglia, and periventricular white matter (17) and is thought to be a major cause of prolonged coma and morbidity in pediatric TBI (18). TAI also appears to be common in victims of nonaccidental trauma (19). The pediatric population is thought to be at a higher risk for TAI due to the incomplete myelinization of axons and the higher ratio of head to body mass, which makes children more susceptible to angular forces.

■ DIFFERENTIAL DIAGNOSIS

As a pediatric patient with severe TBI is evaluated, management must focus on ABCs (airway, breathing, circulation) and recognition of the signs and symptoms of life-threatening intracranial hemorrhages and mass occupying lesions producing intracranial hypertension. It is important to note that infants can lose significant portions of their blood volume through intracranial and extracranial bleeding resulting in circulatory compromise and shock.

TBI injury may be penetrating or closed head. Vascular injuries are more common with penetrating than closed head injury. The following is a summary of the intracranial hemorrhage types.

Epidural hematomas: An accumulation of blood between the inner table of the calvarium and the dura (Figure 7.1). The leading causes of epidural hematomas in the pediatric population are falls (49%) and traffic-related accidents (34%) (20,21). Epidural bleeding has been historically attributed to injury to the middle meningeal artery, but can also result from injury to the middle meningeal vein, the diploic veins, or the venous sinuses. In report of a 102 pediatric patients, arterial bleeding was found in 18% of epidural hematomas while 32% were associated with venous bleeding and 31% had no identifiable source (22). The most frequent locations of epidural hematomas are the temporoparietal and temporal regions (21,22).

Subdural hematomas: An accumulation of blood between the dura and the brain parenchyma, usually the result of injury to the cortical bridging veins. They are more common in infancy and the incidence decreases

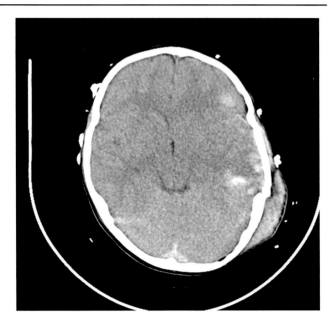

FIGURE 7.2 CT scan of 10-year-old struck by automobile with multiple parenchymal contusions.

with age (23). Acute subdural hematomas are usually the result of high velocity injuries and are associated with primary brain parenchyma injuries with tearing of bridging veins such as contusions or TAI (24). In infants without a clear history or mechanism for accidental trauma or with concurrent interhemispheric bleeding, further evaluation for inflicted trauma is required.

Subarachnoid hemorrhage: An accumulation of blood within the subarachnoid space. Subarachnoid hemorrhage occurs after injury to the small vessels traversing the subarachnoid space. It does not typically require emergent intervention, unless it causes cerebrospinal fluid (CSF) flow obstruction leading to hydrocephalus, which suggests there may be associated significant brain parenchymal injury.

Intraparenchymal hemorrhage: Hemorrhagic contusions are common after pediatric head injury (Figure 7.2), but large intracerebral hemorrhages are rare (25). Contusions result from the brain impacting the adjacent skull.

■ **EVALUATION**

History

Details on the timing and mechanism of injury, resuscitative efforts, and therapeutic interventions implemented and attempted from witnesses at the scene as

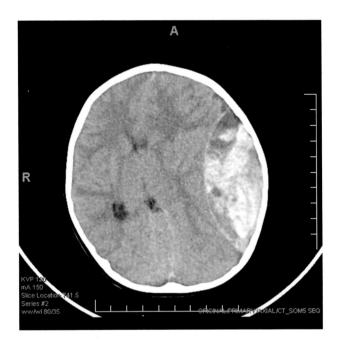

FIGURE 7.1 Computed tomographic (CT) scan of an 18-month-old with large left epidural hematoma. Note the swirling nature of the hematoma indicating active bleeding.

■ **Table 7.1** Herniation Syndromes			
Herniation Type	**Eye Findings**	**Gross Motor**	**Respiration**
Uncal	Unilateral fixed dilated pupil with unilateral ptosis	Hemiparesis	
Diencephalic	Small midpoint pupils, but reactive to light	Decorticate posturing, hypertonia	Cheyne-Stokes
Midbrain	Midpoint fixed pupils	Decerebrate posturing	Hyperventilation
Medullary	Dilated and fixed pupils	No response to pain	Irregular or gasping

well as from emergency medical personnel are essential. The use of the "AMPLE" mnemonic (allergies, medications currently used, past illnesses, last meal, and events/environment related to the injury) may be helpful for practitioners to quickly acquire the necessary information to improve understanding of the patient's current physiologic state (26). Presentation symptoms have little or no correlation with injury severity and the practitioner must rely on physical examination (27).

Physical Examination

Adequacy of the ABCs and the patient's neurologic status must be rapidly assessed. Immediate evaluation for life-threatening signs and symptoms of intracranial hypertension or impending herniation is essential. These symptoms include altered level of consciousness, pupillary dysfunction, lateralizing extremity weakness, Cushing triad (hypertension, bradycardia, and irregular respirations), or herniation syndromes (Table 7.1).

If the patient is intubated, capnography permits rapid assessment for esophageal intubation (28–30) as well as optimization of arterial carbon dioxide. The head and spine should be thoroughly examined for any external evidence of injury such as scalp lacerations and skull depressions that may indicate underlying skull fracture and severe intracranial injury. In the infant, a bulging fontanelle may be a sign of increased intracranial pressure (ICP), although a flat fontanelle does not preclude intracranial hypertension (6). Mastoid (Battle sign) and periorbital (raccoon eyes) bruising due to dissection of blood, hemotympanum, and clear rhinorrhea are all signs of possible basilar skull fracture. A basilar skull fracture would be a contraindication to a nasal tube.

It is important that a rapid but detailed and easily reproducible neurologic assessment be performed and documented (27). The Glasgow Coma Scale (GCS) is the most widely used method to quantify initial neurologic assessment in older children and adults (Table 7.2) (31). In younger pediatric patients, the Children's Coma Scale

is often utilized (Table 7.3) (32). It is critical that the GCS be recorded on the initial medical record and repeated regularly to detect changes in GCS indicative of progressive injury.

The pupillary exam is vital when assessing the neurologic status of the head-injured child. The size, shape, and reactivity to light provide critical insight into the balance of sympathetic and parasympathetic influences. Evaluation of eye movements and brainstem reflexes can help localize intracranial lesions. Dysfunction of all three cranial nerves in eye movement (oculomotor, trochlear, and abducens nerves) can be the result of injury to the ipsilateral cavernous sinus. Cough and gag reflexes detect glossopharyngeal and vagus nerve function. Abnormalities in the respiratory pattern may also assist in localizing brain injury and herniation syndromes (Table 7.1). Deep tendon reflexes (DTRs) are typically exaggerated in head-injured patents due to the lack of cortical inhibition. However, decreased DTRs may

■ **Table 7.2** Glasgow Coma Scale	
Eye opening	
Spontaneous	4
To speech	3
To painful stimuli	2
None	1
Verbal	
Oriented	5
Confused	4
Inappropriate	3
Incomprehensible	2
None	1
Motor	
Obeys commands	6
Localizes to pain	5
Withdraws from pain	4
Flexion to pain (decorticate response)	3
Extension to pain (decerebrate response)	2
None	1

■ **Table 7.3** Modified Children's Coma Scale	
Eye opening	
Spontaneous	4
To speech	3
To pain	2
None	1
Verbal	
Coos, babbles	5
Irritable	4
Cries to pain	3
Moans to pain	2
None	1
Motor	
Normal spontaneous movements	6
Withdraws to touch	5
Withdraws to pain	4
Abnormal flexion	3
Abnormal extension	2
Flaccid	1

suggest a spinal cord injury. The presence of Cushing triad (systemic hypertension, bradycardia, and irregular respirations) due to compression of the cardiorespiratory centers in the brainstem is a late and ominous sign for herniation.

Diagnostic Studies

The ABCs are first addressed with a chest x-ray to rule out any associated thoracic injuries and appropriate endotracheal tube placement. Likewise, the spine is immobilized presumptively until those injuries are ruled out. Computed tomography (CT) is the mainstay of the diagnostic evaluation of the severely head-injured pediatric patient. For intubated patients, continuous capnometry is vital for titrating treatment of intracranial hypertension (see below). A chemistry panel should be sent to assess electrolyte abnormalities and renal function, especially if hyperosmolar therapy may be instituted (33). Liver enzymes and pancreatic function should also be evaluated for possible blunt trauma and especially if nonaccidental trauma is suspected. A complete blood count and a coagulation profile should be evaluated in patients with intracranial hemorrhage. In one prospective observational study, 22% of children with severe head injury had laboratory evidence of disseminated intravascular coagulation (34). Repeated measurements may be needed since coagulopathy or thrombocytopenia

may develop over time (35). In the adolescent population, where there are increased rates of high impact injuries from motor vehicle crashes, a toxicology screen should also be considered (36).

Imaging with plain films of the cervical spine should be performed to assess for associated cervical spine injury or instability that may require urgent immobilization and management. Chest radiographs may identify rib fractures, pneumothoracis, and widened mediastinum, and are needed for intubated patients to evaluate for right mainstem intubations. Pelvic radiographs should be considered if pelvic injuries are suspected. Other radiographs should be performed based on the results of the secondary survey. If nonaccidental injury is suspected then a full skeletal survey may be indicated. If there is no clear history or mechanism of accidental trauma, especially in infants and early toddlers, further investigation for other occult injuries, such as abdominal injuries, skeletal injuries, or retinal hemorrhages (which are commonly associated with shaken-baby or shaken-impact syndrome) should be sought (37). However, this workup should not take precedence over life-threatening issues such as hypoxemia, hypotension, and intracranial hypertension.

In pediatric patients with moderate and severe TBI, CT scans are the imaging modality of choice and can rapidly detect skull fractures, intracranial hematomas, intraparenchymal contusions, cerebral edema, and obliteration of the basal cisterns. CT scan has widespread availability and rapid imaging time which makes it very useful in the emergency and critical care settings. Several early CT scan findings have been associated with outcome including the status of the basal cisterns, midline shift, and presence of subarachnoid hemorrhage in the basal cisterns (38–40). The basal cisterns are evaluated at the level of the midbrain—compressed or absent cisterns increase the risk of intracranial hypertension and poor outcome (40,41). The degree of midline shift at the foramen of Monro is inversely related to prognosis (38, 40,41). The presence of traumatic subarachnoid hemorrhage in severe TBI increases mortality and its presence in the basal cisterns is a predictor of poor outcome (38, 40,41).

Magnetic resonance imaging (MRI) has demonstrated superiority to CT for detection of TAI and its correlation with long-term outcome. However, MRI is of limited use during the initial stabilization and management of pediatric TBI patients due to limited availability, long time required for image acquisition, and limited physiologic monitoring availability in the MRI suite (42–44). In summary, pediatric patients with moderate and severe TBI should have CT imaging as soon as possible, but not before physiologic stabilization has occurred (ABCs) and appropriate monitoring has been placed (such as end-tidal CO_2).

■ MANAGEMENT

Initial Stabilization

Hypoxemia and hypotension should be avoided and managed to prevent or minimize secondary hypoxic-ischemic brain injury, which may promote cerebral swelling and elevated ICP. Thus, the first step in treating the head-injured pediatric patient is always to promote adequate oxygenation and ventilation, and to prevent or treat shock.

Criteria for tracheal intubation include: hypoxemia not resolved with supplemental oxygen, apnea, hypercarbia ($Paco_2 > 45$ mmHg), GCS ≤ 8, a decrease in GCS > 3 independent of the initial GCS, anisocoria > 1 mm, cervical spine injury compromising ventilation, loss of pharyngeal reflex, and any clinical evidence of a herniation syndrome or Cushing triad (6).

Intubation should be performed utilizing a cerebro-protective, rapid-sequence induction and all patients should be assumed to have a full stomach and cervical spine injury. Supplemental oxygen should be delivered by face mask to allow nitrogen washout from the patient's functional residual capacity to allow sufficient oxygenation prior to intubation of the trachea. Bag-valve-mask ventilation should not be done, unless the patient has signs and symptoms of impending herniation, apnea, or hypoxemia (45). As a general rule, the proper tracheal tube size for children older than 6 months of age (as described by the inner diameter measured in millimeters) = (16 + age [in years]) divided by 4, but this is only a starting estimate. Tracheal tubes that are one size smaller and larger should always be available. Orotracheal intubation by direct laryngoscopy is the preferred method. Nasotracheal intubation should be avoided since it may require excessive movement of the cervical spine and could result in direct intracranial damage in a patient with a basilar skull fracture. The endotracheal tube should be secured with tape, but this adhesive tape should not pass around the neck as venous return from the brain can be compromised.

Because endotracheal intubation is a noxious stimulus and can increase ICP, appropriate medications should be used during rapid-sequence induction. A combination of medications to sedate and paralyze the patient are required. Medications and doses must be chosen to ensure intubation occurs quickly and safely and episodes hypoxemia and hypotension are avoided. The hemodynamic and neurologic status of the patient dictates drug choice. For the patient in cardiopulmonary arrest, no medications are needed for tracheal intubation. All the other patients usually receive lidocaine (1–1.5 mg/kg) intravenously (IV) 3 minutes before intubation to help blunt the rise in ICP that occurs during direct laryngoscopy (46). For the hemodynamically unstable patient, the combination of lidocaine, etomidate (0.2–0.6 mg/kg), and neuromuscular blockade with rocuronium (1 mg/kg) or vecuronium (0.3 mg/kg) IV is a popular choice. An alternative is the combination of lidocaine, fentanyl (2–4 micrograms/kg), and rocuronium or vecuronium. In the hemodynamically stable patient, either of the above combinations in addition to the fast-acting benzodiazepine midazolam (0.1–0.2 mg/kg) can utilized. Another alternative in the hemodynamically stable patient is the combination of thiopental (3–5 mg/kg), lidocaine, and rocuronium or vecuronium. Thiopental and etomidate are ultrafast acting and quickly reduce cerebral metabolism, which ameliorates the increased ICP associated with direct laryngoscopy. In addition, the short-acting narcotic fentanyl, when used with lidocaine, can decrease the catecholamine release associated with direct laryngoscopy (45).

Unless the patient has signs or symptoms of herniation and a more definitive therapy such as neurosurgical intervention is being instituted, prophylactic hyperventilation ($Paco_2 < 35$ mmHg) should be avoided. Hyperventilation causes cerebral vasoconstriction, which decreases CBF and subsequent cerebral blood volume. Thus, while ICP may be reduced temporarily, ischemia can occur (47), and this could lead to further secondary injury and ICP elevation. Furthermore, respiratory alkalosis caused by hyperventilation shifts the hemoglobin-oxygen curve to the left, leading to less oxygen release in the brain.

Assessment of the patient's circulatory status (central and peripheral pulse quality, capillary refill, heart rate, blood pressure) is critical as hypotension after pediatric TBI is associated with increase in morbidity and mortality (1,48,49). The most common cause for compensated or "early" shock (tachycardia with normal blood pressure) and uncompensated or "late" shock (low blood pressure) in the trauma patient is hypovolemic (ie, hemorrhagic) shock. Rapid IV fluid resuscitation is needed for hypovolemic shock. Isotonic solutions, such as 0.9% NaCl solution and/or packed red blood cells can be administered. Hypotonic fluids can worsen cerebral edema and should be avoided. Although its efficacy has not been studied in a clinical trial, resuscitation with hypertonic saline (3% saline) is generally indicated in the severely brain injured child with initial signs and symptoms of both hypovolemic shock and intracranial hypertension, and is further discussed in the "Intracranial Hypertension Management: First-Tier Therapies" section below. If hypotension is present and cervical-thoracic spine injuries are present or suspected then special consideration must be given to spinal (neurogenic) shock. These patients may also be bradycardic. Both spinal shock and bradycardia can be treated with isotonic fluid and/or blood resuscitation to ensure adequate circulation and prevent further ischemia. In spinal shock, α-adrenergic agonists, such as IV phenylephrine, are also needed to treat the vasodilatation that results from injury to the sympathetic outflow tract.

Prophylactic "brain-specific" interventions (such as hyperventilation and hyperosmolar therapy with mannitol or 3% saline) in the absence of signs and symptoms of herniation or other neurologic deterioration, are not recommended. However, in the presence of signs and symptoms of herniation, such as Cushing triad (irregular respirations, bradycardia, systemic hypertension), pupillary dysfunction, lateralizing extremity weakness, or extensor posturing, emergent treatment is needed and is discussed further in the "Herniation" section below.

Herniation

While the ABCs are being addressed, signs and symptoms of impending herniation such as Cushing triad or one of the herniation syndromes must also be immediately treated. Early consultation with a neurosurgeon is important. In one study, mass lesions occurred in 30% of children with severe TBI (50). Hyperventilation with 100% oxygen can be lifesaving in the setting of impending herniation, such as a child who has a rapidly expanding epidural hematoma with pupillary dilatation, bradycardia, systemic hypertension, and extensor posturing. Elevating the head to 30° increases venous drainage and lowers ICP (51). Furthermore, the head should be midline to prevent obstruction of venous return from the brain. If these

maneuvers do not relieve the signs and symptoms of herniation, hyperosmolar therapy (mannitol or 3% saline) should be instituted (see the "Intracranial Hypertension Management: First-Tier Therapies" section below). In addition, intubating doses of short acting medications, such as thiopental or etomidate, as described previously, can be administered emergently in this setting (6). During this time, the patient usually undergoes CT imaging and/or is taken directly to the neurosurgical operating room for definitive therapy. Surgical evacuation of hemorrhagic lesions or craniotomy to reduce ICP may terminate herniation and be lifesaving.

Besides expanding mass lesions, diffuse cerebral swelling may also lead to herniation. Diffuse swelling is more common in pediatric than adult TBI (52). As a result, secondary causes of brain injury, such as hypoxemia, hypercarbia, hypotension, excessive fluid administration (especially hypotonic fluids), or seizures that can precipitate herniation must be prevented or immediately treated. Craniotomy may be useful for severe cerebral edema, especially if it is focal or hemispheric.

ICP, Autoregulation, and Cerebral Perfusion

Once the initial resuscitation with attention to the ABCs is completed and issues of herniation or expanding hemorrhages have been medically and surgically addressed, further management is aimed at preventing or treating causes of secondary brain injury. These include hypoxemia, hypotension, intracranial hypertension, hypercarbia, hyperglycemia or hypoglycemia, electrolyte abnormalities, enlarging hematomas, coagulopathy, seizures, and hyperthermia.

One of the most important consequences of secondary brain injury is the development of intracranial hypertension. First described in the Monroe-Kellie doctrine, the intracranial vault is a fixed volume of brain, CSF, and blood (6). An enlarging space occupying lesion, such as an expanding epidural hematoma or worsening cerebral edema, will not initially cause intracranial hypertension since initial compensatory mechanisms including displacement of CSF to the spinal canal and venous blood to the jugular veins is sufficient to prevent elevated ICP. However, once these compensatory mechanisms are exhausted, even a small increase in the size of the hematoma or cerebral edema will lead to increased ICP. As ICP approaches mean arterial pressure (MAP), cerebral perfusion is compromised. This leads to ischemia which worsens cerebral edema, further elevating ICP and reducing cerebral perfusion, and this cycle may ultimately lead to herniation.

Under normal conditions, cerebral autoregulation provides constant CBF over a wide range of CPPs and is "coupled" to the metabolic demands of the brain. CPP is the defined as the difference between MAP and ICP. Thus, CPP = MAP – ICP (6). After TBI, cerebral autoregulation can become "uncoupled" from the metabolic demands of the brain. Without autoregulation, reduction in CPP due to either elevated ICP or reduced MAP may result in CBF fluctuations, potentially leading to cerebral ischemia. In contrast, increased CPP due to a decrease in ICP or increased MAP may increase CBF and result in hyperemia. A study utilizing xenon CBF-CT studies in children after TBI demonstrated that marked reductions in CBF within the first 24 hours after injury was associated with poor outcome, while high CBF 24 hours after the injury was associated with improved outcome (8). However, because this type of study cannot measure minute-to-minute assessment of CBF fluctuations, and due to the potential risk of transporting and performing prolonged studies in critically-ill patients, most institutions continuously measure ICP and MAP to calculate CPP, which is used as an estimate of CBF.

In general, after initial stabilization and resuscitation, an ICP monitor is placed by the neurosurgeon in children with an initial GCS ≤ 8 for treatment of potential intracranial hypertension. Since clinical signs and symptoms of herniation are very late signs of intracranial hypertension, the use of ICP monitors allows early detection of intracranial hypertension, often well before signs and symptoms of herniation are observed (53). An additional benefit is that if the ventricles are not compressed due to severe cerebral swelling, ICP monitoring by ventricular catheter permits therapeutic CSF drainage if needed. However, ICP monitors can rarely cause hemorrhage and infection. Coagulopathy needs to be corrected before ICP monitor placement and some centers administer prophylactic antibiotics. Placement of an intracranial monitor should be performed with adequate anesthesia.

Treatment for intracranial hypertension should begin at an ICP ≥ 20 mmHg, as most pediatric TBI studies show poor outcome with ICP > 20 mmHg, and aggressive treatment of intracranial hypertension is associated with improved outcomes in some studies (54–57). However, further studies are needed to determine an age-appropriate treatment for intracranial hypertension in infants and young children. Younger children have a lower MAP, and thus may require a lower ICP

treatment threshold if CPP is to be maintained. The optimal CPP for pediatric TBI is unknown and there is no evidence that targeting a specific CPP improves outcome. However, there are pediatric TBI studies that show that a CPP < 40 mmHg is associated with poor outcome (58,59). As a result, the pediatric guidelines recommend the option of maintaining an "age-related continuum" of CPP from 40 to 65 mmHg in infants to adolescents, respectively (1). Further studies are needed to determine the age-appropriate CPP.

Lowering ICP or raising MAP will increase CPP. Most treatments are aimed at lowering ICP, maintaining normal MAP, and maintaining euvolemia. If the treatments fail to lower ICP, then vasopressors are commonly added to augment MAP and thus increase the CPP. However, this mechanism only works if cerebral autoregulation is at least partially intact. Otherwise, as the MAP is increased, the ICP will also increase, and there is no net augmentation in CPP. If the child is hypotensive, isotonic fluid boluses and/or vasopressors can be administered to augment the MAP in the hopes of improving CPP.

Intracranial Hypertension Management: First-Tier Therapies

A general approach to first-tier treatments for established intracranial hypertension in pediatric TBI was provided in the "Guidelines for the management of severe TBI in infants, children, and adolescents" (1). As discussed below, first-tier therapies include head position; sedation, analgesia, and neuromuscular blockade; ventricular CSF drainage; hyperosmolar therapy; and mild hyperventilation.

Head Position

Elevating the head to 30° has been shown to reduce ICP without decreasing CPP in adults after severe TBI (51). While pediatric studies are lacking, the same degree of head elevation with midline position may promote venous drainage. There are some patients who may have a more optimal CPP at angles other than 30°. This angle will change day to day, and may be greater or less than 30°. Optimally, the head position will be individualized and titrated to CPP or CBF monitors (60). Head elevation may also reduce ventilator associated pneumonias. In some centers, practitioners avoid placing a central venous catheter in the internal jugular vein to maximize venous drainage from the brain.

Sedation, Analgesia, and Neuromuscular Blockade

If there is continued ICP elevation, sedation, analgesia, and neuromuscular blockade can be administered. Anxiety, stress, and pain can increase cerebral metabolic demands, which can pathologically increase cerebral blood volume and increase ICP. Narcotics, benzodiazepines, or barbiturates are commonly used. There are few studies of the use of sedatives in pediatric patients with severe TBI. However, the goal should be to use the lowest possible doses to lower ICP without causing side effects such as hypotension. In addition, potentially noxious stimulus such as endotracheal tube suctioning should be pretreated with sedation and/or analgesics, and lidocaine (1 mg/kg IV) may be utilized to blunt rises in ICP.

Ketamine has been associated with increasing cerebral blood volume and increased ICP, and thus has been considered contraindicated in patients with increased ICP (61). More recently, ketamine administration in mechanically ventilated pediatric TBI patients has been reported to decrease ICP (62). Further study of ketamine is needed.

A number of non-TBI and one TBI case report have reported metabolic acidosis and death in pediatric patients on prolonged (24 hours) continuous infusion of propofol (63–66). Based on recommendations of the Food and Drug Administration, the pediatric guidelines state: "continuous infusion of propofol is not recommended in the treatment of pediatric traumatic brain injury" (1).

Neuromuscular blocking agents are thought to reduce ICP by reducing airway and intrathoracic pressure with improved cerebral venous outflow and by preventing shivering, coughing, posturing, or ventilator-patient asynchrony (67). Risks of neuromuscular blockade include hypoxemia and hypercarbia due to inadvertent extubation, masking of seizures, nosocomial pneumonia (shown to occur in adults with severe TBI), immobilization stress due to inadequate sedation and analgesia, increased ICU stay duration, and myopathy of critical illness (67). The loss of clinical exam should be less concerning if ICP monitoring is used, as increases in ICP usually occur before changes in clinical exam.

Ventricular Cerebrospinal Drainage

Removal of CSF may decrease ICP in a patient with intracranial hypertension. The placement of a ventricular ICP monitor provides diagnostic information as well as a therapeutic intervention (CSF drainage). Small ventricles due to diffuse cerebral edema or intracranial bleeding may make catheter placement difficult.

Hyperosmolar Therapy

Two agents are generally considered for hyperosmolar therapy: mannitol and 3% normal saline. While mannitol has been traditionally administered, 3% saline is also gaining favor. However, there is no literature to support the superiority of one over the other in severe pediatric TBI. Mannitol reduces ICP by two mechanisms. First, mannitol rapidly reduces blood viscosity which promotes reflex vasoconstriction of the arterioles by autoregulation, thus decreasing cerebral blood volume and ICP. In addition to decreasing intracranial blood volume, it may enhance flow dependent vasodilation, improving CBF overall. This mechanism is rapid but transient, lasting about 75 minutes, and it requires an intact autoregulation (68,69). Second, mannitol has an osmotic effect. By increasing serum osmolality, mannitol causes a shift of water from the brain cells into the intravascular space, and thus decreases cellular or cytotoxic edema. While this effect is slower in onset (15–30 minutes), the osmotic effect lasts up to 6 hours. Importantly, if the blood-brain barrier is not intact, which is often the case in children with severe TBI, over time mannitol may accumulate in injured brain regions and cause a shift in fluid from the intravascular space to the brain parenchyma and thus worsen ICP. This problem is reported when mannitol is present in the circulation for extended periods, supporting the use of intermittent boluses (70,71). Furthermore, mannitol is a potent osmotic diuretic and may precipitate hypotension and renal failure if the patient becomes hypovolemic and the serum osmolality is > 320 mOsm/L (72–74). Mannitol is administered in bolus doses of 0.25 g/kg to 1 g/kg IV (72).

More recently, hypertonic saline has been used for hyperosmolar therapy in pediatric TBI. The main mechanism of action is the osmotic effect similar to mannitol, but its main theoretical advantage over mannitol is that hypertonic saline can be administered in a hemodynamically unstable patient with impending herniation, as hypertonic saline is thought to preserve intravascular volume status (75–78). Mannitol is an osmotic diuretic and may worsen intravascular depletion and hypotension. Hypertonic saline exhibits several other theoretical benefits such as restoration of normal cellular resting membrane potential and cell volume, inhibition of inflammation, stimulation of atrial natriuretic peptide release, and enhancement of cardiac output (78–81). Hypertonic saline, as 3% saline, can be administered as a bolus IV dose. While not well studied, 1–6 mL/kg

IV is an often used dose. Three percent saline continuous infusions of 0.1 to 1 mL/kg/hour titrated to maintain ICP < 20 mmHg have been used (82,83). Caution should be exercised if the serum osmolality approaches 320 mOsm/L as there have been reports of renal insufficiency (33). Another potential concern with the use of hypertonic saline is myelinosis, which may be central pontine (demyelination of the pons) or extrapontine (demyelination of the thalamus, basal ganglia, and cerebellum). Myelinosis occurs with hypernatremia and/or its correction (84), although this has not been clinically reported in pediatric TBI management. Rebound intracranial hypertension has been described with the use of hypertonic saline bolus administration or after stopping the continuous infusion (82,85). Further studies evaluating optimal dosing and long-term outcome are needed to compare mannitol administration with 3% saline.

Hyperventilation

Hyperventilation may rapidly lower ICP. However, without signs of herniation, mild or prophylactic hyperventilation ($Paco_2$ < 35 mmHg) in children should be avoided. Mild hyperventilation ($Paco_2$ 30–35 mmHg) may be considered as a first-tier option for longer periods of intracranial hypertension refractory to all the above measures (sedation, analgesia, neuromuscular blockade, CSF drainage, and hyperosmolar therapy) (1). This rationale is based on studies that CBF may be decreased early following pediatric TBI and may be associated with poor outcome, and that prophylactic hyperventilation may cause further ischemia and hypoperfusion (47). Aggressive hyperventilation ($Paco_2$ < 30 mmHg) may be considered as a second tier option in the setting of refractory intracranial hypertension. CBF, jugular venous oxygen saturation, or brain tissue oxygen monitoring to help identify cerebral ischemia is suggested (86,87).

Intracranial Hypertension Management: Second-Tier Therapies

Refractory intracranial hypertension occurs in as many as 42% of cases of severe pediatric TBI and is associated with mortality rates between 29% and 100% (88–91). Repeat CT scan should be performed to rule out a surgically correctable etiology for persistent, refractory intracranial hypertension. If there is no surgical lesion, then the guidelines recommend second-tier therapies, which

includes aggressive hyperventilation, barbiturates, hypothermia, decompressive craniectomy, and lumbar CSF drainage (1). There is less data for these therapies compared to first-tier therapies.

Barbiturates

Barbiturates reduce ICP by decreasing the cerebral metabolic rate (92–94). An electroencephalogram (EEG) should be used to assess the cerebral metabolic response to barbiturate treatment. Pentobarbital or thiopental is often administered to achieve burst suppression on the EEG, although the optimal degree of burst suppression is unknown. Side effects include decreased cardiac output, decreased systemic vascular resistance, and hypotension (89). As a result, if high-dose barbiturate therapy is used to treat refractory intracranial hypertension, then appropriate hemodynamic monitoring and cardiovascular support is required.

Hypothermia

In animal studies of experimental TBI, hyperthermia has been shown to exacerbate neuronal cell death. Further, therapeutic hypothermia was found to be neuroprotective by ameliorating mechanisms of secondary brain injury, such as decreasing cerebral metabolism, inflammation, lipid peroxidation, and excitotoxicity (95). While most agree that hyperthermia should be avoided in children with severe TBI, the role of hypothermia is unclear. A recent randomized controlled clinical trial did not show any benefit to 24 hours of hypothermia and there was a trend toward poorer outcome in the hypothermia group (96). Until further clinical studies are done, moderate hypothermia is reserved for patients with persistent intracranial hypertension refractory to other medical interventions, if no medical contraindications exist (1). Potential complications associated with hypothermia include hypovolemia (due to cold-induced dieresis), electrolyte disturbances such as hypokalemia with consequent arrhythmias, coagulopathy, and increased susceptibility to infection.

Decompressive Craniectomy

The main goal of decompressive craniectomy is to reduce ICP and thus maintain CPP, thereby preventing herniation due to refractory cerebral swelling. This surgical option is considered a second-tier therapy for pediatric TBI patients with refractory intracranial hypertension and may be particularly appropriate in patients who have a potentially recoverable brain injury. Other indications for decompressive craniectomy include secondary clinical deterioration or evolving cerebral herniation syndrome within 48 hours of injury (1). Decompressive craniectomy should be considered in the treatment of severe TBI and refractory intracranial hypertension in infants and young children with nonaccidental head trauma, as these patients had improved survival and neurologic outcomes compared to those undergoing medical management alone (97). However, there are concerns that this procedure may exacerbate hemorrhage and cerebral edema formation, so further studies addressing the safety, efficacy, and impact on long-term outcome of this surgical procedure are needed.

Lumbar CSF Drainage

Although not commonly used, lumbar CSF drainage has been shown to be successful in treating refractory intracranial hypertension following pediatric TBI (98). However, to avoid the risk of herniation, the child must already have a functional ventriculostomy drain and open basal cisterns, and no mass effect or shift on concurrent CT. Care is required to avoid herniation as pressure below the brain is lowered by lumbar CSF drainage.

Seizures

Seizures should be aggressively treated as seizures can elevate ICP and induce metabolic distress (99), potentially leading to worsened secondary brain injury. Note that many seizures may not have any clinical correlate and may be nonconvulsive, also referred to as subclinical or electrographic only seizures. Children with TBI may have nonconvulsive seizures, even when not paralyzed, and these can only be detected using continuous EEG monitoring (100). Studies are needed to determine whether detection and management of nonconvulsive seizures improves outcome.

While prophylactic anticonvulsants may be considered a treatment option to prevent early posttraumatic seizures (occurring within 7 days following injury) in infants and young children, prophylactic anticonvulsants are not recommended for preventing late posttraumatic seizures (occurring after 7 days), as they have not been shown to improve outcome (101,102). If clinical seizures are detected, most would treat with standard anticonvulsants. If nonconvulsive seizures are detected,

most neurologists would treat using standard anticonvulsants (103), although further study is needed.

■ CONCLUSIONS

Resuscitation of the child with severe TBI should focus on prompt stabilization and avoidance of hypoxemia and hypotension. Early evaluation to determine the need for surgical intervention is critical. Care in the ICU setting should focus on the prevention or amelioration of secondary brain injury including optimization of CPP and reduction of intracranial hypertension. Further research is needed on the optimization of pediatric neurointensive care for the child with severe TBI, as well as the development of novel therapeutics aimed at the cellular and subcellular level to promote neuron recovery.

■ REFERENCES

1. Adelson PD et al. Guidelines for the acute medical management of severe traumatic brain injury in infants, children, and adolescents. *Pediatr Crit Care Med.* 2003;4:S1–S75.
2. Langlois J, Rutland-Brown W, Thomas K. *Brain Injury in the United States: Emergency Department Visits, Hospitalizations, and Deaths.* Centers fot Disease Control and Prevention, National Center for Injury Prevention and Control. Atlanta, GA; 2004:1–32.
3. Schneier AJ et al. Incidence of pediatric traumatic brain injury and associated hospital resource utilization in the United States. *Pediatrics.* 2006;118(2):483–492.
4. Keenan HT et al. A population-based study of inflicted traumatic brain injury in young children. *JAMA.* 2003;290:621–626.
5. Fisher MD. Pediatric traumatic brain injury. *Crit Care Nursing.* 1997;20:36–51.
6. Kochanek PM et al. Severe traumatic brain injury in infants and children. In: Fuhrman BP, Zimmerman JJ, eds. *Pediatric Critical Care.* Philadelpia: Mosby; 2006:1595–1617. Textbook.
7. Lenzlinger PM et al. Overview of basic mechanisms underlying neuropathological consequences of head trauma. In: Miller, Hayes C, eds. *Head Trauma—Basic, Preclinical, and Clinical Directions.* Hoboken, NJ, Wiley-Liss; 2001:3–36. Review.
8. Adelson PD et al. Cerebrovascular response in infants and young children following severe traumatic brain injury: a preliminary report. *Pediatr Neurosurg.* 1997;26:200–207.
9. Armstead WM. Cerebral hemodynamics after traumatic brain injury of immature brain. *Exp Toxicol Pathol.* 1999;51: 137–142.
10. Armstead WM. Superoxide generation links protein kinase C activation to impaired ATP sensitive K-channel function after brain injury. *Stroke.* 1999;30:153–159.

11. Armstead WM. Brain injury impairs prostaglandin cerebro-vasodilation. *J Neurotrauma*. 1998;15:721–729.

12. Armstead WM. Role of endothelin-1 in age-dependent cerebrovascular hypotensive responses after brain injury. *Am J Physiol*. 1999;277:111884–111894.

13. Choi DW. Ionic dependence of glutamate neurotoxicity. *J Neurosci*. 1987;7:369–379.

14. Kochanek PM et al. Biochemical, cellular, and molecular mechanisms in the evolution of secondary damage after severe traumatic brain injury in infants and children: Lessons learned from the bedside. *Pediatr Crit Care Med*. 2000;1(1):4–19.

15. Barzo P et al. Contribution of vasogenic and cellular edema to traumatic brain swelling measured by diffusion-weighted imaging. *J Neurosurg*. 1997;87(6):900–907.

16. Povlishock JT, Christian CW. The pathobiology of traumatically induced axonal injury in animals and humans: a review of current thoughts. In: Bandak FA, Eppinger RH, Ommaya AK, eds. *Traumatic Brain Injury: Bioscience and Mechanics*. New York, NY: Mary Ann Liebert; 1996:51–60. Review.

17. Adams JH et al. Diffuse axonal injury due to nonmissile head injury in humans: an analysis of 45 cases. *Ann Neurol*. 1982;12(6):557–563.

18. Chiaretti A et al. [Diffuse axonal lesions in childhood]. *Pediatr Med Chir*. 1998;20(6):393–397.

19. Shannon P et al. Axonal injury and the neuropathology of shaken baby syndrome. *Acta Neuropathol (Berl)*. 1998;95(6):625–631.

20. Ben Abraham R et al. Metabolic and clinical markers of prognosis in the era of CT imaging in children with acute epidural hematomas. *Pediatr Neurosurg*. 2000;33(2):70–75.

21. Maggi G et al. Extradural hematomas in children. *J Neruosurg Sci*. 1998;42(2):95–99.

22. Mohanty A et al. Prognosis of extradural hematomas in children. *Pediatr Neurosurg*. 1995;23(2):57–63.

23. Hahn YS et al. Head injuries in children under 36 months of age. Demography and outcome. *Childs Nerv Syst*. 1988;4(1):34–40.

24. Fell DA, Fitzgerald S, Moiel RH. Acute subdural hematomas: review of 144 cases. *J Neurosurg*. 1975;42:37.

25. Kang JK et al. Traumatic isolated intracerebral hemorrhage in children. *Childs Nerv Syst*. 1989;5(5):303–306.

26. *ATLS: Advanced Trauma Life Support for Doctors*. 7th ed. Chicago, IL: American College of Surgeons; 2004. Textbook.

27. Falk AC et al. Management and classification of children with head injury. *Childs Nerv Syst*. 20005;21(6):430–436.

28. Repetto J et al. Use of capnography in the delivery room for assessment of endotracheal tube placement. *J Perinat*. 2001;21(5):284–287.

29. Roberts WA et al. The use of capnography for recognition of esophageal intubation in the neonatal intensive care unit. *Pediatr Pulmonol*. 1995;19(5):262–268.

30. Silvestri S et al. The effectiveness of out-of-hospital use of continuous end-tidal carbon dioxdie monitoring on the rate of unrecognized misplaced intubation within a regional emergency medical services system. *Ann Emerg Med*. 2005;45:497–503.

31. Teasdale G, Jennett B. Assessment of coma and impaired consciousness. A practical scale. *Lancet*. 1974;13:81–84.

32. Reilly PL et al. Assessing the conscious level in infants and young children: a pediatric version of the Glasgow Coma Scale. *Childs Nerv Syst*. 1988;4(1):30–33.

33. Dominguez TE, Priestley MA, Huh JW. Caution should be exercised when maintaining a serum sodium level >160 meq/L. *Crit Care Med*. 2004;32(6):1438–1439.

34. Chiaretti A et al. The influence of hemocoagulative disorders on the outcome of children with head injury. *Pediatr Neurosurg*. 2001;34:131–137.

35. Carrick MM et al. Subsequent development of thrombocytopenia and coagulopathy in moderate and severe head injury: support for serial laboratory examination. *J Trauma*. 2005;58:725–730.

36. Keenan HT, Bratton SL. Epidemiology and outcomes of pediatric traumatic brain injury. *Dev Neurosci*. 2006;28:256–263.

37. Duhaime AC et al. Nonaccidental head injury in infants—the "shaken-baby syndrome". *N Engl J Med*. 1998;338:1822–1829.

38. Hiler M et al. Predictive value of initial computerized tomography scan, intracranial pressure, and state of autoregulation in patients with traumatic brain injury. *J Neurosurg*. 2006;104(5):731–737.

39. Pillai S et al. Prognostic factors in children with severe diffuse brain injuries: a study of 74 patients. *Pediatr Neurosurg*. 2001;34(2):98–103.

40. Bullock MR et al. Appendix II: evaluation of relevant computed tomographic scan findings. *Neurosurgery*. 2006;58(3):S62.

41. Maas AI et al. Prognostic value of computerized tomography scan characteristics in traumatic brain injury: results from the IMPACT study. *J Neurotrauma*. 2007;24(2):303–314.

42. Ashwal S et al. Susceptibility-weighted imaging and proton magnetic resonance spectroscopy in assessment of outcome after pediatric traumatic brain injury. *Arch Phys Med Rehabil*. 2006;87:850–858.

43. Ashwal S, Holshouser BA, Tong KA. Use of advanced neuroimaging techniques in the evaluation of pediatric traumatic brain injury. *Dev Neurosci*. 2006;28:309–326.

44. Wilde EA et al. Diffusion tensor imaging in the corpus callosum in childre n after moderate to severe traumatic brain injury. *J Neurotrauma*. 2006;23:1412–1426.

45. Mansfield RT, Kochanek PM. Traumatic head or spinal injury. In: McCloskey O, ed. *Textbook of Pediatric Transport Medicine*. Philadelphia, PA: Mosby; 1995.

46. Lev R, Rosen P. Prophylactic lidocaine use preintubation: a review. *J Emerg Med*. 1994;12(4):499–506.

47. Skippen P et al. Effect of hyperventilation on regional cerebral blood flow in head-injured children. *Crit Care Med*. 1997;25(8):1402–1409.

48. Coates BM et al. Influence of definition and location of hypotension on outcome following severe pediatric traumatic brain injury. *Crit Care Med*. 2005;33(11):2645–2650.

49. Ducrocq SC et al. Epidemiology and early predictive factors of mortality and outcome in children with traumatic severe brain injury: experience of a French pediatric trauma center. *Pediatr Crit Care Med*. 2006;7(5):461–467.

50. Anderson VA et al. Identifying factors contributing to child and family outcome 30 months after traumatic brain injury in children. *J Neurol Neurosurg Psychiatry*. 2005;76(3):401–408.

51. Feldman Z et al. Effect of head elevation on intracranial pressure, cerebral perfusion pressure, and cerebral blood flow in head-injured patients. *J Neurosurg*. 1992;76(2):207–211.

52. Aldrich EF et al. Diffuse brain swelling in severely head-injured children. A report from the NIH Traumatic Coma Data Bank. *J Neurosurg*. 1992;76(3):450–454.

53. Lundberg N. Continuous recording and control of ventricular fluid pressure in neurosurgical practice. *Acta Psychiatr Scand Suppl.* 1960;36(149):1–193.
54. Pfenninger J et al. Treatment and outcome of the severely head injured child. *Intensive Care Med.* 1983;9(1):13–16.
55. Esparza J et al. Outcome in children with severe head injuries. *Childs Nerv Syst.* 1985;1(2):109–114.
56. Sharples PM et al. Cerebral blood flow and metabolism in children with severe head injury. Part 1: relation to age, Glasgow Coma Score, outcome, intracranial pressure, and time after injury. *J Neurol Neurosurg Psychiatry.* Feb 1995;58(2):145–152.
57. Shapiro K, Marmarou A. Clinical applications of the pressure-volume index in treatment of pediatric head injuries. *J Neurosurg.* 1982;56(6):819–825.
58. Elias-Jones AC et al. Management and outcome of severe head injuries in the Trent region 1985-90. *Arch Dis Child.* 1992;67:1430–1435.
59. Downard C et al. Relationship of cerebral perfusion pressure and survival in pediatric brain-injured patients. *J Trauma.* 2000;49:654–658.
60. Schneider GH et al. Influence of body position on jugular venous oxygen saturation, intracranial pressure and cerebral perfusion pressure. *Acta Neurochir Suppl (Wien).* 1993;59:107–112.
61. Silvay G. Ketamine. *Mt Sinai J Med.* 1983;50(4):300–304.
62. Bar-Joseph G et al. Effectiveness of ketamine in decreasing intracranial pressure in children with intracranial hypertension. *J Neurosurg Pediatr.* 2009;4(1):40–46.
63. Bray RJ. Propofol infusion syndrome in children. *Paediatr Anaesth.* 1998;8(6):491–499.
64. Cray SH, Robinson BH, Cox PN. Lactic acidemia and bradyarrhythmia in a child sedated with propofol. *Crit Care Med.* 1998;26(12):2087–2092.
65. Parke TJ et al. Metabolic acidosis and fatal myocardial failure after propofol infusion in children: five case reports. *BMJ.* 1992;305(6854):613–616.
66. Canivet JL et al. Massive ketonuria during sedation with propofol in a 12 year old girl with severe head trauma. *Acta Anaesthesiol Belg.* 1994;45(1):19–22.
67. Hsiang JK et al. Early, routine paralysis for intracranial pressure control in severe head injury: is it necessary? *Crit Care Med.* 1994;22(9):1471–1476.
68. Muizelaar JP, Lutz HA III, Becker DP. Effect of mannitol on ICP and CBF and correlation with pressure autoregulation in severely head-injured patients. *J Neurosurg.* 1984;61(4):700–706.
69. Muizelaar JP et al. Mannitol causes compensatory cerebral vasoconstriction and vasodilation in response to blood viscosity changes. *J Neurosurg.* 1983;59(5):822–828.
70. James HE. Methodology for the control of intracranial pressure with hypertonic mannitol. *Acta Neurochir (Wien).* 1980;51(3-4):161–172.
71. Kaufmann AM, Cardoso ER. Aggravation of vasogenic cerebral edema by multiple-dose mannitol. *J Neurosurg.* 1992;77(4):584–589.
72. Bullock RM, Chesnut RM, Clifton GL, Ghajar J, Marion DW, Narayan RK, Newell DW, Pitts LH, Rosner MJ, Walters BC, Wilberger JE. Management and prognosis of severe traumatic brain injury. part 1: guidelines for the management of severe traumatic brain injury. Use of mannitol. *J Neurotrauma.* 2000;17:521–525.
73. Becker DP, Vries JK. The alleviation of increased intracranial pressure by the chronic administration of osmotic agents. In: Brook M, Dietz H, eds. *Intracranial Pressure.* Berlin, Germany: Springer; 1972:309–315.
74. Feig PU, McCurdy DK. The hypertonic state. *N Engl J Med.* 1977;297(26):1444–1454.
75. Prough DS et al. Regional cerebral blood flow following resuscitation from hemorrhagic shock with hypertonic saline. Influence of a subdural mass. *Anesthesiology.* 1991;75(2):319–327.
76. Shackford SR et al. Hypertonic saline resuscitation of patients with head injury: a prospective, randomized clinical trial. *J Trauma.* 1998;44(1):50–58.
77. Walsh JC, Zhuang J, Shackford SR. A comparison of hypertonic to isotonic fluid in the resuscitation of brain injury and hemorrhagic shock. *J Surg Res.* 1991;50(3):284–292.
78. Qureshi AI, Suarez JI. Use of hypertonic saline solutions in treatment of cerebral edema and intracranial hypertension. *Crit Care Med.* 2000;28(9):3301–3313.
79. Nakayama S et al. Infusion of very hypertonic saline to bled rats: membrane potentials and fluid shifts. *J Surg Res.* 1985;38(2):180–186.
80. Arjamaa O et al. Plasma ANP during hypertonic NaCl infusion in man. *Acta Physiol Scand.* 1992;144(2):113–119.
81. Moss GS, Gould SA. Plasma expanders. An update. *Am J Surg.* 1988;155(3):425–434.
82. Peterson B et al. Prolonged hypernatremia controls elevated intracranial pressure in head-injured pediatric patients. *Crit Care Med.* 2000;28(4):1136–1143.
83. Khanna S et al. Use of hypertonic saline in the treatment of severe refractory posttraumatic intracranial hypertension in pediatric traumatic brain injury. *Crit Care Med.* 2000;28(4):1144–1151.
84. Sterns RH, Riggs JE, Schochet SS Jr. Osmotic demyelination syndrome following correction of hyponatremia. *N Engl J Med.* 1986;314(24):1535–1542.
85. Qureshi AI, Suarez JI, Bhardwaj A. Malignant cerebral edema in patients with hypertensive intracerebral hemorrhage associated with hypertonic saline infusion: a rebound phenomenon? *J Neurosurg Anesthesiol.* 1998;10(3):188–192.
86. Cruz J et al. Cerebral extraction of oxygen and intracranial hypertension in severe, acute, pediatric brain trauma: preliminary novel management strategies. *Neurosurgery.* 2002;50(4):774–779; discussion 779–780.
87. Stiefel MF et al. Brain tissue oxygen monitoring in pediatric patients with severe traumatic brain injury. *J Neurosurg.* 2006;105(4 suppl):281–286.
88. Cordobes F et al. Post-traumatic diffuse brain swelling: isolated or associated with cerebral axonal injury. Clinical course and intracranial pressure in 18 children. *Childs Nerv Syst.* 1987;3(4):235–238.
89. Kasoff SS et al. Aggressive physiologic monitoring of pediatric head trauma patients with elevated intracranial pressure. *Pediatr Neurosci.* 1988;14(5):241–249.
90. Bruce DA et al. Outcome following severe head injuries in children. *J Neurosurg.* 1978;48(5):679–688.
91. Berger MS et al. Outcome from severe head injury in children and adolescents. *J Neurosurg.* 1985;62(2):194–199.
92. Piatt JH Jr, Schiff SJ. High dose barbiturate therapy in neurosurgery and intensive care. *Neurosurgery.* 1984;15(3):427–444.
93. Demopoulos HB et al. The free radical pathology and the microcirculation in the major central nervous system disorders. *Acta Physiol Scand Suppl.* 1980;492:91–119.

94. Kassell NF et al. Alterations in cerebral blood flow, oxygen metabolism, and electrical activity produced by high dose sodium thiopental. *Neurosurgery*. 1980;7(6):598–603.

95. Marion DW et al. The use of moderate therapeutic hypothermia for patients with severe head injuries: a preliminary report. *J Neurosurg*. 1993;79(3):354–362.

96. Hutchison JS et al. Hypothermia therapy after traumatic brain injury in children. *N Engl J Med*. 2008;358(23): 2447–2456.

97. Cho DY, Wang YC, Chi CS. Decompressive craniotomy for acute shaken/impact baby syndrome. *Pediatr Neurosurg*. 1995;23(4):192–198.

98. Levy DI et al. Controlled lumbar drainage in pediatric head injury. *J Neurosurg*. 1995;83(3):453–460.

99. Vespa PM et al. Nonconvulsive electrographic seizures after traumatic brain injury result in a delayed, prolonged increase in intracranial pressure and metabolic crisis. *Crit Care Med*. 2007;35(12):2830–2836.

100. Abend NS et al. Non-convulsive seizures are common in critically ill children. *Neurology*. 2011;76(12):1071–1077.

101. Young B et al. Failure of prophylactically administered phenytoin to prevent post-traumatic seizures in children. *Childs Brain*. 1983;10(3):185–192.

102. Lewis RJ et al. Clinical predictors of post-traumatic seizures in children with head trauma. *Ann Emerg Med*. 993;22(7):1114–1118.

103. Abend NS et al. Use of EEG monitoring and management of non-convulsive seizures in critically ill patients: a survey of neurologists. *Neurocrit Care*. 2010;12(3):382–389.

8 | Status Epilepticus and Seizures

JOSHUA L. GOLDSTEIN and MELISSA G. CHUNG

■ INTRODUCTION

Seizures and status epilepticus (SE) have been described as early as 600 to 700 BC (1). In medical writings from the early 1700s, writers acknowledged the often fatal outcome of SE (1). Despite advances in medical treatment since that time, SE remains a neurologic emergency, and it is a common cause of admission to the intensive care unit (ICU). Furthermore, physicians must be vigilant about monitoring for seizures in the ICU due to the multiple risk factors that critically ill children have for convulsive and nonconvulsive seizures. This chapter focuses on SE and seizures in critically ill children above one month of age except when noted otherwise.

The precise definition of SE has evolved over the years and physicians still debate the required duration of a seizure (2). The International League Against Epilepsy defines SE as "a seizure that persists for a sufficient length of time or is repeated frequently enough that recovery between attacks does not occur" (3). For the purposes of this chapter, SE is defined as a seizure lasting more than 30 minutes or a series of seizures without return to baseline over a 30 minute period, which is the most common criteria used in studies published over the last three decades.

■ EPIDEMIOLOGY AND RISK FACTORS FOR CONVULSIVE SE

Children have a predilection for prolonged seizures; approximately 12% of first unprovoked seizures last more than 30 minutes (4). SE is a common neurologic problem in the pediatric age group with a reported incidence of 10:100,000 to 58:100,000 (5–11). Younger children are at higher risk for convulsive SE than older children or adults; the incidence in the first year of life may be as high as 1:1,000 (6,7).

The most common cause of SE in children is an acute symptomatic etiology. Acute symptomatic seizures are defined as seizures occurring at the time of a systemic insult or in close temporal association with a documented brain insult (12). Common acute symptomatic etiologies include fever, hypoxic-ischemic injury, cerebrovascular disease, systemic infection, and central nervous system (CNS) infection (Table 8.1). Studies report that acute symptomatic seizures, including febrile seizures, are responsible for 30% to over 50% of episodes of SE in children (6,7,11,13–15). A meta-analysis of studies from 1970 to 2005 concluded that SE in children is due to acute symptomatic seizures in 26%, febrile seizures in 22%, and remote symptomatic etiologies in 33% (16). The reported incidence is similar in most non-Western countries (11,17,18). However, some developing countries, such as Kenya, report a higher incidence of acute symptomatic seizures due to infection (19). Acute symptomatic etiologies also are more commonly seen in children under the age of 2 than in older children (11,20,21). Remote symptomatic etiologies such as a history of birth injury, cortical malformation, or preexisting neurologic abnormalities also increase the risk of SE (7,10).

A large number of children with epilepsy will develop SE at least once. A community-based cohort of 613 children with epilepsy in Connecticut reported that 7.3% had at least 1 episode of unprovoked SE. Further, in 16 of the 45 children, SE was their initial seizure type (22). A Dutch

■ **Table 8.1** Common Etiologies for Status Epilepticus and Seizures in the Pediatric Intensive Care Unit

Acute symptomatic	Febrile	Remote symptomatic	Structural lesion
	Cerebrovascular disease		Perinatal/prenatal injury
	Ischemic stroke		Prior traumatic brain injury
	Hemorrhagic stroke		Prior stroke
	Sinovenous thrombosis		**Genetic/chromosomal disorder**
	Hypoxia/anoxia		*With acute provocation*
	Traumatic brain injury		Medication nonadherence
	Provoked		Acute illness/fever
	Nonaccidental trauma		Subtherapeutic antiepileptic
	CNS infection		drug levels
	Non-CNS infection	Progressive neurologic	*Metabolic disorders*
	Upper respiratory		Amino and organic acidopathies
	Gastroenteritis		Storage disorders
	Sepsis		**Mitochondrial disorders**
	Hypertensive encephalopathy		**Leukodystrophy**
	Toxic		*Tumor*
	Chemotherapy		Primary CNS
	Immunosuppression		Metastatic to CNS
	Theophyline		*Autoimmune*
	Tricyclic antidepressants		Limbic encephalitis
	Cocaine		CNS vasculitis (primary or
	Electrolyte abnormalities		secondary)
	Withdrawal	Epilepsy syndromes	Benign focal epilepsies of
	Benzodiazepines		childhood
	Alcohol		Panayiotopoulos syndrome
	Baclofen		Benign rolandic epilepsy
	Postinfectious/Autoimmune		Absence status epilepticus
	Acute demyelinating		
	encephalomyelitis		

Abbreviation: CNS, central nervous system.

cohort reported similar numbers, with 9.5% of children with epilepsy having at least 1 episode of unprovoked SE (23). However a Finnish population based study reports a much higher incidence of 27% (24). The greatest risk for prolonged seizures is during the first 2 years after diagnosis of epilepsy (24). Other risk factors for SE in children with preexisting epilepsy include focal seizures and/or focal electroencephalography (EEG) abnormalities (odds ratio [OR], 2.2–6.51), recent intracranial procedures (OR, 22.1), and presentation with SE as their first seizure (22,25). Children with some specific epilepsy syndromes, including Dravet syndrome (severe myoclonic epilepsy of infancy) and Panayiotopoulos syndrome (benign childhood autonomic epilepsy), are at higher risk of prolonged seizures (Figure 8.1) (15). Genetics may contribute to risk of SE as well; monozygotic twins have a higher concordance rate for SE than dizygotic twins (26).

Many children that present with SE do not have a history of seizures or epilepsy. Singh et al (13) reported that 10% of children present with SE as their first seizure. In the ICU, the percentage of children with SE as their first seizure is even higher; one study found that 71% of children admitted to the pediatric ICU (PICU) with a diagnosis of SE do not have a prior history of seizures (20). The discrepancy in these numbers may be due to the bias towards more serious acute symptomatic etiologies in critical care populations.

In addition, children with SE often require care in the PICU (20,27–29). A retrospective review of admissions to a tertiary care hospital PICU in Canada revealed that 1.6% of all admissions between 1976 and 1986 were for SE (29). The absolute number of admissions varies between tertiary care centers due to location and size of the ICU. Over a 5 year period in three different

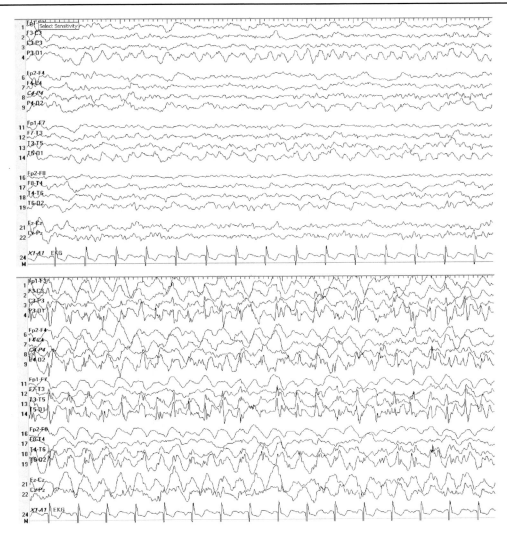

FIGURE 8.1 Five-year-old boy with a history of febrile seizures admitted with refractory status epilepticus with clinical seizures characterized by right sided jerking that required a midazolam drip for control. Electroencephalogram (EEG) showed occipital lobe seizures and stereotyped occipital discharges consistent with a diagnosis of benign occipital epilepsy of childhood. This image shows a left occipital lobe seizure (displayed at a sensitivity of 15 µV) that spreads to the right occipital lobe as the seizure progresses.

institutions, the absolute number of reported admissions for SE ranged from 25 to 218 (20,27,28). Admission to the PICU for any type of seizure is even higher; a total of 554 admissions to the PICU were reported over a 5 year period at one tertiary care center (20). Of note, these numbers do not include the number of children who developed SE or seizures after admission to the hospital.

The true incidence of seizures and SE in the PICU is even higher when nonconvulsive seizures are included. Over the last decade, the use of continuous EEG has led to an increased awareness of the prevalence of nonconvulsive seizures and nonconvulsive SE in critically ill children. Some children have preceding clinical seizures (Figure 8.2) but others may present only with nonspecific changes in mental status or coma. In a retrospective study of 236 patients admitted to the ICU with coma (11% were children aged 1 month through 15 years), 8% of patients had nonconvulsive SE (30). In another large retrospective study at a tertiary care hospital, 16.3% of children monitored with video EEG over 3 years had nonconvulsive seizures; none of these children presented first with convulsive seizures during

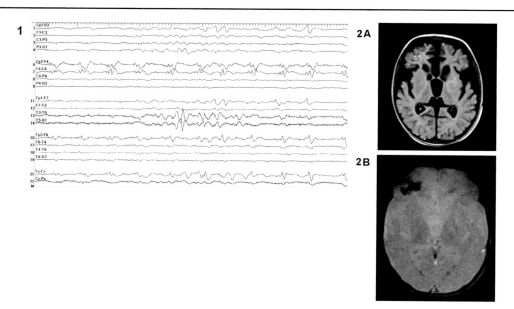

FIGURE 8.2 Seven-week-old boy with cardiorespiratory failure due to pertussis who was placed on extracorporeal membrane oxygenation. Patient initially had clinical seizures with right hand clonic movements. After convulsive seizures abated, continuous EEG (sensitivity 5 μV) revealed nonconvulsive seizures from the right frontal lobe that required a midazolam drip for cessation. MRI brain done 1 month later showed diffuse atrophy, ex vacuo hydrocephalus, and focal encephalomalacia on axial FLAIR (fluid-attenuated inversion recovery) images (A) and multifocal gradient susceptibility consistent with prior hemorrhage, most notable in the right frontal lobe (B).

that admission and 43% had no preexisting neurologic conditions (31). Similarly, 2 studies concluded that approximately 45% of children monitored by continuous EEG have nonconvulsive seizures and 69% to 75% of them only have electrographic seizures, and thus would not be detected without EEG monitoring. Common etiologies for isolated electrographic seizures include acute infarcts, cerebral edema, and diffuse hypoxic-ischemic encephalopathy (32,33). Even these numbers may underestimate the incidence of nonconvulsive seizures because some electrographic seizures are detectable only on intracortical EEG (34).

■ CRITICALLY ILL CHILDREN WITH INCREASED RISK FOR SEIZURES

Hypoxic-Ischemic Encephalopathy

Hypoxic injury is a common cause for SE in adults; 15% to 44% of adults with cardiac arrest will have seizures or postanoxic myoclonus (35). Anoxia is a less common reason for seizures in children, likely due to the lower

incidence of cardiac arrest in the PICU than in adult ICU (6). Nonetheless, children with global hypoxia-anoxia (e.g., cardiopulmonary arrest) are at increased risk for seizures. EEG monitoring of 19 children during hypothermia after cardiac arrest revealed that 47% of the patients developed seizures, approximately two-thirds of which were nonconvulsive (36).

Extracorporeal Membrane Oxygenation

Children placed on extracorporeal membrane oxygenation (ECMO) are an important group of patients in the PICU that are at high risk for seizures. Complications of ECMO include intracranial hemorrhage, infarction, hypoperfusion, microemboli, and electrolyte abnormalities which all may be symptomatic etiologies for seizures. Furthermore, children who require ECMO usually have a diagnosis that increases the risk of seizures such as cardiac failure, respiratory failure, or sepsis. Approximately 40% of children who survive ECMO as a neonate have a history of acute symptomatic seizures (37). One study reported that 11.5% of pediatric patients older than 1 month of age placed on ECMO developed seizures during the acute period (38). However, the incidence of seizures was higher in children with sepsis as well, so it is difficult to discern the effect of ECMO versus infection as risk factors for seizures (38).

Traumatic Brain Injury

Children are twice as likely as adults to experience early posttraumatic seizures, which are defined as seizures occurring less than 7 days after injury (39). The risk of seizures rises with increasing severity of injury, from 1% to 2% in mild traumatic brain injury to 20% to 39% in severe injuries (39–43). Children under 2 years of age are at greatest risk for developing seizures (OR, 2.96 for children < 2 years compared to children > 12 years of age) (43). Early recognition and treatment of seizures is important to minimize cerebral metabolic demand, prevent hyperthermia, and prevent elevation of intracranial pressure. The use of prophylactic antiepileptics (AEDs) to prevent early posttraumatic seizures in pediatric patients "may be considered" in severe traumatic brain injury according to a consensus guideline; however prophylactic AEDs are not recommended to prevent late posttraumatic seizures (after 7 days from injury) as there is no evidence that this tactic is effective (44). During early resuscitation in the PICU, controlling seizures can improve management and stability, but beyond early stabilization, this approach is likely unnecessary (45).

Children with a history of nonaccidental (inflicted) trauma are at particularly high risk for posttraumatic seizures, possibly due to the multiple mechanisms of possible injury (shear injury, diffuse axonal injury, ischemic infarct from vascular injury, hemorrhage, contusions, anoxia). In a study of 14 children with varying degrees of intracranial injury, 79% had posttraumatic seizures within the first 72 hours of admission. Seizures in 8 of the children were considered "difficult to control" (46). A large French study also reported that 73% of children with shaken baby syndrome presented with or developed seizures during the acute period (47).

Infection

One of the most common neurologic complications of CNS infections is acute symptomatic seizures. In addition to direct invasion by the pathogen and increased inflammation, CNS infection increases the risk of seizures by causing intracranial abnormalities (eg, hydrocephalus, abscess, ischemia, hemorrhage, sinus venous thrombosis), electrolyte abnormalities (eg, hyponatremia from syndrome of inappropriate antidiuretic hormone

hypersecretion, cerebral salt wasting), and/or fever. Approximately a quarter of patients with any type of CNS infection (meningitis, encephalitis, brain abscess, empyema) develop provoked seizures (48,49). Thirty-one percent to 50% of infants and children have seizures during acute bacterial meningitis (Figure 8.3) and one study reported that 13% of children in the PICU with meningitis developed SE (29). Acute seizures in bacterial meningitis are predictive of poor outcome and as is the development of late seizures (50,51). One contributing factor to these findings is that children with acute seizures are more likely to have structural lesions than those without seizures (50,51).

Seizures and SE also frequently occur with viral encephalitis. In one study, 40% of children in the PICU with viral encephalitis developed SE (29). Most of the research on seizures in the setting of viral encephalitis focuses on herpes simplex virus (HSV) encephalitis, which has a predilection for the temporal lobe. Most studies estimate that 40% to 60% of patients with HSV will have seizures acutely (52,53). However, one case series from India reported that as many as 89% of patients will have seizures (54). The predictive value of provoked seizures in children with viral encephalitis is controversial. Some studies conclude that multiple acute symptomatic seizures and SE are poor prognostic factors in children with viral encephalitis whereas other researchers report that there is no difference in outcome between patients with and without seizures (55,56).

Influenza infections are frequently seen in the PICU, and a small percentage of children with influenza, with or without encephalopathy, develop seizures. One study reported that 6.5% of children admitted with influenza over a 4 year period developed seizures; approximately 50% of them were deemed febrile seizures, 14% were acute symptomatic, and 37% occurred in children with preexisting neurologic problems (remote symptomatic with acute provocation) (57). A similar incidence (6%) of seizures was reported in children admitted to a Chinese hospital in 2009 with H1N1; children in the ICU are more likely to experience seizures, presumably because these children are the sickest (58). However, the overall incidence of seizures with influenza infection is lower than reported in these studies since most children do not require admission for influenza infection; a Morbidity and Mortality Weekly Report from 2009 reported that only 2.7% of children in Dallas with influenza had acute symptomatic seizures, 50% of which were due to influenza encephalopathy (59).

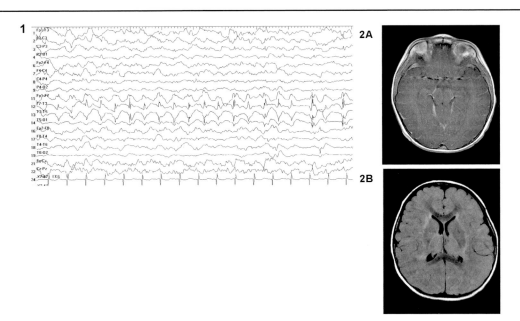

FIGURE 8.3 Twenty-month-old boy with meningitis who developed refractory status epilepticus. Patient initially had clinical seizures with nystagmus, upper extremity jerking which evolved into subtle clinical seizures with nystagmus alone. After clinical seizures stopped on a midazolam drip, continuous EEG (sensitivity 15 μV) shows right occipital lobe spikes and slow wave discharges consistent with an electrographic seizure; (2) MRI of the brain with and without contrast revealed on axial FLAIR images, diffuse patchy areas of increased signal in the subcortical and periventricular white matter, internal and external capsules, and thalami (A) and on axial postcontrast T1 images, diffuse leptomeningeal enhancement (B).

The risk of seizures is not confined to the period of acute infection, and may extend to the postinfectious period. Seventeen percent to 47% of children with acute disseminated encephalomyelitis have seizures at some point in their disease course and many present with seizures. One study has documented prolonged focal motor seizures in 70% of the younger patients, with 82% of these patients going on to develop SE (60,61).

Cerebrovascular Disease

Stroke is less prevalent in children than in adults; however, children are more likely to present with seizures or develop early seizures after cerebral ischemia (Figure 8.4). A population based study in the Greater Cincinnati area reported that 3.1% of adults experienced acute seizures with ischemic stroke; in contrast, a population based study of children (excluding neonates) in the same region reported an incidence of acute seizures in 58% of children (62,63). The incidence of seizures is higher with hemorrhagic than ischemic stroke.

Children with sickle cell disease are a high risk group for cerebrovascular disease including ischemic stroke, hemorrhage stroke, transient ischemic attacks, and cerebral sinus venous thrombosis. They are approximately 10 times more likely than the general population to have seizures (12%–14% of patients) (64–66). Children with seizures are more likely to have cerebral hypoperfusion and vasculopathy. Seizures can be secondary to remote symptomatic epilepsy related to prior cerebral injury but in up to one-third of sickle cell patients, seizures are the presenting symptom of acute stroke (65).

Children with cerebral venous thrombosis also are at high risk for seizures. The seizures may be the heralding sign of a cerebral venous thrombosis in approximately 30% to 50% of adults (67–69). In several multicenter studies, another 7% to 10% of patients had early seizures within 2 weeks of diagnosis (67–69). Studies report a higher incidence of seizures as a presenting symptom in infants than children with cerebral venous thrombosis (50%–60%) (70–73). Since a large percentage of critically ill children have risk factors for cerebral venous thrombosis (eg, dehydration, infection), clinicians should consider cerebral venous thrombosis as a possible etiology for new onset seizures in the PICU.

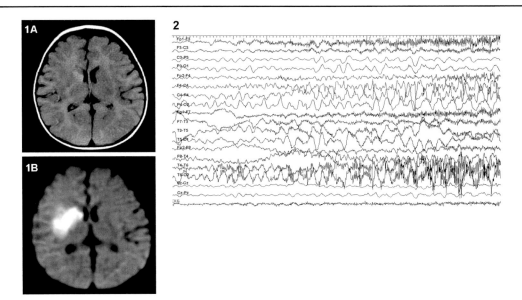

FIGURE 8.4 Six-month-old girl with a right middle cerebral artery stroke with periods of decreased responsiveness. MRI imaging showed (1), Increased FLAIR signal in the right basal ganglia (A) and diffusion restriction in a right middle cerebral artery distribution (B). (2), Continuous EEG monitoring (sensitivity of 20 μV) found that these episodes correlated with electrographic seizures.

Congenital Heart Defects

Children with congenital heart defects often have multiple risk factors for seizure including chronic hypoxia with risk of acute hypoxia during bypass surgery or periods of cardiac decompensation, hemorrhage, prematurity, thromboemboli, and metabolic disturbances. They are most vulnerable during the postoperative period. A study in San Francisco found that 13% of 114 infants had EEG seizures in the postoperative period after repair of a congenital heart defect; 22% of infants with hypoplastic left heart syndrome had postoperative seizures (74). A similar incidence is reported in a Philadelphia cohort and the Boston Circulatory Arrest study (75,76). Nonconvulsive seizures also occur frequently in this patient population (31).

Hypertensive Encephalopathy

Hypertension is a common problem in the critical care unit, and is often secondary to medications (steroids, chemotherapy/immunosuppressant medications), renal disease, or other primary medical problems. Children with hypertensive encephalopathy or posterior reversible encephalopathy syndrome often present with seizures along with encephalopathy, visual changes, headache, or other neurologic dysfunction (Figure 8.5). Seizures may be single, multiple, focal, or generalized (77,78).

■ TREATMENT

Evaluation of the patient's vital signs and an assessment of airway, breathing, and circulation (with appropriate interventions) should occur at the same time as AED treatment is initiated. Oxygenation should be maintained with supplemental oxygen when appropriate. There is no consensus as to a treatment approach for SE with respect to either medication selection or dosing, and therapy is highly variable between institutions and practitioners. A guiding general principle in the medical treatment of SE with AEDs is to rapidly administer appropriate medications at appropriate doses. Common errors include medication underdosing, excessive intervals between medications, and inappropriate medication choices and routes of administration. AEDs may impact the airway, breathing, and circulation, so close monitoring is essential. Our management pathway is provided in Figures 8.6A and 8.6B.

Benzodiazepines including diazepam, midazolam, and lorazepam are the most commonly used first-line AEDs for SE. Intravenous or rectal routes of administration are usually preferred for these drugs given their more rapid onset of action. Dosing recommendations are highly variable as are the number of repeated doses, although most will give 2 or 3 total doses of a benzodiazepine. Frequent dosing of small or inadequate

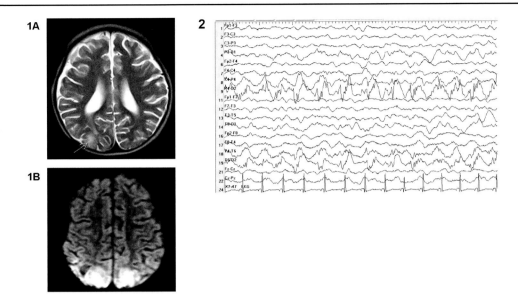

FIGURE 8.5 Three-year-old girl status post stem cell transplant for clear cell carcinoma and central nervous system metastases who presented hypertension after cyclosporine, altered mental status, and visual problems. Imaging findings were compatible with a diagnosis of posterior reversible encephalopathy syndrome. (1), MRI of the brain: T2 sequence shows areas of increased signal in the bilateral parietal occipital lobes, predominantly on the right side (A); diffusion weight imaging also shows diffusion restriction in a similar distribution (B). (2), Continuous EEG monitoring (10–20 international system convention) shows right occipital electrographic seizures without clinical correlate (displayed at sensitivity of 15 µV).

individual doses should be avoided as this practice only prolongs the time to achieving a therapeutic level of the AED. Rather, higher individual doses should be used either once or twice to allow for the more timely institution of a second AED if needed.

Fosphenytoin is often considered the second AED for SE treatment. This prodrug of phenytoin converts to phenytoin within 15 minutes of infusion. Care in dosing is important as it is dosed in phenytoin equivalents (PE) rather than milligrams. A standard initial loading dose for SE is 20 PE/kg, although some use lower doses. Advantages of fosphenytoin over phenytoin include a lower risk of cardiac dysfunction with acute infusion, lower rates of phlebitis, and less severe tissue necrosis if the medication extravasates from the vein during infusion. Although it can be infused at a significantly faster rate than phenytoin, fosphenytoin should not be infused at a rate greater than 3 PE/kg/minute (or, over 7 minutes for a 20 PE unit/kg load). A loading dose of 20 PE units/kg often provides a serum phenytoin level of around 20 µg/mL. A second dose of 10 PE/kg (to a total of 30 PE/kg) is often given if the first loading dose fails to terminate SE. The rapidity of the administration of the AED is critical and delays should be strictly avoided.

At our institution, we aim to administer fosphenytoin within 20 minutes of treatment initiation.

Phenobarbital is commonly chosen as the next AED for refractory SE given its long history of use, good efficacy, and the practitioner comfort level with it as a familiar medication. Phenobarbital is given via intravenous infusion at an initial dose of 20 mg/kg. While it is often highly effective, potential adverse effects include substantial respiratory suppression, especially after benzodiazepines have been given, often requiring ventilatory support. Phenobarbital's half-life of 24 to 72 hours also makes the ongoing assessment of clinical neurologic function difficult for a prolonged period. For these reasons many clinicians are now avoiding its use in refractory SE, opting for some of the treatments discussed below. In the infant, many sites use phenobarbital in place of fosphenytoin as a second-line medication based primarily on its long history of use and not any formal study.

After appropriate doses of benzodiazepines and fosphenytoin and sometimes phenobarbital have been given, the selection of subsequent AEDs is even more varied. At this point, having persisting SE despite administration of adequate doses of two AEDs, the patient

A

TIME

0

3 min

8 min

20 min

Witnessed or suspected seizure
Goal is to intervene for seizures lasting more than 5 minutes

STABILIZE AND ASSESS THE PATIENT
1. **Check ABCs**
   Evaluate and maintain the airway - (reposition patient's head/suction)
   Provide 100% oxygen (non-rebreather). Place pulse oximeter.
   Assess and support ventilation
   Check and establish monitoring of vital signs
   (RR, BP, pulse, temperature, pulse oximetry)
2. **Request for Crash Cart and Seizure Medication Box**
   (Note: Fosphenytoin and Lorazepam are stored in the medication refridgerator)
3. **Check vascular access**
4. **Note the time and check time of seizure onset**
5. **Check bedside glucose**
   If glucose < 40 mg/dl., administer 5 ml/kg D10%W
6. **Administer antipyretics as indicated**

SEIZURE DURATION NOW 5 MINUTES
START INITIAL IV OR PR THERAPY
RE-ASSESS ABCs
1. **LORAZEPAM 0.1** mg/kg **IV (Rate 2 mg/min)**
                    OR
2. **DIAZEPAM PR**   Maximum: 20 mg

   Ages 2 - 5 yr: 0.5 mg/kg PR
   Ages 6 - 11 yr: 0.3 mg/kg PR
   Age > 12 yr   0.2 mg/kg PR

   WAIT 3-5 minutes

SEIZURES CONTINUE

1. **LOAD Fosphenytoin 20 mg PE/kg IV**
   RATE = 3 mg PE/kg/minute.
   If patient is already on PHT, give 10 mg PE/kg
2. RE-ASSESS ABCs
3. **CALL PICU and PAGE NEUROLOGY**

SEIZURES CONTINUE

1. **Fosphenytoin 10 mg mg PE/kg IV or Phenobarbital (neonates) up to total of 40 mg/kg IV**
2. **CALL PICU or NICU**
3. Maintain airway, re-assess ABCs.

General Principles
1. Assess ABCs at each step
2. Get a good history and description from a witness
3. Determine **time of onset** of seizure and **whether this is a seizure**
4. Follow sequence of benzodiazepine, Fosphenytoin, Midazolam.
5. **Substitute Phenobarbital for Fosphenytoin in neonates.**
6. Assess risk of morbidity (see page 2)

Keys to effective treatment
1. Begin treatment early, within 3-5 minutes of seizure onset if possible
2. Use adequate doses of effective drugs.

Select Initial labs
1. Electrolytes (Glucose, Na, Ca, Mg)
2. Antiepileptic drug levels
3. CBC

Neonates < 1 month age
1. Load with Phenobarb 20mg/kg IV
2. RE-ASSESS ABCs
3. **Call NICU and page Neurology**
4. Repeat up to 40 mg/kg total dose

SEIZURES STOPPED

1. **Check vital signs**
2. **Additional diagnostic testing**
3. **Consider maintenance Fosphenytoin:**
      5 mg PE/kg/d ÷ q8 hr
   or Phenobarbital
      3-5 mg/kg/d

Figure 8.6 (A) Inpatient Guidelines for management and evaluation of status epilepticus. (*Continued.*)

B

SEIZURES CONTINUE AFTER -
a) 30 Mg PE/Kg Fosphenytoin
OR
b) 40 mg/kg Phenobarbital

Notify Neurology
if not yet paged

TRANSFER
TO ICU

Notify primary
attending if not
yet paged

1. Load with Midazolam IV 100-200 mcg/kg
Should be given in ICU or ER with
cardiopulmonary monitoring
2. Start continuous infusion 100 mcg/kg/hr
3. Increase dose every 15-30 minutes by 25-50
mcg/kg/hr
4. Titrate to cessation of clinical seizure activity
5. Manage these patients with continuous EEG
monitoring

1. If Midazolam contra indicated (allergy or history
of seizure exacerbation) use IV Valproic acid (VPA)
2. Loading Dose 25 mg/kg IV
    Do not use in liver or mitochondrial disease
3. Divide loading dose in 2 over 4hr if >800 mg
4. Maintenance dosing 15 - 60 mg/kg/day

Selected Laboratory Studies

1. Electrolytes
2. Toxicology (serum/urine)
3. LFTs, Coags, Albumin
4. Metabolic screens
    Lactate, Pyr, CPK, ketones, **NH3,**
acylcarntine, amino, organic acids
5. Blood and urine cultures
6. CSF (meninoencephalitis panel, **HHV6,**
EBV, CMV, cytology, lactate)
7. Antiepileptic levels
8. Imaging as indicated (CT, **CTV, MRI,**
MRS, MRV, Diffusion weighting; contrast
enhancement)

Refractory Status Epilepticus in
Neonates
1. Midazolam (see dosing)
2. 50-100 mg **pyridoxine IV** with EEG
monitoring. If no response, then:
3. Add empirically Pyridoxal phosphate 30
mg/kg/d po or ng
Obtain serum and urine and organic acids
pre and post treatment
4. Leucovorin (Folinic acid)

RISK ASSESSMENT FOR MORBIDITY WITH STATUS EPILEPTICUS

1. Acute Symptomatic SE (eg TBI, Meningitis, ICH, Stroke, Encephalitis, Toxin
        Highest mortality and morbidity
2. Febrile Status Epilepticus or Complex Febrile Seizures
        Increased long-term risk of mesial temporal sclerosis
3. Remote Symptomatic Epilepsy - history of previous neurologic injury with new onset seizures
4. Known Epilepsy
        Low mortality and morbidity
5. First Seizure in Idiopathic Epilepsy

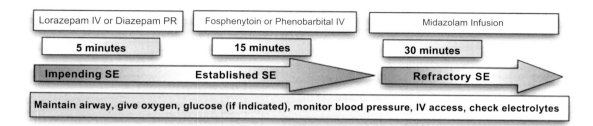

Lorazepam IV or Diazepam PR | Fosphenytoin or Phenobarbital IV | Midazolam Infusion

5 minutes | **15 minutes** | **30 minutes**

Impending SE | **Established SE** | **Refractory SE**

Maintain airway, give oxygen, glucose (if indicated), monitor blood pressure, IV access, check electrolytes

FIGURE 8.6 (B) refractory status epilipticus.

has met the criteria for refractory SE and a neurologist should be consulted if available. Commonly used treatments for refractory SE include valproic acid (Depacon), levetiracetam (Keppra), intravenous anesthetic agents (propofol), potent inhalational anesthetics (isoflurane), and continuous infusions of barbiturates (pentobarbital) or benzodiazepines (midazolam).

Midazolam continuous infusions are usually started at 50 to 100 µg/kg/h and titrated upwards to a range of 600 to 1,200 µg/kg/h. To avoid tachyphylaxis, the infusion rate increases should be aggressive, reaching a maximal dose a few hours after initiation. One commonly used protocol increases the rate by increments of 50 to 100 µg/kg/h every 15 to 20 minutes. Continuous EEG should be instituted if available when continuous infusions of AEDs are used to ensure that nonconvulsive seizures do not persist after convulsive seizures terminate.

Like midazolam, pentobarbital can also be administered as a continuous infusion for refractory SE. It is usually initiated with a loading dose of 6 to 8 mg/kg followed by a continuing infusion at a rate of 0.5 to 1 mg/kg/h and then increased as needed to 3 to 5 mg/kg/h. Pentobarbital, like phenobarbital, is extremely sedating and has a higher associated rate of hypotension than midazolam, often requiring pressor support.

Intravenous valproic acid and levetiracetam have some evidence for their efficacy in SE and many centers are investigating their use in SE treatment. There are some theoretical advantages to these medications. Valproic acid and levetiracetam are considered broad spectrum AEDs and should not exacerbate primary generalized epilepsy as can phenytoin or fosphenytoin. They also are considered less sedating than the benzodiazepines, phenobarbital, or phenytoin, thereby allowing for more precise ongoing neurologic examinations. Valproic acid is most commonly dosed intravenously between 20 and 60 mg/kg (79). A second dose may be given. Levetiracetam is also administered intravenously and doses range from 20 mg/kg to 60 mg/kg or higher (80,81).

The use of anesthetic agents in the treatment of refractory SE is rapidly gaining popularity in adult neurology but has yet to gain as widespread acceptance in the pediatric population (82,83). The most commonly used anesthetic is propofol. This medication has the advantage of a short half-life, allowing reexaminations. Propofol may cause "propofol syndrome" manifest by acidosis, rhabdomyolysis, and cardiac/renal failure. This is more frequent in children than adults, and this risk limits the

duration propofol can be administered. Thiopental has also been utilized for refractory SE with good efficacy. As escalating doses of drugs are used to treat SE, often, protective airway reflexes are lost, and intubation and mechanical ventilation become necessary. For SE not responsive to the above AEDs, potent inhalational anesthetics such as isoflurane have been utilized (84,85).

■ PRIMARY SYSTEMIC COMPLICATIONS FROM SE

Seizures and SE cause local neuronal inflammation/injury, calcium related injury, cytotoxic injury, alterations in glutaminergic and γ-aminobutyric acid receptors, and other changes in the neuronal cell environment. These changes in the neuronal network, the activation of the autonomic nervous system, changes in metabolic state, and the strain of repetitive convulsions can lead to systemic complications (86–92).

The continuous contraction and relaxation of muscles with convulsive SE can lead to muscle breakdown, fever, rhabdomyolysis, and subsequent renal failure (93–97). Fever increases metabolic demand of the brain and augments excitotoxicity and neuroinflammation, worsening ongoing brain injury in acute symptomatic etiologies. Convulsions also increase metabolic demand in the muscle; eventually muscle changes from aerobic to anaerobic respiration, with the production of lactic acid and acidosis (98). Thus, maintenance of adequate hydration is extremely important. Ultimately, muscle relaxants and active cooling may be required. Seizures also alter autonomic and cardiac function. Some patients develop ictal tachycardia, ictal bradycardia, and postictal changes in heart rate variability, while some AEDs induce prolonged corrected QT interval (97,99,100).

Blood pressure usually rises in the acute stage of SE but falls with more prolonged convulsive seizure activity (usually after 30–40 minutes in animal models) (101, 102). Patients with SE also are at increased risk for cardiac failure and arrhythmias. Some patients may display gradual compromise of cardiovascular function with decreased blood pressure and/or heart rate prior to death but acute cardiac decompensation occurs in other patients (103). Cardiac myofilament damage, myocardiac stunning, and myocardiac contraction bands have been described in animal models of SE as well as autopsy of patients who died from SE (104–106). Cardiac injury is suspected to be secondary to unopposed sympathetic activation in SE.

Independent of medication side effects, seizures can affect respiratory status. Ictal hypoxia occurs in 40% or greater of children with generalized seizures (107–109). Neurogenic pulmonary edema is a less common complication (110,111).

Brain metabolism is affected by SE. Initially blood glucose rises with release of catecholamines but glucose normalizes or decreases after 30 to 40 minutes (101,112). Cerebrovascular reserve and blood flow may increase initially but these changes cannot be maintained over time (112–114). With prolonged seizures, cerebral energy demands remain high but stores of oxygen and glucose become depleted; this inequity contributes to cerebral injury in animal models (102,112). Cerebral edema can develop, likely due to the ongoing CNS inflammation but also from an increase in vascularity and compromise of the blood-brain barrier (113,115–117).

■ COMPLICATIONS SECONDARY TO SE TREATMENT

Side effects from AEDs are a common cause of morbidity in children with SE. Respiratory compromise with seizures is a common reason for admission to the PICU; Hussain et al (27) found that 13% of children admitted to the PICU with a diagnosis of seizures required ventilator support. Many of the medications, particularly the first-line benzodiazepines and phenobarbital, are respiratory depressants. In addition, many of the medications, especially when given quickly, cause hypotension which further compromises the child's cardiorespiratory status. Individual AEDs have unique side effects which should be taken to account when choosing an agent and selecting monitoring parameters (Table 8.2). Many AEDs are processed through the hepatic p450 system and may interact with other medications that the patient is receiving; careful attention should be paid to dosing of medications in patients with either liver or renal failure.

Propofol and the risk of fatality with its use deserves special attention. Although propofol is commonly used in the adult ICUs for sedation and burst suppression, children are at high risk for developing propofol infusion syndrome. This syndrome is characterized by rhabdomyolysis, hyperkalemia, liver, cardiac, and renal

failure, and metabolic acidosis (118). Alternative agents should be considered for control of SE; if the medication is used, then children should be carefully monitored for signs and symptoms of propofol infusion syndrome with discontinuation of the drug immediately if they develop.

In some children, valproate may lead to hyperammonia and hepatic encephalopathy. The increase in serum ammonium level is due to several mechanisms, the most important one appearing to be the inhibition of carbamoyl phosphate synthetase I, the enzyme that begins the urea cycle. In these susceptible patients, carnitine can avoid and treat this complication (118).

In children with refractory SE, prolonged sedation/coma compromises hemodynamic function and respiratory drive but the period of immobility may also have complications. The risk of deep venous thrombosis and pulmonary embolism should be considered. Infections, especially pneumonia or tracheitis, are common.

■ MORTALITY RELATED TO SE

Since Louis Calmeil's early clinical description differentiating SE (*état de mal*) from brief seizures in 1824, SE has been viewed as a significant source of mortality. However, short-term mortality (death within the first 30 days of SE) in the pediatric population is much lower than in adults (7,119). Most studies in children report an incidence of short-term mortality of less than 10% (7,14,17,20,21,28,120–124). A systematic review found that short-term mortality in children is approximately 2.7% to 5.2% though the incidence is slightly higher in the PICU (125). Usually, mortality during hospitalization or within 30 days is due to comorbidities and the underlying disease process that led to seizures rather than a direct effect of the seizures. A few rare cases are reported in the studies in which patients died from SE (0%–2%) but the cases included children whose parents elected to defer or limit medical intervention, such as intubation.

■ LONG-TERM SEQUELAE OF SE

In a landmark study of children with SE, Aicardi and Chevrie (126) wrote that "the prognosis of symptomatic status is uniformly poor, whatever the age." Overall,

■ **Table 8.2** Important Side Effects of Antiepileptic Medications

	Side Effect	Medications
Respiratory	Respiratory depression	Phenobarbital, benzodiazepines (clonazepam, diazepam, midazolam, lorazepam), pentobarbital, propofol
	Dyspnea	Valproic acid, lamotrigine, tiagabine
Cardiac	Chest pain	Lamotrigine, tiagabine, pregabalin
	Arrhythmias	Phenytoin, pentobarbital
	Heart block	Carbamazepine
	Prolonged QTc	Phenytoin, fosphenytoin, felbamate
	Shortened QTc	Rufinamide
	Congestive heart failure	Carbamazepine
	Hypotension	Phenytoin, fosphenytoin, phenobarbital, benzodiazepines, pentobarbital, propofol
	Hypertension	Valproic acid, tiagabine
	Bradycardia	Phenytoin, fosphenytoin, phenobarbital, pentobarbital, phenytoin, propofol
	Tachycardia	Phenytoin, fosphenytoin, valproic acid, felbamate, tiagabine
Temperature regulation	Oligohydrosis/hyperthermia	Topiramate, zonisamide
	Hypothermia	Pentobarbital
Electrolyte disturbances	Metabolic acidosis	Topiramate, zonisamide, high dose midazolam (possibly due to solvent), phenytoin, propofol (may be fatal)
	Hyperglycemia	Fosphenytoin
	Hypokalemia	Topiramate
	Hyponatremia	Carbamazepine, oxcarbazepine, valproic acid
Genitourinary	Nephrolithiasis	Topiramate, zonisamide
	Oliguria	Pentobarbital
	Urinary retention	Carbamazepine
	Urinary frequency	Lamotrigine
Gastrointestinal	Liver toxicity	Valproic acid (special caution in mitochondrial disorders), phenytoin, carbamazepine, valproic acid, propofol, felbamate (potentially fatal acute liver failure)
	Hyperammonemia	Valproic acid, topiramate
	Pancreatitis	Valproic acid, carbamazepine, oxcarbazepine
Hematologic	Blood dyscrasias	Phenytoin, fosphenytoin, primidone (megaloblastic anemia, leukopenia), carbamazepine, valproic acid (thrombocytopenia), felbamate (aplastic anemia—100-fold risk), rufinamide (leucopenia), vigabatrin, phenobarbital (megaloblastic anemia)
CNS	Dizziness, ataxia, CNS depression	Phenobarbital, phenytoin, fosphenytoin, primidone, ethosuximide, carbamazepine, valproic acid, felbamate, gabapentin, lamotrigine, topiramate, tiagabine, levetiracetam, oxcarbazepine, zonisamide, pregabalin, rufinamide, pentobarbital

(continued)

■ **Table 8.2** Important Side Effects of Antiepileptic Medications (*continued*)

	Side Effect	Medications
Other	Acute angle closure glaucoma	Topiramate
	Drug induced lupus	Primidone, ethosuximide, phenytoin
	Tissue necrosis with extravasation/local reaction	Phenobarbital, phenytoin, pentobarbital (arterial spasm, thrombophlebitis, gangrene), valproic acid, propofol
	High risk of hypersensitivity reaction	Carbamazepine, valproic acid, lamotrigine, rufinamide, oxcarbazepine

Abbreviation: QTc, QT corrected for heart rate.

Aicardi reported that 11% of patients died during their first episode of SE and 50% of these deaths were related to the seizures. Of survivors, 37% developed permanent neurologic signs and 48% had mental retardation. Of note, Aicardi defined SE as seizures lasting for more than an hour rather than 30 minutes which may have affected outcome. However, a number of studies in the last decade have suggested that the outcome of SE in children may be less dire than previously thought.

At least 50% of children with one episode of SE will have recurrent prolonged seizures even while on prophylactic AEDs. The incidence of recurrence varies in studies, likely due to variability in inclusion criteria and time to follow-up, with incidences ranging from 3% to 56% (5,7,14,15,23,24,125,127–129). Most children who will have recurrence of SE will do so within the first 2 years (24,125). Risk factors for repeated episodes of SE include young age, progressive encephalopathy, and remote symptomatic etiology. Children with preexisting neurologic abnormalities are almost 24 times more likely to have recurrent status than previously healthy children (7,125,128). Certain epilepsy syndromes also are associated with an increased risk of prolonged seizures. Eighty-one percent of children with Panayiotopoulos syndrome and approximately two-thirds of children with severe myoclonic epilepsy of infancy (Dravet syndrome) will have at least 1 more episode of SE (15).

Children with a history of SE are at increased risk of developing epilepsy. The incidence of subsequent diagnosis of epilepsy in patients varies in studies from 13% to 74%, which is most likely secondary to differences in sample selection, length of follow-up after SE, and whether patients with febrile status were included (14,28,122, 25,130). However, the incidence of subsequent epilepsy likely reflects underlying cause for the SE because duration of the first unprovoked seizures does not increase the risk of developing subsequent epilepsy (131–133). In patients with a history of SE, including adults, the risk of developing subsequent epilepsy is highest in patients with anoxia (risk ratio of 19.9) or with structural lesions (risk ratio of 7.1) (130). Among children only, patients with focal SE are the most likely to go on to develop epilepsy, which may be partially due to the fact that this subgroup includes patients with structural lesions (125).

Whether SE leads to new or worsened neurologic deficits and behavioral and cognitive problems is a controversial topic. Animal studies and autopsies of patients who died after SE provide evidence of neuronal injury and cerebral atrophy after prolonged seizures (101,134). However, it is unclear whether these pathologic changes have clinical significance. Some studies conclude that SE does not convey any significant morbidity beyond that expected for the underlying disease process nor a difference between patients with SE compared to other children with childhood onset epilepsy (24). However other studies report that children often develop new neurologic deficits after SE. This discrepancy in results likely relates to the heterogeneity of length of follow-up and outcome measures used in the literature. Overall, it appears that most children return to their neurologic baseline except for those with an acute symptomatic etiology; neurologic deterioration more likely is related to the underlying disease process (14,27,28,120,135,136).

The impact of SE on cognitive outcome is more difficult to evaluate especially since well-documented baseline cognitive testing and formal cognitive testing are rare in studies. Some studies report no difference in mental abilities or intelligence quotient in children with epilepsy with and without SE (120,137,138). However, other studies report that up to 37% of children who were neurologically normal prior to SE developed mental disabilities (139). Of note, this percentage is similar to the percentage of children with SE with acute symptomatic etiologies, so the causal relationship might be with the neurologic disease rather than with the occurrence of SE. A meta-analysis in 1990 concluded that general SE has a "slight adverse effect" upon mental abilities (140). Overall, cognitive and neurologic outcome after SE needs to be addressed on an individual basis, taking into account the child's comorbidities.

Children with a history of refractory SE from acute symptomatic etiologies require special consideration. These patients may have a significantly worse outcome; 100% of patients in one small case series of seven patients with refractory SE went on to develop intractable epilepsy and new neurologic deficits (122).

■ DIAGNOSTIC EVALUATION OF A CHILD WITH SE

In 2006, the American Academy of Neurology (AAN) and the Child Neurology Society published a practice parameter on the assessment of a child with SE (16). Only one of the recommendations is a Level B recommendation, though there are few definitive guidelines for studies. In this section, we offer some suggestions for testing in a patient that presents with SE based upon both the practice parameter and clinical practice at our institution, which is a tertiary care center with a 45-bed PICU with an independent neurocritical care consultation service.

General Guidelines

The AAN and Child Neurology Society guidelines state that obtaining a complete blood count and electrolytes is "common practice," so this basic laboratory evaluation should be completed in all patients. An EEG also may be considered in a child with SE as it may be helpful. In most situations, we would recommend that an EEG be obtained in children with new onset SE, new onset seizures, or if there is concern for nonconvulsive seizures. The use of emergent EEG should be considered if available in situations where there is concern for nonconvulsive seizures, such as when the patients has not experienced ongoing improvement in mental status and/or in the paralyzed patient.

Febrile Child, Without History of Epilepsy

The diagnosis of febrile SE is high on the differential diagnosis for an otherwise healthy child between 6 months and 5 years of age who presents with a prolonged generalized tonic-clonic seizure. Unlike with simple febrile seizures, detailed recommendations have not been published for febrile SE. Certainly, an evaluation should be done for the source of infection/fever. According to the AAN/Child Neurology Society guidelines for SE, blood cultures and lumbar puncture are commonly done if there is a suspicion of systemic or CNS infection, but there is inadequate data to determine whether these studies should or should not be done. In children with a prolonged postictal state, encephalopathy, meningismus, age under 18 months, refractory SE, or focal findings on examination, we recommend that a lumbar puncture be strongly considered to test for bacterial as well as viral (especially HSV) infection. If the child is obtunded or has focal findings on examination, then head imaging should be considered to evaluate for a mass lesion prior to lumbar puncture. A magnetic resonance imaging (MRI) of the brain with and without contrast including imaging of the venous structures is recommended in children with persistent encephalopathy, focal findings on examination, or evidence of increased pressure (including elevated opening pressure on lumbar puncture or papilledema) to evaluate for an intracranial etiology for seizures (such as inflammation, ischemic or hemorrhagic injury, sinus venous thrombosis, or subdural empyema). An EEG is useful to help evaluate for interictal abnormalities or nonconvulsive seizures. If a systemic or CNS infection is suspected, appropriate antimicrobial drugs should not be delayed for definitive diagnosis.

If a child has prolonged hemiconvulsions, especially if recurrent, then the clinician should consider testing of SCN1a (voltage-gated sodium channels) for Dravet syndrome (141). Females (usually with a family history of epilepsy) and a Dravet-like phenotype but negative SCN1a testing also can be tested for protocadherin 19 (epilepsy and mental retardation in females) (142). If a child has fever and other signs of autonomic instability without any other infectious symptoms and the initial diagnostic evaluation is negative, then inflammatory/autoimmune etiologies should be considered. Rheumatologic disorders such as systemic lupus erythematosus can be associated with seizures (85).

Children with limbic encephalitis (eg, due to anti-N-methyl-D-aspartic acid receptor encephalitis) may present with seizures, fever, and cerebral spinal fluid leukocytosis. The leukocytosis may lead to a misdiagnosis of viral encephalitis. These children often will have other signs and symptoms of neurologic dysfunction including behavioral problems and movement disorders

(143). Studies to consider testing for include (but are not limited to) erythrocyte sedimentation rate, C-reactive protein, neopterin, anti-NMDA receptor antibodies, antinuclear antibodies, double-stranded DNA antibodies, antithyroid antibodies, complements, antiphospholipid antibodies, and a paraneoplastic panel including voltage gated potassium channels.

Child With Known History of Epilepsy

As noted earlier in this chapter, children with known epilepsy, particularly those with history of SE, often will have prolonged seizures. Initial evaluation should focus on identifying provoking factors including missed AED doses, sleep deprivation, intercurrent illness, new medications that interact or interfere with AEDs, or hormonal changes. The AAN/Child Neurology Society guidelines recommend that AED levels be considered when a child with epilepsy develops SE (Level B recommendation) (16). If the child also is febrile, then the source of illness should be investigated to look for treatable causes of fever. Lumbar puncture likely may be deferred unless the child is immunosuppressed, has a prolonged postictal period, or has signs/symptoms of CNS infection. If a CNS infection is suspected, it should be treated presumptively.

In general, head imaging does not need to be done routinely. Exceptions to this rule include the following:

1. Patients with a history of or risk for hydrocephalus, especially those with a ventriculoperitoneal shunt, should be evaluated for worsening hydrocephalus and/or shunt malfunction. Standard practice includes a shunt series to ensure that the shunt is intact and head imaging (computed tomography [CT] or MRI) to evaluate size of the ventricles. A neurosurgical consult may be necessary, especially if the child has any other signs or symptoms of increased intracranial pressure.
2. Children at risk for intracranial hemorrhage, such as those with clotting disorders, on anticoagulation, with known history of a vascular malformation, neoplasms (especially known intracranial disease), recent ischemic stroke, or known sinus venous thrombosis. CT scan (and a coagulation profile) should be obtained, especially if there are signs or symptoms of increased intracranial pressure and/or new focal findings on examination.
3. Children with a history of ischemia with continued risk for further strokes. Children at high risk for cerebrovascular disease include those with known

hypercoagulable states (including antiphospholipid syndrome), congenital heart defects, trisomy 21 (from moyamoya syndrome), or sickle cell disease. CT is inadequate for evaluating for ischemic injury; MRI of the brain with diffusion weighted image should be done if the history and examination are concerning for possible ischemic stroke.
4. Children who manifest clinical evidence of increased intracranial pressure such as Cushing triad (hypertension, bradycardia, and abnormal respirations).

Child Without Fever or History of Epilepsy

The AAN, Child Neurology Society, and American Epilepsy Society published guidelines for evaluation of the first nonfebrile seizure in children in 2000 (144). This guideline recommends that an EEG be done and states that MRI of the brain is the preferred imaging modality if imaging is needed. If a child has prolonged Todd paralysis or is not returning to baseline within several hours, then emergent imaging of the brain should be obtained. The guidelines suggest that the clinician strongly consider nonurgent MRI imaging in children with "a significant cognitive or motor impairment of unknown etiology, unexplained abnormalities on neurologic examination, a seizure of partial (focal) onset with or without secondary generalization, an EEG that does not represent a benign partial epilepsy or childhood or primary generalized epilepsy, or in children under 1 year of age." Lumbar puncture is not routinely recommended unless there is suspicion of CNS infection. Toxicology testing and labs can be sent on a case by case basis. The AAN/Child Neurology Society guidelines on SE concur that toxicology testing is a reasonable consideration, though targeted testing is more likely to be helpful than a urine drug screen. There are no other formal guidelines published. A careful neurologic history review of symptoms and family history and physical examination (that includes ophthalmologic examination and evaluation of the skin, including with a Wood lamp) can help direct further testing. For a child without preexisting neurologic deficits, with relatively normal development and history, and with rapid return to baseline, baseline testing often is sufficient.

In some cases, an acute symptomatic etiology may be obvious, such as a recent history of traumatic brain injury, recent stroke, or CNS infection. If there is a clear explanation for seizures, then the baseline testing (electrolytes, EEG, MRI if not previously obtained) might be sufficient for diagnostic studies.

For a child with a known static neurologic disorder without risk of progression (remote symptomatic etiology), such as hypoxic-ischemic encephalopathy, perinatal/prenatal stroke, congenital CNS malformation, or chromosomal abnormality, an EEG, complete blood count, and chemistries should be obtained. A nonurgent MRI of the brain should be considered if the child has not been imaged previously. An emergent CT is indicated if there is a new focal neurologic finding or signs/symptoms of increased intracranial pressure, the child is unstable, or a MRI is not planned or feasible in the near future.

In a previously healthy child, especially infants, with an unrevealing MRI and continued encephalopathy despite control of seizures, the clinician should strongly consider evaluation for CNS infection, especially HSV encephalitis, even in the absence of meningismus or fever. In addition, in the presence of ongoing encephalopathy, an autoimmune encephalopathy should be considered and evaluated as described above.

The AAN/Child Neurology Society states that a clinician may consider testing for inborn errors of metabolism in children with SE when there is clinical indications or initial studies are negative (Class C evidence). A reasonable approach would be to pursue testing for inborn errors of metabolic disorders, specific genetic disorders, and/or mitochondrial testing if the EEG, head imaging, history, and examination do not yield a clear diagnosis and the child has a history of significant developmental delays or other unexplained neurologic problems; alternatively a clinician may elect to start the evaluation immediately if the patient has a history strongly suggestive of a metabolic or genetic problem (especially recurrent episodes of encephalopathy and emesis) or very young age (< 6–9 months). A reasonable first round of testing would be general screening tests for amino acidopathies, urine organic acidopathies, disorders of fatty acid oxidation, and mitochondrial disorders (serum amino acids, urine organic acids, ammonia, urine dip for ketones and reducing substances, liver function testing, acylcarnitine profile, carnitine profile, lactate-pyruvate ratio—serum and also spinal fluid if obtained, Creatine kinase). The clinician should verify that infants had a negative newborn screen if they were born in the United States. A microarray may be helpful as well, particularly if the child has any other dysmorphic features or chronic medical problems in other organ systems. For these children, we often will obtain a magnetic resonance (MR) spectroscopy when the initial MRI is done to avoid repeating head imaging (and associated sedation) unnecessarily. A dilated ophthalmologic examination may yield clues to a diagnosis, such as mitochondrial disease, storage disorders, etc and guide further testing if initial screening studies are negative. A reasonable approach is to approach testing in a stepwise manner after discharge from the hospital. We have been more aggressive with inpatient testing in young infants, explosive onset of epilepsy, or refractory SE without obvious cause.

Mitochondrial disorders deserve special consideration. Even if the lactic acid to pyruvate ratio is normal, testing for a mitochondrial disorder should be strongly considered in children with risk factors including: personal history or family history of sensorineural hearing loss, optic atrophy, short stature/failure to thrive, cardiac disease (especially cardiomyopathy or arrhythmias), diabetes mellitus type I, exercise intolerance, liver disease, ataxia, epilepsia partialis continua, and migraines. If several of these indicators are found in the history (or if characteristic changes are seen on the MRI), then clinicians can consider performing a dilated ophthalmologic examination, echocardiogram, and electrocardiograph for further evidence of mitochondrial disorders. In a child with history that strongly suggests a mitochondrial disorder, early testing with serum studies, such as the mitochondrial common point mutation and deletion panel, and testing for POL-G mutations is reasonable.

A large number of other genetic disorders, such as Rett, aristaless related homeobox, and cyclin-dependent kinase-like 5, may cause SE and developmental delay but we would not recommend routine testing; instead testing for specific genetic disorders should be tailored to the individual patient based on their history and presence/absence of characteristic phenotype.

■ DIAGNOSTIC EVALUATION OF SEIZURES FOR SELECTION PATIENT POPULATIONS IN THE ICU

Children with congenital heart defects are at high risk for seizures. These children may develop cerebrovascular disease (hemorrhagic or ischemic), diffuse hypoxic injury from arrhythmia or poor cardiac function, and electrolyte abnormalities. Emergent MRI of the brain with diffusion weight imaging and gradient echo sequences (or if contraindicated, head CT) should be strongly considered, especially in children with focal seizures, new neurologic findings on examination, or history of recent cardiac surgery or cardiac catheterization.

Children with sickle cell disease also require urgent attention when they present with new onset seizures or seizures with focal deficits because the seizures may secondary to acute stroke (ischemic or hemorrhagic) (65). Any child with sickle cell disease should have emergent head imaging. Head CT can be done first if there is clinical concern for intracranial hemorrhage but an emergent MRI, including diffusion weight imaging, gradient echo sequences, and MR arteriography is strongly recommended to evaluate for an acute ischemic stroke. MR venogram should be considered, particularly if the child has risk factors for or signs and symptoms of dehydration. If an EEG is performed, hyperventilation, which is often utilized as a standard activating procedure, is contraindicated (145).

We also suggest pursuing a more extensive initial evaluation in infants, especially if they are under 6 months of age. Nonaccidental trauma should be considered in the differential and head imaging should be ordered early on if there is high clinical suspicion based on the patient's history or if there is evidence of bruising and/or retinal hemorrhages. For an infant with frequent seizures and normal MRI, consider an intravenous pyridoxine trial to evaluate for pyridoxine dependent seizures. In very young infants with frequent seizures and negative initial studies, the clinician should consider not only the standard metabolic testing (discussed above) but also lumbar puncture since spinal fluid may be useful in the diagnosis of neurotransmitter disorders (neurotransmitters, biopterin/neopterin panel, pyridoxal-5-phosphate level), nonketotic hyperglycinemia (requires simultaneous serum and cerebral spinal fluid amino acids testing), and GLUT-1 deficiency (cerebral spinal fluid glucose-serum glucose ratio).

Evaluation of seizures in children with known oncologic disease must take into account their risk for CNS involvement of their disease, infection (including CNS infections) due to immunosuppression, side effects of their medication, risk of intracranial hemorrhage (from thrombocytopenia), and hypercoagulable state. Head CT should be obtained emergently if the child is coagulopathic or has sudden deterioration in mental status. Ultimately, MRI of the brain with and without contrast should be done; imaging of the venous structures is recommended if the child has been dehydrated or recently received PEG-asparaginase. In the absence of contraindications, clinicians should have a low threshold to do a lumbar puncture for evaluation of CNS infection if the child is currently immunosuppressed; in addition to

routine bacterial testing, testing should include cytology, human herpesvirus 6, HSV, fungal culture, John Cunningham (JC) virus, and cryptococcus. Medication toxicity from chemotherapy, especially methotrexate, may cause seizures so the medication list should be carefully reviewed. If the child has an elevated blood pressure (especially if on high dose steroids, cyclosporine, or tacrolimus), hypertensive encephalopathy is a common diagnosis; posterior reversible encephalopathy will have characteristic changes on MRI. Other symptoms that support this diagnosis are encephalopathy, visual problems, and headache. Evaluation of immunosuppressed children for nononcologic reasons similarly should address the risk of infection and medication side effects.

Children with known CNS infection may present with seizures after admission. Electrolyte abnormalities, especially hyponatremia, may be evident on baseline labs. However, if neuroimaging has not been obtained, we recommend obtaining a MRI of the brain with and without contrast, including evaluation of the venous and arterial structures. Emergent CT should be performed if there are symptoms or signs of increased intracranial pressure.

As mentioned previously, children with global anoxia/hypoxia and those with traumatic brain injury are at high risk for seizures. If clinically indicated, evaluation for increased intracranial pressure should be done due to the risk of cerebral edema. For children admitted with sudden cardiorespiratory failure without a clear etiology, though, testing for inborn errors of metabolism is reasonable using the approach described in the preceding section.

Children on ECMO are at risk for electrolyte abnormalities, cardioembolic events, and hemorrhage in addition to hypoxic injury. Electrolytes and coagulation profile should be checked. If feasible, head ultrasound (infants) and/or portable head CT are useful studies to evaluate for large hemorrhages, though ischemic injury cannot be assessed by an early CT scan.

In all situations, maintaining cardiorespiratory stability is the most important goal, so suggested imaging, especially MRI, may need to be deferred if the child is unstable. If the child cannot tolerate sedation or a prolonged scan but there is concern for acute ischemia, then we recommend that the clinician discuss appropriate plans with the neuroradiologists since a limited MRI scan can be obtained (T2 sequence, diffusion weighted images, and apparent diffusion map).

Overall, these broad recommendations reflect our clinical practice and experience and are meant to help guide initial evaluation but ultimately evaluation for the underlying etiology should be tailored in each case to the individual patient.

■ CONCLUSIONS

Seizures and SE are common neurologic emergencies which may lead to PICU admission or occur in the context of other critical illnesses. These may occur in children with epilepsy, but generally should be considered as symptomatic of an underlying acute encephalopathy until proven otherwise. Care involves simultaneous monitoring and support of systemic functions including airways, breathing, and circulation, intervention with appropriate doses of rapidly administered AEDs, and evaluation to identify the underlying etiology.

■ REFERENCES

1. Neligan A, Shorvon SD. The history of status epilepticus and its treatment. *Epilepsia*. 2009;50(suppl 3):56–68.
2. Lowenstein DH, Bleck T, Macdonald RL. It's time to revise the definition of status epilepticus. *Epilepsia*. 1999;40(1):120–122.
3. Proposal for revised clinical and electroencephalographic classification of epileptic seizures. From the Commission on Classification and Terminology of the International League Against Epilepsy. *Epilepsia*. 1981;22(4):489–501.
4. Shinnar S et al. How long do new-onset seizures in children last? *Ann Neurol*. 2001;49(5):659–664.
5. Verity CM, Ross EM, Golding, J. Outcome of childhood status epilepticus and lengthy febrile convulsions: findings of national cohort study. *BMJ*. 1993;307(6898):225–228.
6. Hesdorffer DC et al. Incidence of status epilepticus in Rochester, Minnesota, 1965-1984. *Neurology*. 1998;50(3):735–741.
7. DeLorenzo RJ et al. Status epilepticus in children, adults, and the elderly. *Epilepsia*. 1992;33(suppl 4):S15–S25.
8. Coeytaux A et al. Incidence of status epilepticus in French-speaking Switzerland: (EPISTAR). *Neurology*. 2000;55(5):693–697.
9. Wu YW et al. Incidence and mortality of generalized convulsive status epilepticus in California. *Neurology*. 2002;58(7):1070–1076.
10. DeLorenzo RJ et al. Epidemiology of status epilepticus. *J Clin Neurophysiol*. 1995;12(4):316–325.
11. Nishiyama I et al. An epidemiological study of children with status epilepticus in Okayama, Japan. *Epilepsia*. 2007;48(6):1133–1137.
12. Beghi E et al. Recommendation for a definition of acute symptomatic seizure. *Epilepsia*. 2010;51(4):671–675.
13. Singh RK et al. Prospective study of new-onset seizures presenting as status epilepticus in childhood. *Neurology*. 2010;74(8):636–642.
14. Barnard C, Wirrell E. Does status epilepticus in children cause developmental deterioration and exacerbation of epilepsy? *J Child Neurol*. 1999;14(12):787–794.
15. Okanishi T et al. Underlying neurologic disorders and recurrence rates of status epilepticus in childhood. *Brain Dev*. 2008;30(10):624–628.
16. Riviello JJ Jr et al. Practice parameter: diagnostic assessment of the child with status epilepticus (an evidence-based review): report of the Quality Standards Subcommittee of the American Academy of Neurology and the Practice Committee of the Child Neurology Society. *Neurology*. 2006;67(9):1542–1550.
17. Mah JK, Mah MW. Pediatric status epilepticus: a perspective from Saudi Arabia. *Pediatr Neurol*. 1999;20(5):364–369.
18. Huang CC, Chang YC, Wang ST. Acute symptomatic seizure disorders in young children—a population study in southern Taiwan. *Epilepsia*. 1998;39(9):960–964.
19. Idro R et al. The incidence, aetiology and outcome of acute seizures in children admitted to a rural Kenyan district hospital. *BMC Pediatr*. 2008;8:5.
20. Phillips SA, Shanahan RJ. Etiology and mortality of status epilepticus in children. A recent update. *Arch Neurol*. 1989;46(1):74–76.
21. Shinnar S et al. In whom does status epilepticus occur: age-related differences in children. *Epilepsia*. 1997;38(8):907–914.
22. Berg AT et al. Status epilepticus in children with newly diagnosed epilepsy. *Ann Neurol*. 1999; 45(5):618-623.
23. Stroink H et al. Status epilepticus in children with epilepsy: Dutch study of epilepsy in childhood. *Epilepsia*. 2007;48(9):1708–1715.
24. Sillanpaa M, Shinnar S. Status epilepticus in a population-based cohort with childhood-onset epilepsy in Finland. *Ann Neurol*. 2002;52(3):303–310.
25. Novak G et al. Risk factors for status epilepticus in children with symptomatic epilepsy. *Neurology*. 1997;49(2):533–537.
26. Corey LA, Pellock JM, DeLorenzo RJ. Status epilepticus in a population-based Virginia twin sample. *Epilepsia*. 2004;45(2):159–165.
27. Hussain N, Appleton R, Thorburn K. Aetiology, course and outcome of children admitted to paediatric intensive care with convulsive status epilepticus: a retrospective 5-year review. *Seizure*. 2007;16(4):305–312.
28. Kwong KL, Chang K, Lam SY. Features predicting adverse outcomes of status epilepticus in childhood. *Hong Kong Med J*. 2004;10(3):156–159.
29. Lacroix J et al. Admissions to a pediatric intensive care unit for status epilepticus: a 10-year experience. *Crit Care Med*. 1994;22(5):827–832.
30. Towne AR et al. Prevalence of nonconvulsive status epilepticus in comatose patients. *Neurology*. 2000;54(2):340–345.
31. Saengpattrachai M et al. Nonconvulsive seizures in the pediatric intensive care unit: etiology, EEG, and brain imaging findings. *Epilepsia*. 2006;47(9):1510–1518.
32. Abend NS et al. Non-convulsive seizures are common in critically ill children. *Neurology*. 2011;76(12):1071–1077.

33. Jette N et al. Frequency and predictors of nonconvulsive seizures during continuous electroencephalographic monitoring in critically ill children. *Arch Neurol.* 2006;63(12):1750–1755.

34. Waziri A et al. Intracortical electroencephalography in acute brain injury. *Ann Neurol.* 2009;66(3):366–377.

35. Khot S, Tirschwell DL. Long-term neurological complications after hypoxic-ischemic encephalopathy. *Semin Neurol.* 2006;26(4):422–431.

36. Abend NS et al. Electroencephalographic monitoring during hypothermia after pediatric cardiac arrest. *Neurology.* 2009;72(22):1931–1940.

37. Parish AP et al. Seizures as a predictor of long-term neurodevelopmental outcome in survivors of neonatal extracorporeal membrane oxygenation (ECMO). *J Child Neurol.* 2004;19(12):930–934.

38. Meyer DM, Jessen ME. Results of extracorporeal membrane oxygenation in children with sepsis. The Extracorporeal Life Support Organization. *Ann Thorac Surg.* 1997;63(3):756–761.

39. Annegers JF et al. Seizures after head trauma: a population study. *Neurology.* 1980;30(7 pt 1):683–689.

40. Hahn YS et al. Factors influencing posttraumatic seizures in children. *Neurosurgery.* 1988;22(5):864–867.

41. Lewis RJ et al. Clinical predictors of post-traumatic seizures in children with head trauma. *Ann Emerg Med.* 1993;22(7):1114–1118.

42. Asikainen I, Kaste M, Sarna S. Early and late posttraumatic seizures in traumatic brain injury rehabilitation patients: brain injury factors causing late seizures and influence of seizures on long-term outcome. *Epilepsia.* 1999;40(5):584–589.

43. Ratan SK, Kulshreshtha R, Pandey RM. Predictors of post-traumatic convulsions in head-injured children. *Pediatr Neurosurg.* 1999;30(3):127–131.

44. Adelson PD et al. Guidelines for the acute medical management of severe traumatic brain injury in infants, children, and adolescents. Chapter 19. The role of anti-seizure prophylaxis following severe pediatric traumatic brain injury. *Pediatr Crit Care Med.* 2003;4(3 suppl):S72–S75.

45. Schierhout G, Roberts I. Anti-epileptic drugs for preventing seizures following acute traumatic brain injury. *Cochrane Database.* 2001; 4: Art No CD000173.

46. Gilles EE, Nelson MD Jr. Cerebral complications of nonaccidental head injury in childhood. *Pediatr Neurol.* 1998;19(2):119–128.

47. Bourgeois M et al. Epilepsy associated with shaken baby syndrome. *Childs Nerv Syst.* 2008;24(2):169–172; discussion 173.

48. Kim MA et al. Acute symptomatic seizures in CNS infection. *Eur J Neurol.* 2008;15(1):38–41.

49. Misra UK, Kalita J, Nair PP. Status epilepticus in central nervous system infections: an experience from a developing country. *Am J Med.* 2008;121(7):618–623.

50. Chang C-J et al. Seizures complicating infantile and childhood bacterial meningitis. *Pediatric Neurology.* 2004;31(3):165–171.

51. Pomeroy SL et al. Seizures and other neurologic sequelae of bacterial meningitis in children. *N Engl J Med.* 1990;323(24):1651–1657.

52. Misra UK, Tan CT, Kalita J. Viral encephalitis and epilepsy. *Epilepsia.* 2008;49(suppl 6):13–18.

53. Hsieh WB et al. Outcome of herpes simplex encephalitis in children. *J Microbiol Immunol Infect.* 2007;40(1):34–38.

54. Panagariya A et al. Herpes simplex encephalitis in North West India. *Neurol India.* 2001;49(4):360–365.

55. Wang IJ et al. The correlation between neurological evaluations and neurological outcome in acute encephalitis: a hospital-based study. *Eur J Paediatr Neurol.* 2007;11(2):63–69.

56. Fowler A et al. Childhood encephalitis in Sweden: etiology, clinical presentation and outcome. *Eur J Paediatr Neurol.* 2008;12(6):484–490.

57. Newland JG et al. Neurologic complications in children hospitalized with influenza: characteristics, incidence, and risk factors. *J Pediatr.* 2007;150(3):306–310.

58. Zheng Y et al. Hospitalized children with 2009 influenza a (H1N1) infection in Shenzhen, China, November-December 2009. *Pediatr Pulmonol.* 2010;46(3):246–252.

59. Neurologic complications associated with novel influenza A (H1N1) virus infection in children—Dallas, Texas, May 2009. *MMWR Morb Mortal Wkly Rep.* 2009;58(28):773–778.

60. Tenembaum S, Chamoles N, Fejerman N. Acute disseminated encephalomyelitis: a long-term follow-up study of 84 pediatric patients. *Neurology.* 2002;59(8):1224–1231.

61. Tenembaum S et al. Acute disseminated encephalomyelitis. *Neurology.* 2007;68(16 suppl 2):S23–S36.

62. Chadehumbe MA et al. Seizures are common in the acute setting of childhood stroke: a population-based study. *J Child Neurol.* 2009;24(1):9–12.

63. Szaflarski JP et al. Incidence of seizures in the acute phase of stroke: a population-based study. *Epilepsia.* 2008;49(6):974–981.

64. Liu JE, Gzesh DJ, Ballas SK. The spectrum of epilepsy in sickle cell anemia. *J Neurol Sci.* 1994;123(1–2):6–10.

65. Prengler M et al. Sickle cell disease: ischemia and seizures. *Ann Neurol.* 2005;58(2):290–302.

66. Prengler M et al. Sickle cell disease: the neurological complications. *Ann Neurol.* 2002;51(5):543–552.

67. Ferro JM et al. Early seizures in cerebral vein and dural sinus thrombosis: risk factors and role of antiepileptics. *Stroke.* 2008;39(4):1152–1158.

68. Masuhr F et al. Risk and predictors of early epileptic seizures in acute cerebral venous and sinus thrombosis. *Eur J Neurol.* 2006;13(8):852–856.

69. Ferro JM et al. prognosis of cerebral vein and dural sinus thrombosis: results of the International Study on Cerebral Vein and Dural Sinus Thrombosis (ISCVT). *Stroke.* 2004;35(3):664–670.

70. Sébire G et al. Cerebral venous sinus thrombosis in children: risk factors, presentation, diagnosis and outcome. *Brain.* 2005;128(3):477–489.

71. Wasay M et al. Cerebral venous sinus thrombosis in children: a multicenter cohort from the United States. *J Child Neurol.* 2008;23(1):26–31.

72. deVeber G et al. Cerebral sinovenous thrombosis in children. *N Engl J Med.* 2001;345(6):417–423.

73. Vieira JP et al. Cerebral sinovenous thrombosis in children: clinical presentation and extension, localization and recanalization of thrombosis. *Eur J Paediatr Neurol.* 2010;14(1):80–85.

74. Gaynor JW et al. The relationship of postoperative electrographic seizures to neurodevelopmental outcome at 1 year

of age after neonatal and infant cardiac surgery. *J Thorac Cardiovasc Surg*. 2006;131(1):181–189.

75. Clancy RR et al. Risk of seizures in survivors of newborn heart surgery using deep hypothermic circulatory arrest. *Pediatrics*. 2003;111(3):592–601.

76. Rappaport LA et al. Relation of seizures after cardiac surgery in early infancy to neurodevelopmental outcome. Boston Circulatory Arrest Study Group. *Circulation*. 1998;97(8):773–779.

77. Lee VH et al. Clinical spectrum of reversible posterior leukoencephalopathy syndrome. *Arch Neurol*. 2008;65(2):205–210.

78. Gumus H et al. Reversible posterior leukoencephalopathy syndrome in childhood: report of nine cases and review of the literature. *Neurol Sci*. 2010;31(2):125–131.

79. Taylor LM, Farzam F, Cook AM. Clinical utility of a continuous intravenous infusion of valproic acid in pediatric patients. *Pharmacotherapy*. 2007;27:519–525.

80. Abend NS, Bonnemann CG, Licht DJ. Status epilepticus secondary to hypertensive encephalopathy as the presenting manifestation of Guillain-Barre syndrome. *Pediatr Emerg Care*. 2007;23(9):659–661.

81. Kirmani BF, Crisp ED, Kayani S. Role of intravenous levetiracetam in acute seizure management of children. *Pediatr Neurol*. 2009;41:37–39.

82. van Gestel J, Blusse van Oud-Alblas H, Malingre M. Propofol and thiopental for refractory status epilepticus in children. *Neurology*. 2005;65:591–592.

83. Iyer R, Hoel R, Rabinstein A. Propofol infusion syndrome in patients with refractory status epileptics: an 11-year clinical experience. *Crit Care Med*. 2009;37:3024–3030.

84. Mirsattari S, Sharpe M, Young G. Treatment of refractory status epilepticus with inhalational anesthetic agents isoflurane and desflurane. *Arch Neurol*. 2004;61(8):1254–1259.

85. Segura-Bruna N et al. Valproate-induced hyperammonemic encephalopathy. *Acta Neurol Scand*. 2006;114(1):1–7.

86. Ravizza T et al. Inflammatory response and glia activation in developing rat hippocampus after status epilepticus. *Epilepsia*. 2005;46(suppl 5):113–117.

87. Ravizza T, Vezzani A. Status epilepticus induces time-dependent neuronal and astrocytic expression of interleukin-1 receptor type I in the rat limbic system. *Neuroscience*. 2006;137(1):301–308.

88. Vezzani A, Balosso S, Ravizza T. The role of cytokines in the pathophysiology of epilepsy. *Brain Behav Immun*. 2008;22(6):797–803.

89. Bernardino L et al. Inflammatory events in hippocampal slice cultures prime neuronal susceptibility to excitotoxic injury: a crucial role of P2X7 receptor-mediated IL-1beta release. *J Neurochem*. 2008;106(1):271–280.

90. Vezzani A et al. Glia as a source of cytokines: implications for neuronal excitability and survival. *Epilepsia*. 2008;49(suppl 2):24–32.

91. Ravizza T et al. Innate and adaptive immunity during epileptogenesis and spontaneous seizures: evidence from experimental models and human temporal lobe epilepsy. *Neurobiol Dis*. 2008;29(1):142–160.

92. Vezzani A et al. Basic mechanisms of status epilepticus due to infection and inflammation. *Epilepsia*. 2009;50(suppl 12):56–57.

93. Diamond I, Aquino TI. Myoglobinuria following unilateral status epilepticus and ipsilateral rhabdomyolysis:

a clinicopathological report. *N Engl J Med*. 1965;272:834–837.

94. Singhal PC, Chugh KS, Gulati DR. Myoglobinuria and renal failure after status epilepticus. *Neurology*. 1978;28(2):200–201.

95. Guven M et al. Rhabdomyolysis and acute renal failure due to status epilepticus. *Clin Nephrol*. 1998;50(3):204.

96. Sato T et al. Recurrent reversible rhabdomyolysis associated with hyperthermia and status epilepticus. *Acta Paediatr*. 1995;84(9):1083–1085.

97. Sagduyu A, Tarlaci S, Sirin H. Generalized tonic-clonic status epilepticus: causes, treatment, complications and predictors of case fatality. *J Neurol*. 1998;245(10):640–646.

98. Winocour PH et al. Severe, self-limiting lactic acidosis and rhabdomyolysis accompanying convulsions. *Postgrad Med J*. 1989;65(763):321–322.

99. Sevcencu C, Struijk JJ. Autonomic alterations and cardiac changes in epilepsy. *Epilepsia*. 2010;51(5):725–737.

100. Kandler L et al. Early post-convulsive prolongation of QT time in children. *Acta Paediatr*. 2005;94(9):1243–1247.

101. Lothman E. The biochemical basis and pathophysiology of status epilepticus. *Neurology*. 1990;40(5 suppl 2):13–23.

102. Meldrum BS, Brierley JB. Prolonged epileptic seizures in primates. Ischemic cell change and its relation to ictal physiological events. *Arch Neurol*. 1973;28(1):10–17.

103. Boggs JG et al. Hemodynamic monitoring prior to and at the time of death in status epilepticus. *Epilepsy Res*. 1998;31(3):199–209.

104. Metcalf CS et al. Status epilepticus induces cardiac myofilament damage and increased susceptibility to arrhythmias in rats. *Am J Physiol Heart Circ Physiol*. 2009;297(6):H2120–H2127.

105. Shimizu M et al. Neurogenic stunned myocardium associated with status epileptics and postictal catecholamine surge. *Intern Med*. 2008;47(4):269–273.

106. Manno EM et al. Cardiac pathology in status epilepticus. *Ann Neurol*. 2005;58(6):954–957.

107. O'Regan ME, Brown JK. Abnormalities in cardiac and respiratory function observed during seizures in childhood. *Dev Med Child Neurol*. 2005;47(1):4–9.

108. Moseley BD et al. How common is ictal hypoxemia and bradycardia in children with partial complex and generalized convulsive seizures? *Epilepsia*. 2010;51(7):1219–1224.

109. Hewertson J et al. Hypoxaemia and cardiorespiratory changes during epileptic seizures in young children. *Dev Med Child Neurol*. 1996;38(6):511–522.

110. Fredberg U, Botker HE, Romer FK. Acute neurogenic pulmonary oedema following generalized tonic clonic seizure. A case report and a review of the literature. *Eur Heart J*. 1988;9(8):933–936.

111. Swallow RA, Hillier CE, Smith PE. Sudden unexplained death in epilepsy (SUDEP) following previous seizure-related pulmonary oedema: case report and review of possible preventative treatment. *Seizure*. 2002;11(7):446–448.

112. Blennow G et al. Epileptic brain damage: the role of systemic factors that modify cerebral energy metabolism. *Brain*. 1978;101(4):687–700.

113. Sammaritano M et al. Prolonged focal cerebral edema associated with partial status epilepticus. *Epilepsia*. 1985;26(4):334–339.

114. Bek S et al. Cerebral vasomotor reactivity in epilepsy patients. *J Neurol*. 2010;257(5):833–838.

115. Cutler RW, Lorenzo AV, Barlow CF. Changes in blood-brain permeability during pharmacologically induced convulsions. *Prog Brain Res*. 1968;29:367–384.

116. Lorenzo AV et al. Temporary alteration of cerebrovascular permeability to plasma protein during drug-induced seizures. *Am J Physiol*. 1972;223(2):268–277.

117. Lansberg MG et al. MRI abnormalities associated with partial status epilepticus. *Neurology*. 1999;52(5):1021–1027.

118. Roberts RJ et al. Incidence of propofol-related infusion syndrome in critically ill adults: a prospective, multicenter study. *Crit Care*. 2009;13(5):R169.

119. Logroscino G et al. Short-term mortality after a first episode of status epilepticus. *Epilepsia*. 1997;38(12):1344–1349.

120. Dunn DW. Status epilepticus in children: etiology, clinical features, and outcome. *J Child Neurol*. 1988;3(3):167–173.

121. Dunn DW. Status epilepticus in infancy and childhood. *Neurol Clin*. 1990;8(3):647–657.

122. Sahin M et al. Prolonged treatment for acute symptomatic refractory status epilepticus: outcome in children. *Neurology*. 2003;61(3):398–401.

123. Koubeissi M, Alshekhlee A. In-hospital mortality of generalized convulsive status epilepticus: a large US sample. *Neurology*. 2007;69(9):886–893.

124. KarasalIhoGlu S et al. Risk factors of status epilepticus in children. *Pediatr Int*. 2003;45(4):429–434.

125. Raspall-Chaure M et al. Outcome of paediatric convulsive status epilepticus: a systematic review. *Lancet Neurol*. 2006;5(9):769–779.

126. Aicardi J, Chevrie JJ. Convulsive status epilepticus in infants and children. A study of 239 cases. *Epilepsia*. 1970;11(2):187–197.

127. Berg AT et al. Status epilepticus after the initial diagnosis of epilepsy in children. *Neurology*. 2004;63(6):1027–1034.

128. Shinnar S et al. Recurrent status epilepticus in children. *Ann Neurol*. 1992;31(6):598–604.

129. Hesdorffer DC et al. Recurrence of afebrile status epilepticus in a population-based study in Rochester, Minnesota. *Neurology*. 2007;69(1):73–78.

130. Hesdorffer DC et al. Risk of unprovoked seizure after acute symptomatic seizure: effect of status epilepticus. *Ann Neurol*. 1998;44(6):908–912.

131. Hauser WA et al. Seizure recurrence after a first unprovoked seizure. *N Engl J Med*. 1982;307(9):522–528.

132. Shinnar S et al. The risk of seizure recurrence after a first unprovoked afebrile seizure in childhood: an extended follow-up. *Pediatrics*. 1996;98(2 pt 1):216–225.

133. Berg AT, Shinnar S. The risk of seizure recurrence following a first unprovoked seizure: a quantitative review. *Neurology*. 1991;41(7):965–972.

134. Corsellis JA, Bruton CJ. Neuropathology of status epilepticus in humans. *Adv Neurol*. 1983;34:129–139.

135. Sahin M et al. Outcome of severe refractory status epilepticus in children. *Epilepsia*. 2001;42(11):1461–1467.

136. Maytal J et al. Low morbidity and mortality of status epilepticus in children. *Pediatrics*. 1989;83(3):323–331.

137. Ellenberg JH, Hirtz DG, Nelson KB. Do seizures in children cause intellectual deterioration? *N Engl J Med*. 1986;314(17):1085–1088.

138. Ellenberg JH, Nelson KB. Febrile seizures and later intellectual performance. *Arch Neurol*. 1978;35(1):17–21.

139. Fujiwara T et al. Status epilepticus in childhood: a retrospective study of initial convulsive status and subsequent epilepsies. *Folia Psychiatr Neurol Jpn*. 1979;33(3):337–344.

140. Dodrill CB, Wilensky AJ. Intellectual impairment as an outcome of status epilepticus. *Neurology*. 1990;40(5 suppl 2):23–27.

141. Harkin LA et al. The spectrum of SCN1A-related infantile epileptic encephalopathies. *Brain*. 2007;130(pt 3):843–852.

142. Scheffer IE et al. Epilepsy and mental retardation limited to females: an under-recognized disorder. *Brain*. 2008;131(pt 4):918–927.

143. Dalmau J et al. Anti-NMDA-receptor encephalitis: case series and analysis of the effects of antibodies. *Lancet Neurol*. 2008;7(12):1091–1098.

144. Hirtz D et al. Practice parameter: evaluating a first nonfebrile seizure in children: report of the quality standards subcommittee of the American Academy of Neurology, the Child Neurology Society, and the American Epilepsy Society. *Neurology*. 2000;55(5):616–623.

145. Millichap JG. Electroencephalography hyperventilation and stroke in children with sickle cell disease. *Clin EEG Neurosci*. 2006;37(3):190–192.

9
Electroencephalography in Critically Ill Children

NICHOLAS S. ABEND and DENNIS J. DLUGOS

■ INTRODUCTION

The electroencephalogram (EEG) provides a noninvasive and continuous means of assessing and monitoring brain function at the bedside of critically ill children. An EEG tracing has two main components. First, the background brain activity may serve as a marker of global and regional brain function. Second, intermittent events such as electrographic seizures may be identified. This chapter discusses the purposes of EEG in the critical care setting, common background patterns observed in critically ill children, and available data regarding electrographic seizure identification and impact on outcome.

■ PURPOSES OF EEG IN CRITICALLY ILL CHILDREN

Information derived from an EEG may be useful in encephalopathic or comatose children in several ways. First, EEG reflects cerebral cortical activity, as modulated by brainstem and diencephalic inputs, so EEG abnormalities provide objective evidence for brain dysfunction. In some children, subtle or overt EEG abnormalities may develop before clinical symptoms of encephalopathy appear. Thus, EEG may be useful in identifying and differentiating between patients with encephalopathy, psychogenic unresponsiveness, or a locked-in state. Patients with a *neurologic or systemic etiology* for encephalopathy or coma generally have an abnormal EEG, and the most common abnormal patterns are discussed below. Generally, more severely abnormal EEG patterns are associated with "deeper" or more severe encephalopathy, although linear correlations between the degree of EEG abnormality and the degree of encephalopathy are lacking. Patients with *psychogenic unresponsiveness* will generally have a normal EEG. However, medication effects must be considered since some psychiatric medications impact the EEG. For example, benzodiazepines and barbiturates induce beta activity and, at high doses, slowing, disorganization, and attenuation. Patients with *locked-in syndrome* can have a normal EEG or mild abnormalities including mild diffuse slowing, but generally will not have diffuse severe abnormalities. Patients who are unresponsive but have a normal or only mildly abnormal EEG should be carefully evaluated for evidence of a locked-in syndrome with tests of EEG reactivity and careful physical examination of vertical eye movements.

Second, EEG may help identify the general etiology of coma. Although most EEG patterns are nonspecific for an exact etiology and cannot differentiate between acute and chronic encephalopathy (1), EEG features may be useful in differentiating between categories of dysfunction such as focal or multifocal structural lesions, diffuse toxic or metabolic disorders, and seizure related states. *Diffuse structural or toxic-metabolic etiologies* are suggested by diffuse voltage attenuation, slowing, disorganization, beta activity, burst-suppression, or low-voltage featureless patterns. Unfortunately, these features cannot distinguish between permanent structural injury and potentially reversible metabolic-toxic dysfunction. Thus, the clinical context is important and repeat EEG tracings may be useful to assess for interval changes. In some cases, EEG may permit localization of a discrete lesion, since *focal or multifocal structural abnormalities* are suggested by focal EEG abnormalities. These include focal or multifocal voltage attenuation, slowing, disorganization, epileptiform abnormalities including interictal sharps or seizures, focal beta activity, or focal absence of beta activity in a patient receiving benzodiazepines or barbiturates. In patients with lesions resulting in encephalopathy, neuroimaging provides the best detail regarding localization and etiology, but EEG data is particularly useful for patients who are not stable for transport for neuroimaging. Patients with brainstem or diencephalic lesions affecting cortical inputs may have more diffuse abnormalities, while those with cortical lesions may have focal abnormalities. EEG may help localize abnormalities to cortex or subcortical white matter. A traditional distinction, derived largely from animal models, suggests that encephalopathies involving primarily cortex result in amplitude attenuation, epileptiform abnormalities, and seizures while encephalopathies involving white matter produce slowing. However, in clinical practice, many encephalopathies involve cortical and white matter dysfunction or injury, leading to mixed EEG patterns. *Seizure related states* are suggested by epileptiform abnormalities or ongoing electrographic seizures. If the ictal or postictal state is suspected as the encephalopathy etiology, further evaluation of the seizure etiology would still be needed.

Third, EEG assessment is needed to identify nonconvulsive seizures (NCS) and nonconvulsive status epilepticus (NCSE)—electrographically evident seizures without any clinical correlate. These are also referred to as subclinical seizures or electrographic-only seizures. NCS and NCSE have been reported in 10% to 40% of children who underwent long-term EEG monitoring in pediatric intensive care units (PICU) or emergency departments (2–13). NCS and NCSE may occur in response to many types of acute brain injury, thereby representing acute symptomatic seizures, but may also independently cause or contribute to a patient being encephalopathic or comatose. By definition, since these seizures can only be identified on EEG, they would be missed without EEG monitoring.

Fourth, continuous EEG monitoring or serial standard EEGs may be useful for following the evolution of encephalopathic and comatose states and identifying abrupt changes that could require evaluation and intervention. Tracking EEG features over time may help determine the depth of encephalopathy or coma, and thereby may help establish whether brain dysfunction is improving, stable, or worsening. As toxic or metabolic etiologies resolve, EEG patterns should normalize. Abrupt changes in the EEG may suggest evaluation and intervention is needed. Rapid worsening may suggest increasing edema, increasing intracranial pressure, or expanding lesions. Ensuring that EEG data is time locked with medication administration logs is important in differentiating between worsening brain dysfunction and transiently worsened EEG features related to sedative boluses.

Fifth, when the etiology for encephalopathy or coma is known, then EEG features may provide useful prognostic information. As described above, similar EEG patterns can occur in patients with severe anoxic brain injury and intoxication. Thus, EEG features cannot be used to prognosticate in the absence of clinical information. If the coma etiology is metabolic or toxic, then outcome is determined primarily by the etiology. If intoxication resolves over time or metabolic problems are corrected, then the EEG and the patient can be expected to improve. In contrast, if the etiology is known hypoxic-ischemic injury then severely abnormal EEG features such as burst suppression, the attenuated featureless state, or myoclonic status epilepticus are generally associated with unfavorable outcome. Note that while EEGs may be interpreted as "no definite cerebral activity" indicating a severely abnormal, highly attenuated, and featureless pattern, this should not be interpreted as "electrocerebral inactivity" which can only be diagnosed by an EEG performed using brain death evaluation technical criteria (14) in specific circumstances (15).

■ CEREBRAL ACTIVITY OR ARTIFACT?

A central and initial question when interpreting EEG is whether any pattern observed is generated by brain activity or represents artifact (16,17). There are two artifact types: physiologic artifact and nonphysiologic artifact. Physiologic artifacts originate from patient physiology and movement, and these include electrocardiogram artifact derived from the heart's electrical activity, pulse artifact derived from blood vessel movement near an electrode, ballistocardiographic artifact derived from patient movement with heart beats (particularly in small patients), eye/ocular movement artifacts (blink, eyelid flutter, eye movement), face/throat movement artifacts (swallowing, chewing, glossokinetic), and respiratory artifact (breathing, liquid in endotracheal tube). Non-physiologic artifacts derive from electromagnetic fields outside the body. Instrument and electrode artifacts derive from EEG and other electrical equipment and include 60 Hz artifact (from electrical equipment), electrode artifact (from electrodes with poor skin contact), extracorporeal membrane oxygenation artifact, and patting or chest percussion artifact. Some of these patterns are easily identified as artifact but some can be difficult to identify. For example, patting or chest percussion may lead to the abrupt onset of waves visible at multiple electrodes which slowly evolve in frequency, and this may mimic a seizure.

Identification of artifacts is greatly aided by notes made by bedside caregivers and acquisition and review of time-locked video. Going beyond simple identification of artifact to determine the type of artifact and whether or not the artifact is resolvable will ensure the least contamination of cerebral EEG patterns (17). Collaborative efforts with intensivists and critical care nurses are essential in reducing and identifying artifacts. Documentation of events likely to lead to artifact, such as chest percussion, is essential. This can be done by allowing bedside staff to type comments directly onto the EEG tracing, button pads which provide markers in the EEG tracing, or bedside paper event logs. Avoiding contact between bedside equipment and EEG electrodes and wires is helpful. Collaborative solutions are often needed to identify and reduce artifact. For example, suctioning the endotracheal tubing may reduce artifact related to water movement in the tube. Recognizing and minimizing artifact avoids artifact being mistakenly identified as seizures and ensures background brain activity is not obscured by extracerebral patterns.

■ NORMAL EEG PATTERNS

The background activity of the EEG can be described in terms of the predominant frequency, amplitude, symmetry, and reactivity. Frequency is reported in hertz (Hz) and is often categorized as delta activity (< 4 Hz), theta activity (4–7 Hz), alpha activity (8–12 Hz), and beta activity (> 12 Hz). Normally, the background is symmetric and contains a mixture of frequencies, with amplitudes greater than 25 microvolts (μV) while awake, and higher amplitudes during slow wave sleep. With increasing age, the proportion of slow frequencies decrease and faster frequencies increase. In infants, the EEG contains predominantly delta and theta frequencies, with some faster alpha frequencies. In school-age and older children, the EEG contains mostly alpha frequencies and some admixed slower theta and delta frequencies. During the awake and relaxed state, the normal EEG contains an organization referred to as the anterior to

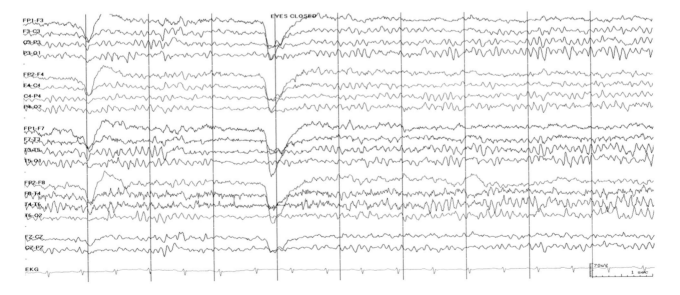

FIGURE 9.1 Normal electroencephalogram (EEG) with a clear 10 Hz posterior dominant rhythm. With eye closure, the posterior dominant rhythm becomes clearer.

posterior amplitude frequency gradient (Figure 9.1). This term describes faster lower amplitude activity in the anterior regions and slower higher amplitude activity in the posterior regions. Normally, the posterior dominant frequency becomes faster with age. Normal posterior dominant frequencies include 3 to 4 Hz at 4 months, 5 to 6 Hz at 1 year, 8 Hz at 3 years, and 9 to 10 Hz by 9 years (18,19).

During drowsiness (early stage 1 sleep) the EEG background develops busts of higher amplitude delta activity (drowsy bursts). These become longer and more persistent, and vertex waves (midline higher amplitude sharply contoured waves) occur. With stage 2 sleep, sleep spindles develop and are generally symmetric between the two hemispheres (Figure 9.2). Stage 3 or slow wave consists of high amplitude delta activity. The normal EEG cycles through the awake and sleep states and demonstrates reactivity, indicating that with auditory or tactile stimulation there is a change in the EEG background.

■ BACKGROUND EEG ABNORMALITIES

Mild Background Slowing

Background slow activity is defined as slowing of the posterior dominant rhythm and/or overall background frequencies. A posterior dominant rhythm may be present, but may contain slower than expected activity in the posterior region. For example, a relaxed and awake teen would be expected to have an alpha frequency activity (8–12 Hz) posterior dominant rhythm, so it would be abnormal for the posterior frequency to be composed of primarily theta frequency activity (4–7 Hz). Alternatively, the overall background may be slower than expected. In this case, some normal frequencies may still be present, but there may be a greater proportion of slower activity than expected for age. For example, a relaxed and awake teen should have very little delta frequency activity while awake and should have primarily faster frequencies. Thus, it would be abnormal for the background activity to contain primarily delta frequency activity. Slowing of the overall background activity or posterior dominant rhythm is a sensitive index of encephalopathy, but is nonspecific in etiology.

Diffuse Slow Activity

Diffuse slow activity may be divided into several categories. Slowing may be continuous or intermittent, and it may be rhythmic or polymorphic. The degree of slowing may be quantified as the predominant frequency. Diffuse continuous slowing describes slower than normal activity without any anterior to posterior amplitude-frequency organization (Figure 9.3). Diffuse intermittent slowing refers to a normal background pattern or mild background slowing with intermittent

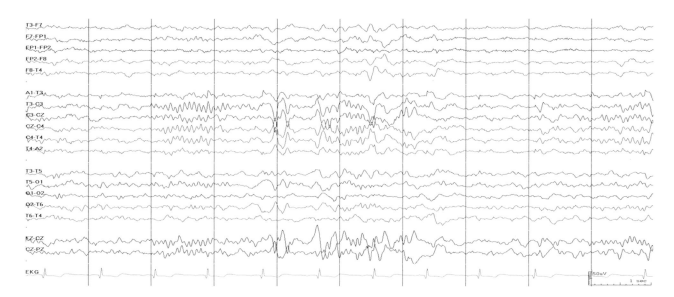

FIGURE 9.2   Normal sleep with sleep spindles and vertex waves.

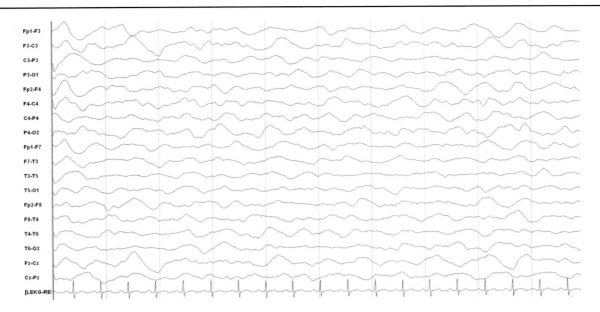

FIGURE 9.3 Diffuse polymorphic delta slowing.

excessive slow activity. Rhythmic slowing refers to bursts of rhythmic slowing and can include frontal intermittent rhythmic delta activity and occipital rhythmic delta activity. Rhythmic slowing may occur with mild background slowing or diffuse continuous slowing.

These types of slowing must be distinguished from the drowsy or sleep states. Drowsy bursts are essentially bursts of diffuse intermittent slowing, and slow wave sleep is essentially diffuse continuous slowing. This issue underscores the importance of knowing the patient's state and medications when interpreting EEG. For example, a patient who is known to be receiving sedative medications with diffuse delta activity would be interpreted as diffuse continuous slowing and not as normal slow-wave sleep. Assessing reactivity may also be important. Normal patients with slow activity as a component of sleep should demonstrate a change in the EEG (often developing faster and lower amplitude frequencies characteristic of the awake state) with stimulation. Tracking an EEG over time is also important, and distinctions may be difficult based on a single brief segment of EEG out of context. If bursts of slowing are seen in a patient transitioning from a normal awake state to stage 1 sleep this will help establish that the slow bursts are drowsy bursts. In contrast, if a patient has a persistently slow record without these normal state transitions then these slow bursts are likely diffuse intermittent slowing.

Diffuse slowing, whether intermittent or continuous, is a nonspecific coma pattern that can occur with metabolic encephalopathy, intoxication, or diffuse or specific focal cerebral lesions. Slowing may persist even after correction of some metabolic abnormalities. For example, after hyponatremia is corrected based on serum levels, disturbances in intracellular and extracellular fluid and electrolyte levels may persist. Diffuse slowing may also occur with diffuse structural lesions or focal lesions in specific regions such as subcortical white matter injury, thalamic, or midbrain tegmental lesions (20). If slowing is focal or multifocal then focal or multifocal lesions or dysfunction should be considered (Figure 9.4). Neuroimaging is generally indicated to establish the etiology of the focal dysfunction. The prognosis of diffuse slowing is dependent on the etiology.

Discontinuity and Burst-Suppression

Discontinuous or burst-suppression EEG patterns describe backgrounds in which there are bursts of activity alternating with periods of lower amplitude suppression (Figure 9.5). Discontinuity refers to periods of activity and suppression that are variable in duration and morphology. Discontinuity is normal in premature neonates and during sleep in term neonates, but beyond that period a normal recording is always continuous. In burst-suppression the appearance is more regular and the EEG

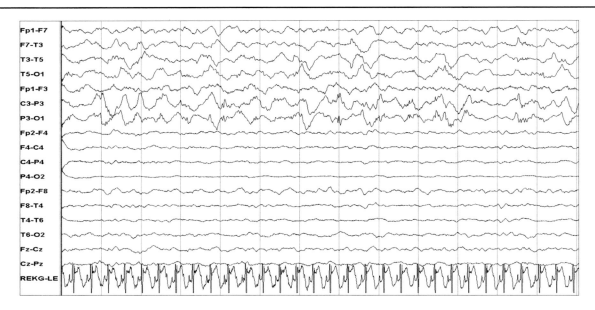

FIGURE 9.4 Diffuse polymorphic delta activity in the left hemisphere with asymmetric amplitude suppression in the right hemisphere.

is invariant (no spontaneous changes including reactivity to external stimulation. The bursts may contain any type of activity, including alpha, theta, delta, and beta activity, and may occur with or without admixed epileptiform discharges. For both discontinuity and burst-suppression, as the encephalopathy deepens the bursts become shorter and the interburst intervals longer. Some

bursts can be separated by extremely long interburst intervals, and this is the basis for the requirement that EEGs being performed to indicate electrocerebral inactivity (ECI) must be at least 30 minutes in duration.

Discontinuity and burst-suppression are nonspecific patterns. Common etiologies include anoxic brain injury, deep hypothermia (lower temperatures than used

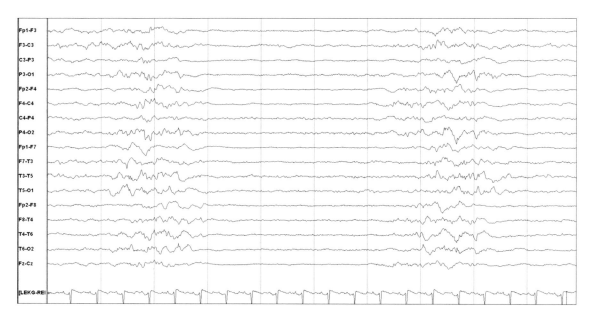

FIGURE 9.5 Burst-suppression with 1- to 2-second bursts and 3- to 4-second interburst intervals.

for therapeutic hypothermia protocols), intoxication with anesthetic and sedative medications, and severe metabolic encephalopathy. Metabolic encephalopathies include hepatic encephalopathy, uremic encephalopathy, sepsis encephalopathy, hypoglycemia, hypothyroidism, Addison disease, porphyria, and Wernicke encephalopathy. Burst-suppression can occur in some epilepsy syndromes, including Ohtahara syndrome (early infantile epileptic encephalopathy) and early infantile myoclonic encephalopathy. Prognosis is dependent on etiology. When burst-suppression occurs with anoxic brain injury it suggests an unfavorable outcome, although this is not absolute and so the full clinical scenario must be considered. As recently reviewed, the burst-suppression pattern with anoxia can either worsen to an isoelectric pattern or improve to diffuse slowing (21). In a recent study of children treated with therapeutic hypothermia after cardiac arrest, the presence of a discontinuous or burst-suppression pattern during hypothermia or upon return to normothermia was associated with unfavorable outcome (22), although the study was small and EEG features were not 100% predictive. Similarly, in adults treated with therapeutic hypothermia after cardiac arrest, burst-suppression as associated with unfavorable prognosis (23). In adults, serum neuron specific enolase was higher in patients with discontinuous and unreactive EEG patterns, indicating that these EEG patterns occur in the context of permanent neuronal damage (24). In contrast, in the context of sedative intoxication, hypothermia, or metabolic encephalopathy, the EEG pattern and the patient may improve over time.

Sedatives may be used to induce a burst-suppression pattern as part of clinical management for refractory status epilepticus and elevated intracranial pressure. While evidence-based protocols to manage refractory status epilepticus are lacking, after failure of several anticonvulsants, pharmacologic suppression is often employed to induce a burst-suppression pattern on EEG. Studies have not explored whether strategies aiming to induce burst-suppression are more effective than strategies aiming for seizure suppression, and the optimal durations for bursts and interburst intervals are unknown. Patients are often maintained in burst-suppression for one or several days, and during this time other anticonvulsants are generally adjusted in an attempt to avoid recurrent seizures as the pharmacologic suppression is weaned (25,26). Second, with refractory intracranial hypertension, inducing a burst-suppression pattern may

reduce metabolic demand and thus serve as a neuroprotective strategy. Again, the optimal durations for bursts and interburst intervals are unknown. It is often stated that administering additional pharmacologic suppression once the EEG is entirely suppressed is likely to provide no additional neuroprotective benefit but may be associated with more sedative adverse effects.

Low Voltage, Slow, Nonreactive Pattern

This nonspecific pattern refers to an EEG with mostly delta frequency activity, amplitude less than 20 µV, and lack of reactivity to auditory or tactile stimulation (Figure 9.6). While some normal individuals may have low-voltage tracings, their tracings are reactive to stimulation and contain posterior alpha frequencies with a normal anterior-posterior amplitude-frequency gradient. A low-voltage, slow, nonreactive pattern is generally seen with diffuse cortical and subcortical damage due to anoxic encephalopathy, severe traumatic brain injury, encephalitis, or diffuse cerebral edema. In these cases, the pattern is generally associated with an unfavorable prognosis. However, this pattern may also occur with high doses of sedating and anesthetic medications that may be associated with a more favorable prognosis.

Reactivity to Stimulation

Reactivity describes an EEG change in response to stimulation. This may occur with standard nursing care, or with specific stimulating procedures such as auditory or tactile stimulation. Generally, a lack of reactivity to stimulation is associated with more severe encephalopathy, and at least in the context of hypoxic-ischemic brain injury is associated with unfavorable outcome in children (22) and adults (23,24,27–30). In a study of 33 EEGs from comatose children of varying etiologies with outcome measured at 1 year, outcome was unfavorable in 29% with reactive EEGs and 65% with nonreactive EEGs (31). In some patients stimulation may induce stimulus induced rhythmic periodic or ictal discharges (SIRPIDs) (32,33), but the physiologic and prognostic implications of SIRPIDs are unknown.

Electrocerebral Inactivity

ECI occurs when there is no identifiable cerebral EEG activity recorded when the EEG is performed according to specific technical criteria. When the amplitude of EEG activity is less than 2 µV, it cannot be differentiated from

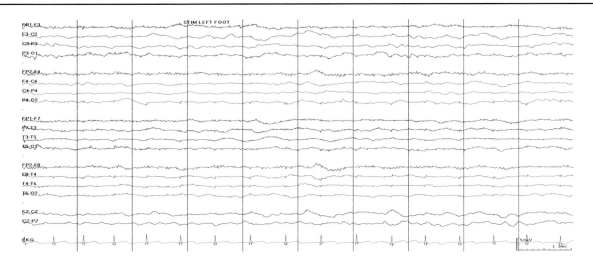

FIGURE 9.6 Low voltage, slow, and unreactive pattern. With stimulation of the foot, there is no change in the EEG (lack of reactivity to stimulation).

electrical noise. The term ECI is not used to describe focal abnormalities; the absence of electrical activity must be global. ECI must persist despite stimulation (lack of reactivity). Artifacts may still be seen on the EEG tracing, most commonly involving electrocardiac, cardioballistic, respiratory, or electrical artifacts, but these must be clearly identified as artifacts. Other terms used to describe ECI include electrocerebral silence and isoelectric EEG.

To interpret an EEG as showing ECI, the EEG must be obtained according to specific technical requirements provided by the American Clinical Neurophysiology Society (14). The EEG recording should demonstrate ECI for a minimum of 30 minutes and show no electrical activity beyond 2 µV at a sensitivity of 2 µV/mm with filter settings at 0.1 or 0.3 second at 70 Hz.

EEG may be used as an ancillary study to diagnose brain death in children. Based on the recently updated guidelines, an ancillary study is required only if (1) any components of the examination or apnea testing cannot be completed, (2) there is uncertainty about the results of the neurologic examination, or (3) a medication effect may be present. Ancillary studies, including an EEG that demonstrates ECI, may also be used to shorten the inter-examination interval required between the two brain death examinations. If the first neurologic examination and an ancillary study both support the diagnosis of brain death, the second neurologic examination and apnea test can be performed at any time (15) (see Brain Death chapter).

While ECI represents a severely abnormal EEG pattern consistent with brain death, it is not synonymous with brain death and the clinical circumstances and physical examination must be considered (15,34). Intoxication with high doses of sedating and anesthetic medications agents (eg, barbiturates, benzodiazepines, narcotics, thiopental, ketamine, halothane, and isoflurane) or hypothermia (35) may produce ECI which could be reversible.

Rhythmic Coma Patterns

Rhythmic coma patterns are reported to occur in as many as 30% of comatose children, and alpha coma is the most common rhythmic coma pattern seen in children (36). Alpha coma describes an EEG that shows predominantly diffuse monomorphic alpha activity (8–13 Hz) that usually has an amplitude of 10–50 µV (Figure 9.7). In contrast to a normal posterior dominant rhythm in which alpha activity is prominent posteriorly, in alpha coma the alpha activity may show a frontal predominance. While it is usually defined as unreactive to stimulation, some patients have reactivity (36,37), and reactivity is associated with more favorable prognosis (37,38). Alpha coma may alternate with other patterns and constitute a mixed alpha-theta or alpha-spindle coma pattern (36,39–41). The pathophysiologic mechanism underlying alpha coma is unknown. One hypothesis is that damage or depression of ascending reticular thalamic pathway produces newly generated and widespread abnormal activity related to cortical synchronization. It is important to differentiate alpha coma from a normal posterior dominant alpha pattern that is reactive to eye opening and closing and which suggests either psychogenic unresponsiveness or a locked-in state related to a brainstem lesion in an unresponsive patient (42,43).

Alpha coma is a nonspecific pattern that may occur with toxic-metabolic encephalopathies including overdoses with a favorable outcome and anoxic brain injury with an unfavorable outcome (37). Intoxications that may produce alpha coma include benzodiazepines, barbiturates, fentanyl, nitrous oxide, isoflurane, propofol, carbamazepine (44), and imipramine (45). Flumazenil, a benzodiazepine receptor antagonist, may reverse alpha coma and improve the clinical state of patients with benzodiazepine intoxication. As intoxication resolves, the EEG evolves to demonstrate reactivity and development of a more posterior dominance alpha rhythm. Alpha coma may occur in metabolic encephalopathy including hepatic encephalopathy (36,46), hyperglycemic hyperosmolar coma (47), and septic encephalopathy (48).

Alpha coma may occur with anoxic brain injury. It is sometimes preceded, accompanied, or followed by a wide range of other EEG patterns including slowing and disorganization, theta coma, low-voltage featureless activity, burst suppression, or ECI (36). Studies have evaluated the prognostic significance of alpha following cardiopulmonary arrest. Only 1% to 3% of patients survive with nearly total or total recovery, 10% survived with neurological sequelae, and about 75% die. Outcome may be better when alpha coma appears shortly after cardiac arrest and resolves within 1 to 2 days, as compared to being detected on or after the second day. The presence of reactivity may also suggest a better prognosis (36,37). In one study, no child with an unreactive pattern had normal neurologic status on follow-up (36). Studies in children have not been conducted in large cohorts or with caregivers blinded to EEG findings. Fewer than 50 children have been described with alpha coma, and all have been as cases or retrospective case series (36,41,43,45,49–58). Studies have not determined whether use of therapeutic hypothermia following cardiac arrest impacts the prognostic significance of alpha coma.

Theta coma is less common than alpha coma in comatose children (36) and less well described. Morphologically, theta coma refers to monotonous diffuse theta (4–7 Hz) activity that is usually unreactive to stimuli. It is often admixed with other rhythmic coma patterns including alpha and spindle coma patterns (36,38–41,59–61). Like alpha coma, theta coma is a nonspecific pattern that may occur with anoxic brain injury signifying a usually unfavorable prognosis or potentially reversible metabolic and intoxication etiologies with a more favorable prognosis. In a study of rhythmic

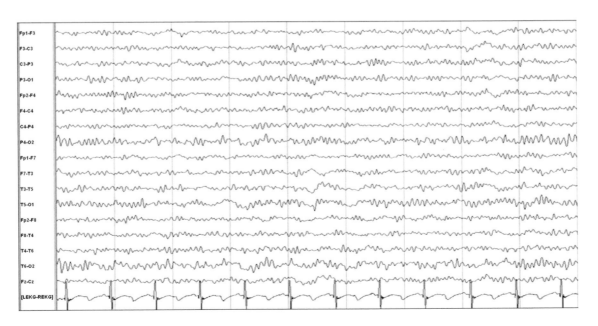

FIGURE 9.7 Alpha coma.

coma patterns in children (alpha, theta, beta, and spindle coma), the frequency of the pattern did not impact outcome (53). A reactive pattern carries a more favorable prognosis (38,39).

Spindle coma is a third type of rhythmic coma pattern (53). Spindle coma may occur in a paroxysmal manner admixed with primarily disorganized and slow theta or delta activity. There are diffuse, synchronous bursts of 11 to 14 Hz activity that is morphologically similar to spindles seen during sleep. Other sleep architecture including vertex waves and K complexes may be present, and on continuous monitoring, patients may cycle through stages of non-REM sleep. Spindle coma may occur admixed with other rhythmic coma patterns including alpha and theta coma patterns (36,39–41,59). The pathophysiologic mechanism of spindle coma is unclear, but some have suggested it may involve dysfunction of the ascending reticular formation leading to a combination of true sleep and coma with relatively intact cerebral hemispheres (62).

Like the other types of rhythmic coma, spindle coma is nonspecific (63,64) and may occur with anoxic encephalopathy, viral encephalitis (65) including measles encephalitis (66), intoxication (67), or metabolic encephalopathy, or with focal lesions in the pontomesencephalic junction and midbrain (68,69). One adult study reported no deaths when spindle coma was related to intoxication or seizures, 15% mortality with traumatic brain injury, 33% mortality with anoxic brain injury, and 73% mortality with brainstem and cerebral infraction and tumors (70). Prognosis is determined by etiology and has not been found to be worse with spindle coma (63,70). Outcome may be worse when brainstem motor function is impaired (64) and better when reactivity is preserved (70). Spindle coma has also been reported with more benign conditions such as vasovagal syncope (71).

Beta coma consists of generalized beta activity (12–16 Hz) that is often bifrontally predominant (Figure 9.8). This beta activity may override slower frequencies including alpha, beta, or delta frequencies. Reactivity may be present or absent. Beta coma is most commonly caused by administration of high doses or overdoses of sedative medications including benzodiazepines and

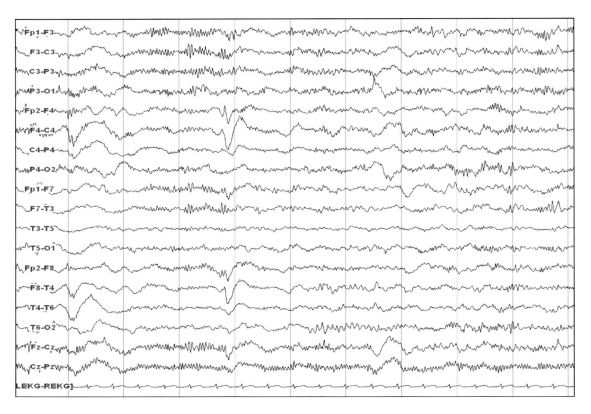

FIGURE 9.8 Beta coma.

barbiturates (72). Medical support is required during the acute intoxication phase, but prognosis is generally favorable. However, beta coma may also occur following anoxic brain injury with an unfavorable prognosis (36) and with acute brainstem lesions (73).

■ SEIZURES AND STATUS EPILEPTICUS

Electrographic seizures describe seizures evident on EEG which may or may not have an associated clinical correlate (Figure 9.9). Clinical correlates may involve clear convulsive seizures or more subtle changes such as eye deviation or vital sign fluctuations. When seizures do not have any clinical change, they are referred to as NCS, and when they constitute a substantial seizure burden are referred to as NCSE. Although there is no clearly accepted definition for NCSE, one definition used in recent studies has been a single seizure lasting more than 30 minutes or recurrent seizures totaling 30 minutes within a 1 hour epoch (50% seizure burden) (74). NCS and NCSE have been reported in 10% to 40% of children who underwent long-term EEG monitoring in PICU or emergency departments

(2–13). The majority of NCS and NCSE are not accompanied by any clinical change, even in nonparalyzed patients (4,9,11–13,74,75).

Studies have described some risk factors for NCS. NCS occurrence may be much lower in children who are comatose without an acute neurologic disorder (9) than children with altered mental status and a known acute neurologic disorder (2). Children may be at increased risk for NCS compared to adults (76). Additional clinical risk factors for NCS in children include younger age (2,11), followed by convulsive status epilepticus (11) or acute seizures (12,75) with structural brain injury (12,75) including traumatic brain injury (11), then cardiac arrest (10). Electrographic risk factors include epileptiform discharges (11,75), periodic epileptiform discharges (PEDs) (4), and lack of background reactivity (4). Given the heterogeneity of risk factors, EEG monitoring is often performed in a large number of patients. In a survey of neurologists, respondents described ordering continuous EEG to screen for NCS in patients with altered mental status with prior convulsions (89%), with altered mental status and no prior convulsive (68%), subtle eye movements (85%), any patient with an acute brain lesion (47%), and any paralyzed neuro-ICU patient (47%) (77).

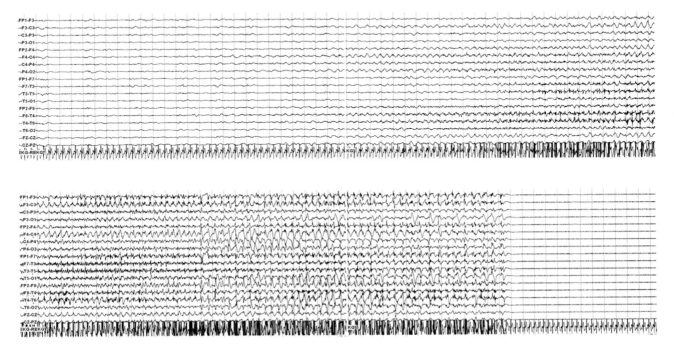

FIGURE 9.9 An electrographic seizure initiates in the right central-temporal area, generalizes, and then terminates. No clinical change was noted, constituting a nonconvulsive seizure.

Studies of critically ill children indicate that about half of patients with seizures are identified in the first hour and about 75% to 90% of children with seizures are identified with 24 hours of EEG monitoring (Figure 9.10) (2,4,5,9,11,12,75,78). This is consistent with large studies of critically ill adults (76). However, these studies may be confounded by the fact that computed-analyzed EEG (cEEG) duration was not predetermined and applied uniformly to all patients. If cEEG duration was longer, NCS may have been detected later in some patients. As expected, given that some seizures occur after the initial 30 to 60 minutes of EEG recording, in critically ill adults continuous EEG monitoring has been found to identify more patients with NCSE than standard EEG recordings (79). A survey of neurologists' current practices related to EEG monitoring in nonneonatal children and adults indicated that the majority monitor for 1 to 2 days if no seizures occur, although there was substantial variability in practice (77).

Studies of children with specific types of acute brain injury and management may better focus the question of the optimal duration of cEEG monitoring. In a prospective study of 19 children undergoing therapeutic hypothermia after cardiac arrest, all of whom underwent urgent initiation of EEG monitoring and continued monitoring for 72 hours, no children had electrographic seizures in the initial 6 hours of monitoring (early hypothermia), one had seizures in the next 6 hours (early hypothermia), four had seizures during the next 12 hours (late hypothermia), and four had seizures in the next 24 hours (rewarming) (10). Similarly, in neonates and infants who underwent repair of congenital heart disease, electrographic seizure onset occurred at a mean of 21 hours (80). These data suggest that in specific populations the durations of cEEG may be tailored to the individual profile of the patients' age, clinical status, and the etiology of the acute encephalopathy.

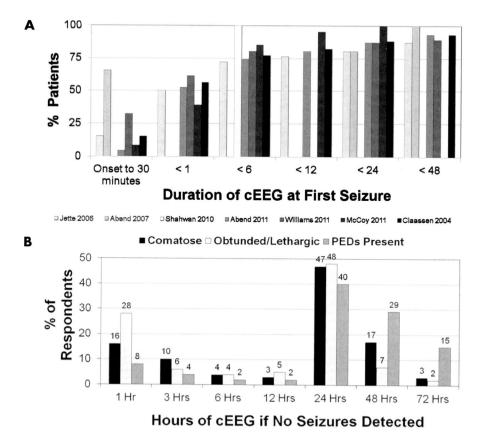

FIGURE 9.10 (A) Compilation of studies showing duration of EEG monitoring at the time of first seizure identification. (B) Survey results showing duration of EEG monitoring performed by neurologists if no seizures are identified. Adapted from Abend NS et al. Use of EEG monitoring and management of non-convulsive seizures in critically ill patients: a survey of neurologists. *Neurocrit Care.* 2010;*12*(3):382–389. PEDs; periodic epileptiform discharges.

The impact of NCS is unclear. While NCS may represent a biomarker of worse brain injury, some evidence suggests NCS or NCSE may independently worsen outcome. More data is available in adults than in children. In adults, longer duration NCSE has been associated with worse outcome (81). NCS have been associated with worse discharge outcome in adults with CNS infection (82) and death or severe neurologic disability in adults in the medical ICU (83). In adults with traumatic brain injury, NCS have been associated with increases in intracranial pressure and metabolic dysfunction in adults with traumatic brain injury (84), and NCS have been associated with later ipsilateral hippocampal atrophy (85). Electrographic seizures have been associated with hemorrhage expansion in adults (86).

Several recent studies have explored the impact of NCS and NCSE on outcome in children. In 75 children, NCS is associated with higher mortality (15% versus 8%) and neurologic morbidity (31% versus 4%) (12). In a second study of 204 critically ill comatose children and neonates, 111 survived to 1 month. Among survivors, worse outcome was associated with clinically evident seizures, electrographic seizures, higher number and longer duration electrographic seizures, and a worse EEG background score. Electrographic seizures were associated with an odds ratio (OR) of 15.4 (4.7–49.7) for worse outcome in a multivariate model that contained etiology, EEG background score, Pediatric Index of Mortality, and Adelaide coma score. Further, no children had favorable outcome if they had more than 139 seizures, more than 759 minutes of total seizures, or any individual seizure lasting longer than 360 minutes (13). A third study evaluated short-term outcome in 200 prospectively enrolled critically ill children who underwent EEG monitoring if they had altered mental status and an acute neurologic problem. Eighty-four (42%) had seizures that were categorized as electrographic seizures in 41 (20.5%) and electrographic status epilepticus in 43 (21.5%). EEGs were scored as no seizures, electrographic seizures, or electrographic status epilepticus. Covariates included age, acute neurologic disorder category, prior neurodevelopmental status, sex, and EEG background category. Outcomes were mortality and worsening of Pediatric Cerebral Performance Category (PCPC) from preadmission to PICU discharge. In multivariable analysis electrographic status epilepticus was associated with an increased risk of mortality (OR, 5.1; 95% confidence interval [CI], 1.4–18; $P = .01$) and PCPC worsening (OR, 17.3; 95% CI, 3.7–80; $P < .001$) while electrographic seizures were not associated with an increased risk of mortality (OR, 1.3; 95% CI, 0.3–5.1; $P = .74$) or PCPC worsening (OR, 1.2; 95% CI, 0.4–3.9; $P = .77$). This suggests that if the seizure burden is high, it is independently associated with worse outcome (87). Further study is needed to determine whether seizure identification and management improves outcome.

If identified, there are few data to guide management of NCS and NCSE. A survey of neurologists reported that the most commonly used medications for NCS and NCSE were lorazepam, phenytoin/fosphenytoin, and levetiracetam. There was substantial variability in practice, and the second and third line medications were these same three in varying combinations. Most physicians reported escalating treatment to include pharmacologic coma induction with intubation if needed, and the most commonly used medications were midazolam and pentobarbital (77). Studies are needed to compare different management regimens and determine whether certain strategies improve outcome.

■ PERIODIC AND RHYTHMIC PATTERNS

EEGs may contain periodic or rhythmic discharges, and in many instances these are of unclear significance. These patterns do not demonstrate the unequivocal evolution in frequency, morphology, or location characteristic of seizures. Rhythmic discharges describe repetition of a waveform with relatively uniform morphology and duration, but without sufficient evolution to constitute electrographic seizures. Their physiologic and prognostic impact is unclear. Periodic discharges describe a pattern with nearly regular interval between waveforms that have a relatively uniform morphology, duration, and interdischarge interval. Common types of periodic discharges are generalized or lateralized periodic epileptiform discharges (PEDs). (Figures 9.11 and 9.12). PEDs have been associated with an increased risk of seizures (4, 10) and worse outcome (83,86,88,89). In a survey of neurologists, 63% would administer anticonvulsants if PEDs are present and occur at a frequency faster than 1.5 Hz, even if they never evolve into a seizure. If an anticonvulsant is administered, the treatment goal is to provide prophylaxis against seizures but not specifically target the PEDs for treatment (66%), aim to reduce PEDs to less than 1.5 Hz (14%), or aim to terminate

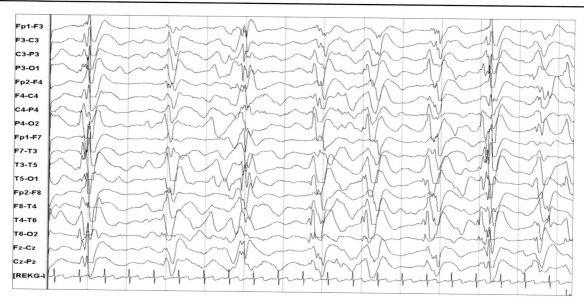

FIGURE 9.11 Bilateral periodic epileptiform discharges.

PEDs (20%) (77). Rhythmic discharges and PEDs are targets of active investigation, and terminology is being developed to improve interrater agreement and foster research on their impact (90).

Triphasic waves are often discussed, although they likely occur less often in children than adults. Triphasic waves are blunt, bilaterally symmetric synchronous, anterior predominant, and often have a frontal-occipital time lag (91). They consist of a high-voltage (100–300 µV) positive wave preceded and followed by lower voltage negative waves, and this morphology provided the triphasic name. The positive wave is the highest in amplitude while the first negative wave is usually the sharpest. Triphasic waves usually occur in the context of a slow background (Figure 9.13). They are a nonspecific sign of encephalopathy and most commonly occur in patients with multiple metabolic abnormalities (92–94). Triphasic waves are reported with hepatic

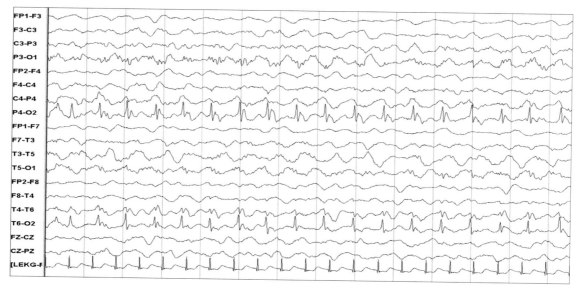

FIGURE 9.12 Focal periodic epileptiform discharges in the right occipital region.

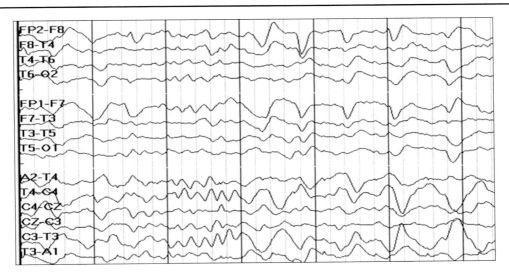

FIGURE 9.13 Triphasic waves.

encephalopathy, renal failure, hyperosmolar state, hypoglycemia, hyponatremia, and hypercalcemia. Less commonly, they are reported with anoxic encephalopathy (94), hyperthyroidism (95,96), sepsis (97), stroke (98,99), cerebral tumors (100,101), carcinomatous meningitis (102), valproate induced hyperammonemia (103), hypothermia (104), chronic dementia (93), and possibly with intoxication with lithium (105), levodopa (106), and levetiracetam (107). The mechanism underlying triphasic waves is not clear, but may involve mesial frontal generators (108). In some situations, triphasic waves may be difficult to distinguish from epileptiform abnormalities and NCSE. Unfortunately, both triphasic waves and epileptiform abnormalities may be abolished by benzodiazepines (109), so this response does not help distinguish between the two.

■ EEG AND PROGNOSIS

Providing prognostic information is often an important aspect of neurocritical care, and although clinical, laboratory, imaging, and neurophysiologic findings may be useful in outcome prediction, few have perfect predictive value (110). EEG can be performed noninvasively at bedside and provides objective data regarding brain function, and thus EEG features have been explored. There are several important considerations regarding the utilization of EEG for prognosis. First, most investigations related to EEG and prognosis has occurred in the context of hypoxic-ischemic encephalopathy, and the predictive value of these features cannot be extrapolated to other types of acute brain injury. EEG features are nonspecific, and if caused by reversible etiologies (ie, toxic or metabolic encephalopathies) they may have little prognostic significance. Second, most studies occurred prior to the utilization of therapeutic hypothermia, but if therapeutic hypothermia is neuroprotective following cardiac arrest, then EEG features may have altered prognostic significance. Third, a fundamental limitation of EEG-based prognosis is the uncertain reproducibility of EEG interpretation in critically ill and comatose patients (90,111–114), although some EEG features in children with hypoxic-ischemic brain injury have substantial interrater agreement (114).

Several studies have investigated comatose children with multiple etiologies. In a study of 48 comatose children who underwent EEGs during the acute phase of their illness, more than half of children with normal or slow activity had good outcomes while all patients in whom the worst EEG demonstrated low amplitude or electrocerebral silence had a poor outcome (115). A second study involved 33 comatose children due to multiple etiologies (hypoxia in 36%). Of 19 children with a nonreactive EEG pattern, 10 (53%) died, 3 (16%) had unfavorable outcome, and 6 (32%) had favorable outcome (although none were normal on follow-up). Of 14 children with a reactive EEG pattern, 3 (21%) were normal at follow-up, an additional 7 (50%) had a favorable outcome, and 4 (29%) died. Lack of reactivity had a 52.6% positive predictive value for mortality (31).

Most studies of EEG and prognosis have focused on hypoxic-ischemic injury. In the prehypothermia period, several EEG classification systems were developed in children (116) and adults (27,29,117,118). An American Academy of Neurology practice parameter focused on outcome prediction in adults after cardiac arrest and, based on data prior to therapeutic hypothermia utilization, described that myoclonic status epilepticus on the first day predicted unfavorable outcome, while diffuse voltage suppression and generalized periodic complexes were strongly but not invariably associated with unfavorable outcome (119). Fewer data are available in children. In 1968 Pampiglione and Harden (120) demonstrated that after circulatory arrest, no patients with periods of burst suppression survived to discharge while if the EEG improved rapidly, few had neurologic impairment. A study of 57 children with hypoxic-ischemic encephalopathy reported that discontinuous activity had a 100% positive predictive outcome for poor outcome (95% CI, 56%–100%), and no reactivity or high voltage slow waves (less than 2 Hz) had a positive predictive value for poor outcome of 96% (95% CI, 76%–100%) (121). Studies have suggested that response to stimulation (a reactive pattern) (122) and normal sleep patterns (122,123) are associated with good prognosis.

When patients are treated with therapeutic hypothermia, many of these prognostic EEG variables seem to retain their prognostic significance, although there have been fewer studies, particularly in children. Lack of electrographic reactivity to stimulation predicts poor prognosis in adults treated with therapeutic hypothermia (27–30). A series of 111 adults treated with therapeutic hypothermia after cardiac arrest found that an unreactive EEG background was a more sensitive predictor of neurologic recovery than clinical signs such as motor responsiveness (30). Similarly, in adults treated with therapeutic hypothermia after cardiac arrest, bispectral index monitoring scores of zero (reflecting a low amplitude, featureless, unreactive EEG) predict unfavorable outcome or death (124–126). In a study of 35 children managed with a standard therapeutic hypothermia algorithm after cardiac arrest, EEG recordings were scored in a standardized manner and categorized. The features which defined each category, reactivity and continuity, were chosen since interpretation has substantial interrater reliability (114). EEG category 1 consisted of continuous and reactive tracings. EEG category 2 consisted of continuous but unreactive tracings. EEG category 3 included those with

any degree of discontinuity, burst suppression, or lack of cerebral activity. The primary outcome was unfavorable short-term outcome defined as PCPC score of 4 to 6 (severe disability, vegetative, death) at hospital discharge. For tracings obtained during hypothermia, patients with EEGs in categories 2 or 3 were far more likely to have poor outcome than those in category 1 (OR, 10.7, P = .023; and OR 35, P = .004, respectively). Similarly, for tracings obtained during normothermia, patients with EEGs in categories 2 or 3 were far more likely to have poor outcomes than those in category 1 (OR, 27, P = .006; and OR, 18, P = .02, respectively). Replication in a larger cohort is needed, but this study suggests that EEGs that are unreactive and discontinuous, even during hypothermia, predict an unfavorable outcome. However, predictions were not perfect, and thus the EEG data must be considered in the context of other information.

■ IMPACT OF EEG ON CLINICAL MANAGEMENT

Several studies have explored whether EEG data impact clinical management. A study of 100 consecutive critically ill children who underwent EEG monitoring if they had acute encephalopathy found that EEG monitoring led to specific changes in clinical management in 59%. These changes included initiating or escalating anticonvulsants due to seizure identification in 43 subjects, determining that a specific event (movement or vital sign change) was not a seizure in 21 subjects, and obtaining urgent neuroimaging in 3 subjects. About one third of subjects in whom specific events were identified as nonepileptic had unrelated electrographic seizures (127). Similarly, a study of seizure occurrence among 122 critically ill children reported that events were found to be nonepileptic in one-quarter (11). These data indicate that when used, EEG monitoring often influences clinical management. Further study is needed to determine whether these changes in management improve outcome.

More data are available in adults. In 25 adults presenting to the emergency department with a mental status change of unknown etiology, a 5 minute EEG was useful in identifying the etiologic category as diffuse encephalopathy, focal abnormality, or seizure related condition (128). A study of 286 emergent EEGs in critically ill adults reported that 62% were rated as clinically useful by physicians (129). A study of 11 emergent EEGs in adults reported that clinicians considered EEG to have contributed to establishing a diagnosis in 78%, confirmed a suspected diagnosis in 36%, and led to patient management modifications in 38%. Further, when NCSE was suspected, it was confirmed in 43% and when EEG was performed after convulsive status epilepticus, NCSE was present in 22% (130). Finally, a study that included 300 consecutive nonelective continuous EEG monitoring studies in 287 adults demonstrated that EEG findings led to anticonvulsant prescribing changes in 52% of studies, including anticonvulsant initiation in 14%, modification in 33%, and discontinuation in 5% (131).

■ INTENSIVIST AND NEUROLOGIST COLLABORATION DURING EEG MONITORING

Collaborative efforts between the critical care, neurology, and neurophysiology services are essential to ensure that EEG monitoring is most beneficial for patients. First, the neurophysiology team must know at least basic information about the patient. While some neurophysiologists may choose to interpret the EEG "blind" to clinical data aside from patient age and medications to avoid any bias, clinical information should be available to ensure the final interpretation is made in the appropriate context and provides the most helpful summary possible for the bedside team. Information that is generally useful is provided in Table 9.1. Understanding the indication for EEG monitoring will allow the neurophysiologist to best tailor their impression to answer the clinical question. Common indication categories are listed in Table 9.1.

Second, it is important to consider that at most institutions EEG is recorded continuously but interpreted only intermittently (77). In a survey of neurologists, when EEG monitoring is being used to screen for NCS it is reviewed once per day by 21%, twice per day by 29%, 3 or 4 times per day by 17%, and almost continuously by only 18% (77). The EEG review schedule in part determines whether identification of ischemia or encephalopathy is feasible for a given patient and condition, and what delay might occur between an EEG change and identification of that change. Given the limited role EEG plays in ischemia identification for most pediatric patients, it is not clear that more frequent review of full array EEG data is indicated. In addition to review of streamlined EEG data, the use of quantitative EEG techniques, such as amplitude integrated EEG and color density spectral array EEG, is an area of active study (132,133).

■ Table 9.1 Clinical Information Provided by Intensive Care Unit to Neurophysiology

Patient age
Medications
Clinical seizures prior to EEG monitoring?
Events of unclear etiology prior to EEG monitoring?
Chronic and past medical problems
Current neurologic and medical diagnoses/problems
Key components of ongoing care (such as paralytic administration, therapeutic hypothermia, ECMO)
Mental status
EEG monitoring indication(s):
    Diagnosis of nonconvulsive seizures
    Monitoring therapy for seizures (ie, prior refractory status epilepticus)
    Characterization of events of unclear etiology
    Assessment of level of sedation
    Management of ICP
    Detection of ischemia
    Monitoring of degree of encephalopathy
    Prognostication

Abbreviations: ECMO, extracorporeal membrane oxygenation; EEG, electroencephalogram; ICP, intracranial pressure.

Third, ongoing collaboration is required to ensure the recording is technically sufficient. As discussed above, many artifacts can occur in the ICU and can obscure the brain generated EEG tracing. When artifact is identified, technologists must often work with nurses to eliminate the artifact safely by adjusting or moving equipment, repositioning the patient, and replacing or adjusting electrodes.

Fourth, continued discussions between the critical care, neurology, and neurophysiology services are essential. First, these discussions ensure that as the clinical situation evolves, the EEG can be interpreted in the appropriate context. Second, these discussions ensure that EEG data is conveyed to the bedside caregivers and interpreted appropriately. While guidelines exist for the overall structure of EEG reports (134), the exact wording is often reader or institution dependent. However, with the increased use of EEG in the ICU setting, reports must be understood by a wider range of practitioners. This communication may occur verbally, via written reports, or usually by a combination of these methods (77).

■ CONCLUSIONS

EEG monitoring provides a continuous monitor of brain function that can be useful in diagnosing encephalopathy, evaluating for interval changes in encephalopathy, establishing broad etiologic categories for encephalopathy, and identifying electrographic seizures. Collaboration between critical care, neurology, and neurophysiology services is essential in obtaining optimal recordings, interpreting these recordings in the appropriate clinical context, and using the EEG data to guide clinical management appropriately.

■ REFERENCES

1. O'Sullivan SS et al. Aetiology and prognosis of encephalopathic patterns on electroencephalogram in a general hospital. *J Clin Neurosci*. 2008;15:637–642.
2. Abend NS et al. Non-convulsive seizures are common in critically ill children. *Neurology*. 2011;76:1071–1077.
3. Hosain SA, Solomon GE, Kobylarz EJ. Electroencephalographic patterns in unresponsive pediatric patients. *Pediatr Neurol*. 2005;32:162–165.
4. Jette N et al. Frequency and predictors of nonconvulsive seizures during continuous electroencephalographic monitoring in critically ill children. *Arch Neurol*. 2006;63:1750–1755.
5. Abend NS, Dlugos DJ. Nonconvulsive status epilepticus in a pediatric intensive care unit. *Pediatr Neurol*. 2007;37:165–170.
6. Alehan FK, Morton LD, Pellock JM. Utility of electroencephalography in the pediatric emergency department. *J Child Neurol*. 2001;16:484–487.
7. Tay SK et al. Nonconvulsive status epilepticus in children: clinical and EEG characteristics. *Epilepsia*. 2006;47:1504–1509.
8. Saengpattrachai M et al. Nonconvulsive seizures in the pediatric intensive care unit: etiology, EEG, and brain imaging findings. *Epilepsia*. 2006;47:1510–1518.
9. Shahwan A et al. The prevalence of seizures in comatose children in the pediatric intensive care unit: a prospective video-EEG study. *Epilepsia*. 2010;51:1198–1204.
10. Abend NS et al. Electroencephalographic monitoring during hypothermia after pediatric cardiac arrest. *Neurology*. 2009;72:1931–1940.
11. Williams K, Jarrar R, Buchhalter J. Continuous video-EEG monitoring in pediatric intensive care units. *Epilepsia*. 2011;52:1130–1136.
12. Greiner HM et al. Nonconvulsive status epilepticus: the encephalopathic pediatric patient. *Pediatrics*. 2012;129:e748–e755.
13. Kirkham FJ et al. Seizures in 204 comatose children: incidence and outcome. *Intensive Care Med*. 2012;38:853–862.
14. Guideline three: minimum technical standards for EEG recording in suspected cerebral death. American Electroencephalographic Society. *J Clin Neurophysiol*. 1994;11:10–13.
15. Nakagawa TA, Ashwal S, Mathur M. Guidelines for the determination of brain death in infants and children: an update of the 1987 task force recommendations. *Crit Care Med*. 2011;39:2139–2155.
16. White DM, Van Cott AC. EEG artifacts in the intensive care unit setting. *Am J Electroneurodiagnostic Technol*. 2010;50:8–25.
17. Tatum WO et al. Artifact: recording EEG in special care units. *J Clin Neurophysiol*. 2011;28:264–277.
18. Kellaway P. Orderly approach to visual analysis: elements of the normal EEG and their characteristics in children and adults. In: Ebersole JS, Pedley TA, eds. *Current Practice of Clinical Electroencephalography*. Philadelphia, PA: Lippincott Williams & Wilkins; 2003:100–159.
19. Petersen I, Eeg-Olofsson O. The development of the electroencephalogram in normal children from the age of 1 through 15 years. Non-paroxysmal activity. *Neuropadiatrie*. 1971;2:247–304.
20. Gloor P, Ball G, Schaul N. Brain lesions that produce delta waves in the EEG. *Neurology*. 1977;27:326–333.
21. Niedermeyer E. The burst-suppression electroencephalogram. *Am J Electroneurodiagnostic Technol*. 2009;49:333–341.
22. Kessler S et al. Short-term outcome prediction by electroencephalographic features in children treated with therapeutic hypothermia after cardiac arrest. *Neurocrit Care*. 2011;14:37–43.
23. Rossetti AO et al. Prognostic value of continuous EEG monitoring during therapeutic hypothermia after cardiac arrest. *Crit Care*. 2010;14:R173.
24. Rossetti AO, Carrera E, Oddo M. Early EEG correlates of neuronal injury after brain anoxia. *Neurology*. 2012;78:796–802.

25. Abend NS, Dlugos DJ. Treatment of refractory status epilepticus: literature review and a proposed protocol. *Pediatr Neurol.* 2008;38:377–390.
26. Shorvon S, Ferlisi M. The treatment of super-refractory status epilepticus: a critical review of available therapies and a clinical treatment protocol. *Brain.* 2011;134:2802–2818.
27. Thenayan EA et al. Electroencephalogram for prognosis after cardiac arrest. *J Crit Care.* 2010;25:300–304.
28. Rossetti AO et al. Predictors of awakening from postanoxic status epilepticus after therapeutic hypothermia. *Neurology.* 2009;72:744–749.
29. Roest A et al. The prognostic value of the EEG in postanoxic coma. *Neurocrit Care.* 2009;10:318–325.
30. Rossetti AO et al. Prognostication after cardiac arrest and hypothermia: a prospective study. *Ann Neurol.* 2010;67:301–307.
31. Ramachandrannair R et al. Reactive EEG patterns in pediatric coma. *Pediatr Neurol.* 2005;33:345–349.
32. Hirsch LJ et al. Stimulus-induced rhythmic, periodic, or ictal discharges (SIRPIDs): a common EEG phenomenon in the critically ill. *Epilepsia.* 2004;45:109–123.
33. Skjei KL, Kessler SK, Abend NS. Stimulus-induced rhythmic, periodic, or ictal discharges in a 13 year old girl after an overdose and respiratory arrest. *Pediatr Neurol.* 2011;45:350–351.
34. Report of special Task Force. Guidelines for the determination of brain death in children. American Academy of Pediatrics Task Force on Brain Death in Children. *Pediatrics.* 1987;80:298–300.
35. Stecker MM et al. Deep hypothermic circulatory arrest: I. Effects of cooling on electroencephalogram and evoked potentials. *Ann Thorac Surg.* 2001;71:14–21.
36. Ramachandrannair R et al. A reappraisal of rhythmic coma patterns in children. *Can J Neurol Sci.* 2005;32:518–523.
37. Kaplan PW et al. Etiology, neurologic correlations, and prognosis in alpha coma. *Clin Neurophysiol.* 1999;110:205–213.
38. Berkhoff M, Donati F, Bassetti C. Postanoxic alpha (theta) coma: a reappraisal of its prognostic significance. *Clin Neurophysiol.* 2000;111:297–304.
39. Young GB et al. Alpha, theta and alpha-theta coma: a clinical outcome study utilizing serial recordings. *Electroencephalogr Clin Neurophysiol.* 1994;91:93–99.
40. Nowack WJ, Beadle B, Janati A. Coexisting alpha pattern coma, theta pattern coma and spindle coma. *Clin Electroencephalogr.* 1987;18:74–80.
41. Sarma GR et al. Post-cardiorespiratory arrest beta-alpha coma: an unusual electroencephalographic phenomenon. *Neurol India.* 2003;51:266–268.
42. Carrai R et al. Transient post-traumatic locked-in syndrome: a case report and a literature review. *Neurophysiol Clin.* 2009;39:95–100.
43. Westmoreland BF et al. Alpha-coma. Electroencephalographic, clinical, pathologic, and etiologic correlations. *Arch Neurol.* 1975;32:713–718.
44. Ono A et al. [A case of carbamazepine intoxication with alpha coma and status epilepticus]. *No To Hattatsu.* 2001;33:528–532.
45. Pulst SM, Lombroso CT. External ophthalmoplegia, alpha and spindle coma in imipramine overdose: case report and review of the literature. *Ann Neurol.* 1983;14:587–590.
46. Das A et al. Alpha coma evolving into spindle coma in a case of acute fulminant hepatic failure: What does it signify? *Ann Indian Acad Neurol.* 2010;13:69–71.
47. Austin EJ, Wilkus RJ, Longstreth WT, Jr. Etiology and prognosis of alpha coma. *Neurology.* 1988;38:773–777.
48. Bragatti JA et al. Alpha coma pattern in a child. *Clin EEG Neurosci.* 2008;39:206–209.
49. Lersch DR, Kaplan AM. Alpha-pattern coma in childhood and adolescence. *Arch Neurol.* 1984;41:68–70.
50. Yamada T, Stevland N, Kimura J. Alpha-pattern coma in a 2-year-old child. *Arch Neurol.* 1979;36:225–227.
51. Homan RW, Jones MG. Alpha-pattern coma in a 2-month-old child. *Ann Neurol.* 1981;9:611–613.
52. Molofsky WJ. Alpha coma in a child. *J Neurol Neurosurg Psychiatry.* 1982;45:95.
53. Horton EJ, Goldie WD, Baram TZ. Rhythmic coma in children. *J Child Neurol.* 1990;5:242–247.
54. Frisher S, Herishanu Y. Mu and alpha rhythm in comatose children. *Childs Nerv Syst.* 1985;1:208–210.
55. Collins AT, Chatrian GE. EEG rhythm of alpha frequency in a 22-month-old child after strangulation. *Neurology.* 1980;30:1316–1319.
56. Zaret BS. Prognostic and neurophysiological implications of concurrent burst suppression and alpha patterns in the EEG of post-anoxic coma. *Electroencephalogr Clin Neurophysiol.* 1985;61:199–209.
57. Ramachandrannair R, Weiss SK. Incomplete alpha coma pattern in a child. *Pediatr Neurol.* 2005;33:127–130.
58. Martinez Bermejo A et al. [Alpha coma: clinical, electroencephalographic and aetiological correlation in childhood]. *Rev Neurol.* 2001;33:1101–1105.
59. Ganji SS, Henry R, Furlow J. Diffuse theta activity and spindle-like bursts during coma after cardiac arrest. *Clin Electroencephalogr.* 1996;27:89–94.
60. Bortone E et al. Post-anoxic theta and alpha pattern coma. *Clin Electroencephalogr.* 1994;25:156–159.
61. Synek VM, Synek BJ. Theta pattern coma, a variant of alpha pattern coma. *Clin Electroencephalogr.* 1984;15:116–121.
62. Nogueira de Melo A, Krauss GL, Niedermeyer E. Spindle coma: observations and thoughts. *Clin Electroencephalogr.* 1990;21:151–161.
63. Hansotia P et al. Spindle coma: incidence, clinicopathologic correlates, and prognostic value. *Neurology.* 1981;31:83–87.
64. Britt CW, Jr. Nontraumatic "spindle coma": clinical, EEG, and prognostic features. *Neurology.* 1981;31:393–397.
65. Dadmehr N, Pakalnis A, Drake ME, Jr. Spindle coma in viral encephalitis. *Clin Electroencephalogr.* 1987;18:34–37.
66. Bortone E et al. Spindle coma and alternating pattern in the course of measles encephalitis. *Clin Electroencephalogr.* 1996;27:210–214.
67. Mouradian MD, Penovich PE. Spindle coma in benzodiazepine toxicity: case report. *Clin Electroencephalogr.* 1985;16:213–218.
68. Seet RC, Lim EC, Wilder-Smith EP. Spindle coma from acute midbrain infarction. *Neurology.* 2005;64:2159–2160.
69. Britt CW, Jr., Raso E, Gerson LP. Spindle coma, secondary to primary traumatic midbrain hemorrhage. *Electroencephalogr Clin Neurophysiol.* 1980;49:406–408.
70. Kaplan PW et al. Clinical correlates and prognosis in early spindle coma. *Clin Neurophysiol.* 2000;111:584–590.

71. Lopez MR, Freeman R, Schomer D. Spindle coma secondary to vasovagal syncope. *Epilepsy Behav.* 2002;3:289–291.

72. Herkes GK et al. Effects of midazolam on electroencephalograms of seriously ill patients. *Mayo Clin Proc.* 1992;67:334–338.

73. Otomo E. Beta wave activity in the electroencephalogram in cases of coma due to acute brain-stem lesions. *J Neurol Neurosurg Psychiatry.* 1966;29:383–390.

74. Abend NS et al. Nonconvulsive seizures are common in critically ill children. *Neurology.* 2011;76:1071–1077.

75. McCoy B et al. Predictors of nonconvulsive seizures among critically ill children. *Epilepsia.* 2011;52:1973–1978.

76. Claassen J et al. Detection of electrographic seizures with continuous EEG monitoring in critically ill patients. *Neurology.* 2004;62:1743–1748.

77. Abend NS et al. Use of EEG monitoring and management of non-convulsive seizures in critically ill patients: a survey of neurologists. *Neurocrit Care.* 2010;12:382–389.

78. Hyllienmark L, Amark P. Continuous EEG monitoring in a paediatric intensive care unit. *Eur J Paediatr Neurol.* 2007;11:70–75.

79. Sutter R et al. Continuous video-EEG monitoring increases detection rate of nonconvulsive status epilepticus in the ICU. *Epilepsia.* 2011;52:453–457.

80. Clancy RR et al. Electrographic neonatal seizures after infant heart surgery. *Epilepsia.* 2005;46:84–90.

81. Young GB, Jordan KG, Doig GS. An assessment of nonconvulsive seizures in the intensive care unit using continuous EEG monitoring: an investigation of variables associated with mortality. *Neurology.* 1996;47:83–89.

82. Carrera E et al. Continuous electroencephalographic monitoring in critically ill patients with central nervous system infections. *Arch Neurol.* 2008;65:1612–1618.

83. Oddo M et al. Continuous electroencephalography in the medical intensive care unit. *Crit Care Med.* 2009;37:2051–2056.

84. Vespa PM et al. Nonconvulsive electrographic seizures after traumatic brain injury result in a delayed, prolonged increase in intracranial pressure and metabolic crisis. *Crit Care Med.* 2007;35:2830–2836.

85. Vespa PM et al. Nonconvulsive seizures after traumatic brain injury are associated with hippocampal atrophy. *Neurology.* 2010;75:792–798.

86. Claassen J et al. Electrographic seizures and periodic discharges after intracerebral hemorrhage. *Neurology.* 2007;69:1356–1365.

87. Topjian AA et al. Electrographic status epilepticus is associated with mortality and worse short-term outcome in critically ill children. *Crit Care Med.* In press.

88. San-Juan OD et al. Periodic epileptiform discharges in hypoxic encephalopathy: BiPLEDs and GPEDs as a poor prognosis for survival. *Seizure.* 2009;18:365–368.

89. Claassen J et al. Prognostic significance of continuous EEG monitoring in patients with poor-grade subarachnoid hemorrhage. *Neurocrit Care.* 2006;4:103–112.

90. Hirsch LJ et al. The ACNS subcommittee on research terminology for continuous EEG monitoring: proposed standardized terminology for rhythmic and periodic EEG patterns encountered in critically ill patients. *J Clin Neurophysiol.* 2005;22:128–135.

91. Brigo F, Storti M. Triphasic waves. *Am J Electroneurodiagnostic Technol.* 2011;51:16–25.

92. Bahamon-Dussan JE, Celesia GG, Grigg-Damberger MM. Prognostic significance of EEG triphasic waves in patients with altered state of consciousness. *J Clin Neurophysiol.* 1989;6:313–319.

93. Sundaram MB, Blume WT. Triphasic waves: clinical correlates and morphology. *Can J Neurol Sci.* 1987;14:136–140.

94. Karnaze DS, Bickford RG. Triphasic waves: a reassessment of their significance. *Electroencephalogr Clin Neurophysiol.* 1984;57:193–198.

95. Scherokman BJ. Triphasic delta waves in a patient with acute hyperthyroidism. *Arch Neurol.* 1980;37:731.

96. Hirano M, Endo M, Kubo T. Triphasic delta waves in a case of hyperthyroidism with psychotic symptoms. *Clin Electroencephalogr.* 1982;13:97–102.

97. Young GB et al. The encephalopathy associated with septic illness. *Clin Invest Med.* 1990;13:297–304.

98. Cherian PJ, Radhakrishnan K. Triphasic waves in a patient with brainstem hemorrhage modified by hemispheric infarct. *Eur J Neurol.* 2004;11:789–790.

99. Townsend JB, Drury I. Triphasic waves in coma from brainstem infarction. *Eur Neurol.* 1991;31:47–49.

100. Ghanem Q. Triphasic waves in a patient with glioblastoma multiforme. *Clin Electroencephalogr.* 1992;23:95–99.

101. Aguglia U et al. Triphasic waves and cerebral tumors. *Eur Neurol.* 1990;30:1–5.

102. Miller B, Brick J. Triphasic sharp waves in a patient with carcinomatous meningitis. *Clin Electroencephalogr.* 1989;20:259–261.

103. Kifune A et al. Valproic acid-induced hyperammonemic encephalopathy with triphasic waves. *Epilepsia.* 2000;41:909–912.

104. Reutens DC, Dunne JW, Gubbay SS. Triphasic waves in accidental hypothermia. *Electroencephalogr Clin Neurophysiol.* 1990;76:370–372.

105. Shibasaki Warabi Y et al. Triphasic waves detected during recovery from lithium intoxication. *Intern Med.* 2003;42:908–909.

106. Neufeld MY. Periodic triphasic waves in levodopa-induced encephalopathy. *Neurology.* 1992;42:444–446.

107. Vulliemoz S et al. Levetiracetam accumulation in renal failure causing myoclonic encephalopathy with triphasic waves. *Seizure.* 2009;18:376–378.

108. Kwon OY et al. Source localization of triphasic waves: implications for the pathophysiological mechanism. *Clin EEG Neurosci.* 2007;38:161–167.

109. Fountain NB, Waldman WA. Effects of benzodiazepines on triphasic waves: implications for nonconvulsive status epilepticus. *J Clin Neurophysiol.* 2001;18:345–352.

110. Abend NS, Licht DJ. Predicting outcome in children with hypoxic ischemic encephalopathy. *Pediatr Crit Care Med.* 2008;9:32–39.

111. Husain AM. Electroencephalographic assessment of coma. *J Clin Neurophysiol.* 2006;23:208–220.

112. Gerber PA et al. Interobserver agreement in the interpretation of EEG patterns in critically ill adults. *J Clin Neurophysiol.* 2008;25:241–249.

113. Ronner HE et al. Inter-observer variability of the EEG diagnosis of seizures in comatose patients. *Seizure.* 2009;18:257–263.

114. Abend NS et al. Interobserver reproducibility of electroencephalogram interpretation in critically ill children. *J Clin Neurophysiol.* 2011;28:15–19.

115. Tasker RC et al. Monitoring in non-traumatic coma. Part II: electroencephalography. *Arch Dis Child*. 1988;63:895–899.
116. Nishisaki A et al. Retrospective analysis of the prognostic value of electroencephalography patterns obtained in pediatric in-hospital cardiac arrest survivors during three years. *Pediatr Crit Care Med*. 2007;8:10–17.
117. Synek VM. Prognostically important EEG coma patterns in diffuse anoxic and traumatic encephalopathies in adults. *J Clin Neurophysiol*. 1988;5:161–174.
118. Young GB et al. An electroencephalographic classification for coma. *Can J Neurol Sci*. 1997;24:320–325.
119. Wijdicks EF et al. Practice parameter: prediction of outcome in comatose survivors after cardiopulmonary resuscitation (an evidence-based review): report of the Quality Standards Subcommittee of the American Academy of Neurology. *Neurology*. 2006;67:203–210.
120. Pampiglione G, Harden A. Resuscitation after cardiocirculatory arrest. Prognostic evaluation of early electroencephalographic findings. *Lancet*. 1968;1:1261–1265.
121. Mandel R et al. Prediction of outcome after hypoxic-ischemic encephalopathy: a prospective clinical and electrophysiologic study. *J Pediatr*. 2002;141:45–50.
122. Cheliout-Heraut F et al. [Cerebral anoxia in near-drowning of children. The prognostic value of EEG]. *Neurophysiol Clin*. 1991;21:121–132.
123. Evans BM, Bartlett JR. Prediction of outcome in severe head injury based on recognition of sleep related activity in the polygraphic electroencephalogram. *J Neurol Neurosurg Psychiatry*. 1995;59:17–25.
124. Leary M et al. Neurologic prognostication and bispectral index monitoring after resuscitation from cardiac arrest. *Resuscitation*, 2010;81:1133–1137.
125. Stammet P et al. Bispectral index (BIS) helps predicting bad neurological outcome in comatose survivors after cardiac arrest and induced therapeutic hypothermia. *Resuscitation*. 2009;80:437–442.
126. Seder DB et al. The bispectral index and suppression ratio are very early predictors of neurological outcome during therapeutic hypothermia after cardiac arrest. *Intensive Care Med*. 2010;36:281–288.
127. Abend NS et al. Impact of continuous EEG monitoring on clinical management in critically ill children. *Neurocrit Care*. 2011;15:70–75.
128. Bautista RE, Godwin S, Caro D. Incorporating abbreviated EEGs in the initial workup of patients who present to the emergency room with mental status changes of unknown etiology. *J Clin Neurophysiol*. 2007;24:16–21.
129. Firosh Khan S et al. Emergent EEG is helpful in neurology critical care practice. *Clin Neurophysiol*. 2005;116:2454–2459.
130. Praline J et al. Emergent EEG in clinical practice. *Clin Neurophysiol*. 2007;118:2149–2155.
131. Kilbride RD, Costello DJ, Chiappa KH. How seizure detection by continuous electroencephalographic monitoring affects the prescribing of antiepileptic medications. *Arch Neurol*. 2009;66:723–728.
132. Stewart CP et al. Seizure identification in the ICU using quantitative EEG displays. *Neurology*. 2010;75:1501–1508.
133. Akman CI et al. Seizure detection using digital trend analysis: Factors affecting utility. *Epilepsy Res*. 2011;93:66–72.
134. Guideline 7: Guideline for writing EEG reports. American Clinical Neurophysiology Society Web site. http://www.acns.org/. Updated 2006. Accessed April 1, 2012.

10 Arterial Ischemic Stroke

DAVID Z. ROSE, SABRINA E. SMITH, and LAUREN A. BESLOW

■ INTRODUCTION AND DEFINITION

In children, as in adults, acute arterial ischemic stroke (AIS) is a significant cause of morbidity and mortality in the United States and around the world. AIS is defined as an acute neurologic deficit due to an infarction in an arterial territory of the brain. A transient ischemic attack (TIA) is also manifested as a focal deficit, but is related to ischemia in a cerebrovascular territory, without evidence of infarction on neuroimaging. Originally, TIA had a time-based definition, with symptoms lasting fewer than 24 hours, but now TIA carries a tissue-based definition: the absence of a correlating infarct must be demonstrated on magnetic resonance imaging (MRI) or head computed tomography (HCT). Obtaining an accurate diagnosis of pediatric AIS and then managing it expeditiously yet thoughtfully may influence outcome. For children, as in adults, outcomes can range from no residual neurologic deficit to severe neurologic impairment or even death.

■ EPIDEMIOLOGY AND RISK FACTORS

In North America, the incidence of childhood AIS ranges between 0.63 and 2.0 per 100,000 person-years (1–3). Recurrence is high; approximately 7% to 20% of all children with AIS may have another stroke by 5 years (1–3). AIS afflicts boys more often than girls, in a 55%-to-45% ratio (2). AIS is also somewhat more prevalent in black children, even when controlling for sickle cell disease (SCD) (2).

The estimated mortality rate for AIS in children ranges from 2% to 11%. Morbidity with persistent neurologic deficits such as hemiplegia or seizures occurs in approximately 70% (4). In the United States, the average cost for treatment of childhood AIS (including rehabilitation services) was estimated between $31,000 and $43,000 in the first year alone (4,73).

The familiar risk factors for adult AIS, such as hypertension, diabetes, hypercholesterolemia, obesity, and smoking, are not generally risk factors for AIS in children, who possess more diverse etiologies. Congenital heart disease, arteriopathy, and SCD comprise the top 3 causes of pediatric AIS. At presentation, about 50% of children with AIS have a known risk factor or another readily apparent underlying reason for the stroke. Further routine workup will identify AIS risk factors in an additional 20% to 40%, which leaves another 10% to 30% classified as cryptogenic. Arteriopathy is one of the most common causes of pediatric stroke (5). The most common arteriopathic risk factor for childhood AIS is focal cerebral arteriopathy (FCA) of childhood, with moyamoya disease and syndrome and arterial dissection being other common causes of pediatric arteriopathy (5). More unusual arteriopathies include vasculitis. Other potential etiologies for pediatric AIS include hypercoagulability (inherited or acquired prothrombotic states), trauma, and infections. Watershed strokes, between the anterior cerebral artery (ACA) and middle cerebral artery (MCA) or MCA and posterior cerebral artery (PCA) territories, for example, can occur during or after cardiac surgery, after cardiac arrest, or from hypovolemic shock. In older teenagers, traditional risk factors for adults start to emerge including AIS related to use of sympathomimetics like cocaine. Lastly, there are rare, inherited mitochondrial, genetic, and/or metabolic abnormalities that may cause pediatric AIS or stroke-like episodes. The treatment of pediatric AIS is based on the most likely etiology of the stroke and on center-based practice and therefore varies; however, there are published consensus guidelines for the evaluation and management of pediatric AIS (6,7,14).

■ ANATOMY OF INTRACRANIAL AND CERVICAL ARTERIES

Figure 10.1 demonstrates normal intracranial arteries. Approximately 75% percent of pediatric AIS occurs in the anterior circulation, which arises from the right and left internal carotid arteries (ICAs). Each ICA comes from its respective common carotid artery, which on the left is a direct branch off the aortic arch and on the right emanates from the brachiocephalic trunk. There are no branches of either ICA until the ICA arrives intracranially. The intracranial branches of the ICAs are the ophthalmic arteries first, then the anterior choroidal arteries, posterior communicating arteries (which connect the anterior and posterior circulations), MCA, and ACA. The circle of Willis connects these arteries across hemispheres via the anterior communicating artery, between the ACAs. The anterior and posterior portions of the circle of Willis are connected

by the left and right posterior communicating arteries that connect to the ICA anteriorly (prior to bifurcation of the ICA into the MCA and ACA) and to the PCA posteriorly. In the posterior circulation, the two posterior cerebral arteries (PCA) each branch from a solitary artery called the basilar artery, which in turn is formed by the joining of the bilateral vertebral arteries. In most people the origin of the PCA is the basilar artery, but in about 15%, it is from the embryological origin, the ICA, referred to as a fetal PCA. The vertebral arteries emanate from the subclavian arteries, which on the right comprises the other half of the brachiocephalic trunk and on the left comes directly off the aortic arch, next to the left common carotid artery.

■ PATHOPHYSIOLOGY OF AIS

There are multiple potential mechanisms that lead to AIS, and there are multiple steps in the chemical cascade during an acute AIS that lead to eventual death of brain tissue. When an artery becomes occluded by a thrombus in the vessel wall or by an embolus from a proximal source, blood flow is cut off to the region supplied by that artery. Alternately, during systemic hypoperfusion from such causes as sepsis or cardiogenic shock or in the case of severe distal carotid stenosis (moyamoya or sickle cell-associated vasculopathy), the border zone between different vascular territories receives less blood flow and can cause "watershed infarcts." Either by thrombus, embolus, or hypoperfusion, the final common pathway is a complex

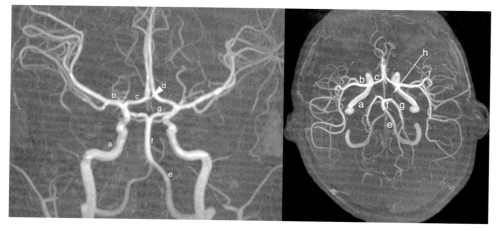

FIGURE 10.1 *Normal intracranial vasculature. Coronal (left panel) and axial (right panel) magnetic resonance angiograms (MRAs) demonstrating normal intracranial vasculature. (a) internal carotid artery; (b) middle cerebral artery; (c) anterior cerebral artery; (d) anterior communicating artery (arrowhead, left panel only); (e) vertebral artery; (f) basilar artery; (g) posterior cerebral artery; (h) posterior communicating artery (arrow, right panel only).*

chain of cellular events. Lack of oxygen and glucose leads to mitochondrial dysfunction, ion pump failure, calcium influx, and glutamate-induced neurotoxicity. Whether cell necrosis or apoptosis occurs depends on a number of factors, including the amount of collateral blood flow available to the injured brain tissue, the oxygen demand in the tissue itself, and the time it takes to restore blood flow to the injured tissue. The time that it takes to restore or improve blood flow to the injured tissue, "time to reperfusion," is a factor that intervention strategies aim to shorten in both pediatric and adult AIS. During a stroke, a core of infarcted tissue in which cells have undergone apoptosis and/or necrosis occurs and is often surrounded by an area that is still salvageable known as the "ischemic penumbra." Without improvement of blood flow into the tissue, irreversible cell death occurs. In theory, a TIA occurs when blood flow in an artery is restored before permanent tissue infarction occurs.

■ CLINICAL PRESENTATIONS AND DIFFERENTIAL DIAGNOSIS

Pediatric AIS is underrecognized within the medical community, despite the considerable and costly long-term disability and residual behavioral, cognitive, emotional, and functional deficits. In one study, the median time to diagnosis of pediatric AIS was over 24 hours (8). Part of the reason for this delay in diagnosis of childhood AIS may be a low index of suspicion by health care professionals. Additionally, the presenting symptoms in children with AIS are more heterogeneous than in adults. Children are much more likely than adults to present with headaches, seizures, or altered mental status as the first sign of stroke. Younger children in particular are more likely than older children to present with an encephalopathy or a decreased level of consciousness; however, a detailed neurologic examination may actually uncover a subtle, new focal deficit. In the study mentioned above, although 86% of children with confirmed AIS had a focal neurologic deficit when first seen by a physician, the presence of a focal deficit was not associated with a more rapid time to stroke confirmation (8).

Hemiparesis is the most common presenting sign of acute AIS in children, and the MCA is the most commonly affected vessel (2,5). Children may also present with focal cortical signs such as aphasia, visual field cuts, or neglect, but deficits depend on both the location of the stroke and the age and developmental stage of the child. For instance, AIS in the posterior circulation can present with ataxia, vertigo, emesis, or cranial nerve palsies. Unfortunately, this symptom complex is often mistaken by families and physicians for a viral infection (8).

If a motor deficit occurs, it is often most pronounced upon presentation but sometimes may exacerbate over minutes or hours. Deficits may even fluctuate with resolution to normal and then back to paresis or plegia. AIS in children with watershed distribution infarction may have weakness that is more proximal than distal.

The differential diagnosis for AIS is broad and includes intracerebral hemorrhage, cerebral venous sinus thrombosis, posterior reversible encephalopathy syndrome, complicated migraine (with or without concurrent headache), seizure with a postictal Todd's paralysis, brain tumor, infections like meningitis, abscess, and encephalitis, and demyelinating diseases like multiple sclerosis, acute disseminated encephalomyelitis, or neurodegenerative diseases, metabolic or mitochondrial diseases, metabolic derangements like hypoglycemia or intoxication, and conversion disorder. In one prospective cohort, 21% of children initially thought to have AIS had stroke mimics (9). Questions about family history of migraines or epilepsy may reveal important clues for the correct diagnosis. Timely triage and neuroimaging studies help to eliminate these alternate diagnoses so that AIS diagnosis and treatment are not delayed.

■ ACUTE DIAGNOSTIC WORKUP AND MANAGEMENT

The emergency room evaluation of a child with suspected AIS should center on diagnosis verification by history and physical examination, vital sign review, laboratory studies, and neuroimaging. The time at which the child was last seen normal should be a crucial part of the history since treatment may vary depending upon the acuity of the stroke. A thorough neurologic examination should be performed, and the Pediatric NIH Stroke Scale score, a measure that has excellent interrater reliability and predictive validity for outcome, should be performed immediately to assess clinical stroke severity (10,11). Acute studies should include electrocardiography, complete blood count with differential, electrolytes, blood urea nitrogen, creatinine, blood glucose, prothrombin time, international normalized ratio, partial thromboplastin time, and toxicology screen. These essential, initial screening tests may rule out stroke mimics and sometimes, as in the case of severe hypoglycemia, reverse the stroke-like symptoms with correction of the underlying problem. As soon as the child is stable, urgent neuroimaging should be performed. A noncontrast HCT should usually be the first image performed since it is fast, does not require sedation in most cases, and is widely available. A HCT is sensitive for acute hemorrhage, and can also be used to rule out large mass lesions. In AIS, noncontrast HCT may be normal early after symptom onset, but occasionally subtle findings of infarction may appear. These include the "hyperdense artery sign" which represents acute clot in an artery (Figure 10.2A), obscuration of the putamen, or

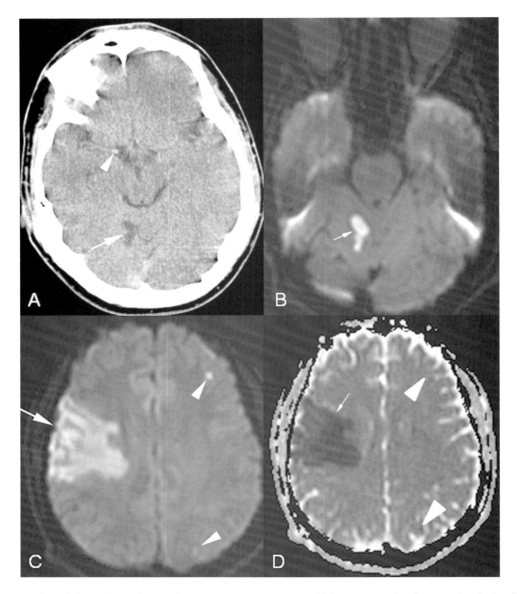

FIGURE 10.2 Cardioembolic stroke and hyperdense artery sign. A 15-year-old boy presented with severe headache, left hemiparesis, hemisensory loss, dysarthria, and neglect 2 days after an episode of dizziness and vomiting. (A), Axial head computed tomography demonstrating subacute cerebellar infarction (arrow) and hyperdense middle cerebral artery (arrowhead) representing acute clot. (B), Axial diffusion weighted imaging (DWI) with restricted diffusion of water (arrow) representing acute infarction corresponding to the area of hypodensity seen in (A). (C), Axial DWI demonstrating acute right middle cerebral artery infarction (arrow) as well as two other punctate areas of infarction on the left (arrowheads). The patient was found to have an intracardiac clot and was treated with heparin. (D), Axial apparent diffusion coefficient (ADC) map corresponding to the areas of restricted diffusion in (C) (arrow and arrowheads).

diminished differentiation of the gray-white matter junction. In one study, an AIS was not detected in 62 of 74 children who had a noncontrast HCT as their first neuroimage. In another study, the stroke was not detected in 47% of acute HCTs (4). However, a normal HCT is still helpful since it excludes hemorrhage or tumor, and acute treatment for presumed AIS can continue while more definitive imaging with MRI is arranged.

Even if subtle findings of AIS are present on HCT, brain MRI with diffusion weighted imaging (DWI) and apparent diffusion coefficient (ADC) is more sensitive for the diagnosis of AIS. In acute AIS hyperintensity is seen on DWI which typically correlates in shape and size with the hypointensity seen on ADC map. These abnormalities on DWI and ADC appear within minutes of AIS onset and may last 7 to 10 days. Figure 10.2 demonstrates a HCT performed 2 days after acute stroke symptoms as well as DWI and ADC sequences on MRI. Other sequences on MRI that should be performed are contrast enhanced images and fluid attenuated inversion recovery sequences which can help to exclude demyelinating lesions as well as infectious processes. AIS may begin to enhance 5 days after the acute event.

In addition to the brain MRI, arterial imaging of the intracranial and cervical vessels should be obtained to evaluate for arteriopathy. Most often, arterial imaging is performed with magnetic resonance angiography (MRA), but CT angiography (CTA) can be performed if a child has a contraindication to an MRI/MRA. If MRA is suspicious for a cervical dissection or if one is suspected but is not seen, a contrast enhanced neck MRA may be helpful, or additional vascular imaging with CTA or even with conventional angiography may be required for a definitive diagnosis. Even in children with a known AIS risk factor such as congenital heart disease, arterial imaging should be obtained since many children with AIS have multiple risk factors.

■ INITIAL SUPPORTIVE CARE AND MANAGEMENT

The ischemic penumbra may become infarcted if perfusion is not restored quickly. Supportive care centers on minimizing metabolic demands of the tissue and avoiding additional insults like seizures, global hypoxia, hypercarbia, hyperthermia, hyperglycemia, or electrolyte disturbances. Thus, initial management principles in pediatric AIS focus on these items, although most data regarding supportive care is from adult AIS (12,13). In the United States, the American Heart Association as well as the American College of Chest Physicians have published guidelines for the management of pediatric stroke, as has the Royal College of Physicians (6,7,14). While there have been no clinical trials in childhood AIS except for stroke prevention in patients with SCD, the consensus guidelines are informed by prospective and retrospective cohort studies. Perhaps one of the most important early interventions is early initiation of speech, physical, and occupational therapy as well as other rehabilitation services in order to generate a recovery plan that fits the child's needs.

Glycemia

Many experts agree that nondiabetic children with AIS should be kept euglycemic with dextrose-free intravenous (IV) fluids while hospitalized (4,7). According to one study, there is a greater mortality rate and a longer length of stay in hyperglycemic children when compared to nonhyperglycemic children for any illness (15). This may be even more pronounced in diabetic children with AIS. Glycemic control has been shown to improve outcomes of critically ill patients in the intensive care unit (ICU), and most children with AIS are admitted to the pediatric ICU, although this is center-specific. Nevertheless, despite strong consensus opinion recommending minimization of hyperglycemia, the degree of morbidity caused by hyperglycemia is unclear in childhood AIS (4).

Blood Pressure and Cerebral Perfusion Pressure

Acutely, when AIS is suspected, the child should be placed supine without pillows to promote blood flow to the injured brain tissue. Additionally, isotonic IV fluids like normal saline should be used at 1 to 1.5 times maintenance for age and weight as tolerated by the child's cardiovascular system in order to augment cerebral perfusion. In rare cases, IV vasopressors may also be required to keep the mean arterial pressure at age-appropriate levels. It is postulated that hypertension is an adaptive response to cerebral ischemia. Unless the child with AIS presents with hypertensive crisis, urgency, or emergency, blood pressure should not routinely be lowered. However, if blood pressure is dangerously elevated, IV labetalol or nicardipine may be considered, based on the child's heart rate, allergies, and other circumstances. The antihypertensive nitroprusside is contraindicated due to its cerebral vasoconstrictive effects. Current guidelines do not delineate precise blood pressure goals for childhood AIS, although many practitioners suggest aiming for mild hypertension with a systolic blood pressure greater than 75% for the child's age.

Fever and Seizure Monitoring

Elevated body temperature and both convulsive and nonconvulsive seizures place significant metabolic demands on any ill child and must be managed immediately. Hyperthermia leads to a hypermetabolic state and portends a poorer prognosis than euthermia, according to animal models of AIS as well as prospective cohort studies in adult AIS (16,17). In an ischemic milieu, this effect may be magnified, causing neuronal injury at a faster rate because fever increases the demand for oxygen and glucose as the body attempts to reduce its temperature. Adult AIS guidelines suggest aggressive reduction of hyperthermia with cooling agents or antipyretics like acetaminophen, but it is still unclear if euthermia improves outcome in adult or pediatric AIS (12). Nevertheless, hyperthermia is associated with longer hospital stay and lower Glasgow Coma Scale in children with traumatic brain injury (18). Parallel studies need to be conducted in childhood AIS. Induced hypothermia is an emerging therapy in adult AIS trials. In the future, induced hypothermia may be studied in children, but at this time there is no recommendation to actively cool children with AIS.

Children with AIS who present with seizure or who have seizures should be treated with an antiepileptic drug, but it is not recommended that children with AIS receive antiepileptic drug prophylaxis in most cases. In a recent study, 22% of children in a cohort presented with seizures (19). Four of these children were monitored with long-term EEG for clinical reasons, and three of these four had electrographic seizures. The findings of this study suggest that nonconvulsive seizures may be underrecognized after acute childhood AIS, but there are no evidence-based recommendations for routine EEG monitoring in children. For children with continued

seizures or altered mental status, continuous EEG monitoring may be helpful.

Intracranial Pressure Monitoring and Treatment

Large infarcts, particularly large middle cerebral artery territory infarcts, are often accompanied by significant cytotoxic edema, midline shift, and mass effect on the ventricles and may require urgent treatment for increased intracranial pressure (ICP). Symptoms of increased ICP may include headache, confusion, depressed mentation, worsening of initial stroke deficits, or coma with herniation. Thus signs and symptoms of increased ICP should be closely observed in a dedicated ICU setting during the first 72 to 96 hours after a large infarct, the peak time for swelling after AIS. Children have less brain atrophy than do adults and therefore may have less of an "anatomic buffer" against brain edema than adults. According to a pilot study evaluating craniectomy and duraplasty for refractory intracranial hypertension in children with traumatic brain injury, timely surgical decompression appeared to be both lifesaving and function-sparing (20).

More thorough evidence and guidelines are needed in the treatment of increased ICP in childhood AIS since current surgical practice is center-dependent and is informed by adult literature. The Royal College of Physicians does recommend early neurosurgical consultation for children with AIS and deteriorating consciousness or other signs of increased ICP (14). A meta-analysis pooling data from 3 adult randomized controlled trials on the topic showed a 71% mortality for medically managed adult AIS patients with early cytotoxic edema compared to 22% for those undergoing decompressive surgical intervention (21). The major caveat from this study is the morbidity: 35% of surgically managed adult AIS survivors were unable either to walk or perform activities of daily living without assistance, compared with 7% of adult AIS patients managed medically (22). However, in a pediatric series of 10 children with malignant middle cerebral artery infarction and Glasgow Coma Scales ranging from 3 to 9, outcome was moderately good following surgical decompression. All 3 who did not receive decompressive craniectomy progressed to brain death. However, the 7 children who had decompressive craniectomy had improvement of their mental status and walked independently at follow-up despite residual hemiparesis (23).

ETIOLOGIES OF PEDIATRIC AIS

Cardiac Sources

Heart conditions that have been associated with childhood AIS include arrhythmias, cardiomyopathies, congenital heart disease, valvular heart disease, Kawasaki disease, extracorporeal membrane oxygenation, cardiac surgery, and cardiac catheterization (7). Evaluation of the child's heart for cardiac sources of emboli including valve abnormalities, vegetations, structural heart disease, or thrombus in the ventricles, atria, or even left atrial appendage should be performed in all children with AIS, particularly if there are strokes in multiple arterial distributions suggesting an embolic source (Figure 10.2). In most pediatric stroke cohorts cardiac disease is identified as a risk factor in a sizeable minority (24), but this estimate was as high as 69% in one series (8). Regardless, most children with AIS due to cardiac emboli already carry a diagnosis of congenital heart disease (25).

For those in whom the mechanism of AIS is unknown, a transthoracic echocardiogram (TTE) with a "bubble study" with agitated saline to look for right-to-left shunting, is usually the initial cardiac imaging modality. If the TTE fails to show any evidence of thrombus, valve abnormalities, vegetations, or other abnormalities, but a cardiac source is still suspected, a transesophageal echocardiogram (TEE) may be indicated. Theoretically, a patent foramen ovale (PFO) can lead to AIS via paradoxical emboli. If a clot were to form in a deep vein and move to the right atrium, it could cross into the left atrium if there is right-to-left shunting and thereby enter the systemic arterial circulation. However, results of a recent clinical trial did not demonstrate a decreased risk of recurrent stroke with PFO closure when compared to medical management (26). The management of AIS with a PFO found on TTE or TEE, especially without evidence of deep venous thrombosis on Doppler ultrasound of the extremities, is unclear at this point in time in both children and adults. Of course, if vegetations are found on the valves in a toxic-appearing child with AIS, infective endocarditis is the likely diagnosis and broad-spectrum antibiotics should be administered as quickly as possible. Blood cultures should be drawn if infective endocarditis is suspected.

Cerebral Arteriopathy

Cerebral arteriopathy is a common, major risk factor for childhood stroke, occurring in as many as 80% of children with AIS (4,27). Not surprisingly, with a recurrence rate of up to 66% at 5 years, it is also a predictor of poor short-term outcome (4,28).

Focal Cerebral Arteriopathy of Childhood and Postvaricella Arteriopathy

FCA, the most common type of arteriopathy seen in children with stroke, is characterized by a unilateral or bilateral focal or multifocal stenosis of the large and/or medium-sized intracranial arteries (Figure 10.3D) that is not attributed to specific diagnoses like moyamoya, arterial dissection, vasculitis, or postvaricella angiopathy (5). The most common location of stenosis is the distal ICA or proximal MCA or ACA, and infarction of the basal ganglia or internal capsule are common locations for the resulting stroke. The stenoses may improve with or without the artery fully returning to normal caliber and size. The stenosis and stroke can be monophasic; however, the stenoses may increase in number, tightness, or length over weeks to months leading to additional strokes and clinical deficits (29). The cause and pathogenesis are unknown, but FCA is likely a heterogeneous illness (5). Some experts believe that the arteriopathy may be due to invasion of the arterial wall by a pathogenic organism (5,29). A search for infectious agents such as varicella, HIV, syphilis, enteroviruses, and even Borrelia is often performed as soon as FCA is suspected. A similar radiologic and clinical picture has been associated with varicella infections, termed postvaricella arteriopathy. For that diagnosis, a varicella infection must be documented within 12 months of the acute AIS, and this may be less common since the advent of the varicella vaccine. A retrospective review of varicella in childhood AIS supports this parainfectious theory since 3-fold more children with AIS had a varicella infection within 1 year when compared to those without childhood AIS (30). Of 525 cases of childhood AIS in the International Pediatric Stroke Study, recent upper respiratory infection had a predictive odds ratio of 2.36 (95% confidence interval [CI], 1.05–5.27) for FCA (5). Therefore, future research for FCA therapy may focus on use of antiviral, antimicrobial, and antiinflammatory agents.

Moyamoya Disease and Syndrome

Translated from Japanese literally as "smoky smoke," moyamoya disease is a noninflammatory vasculopathy that is the second most common childhood arteriopathy (5,31). The name comes from its characteristic appearance during conventional cerebral angiography, like the puff of

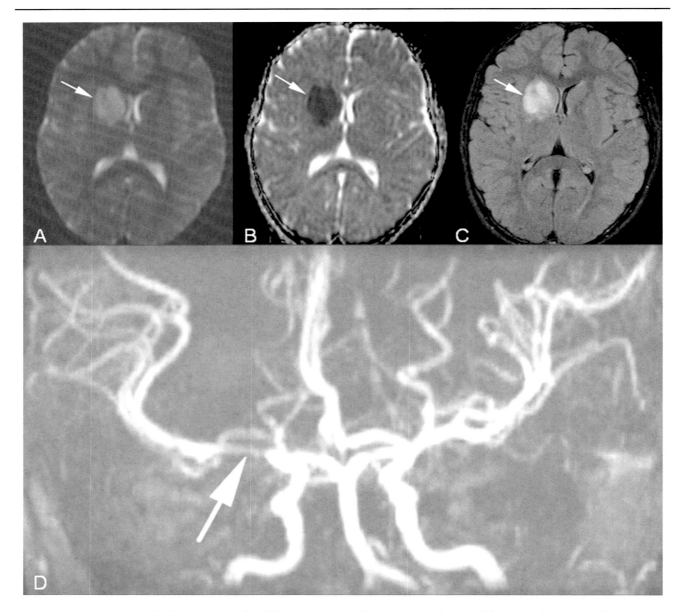

FIGURE 10.3 Focal cerebral arteriopathy of childhood. A 10-year-old girl presented with left facial weakness and left hemichorea. (A), Axial DWI with acute right basal ganglia infarction (arrow). (B), Axial ADC map corresponding to the area of infarction (arrow). (C), Axial fluid attenuated inversion recovery (FLAIR) image with hyperintensity in the right basal ganglia representing infarction (arrow). (D), MRA with focal stenosis of right middle cerebral artery (arrow).

smoke from a cigarette, representing a nebulous pattern of contrast inside progressively smaller, fragile collateral arteries that form as a result of progressive occlusion of both ICAs (Figure 10.4) (31). More common in women than men and in children of Asian descent than in those from other races, idiopathic moyamoya disease classically presents with TIA, AIS, or less commonly with intracerebral or subarachnoid hemorrhage. There are two separate

incidence peaks: one around age 5 years and another in the mid-40s. Other presentations include chorea or headache.

Moyamoya syndrome, unlike the idiopathic disease, is secondary to an associated condition such as SCD, trisomy 21, Williams syndrome (chromosome 7q deletion), neurofibromatosis type 1 (chromosome 17 mutation), and Alagille syndrome, or even cranial irradiation, regardless of dose or duration (31).

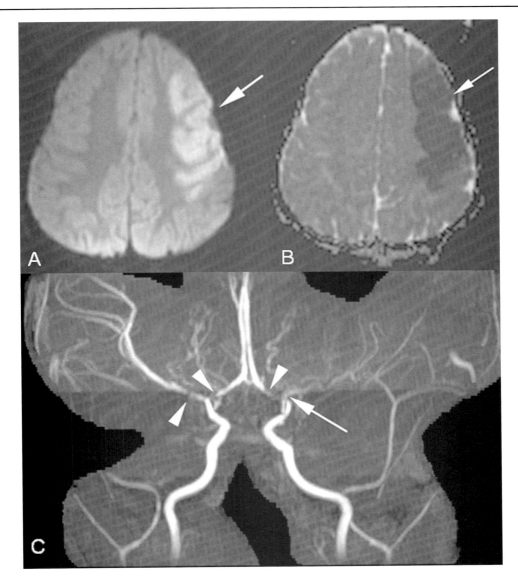

FIGURE 10.4 Moyamoya disease. This 2-year-old healthy male presented with a right sided complex partial seizure. (A), Axial DWI image with acute left middle cerebral artery stroke (arrow). (B), Axial ADC map corresponds to area of abnormality on DWI (arrow). (C), MRA demonstrates severe stenosis of the left middle cerebral artery (arrow) and stenoses of the bilateral supraclinoid internal carotid arteries involving both A1 segments of the anterior cerebral arteries and the right middle cerebral artery (arrowheads).

While in adults moyamoya is usually considered a bilateral disease, some children may have unilateral moyamoya and even involvement of the posterior circulation (Figure 10.5). To date, there is no known acute therapy to reverse the primary disease process, but experts recommend that children with AIS or TIA from moyamoya receive aggressive IV hydration and oxygenation as well as avoid hyperventilation and hypotension (31). Aspirin should be given to lessen the likelihood of microthrombi formation at sites of arterial stenosis. In most patients with AIS or TIA from moyamoya, a neurosurgical revascularization procedure should be considered because there is a high risk of recurrent AIS, and risk of intracerebral or subarachnoid hemorrhage increases over time. There are both direct and indirect bypass procedures available to help improve blood flow to the affected cerebral hemisphere(s). The indirect neurosurgical bypasses, such as encephaloduroarteriomyosynangiosis (EDMS) and encephaloduroarteriosynangiosis (EDAS), have

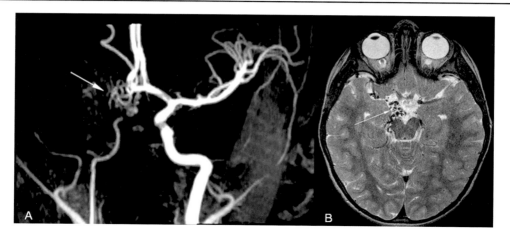

FIGURE 10.5 Unilateral moyamoya disease. This 3-year-old healthy female child presented with left hemichorea. (A), MRA demonstrates unilateral moyamoya disease on the right (arrow). (B), Axial T2-weighted MRI with multiple collaterals (arrow) typical of moyamoya disease.

demonstrated adequate collateralization with resulting resolution of symptoms in as many as 84% of patients (32,33). Direct bypass procedures, such as a superficial temporal artery-to-MCA anastomosis, have also shown effective collateralization and resolution of symptoms but may be more technically challenging than EDMS or EDAS, especially in children (34). There are no randomized prospective trials comparing surgical techniques, and hence the best strategy for revascularization remains uncertain and may depend on factors like surgeon experience with each procedure and the patient's size and vasculature. Additionally, many patients with moyamoya develop intractable migraines; some experts believe that calcium-channel blockers may not only ameliorate these headaches but may also be effective in reducing both the frequency and the severity of refractory TIAs (31). In preparation for a revascularization surgery, a conventional angiogram of both the external carotid arteries and ICAs is usually required. When possible, revascularization is performed weeks after an acute stroke or a flurry of TIAs to minimize the perioperative stroke risk, but in patients with frequent symptoms, waiting may not be possible. Additionally, sedation or anesthesia procedures must be performed carefully to avoid hyperventilation and hypotension that can lead to additional infarction.

Sickle Cell Disease

When compared to the general pediatric population, children with untreated SCD are at an alarming 100-fold increased risk of stroke because of sludging from sickled red blood cells and from arteriopathy (35). Red blood cells can sickle in patients with SCD in the setting of dehydration, infection, acidosis, or deoxygenation. Sickled cells can adhere tightly to endothelium and cause thrombus formation and AIS. About 12% of all SCD-related deaths are associated with an AIS event, according to one study. The cumulative risk of stroke for children with SCD increases with age, and by age 20 years, greater than 20% will have evidence of stroke-related damage on brain MRI (36). Besides AIS, neurologic sequelae of SCD in children may include primary intracerebral or subarachnoid hemorrhage, but AIS is more common. AIS often presents between age 2 and 5 years with hemiparesis, headache, or seizure. However, many children with SCD endure "clinically silent" infarctions, typically in the deep white matter, without overt neurologic deficits (37). Progressive occlusion of the small arteries supplying these territories can lead to a substantial accumulation of injury on MRI, which may result in cognitive deficits and behavioral dysfunction (37).

Children with symptomatic AIS from SCD often have a large vessel arteriopathy involving the supraclinoid ICA and its intracranial branches. This arteriopathy often progresses to ICA occlusions and formation of collateral vessels similar to the classic moyamoya appearance (31,37). Additionally, this large artery arteriopathy in children with SCD can lead to AIS in an anterior watershed pattern or lead to the formation of aneurysms, principally in the vertebrobasilar system (38). If symptomatic, extraordinarily large, or with precarious features, these aneurysms may need to be addressed either surgically or endovascularly.

Stroke risk for children with SCD can be forecasted by detection of increased blood flow velocity on transcranial Doppler ultrasonography (TCD), with high-risk children having an annual stroke risk of up to 10% per year. All 3 sets of pediatric stroke guidelines recommend that all children over 2 years of age with SCD obtain an annual TCD; those at highest risk of AIS by TCD (having a markedly increased velocity of intracranial arterial blood flow) should get chronic transfusion therapy (6,7,14). According to a landmark multicenter, randomized controlled study, 130 children meeting TCD criteria for increased intracranial arterial velocities with no history of prior stroke were randomized to transfusions (simple or exchange) that reduced hemoglobin S to less than 30% of total hemoglobin (experimental group) versus no intervention (standard care group) (39,40). Chronic transfusion reduced the risk of a first stroke by over 90% compared to a risk of 10% per year in the standard care group (40). Additionally, those with abnormal TCDs should have routine MRI/MRA to evaluate for vasculopathy and silent infarcts.

In the acute stroke setting, urgent erythrocyte exchange transfusion or simple transfusion that reduces hemoglobin S percent to less than 30% of total hemoglobin is also recommended, together with administration of IV hydration, supplementary oxygen, and packed red blood cell transfusion if the total hemoglobin concentration is less than 10g/dL (7,14,41). Notably, this practice has not been studied in a randomized trial. Revascularization procedures are normally reserved for children with large vessel arteriopathy associated with SCD who have continued strokes despite maximal medical therapy, including long-term transfusion therapy and hydroxyurea (7). In children who cannot undergo chronic transfusion therapy or who are refractory to transfusions, hydroxyurea is sometimes used (7).

Arterial Dissection

Stroke from arterial dissection, a common cause of arteriopathy in children, is caused by a tearing of the inner wall of an artery in the head (affecting the intracranial vessels) or neck (involving the carotid or vertebral arteries). A "false lumen" pocket may form in the torn vessel and pool blood that can coagulate and then embolize distally, causing an AIS. A pseudoaneurysm may also develop as a result of the tear and also can lead to an AIS by reducing cerebral blood flow or by rupturing. Either minor or major trauma may be the initial insult to provoke an arterial dissection, but patients with connective tissue disorders such as Marfan syndrome or Ehlers-Danlos syndrome may be prone to developing spontaneous arterial dissections without trauma. Often a prior trauma is never identified, even in previously healthy children. Regardless, dedicated arterial imaging of the head and neck is essential if dissection is the suspected diagnosis. Besides focal neurologic deficits, headache is the dominant symptom in about half of all children with dissection (42).

In children the anterior circulation is more likely to be involved than the posterior circulation (42,43). A systematic, retrospective review of 79 studies and case reports published between 1964 and 2000 identified 118 children with stroke from dissection (42). Many of the reports found a significant male predominance for both anterior and posterior circulation dissection and attributed this to a higher incidence of trauma among boys (42). However, in the systematic review, 74% of children with anterior circulation dissections and 87% of posterior circulation dissections were male, and the male predominance remained even after excluding children with preceding trauma. Of children with anterior circulation dissections, 60% were intracranial, unlike adult data in which intracranial dissections are rare (42). Children with intracranial dissections were more likely to be idiopathic or spontaneous and less likely to have had preceding trauma than those with extracranial dissections (42). The most common location for posterior circulation dissection is the vertebral artery at the C1-C2 vertebral body level (Figure 10.6), the segment most susceptible to dissection in adults' posterior circulation as well. Recurrent AIS and TIA were reported more frequently after posterior circulation dissections than after anterior dissection, yet of the 10% of children with one dissection who had a dissection in a second vessel, all were in the anterior circulation (42).

A more aggressive approach to antithrombotics is usually considered in children with dissection. In one study that investigated the clinical and radiographic presentation and outcome of craniocervical arterial dissection in children, about 14% had multiple ischemic events prior to definitive diagnosis of dissection and 9% had recurrent ischemic events after the diagnosis (42). In another series of 16 consecutive patients with AIS from dissection, 12.5% had stroke recurrence (43). Hence, the three guidelines all state that systemic anticoagulation for cervical dissection should be considered or used (6,7,14). However, there have been no studies comparing anticoagulation to antiplatelet agents in children, so the

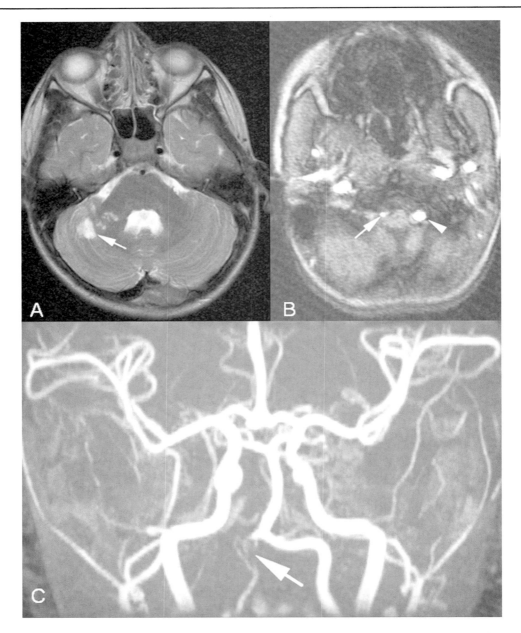

FIGURE 10.6 Verterbral artery dissection. This 8-year-old boy had acute onset of ataxia. Head computed tomography (HCT) was normal, and he was sent home without further workup. He returned to the emergency department 1 week later with new symptoms and was found to have multiple posterior circulation strokes. (A), Axial T2-weighted MRI with subacute right cerebellar strokes in the territory of the right superior cerebellar artery. (B), Axial MRA with narrow right verterbral artery (arrow) compared to normal caliber left vertebral artery (arrowhead). (C), MRA with diffuse narrowing of right vertebral artery (arrow).

American Heart Association (AHA) guidelines state that anticoagulation is reasonable in craniocervical dissection (7). Furthermore, more recent adult cohorts have not shown a difference between recurrent stroke risk in those treated with aspirin versus anticoagulation (44).

Primary and Secondary Central Nervous System Vasculitis

A rare cause of childhood stroke, central nervous system (CNS) vasculitis, is an inflammatory arteriopathy of the brain and meninges. Diagnosis can be difficult and may be aided by a conventional catheter angiography showing the characteristic beaded appearance of the vessels and/or with a biopsy of the brain and leptomeninges revealing inflammatory cell infiltration (typically a lymphocytic transmural infiltrate of T cells) (45). It is considered "primary" when the vasculitis is isolated to the central nervous system and cannot be explained by another process. Vasculitis is termed "secondary" when investigators find evidence of another comorbidity that may provoke inflammation of large-, medium-, or small-caliber vessels, such as rheumatologic (systemic lupus erythematosus, Takayasu arteritis, polyarteritis nodosa), oncologic, or infectious diseases (HIV) (45). Thus evaluation includes testing for infection with blood and urine cultures and for systemic causes of vasculitis with erythrocyte sedimentation rate, C-reactive protein, double-stranded DNA and antinuclear antibody (ANA) profile, anticardiolipin immunoglobulin G and immunoglobulin M, dilute Russell viper venom time, anti-Sjögren's syndrome A (SS-A) antibody, anti-Sjögren's syndrome B (SS-B) antibody, and angiotensin converting enzyme level. Spinal fluid analysis from a lumbar puncture may reveal a mild pleocytosis, elevated protein, or elevated pressure, but the spinal fluid can be normal. A thorough review of the patient's medications (and social history) must be performed because some drugs such as amphetamines have also been associated with secondary CNS vasculitis. Primary CNS vasculitis can present with AIS or hemorrhage, but should be considered in children with a protracted clinical course, with multifocal or diffuse deficits not referable to a single cerebral arterial territory, with both white and gray matter affected on neuroimaging, or with sy stemic symptoms like fever and weight loss (45). Children with primary CNS vasculitis may be classified into one of the following three groups: "progressive" with recurrent AIS, "nonprogressive, monophasic" likely due to large-vessel stenosis, or "small vessel" with unremarkable vascular imaging (45). The progressive form seems to be associated with neurocognitive changes, multifocal strokes, and bilateral or distal stenoses on vascular imaging. Since most children whose vascular imaging is consistent with vasculitis do not undergo biopsy, distinguishing true focal vasculitis from vasculopathy is not easy, and the nonprogressive form may overlap with the FCA. The course of CNS vasculitis and its treatment depend on the underlying etiology, but systemic immunosuppression with IV steroids and cyclophosphamide, cytoxan, or other agents is usually required in addition to antithrombotic therapy.

Hypercoagulability

Hypercoagulability is also an important risk factor for pediatric AIS (46). In a 5-year study of risk factors for recurrent stroke during childhood, a high prevalence of thrombophilia was identified (47). Indeed, prothrombotic abnormalities exist in 30% to 50% of childhood AIS cases, second in prevalence only to arteriopathy. Thus, evaluation for prothrombotic states should be performed when a diagnosis of AIS is confirmed. Protein C and S activity, factor V Leiden gene mutation, antithrombin III activity, antiphospholipid antibodies (anticardiolipin antibodies, β2 glycoprotein antibodies, dilute Russell viper venom time), prothrombin gene mutation, lipoprotein (a), homocysteine, and factor VIII activity are the most common coagulopathies. If routine hypercoagulable studies return negative or inconclusive and thrombophilia is still suspected due to unprovoked or multiple systemic arterial or venous blood clots, a hematology consultation should be considered. The presence of one prothrombotic condition confers only a modestly increased risk for AIS, and hence does not always offer a full explanation for a stroke in a child, although the risk conferred by different hypercoagulable states varies (4). Anticoagulation for hypercoagulable states may be indicated in circumstances when multiple unprovoked clots are found.

Mitochondrial/Metabolic

In some children, the stroke is not caused by arterial occlusion and is characterized by energy failure due to a primary metabolic or mitochondrial disease (7). While such lesions are not actually "strokes," these mimics can masquerade as AIS and can be more difficult to differentiate from AIS than other stroke mimics. Clues to an underlying metabolic or mitochondrial disease include failure of the stroke to evolve in a typical manner on neuroimaging, strokes that cross typical vascular boundaries, basal ganglia calcification, intractable seizures, concomitant neuropathy, hearing abnormalities, growth retardation, or cold or exercise intolerance. Specific diseases that have been associated with metabolic stroke include MELAS (mitochondrial encephalopathy with lactic acidosis and stroke-like episodes) and propionic acidemia. If such an underlying disease is suspected, consultation with an expert in metabolic disorders should be considered. A serum lactate and pyruvate may be helpful, but specific testing may also be required. There is some evidence that stroke-like episodes due to MELAS are improved with supplementation of L-arginine (48).

Genetic Disorders Associated With Stroke

Several rare conditions exist that are associated with stroke (49). Fabry disease is an X-linked lysosomal storage disease with a high penetrance in females (50). The disease is caused by α-galactosidase A deficiency which causes accumulation of globotriaosylceramide in lysosomes, including in the vascular endothelium. In childhood, symptoms like diarrhea, anhydrosis, and febrile crises are more common than stroke, which is more common in adulthood. The treatment is with enzyme replacement therapy.

Hereditary homocystinuria is an autosomal recessive disease of methionine metabolism. Most cases are due to a deficiency of cystathionine β-synthase that converts homocysteine to cystathione. Homocysteine accumulates in the serum which causes endothelial dysfunction and smooth muscle cell proliferation. Strokes occur due to accelerated atherosclerosis.

CADASIL (cerebral autosomal dominant arteriopathy with subcortical infarcts and leukoencephalopathy) is caused by a mutation in the Notch 3 gene on chromosome 19 (51). Although this disorder does not generally present in childhood, the presentation can include TIA and strokes as well as migraine. There is currently no specific treatment for this disorder although patients may be placed on antiplatelet therapy.

■ TREATMENT

Thrombolysis

Tissue plasminogen activator (tPA), an intrinsic activator of the fibrinolytic system, is used in adult AIS as an acute thrombolytic agent. tPA converts endogenous plasminogen to plasmin and is used as a profibrinolytic agent to lyse intracerebral clots with the goal of restoring blood flow to injured and at-risk brain tissue. In the National Institute of Neurological Diseases and Stroke (NINDS) trial from 1995, IV tPA reduced morbidity and mortality when given up to 3 hours after stroke onset (12,52). Based on new randomized controlled trials, adult patients are now routinely given IV tPA when presenting within 4.5 hours of stroke onset (53), and an American Heart Association scientific advisory statement supports this practice with certain exclusions (53,54). In adults, a tPA dose of 0.9 mg/kg (maximum dose 90 mg) is fractionated into 10% given as an IV bolus over the first minute, and the remaining 90% given as a 1-hour IV infusion.

The potential benefits of tPA must be balanced against its risk. The original NINDS trial revealed a 10-times

greater risk for symptomatic intracerebral hemorrhage in patients treated with IV tPA (6.4%) versus those who did not receive the medication (0.6%). Nevertheless, those patients treated with IV tPA did experience better neurologic outcomes at 3 months, even with this increased risk of bleeding (52). The risk for hemorrhage and the benefit of IV tPA in children are unknown.

Alternative AIS therapies in adults, administered by trained neurointerventionalists, include intraarterial (IA) tPA and/or endovascular clot retrieval and suctioning. Although not officially Food and Drug Administration approved, these IA approaches can directly chemically lyse clots and/or mechanically remove them from cerebral arteries, thus extending the potential tPA time window to 6–8 hours for anterior circulation strokes, and 12 to 24 hours for devastating posterior circulation strokes. The best candidates for such therapy are patients who do not improve after acute administration of IV tPA or who arrive to the hospital too late (beyond the 4.5 hour window) for IV therapy. The PROACT study, a randomized controlled trial that enrolled patients in these later windows with an MCA occlusion found a 10.9% rate of hemorrhage with IA thrombolysis versus a 3.1% rate in the IV heparin control group (55). Benefit in those who received IA thrombolysis was seen in the form of increased rate of arterial recanalization, from 18% to 66%, and a superior modified Rankin score at 90 days versus those who did not receive thrombolytic therapy (55). However, interventional procedures should only be performed by experienced neurointerventionalists.

Whether the risk-benefit ratio would similarly favor tPA for pediatric AIS is unknown. The American Heart Association guidelines for the management of childhood stroke currently do not recommend the routine use of tPA in children outside of a clinical trial (7). To date, no randomized controlled trials with IV tPA or IA tPA in childhood AIS have been completed, but a current clinical trial, Thrombolysis In Pediatric Stroke (TIPS), will assess the safety of IV tPA in children up to 4.5 hours from stroke symptom onset (56). However, some children with AIS have received tPA outside the setting of a clinical trial. Between 2000 and 2003, 46 of 2,904 children (1.6%) with International Classification of Disease book 9 (ICD-9) codes for stroke in the United States National Inpatient Sample concomitantly received a procedure code for thrombolytic therapy and ischemic stroke (57). Another study demonstrated that of children enrolled in the International Pediatric Stroke Study, many were administered IV or IA thrombolytics outside the safety time windows established by AHA guidelines in adult AIS. One child received IV tPA 52 hours after the acute stroke (58). In addition to rapidly confirming AIS by HCT or MRI and establishing an arterial occlusion by CTA or MRA, adhering to a firmly set time window will be crucial in the first pilot safety trials of thrombolysis in pediatric stroke (59).

Antiplatelet Agents

Antithrombotic agents are a standard treatment in both children and adults for prevention of stroke recurrence. Aspirin is the most widely used antiplatelet therapy in childhood AIS. The antithrombotic effect of aspirin results largely from irreversible inhibition of the cyclooxygenase-1 enzyme in platelets, leading to impaired platelet aggregation and activation. Other antiplatelet agents, such as dipyridamole, clopidogrel, and glycoprotein IIb/IIIa antagonists, are infrequently used for childhood AIS, but are available options when there is a concern for aspirin allergy or gastritis. Use of aspirin at the time of a varicella or influenza infection may be avoided due to concerns for Reye syndrome (7).

In the acute setting for adult AIS, two large multicenter trials, CAST and IST, evaluated the efficacy of aspirin when given within 48 hours of symptom onset (60,61). When analyzed together, these trials demonstrate a significant protective effect of aspirin against AIS recurrence with an absolute risk reduction of 7 per 1,000 adult AIS patients balanced against a hemorrhagic transformation (HT) or hemorrhagic stroke increase of 2 in 1,000. Thus, the adult AHA recommendations include the administration of aspirin 325 mg within 24 to 48 hours of symptom onset unless the patient has received thrombolytic therapy or has other contraindications (12). Although no trials have evaluated the efficacy of aspirin or any other antiplatelet therapies in acute childhood AIS, guidelines suggest that aspirin at a dose of 3 to 5 mg/kg per day (maximum 325 mg) be administered to children with AIS (7,14), although dosing can be lowered to 1 to 3 mg/kg per day if there is significant gastritis or bleeding (7). The choice between aspirin and systemic anticoagulation is often center-dependent.

Anticoagulation

Anticoagulation is recommended or suggested as reasonable by the three guidelines for childhood AIS when AIS is due to cardioembolism or dissection since these causes may have an increased risk of recurrence (6,7,14). In adult AIS, no net benefit has been established for acute systemic anticoagulation compared with aspirin, even with cardioembolic stroke, mostly due to an increased risk of HT (60,62,63). As noted in the section on arterial dissection, there is emerging evidence in adult cervical artery dissection that anticoagulation is not superior to aspirin for the prevention of recurrent stroke (44). However, some pediatric stroke neurologists believe that systemic anticoagulation should begin acutely in all children with AIS without large HT until a major prothrombotic state, a cardioembolic source, or a dissection has been excluded since these stroke risk factors are more common in childhood stroke.

For children with nonmoyamoya arteriopathy, which carries a 14% cumulative risk of recurrent AIS at 1 year, studies have shown that anticoagulation can be safely administered (47,64). One study found that children with AIS and acute nonmoyamoya arteriopathy treated with anticoagulation for 4 weeks or longer, for a cumulative anticoagulation duration of 1,329 patient-months, had no major bleeding episodes and only two "clinically relevant" bleeding episodes (64). This low hemorrhage rate compares nicely with the 5% incidence of major bleeding in children on therapeutic enoxaparin for deep venous thrombosis (65). A recent cohort study did not demonstrate a difference in HT among children treated with anticoagulation versus those treated with aspirin, although the study was not powered to look at this outcome (66).

Since many children have prothrombotic abnormalities, cardioembolic etiologies, or arterial dissection as risk factors for AIS, and since safety data for acute anticoagulation in children with AIS have been reassuring, the American College of Chest Physicians guidelines suggest empiric treatment with unfractionated heparin, low molecular weight heparin, or aspirin until cardioembolism or vascular dissection have been excluded (6). However, this is controversial advice, and the Royal College of Physicians recommends initial treatment of childhood AIS with aspirin at a dose of 5 mg/kg per day until a valid indication for anticoagulation is identified (14).

■ OUTCOME AND STROKE RECURRENCE

Case fatality rates for ischemic stroke have been estimated at 16% to 20%, but these estimates are based on older data from 1970 to 2003 (2,67). Mortality

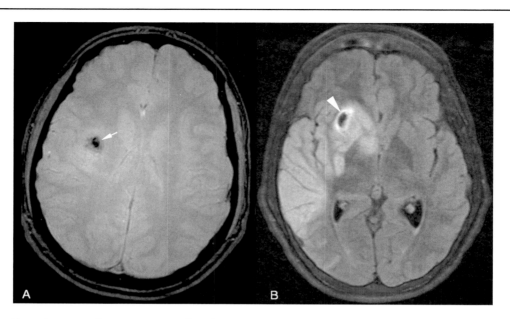

FIGURE 10.7   Hemorrhagic transformation. (A), Axial gradient echo MRI sequence from patient featured in Figure 10.2 with area of hemorrhagic transformation within the area of right middle cerebral artery infarction (arrow). (B), Axial FLAIR image from a different patient with a large right middle cerebral artery stroke with hemorrhagic transformation within the right caudate nucleus (arrowhead).

from childhood stroke has decreased over time (68). However, neurologic deficits including motor and cognitive impairment are present in greater than half of children after AIS (69,70). Predictors of poor outcome are incompletely understood. Young age, male sex, and bihemispheric infarction have been associated with poor outcome (71). In two studies, larger volume of AIS has been found to predict poorer outcome (66,72). In one of these studies, larger stroke volume was associated with HT of the stroke (Figure 10.7), but in multivariable analysis, only supratentorial stroke volume ≥ 5% of supratentorial brain volume was associated with worse score on the Pediatric Stroke Outcome Measure (66). This finding expanded on a previous study in which stroke volume > 10% of supratentorial intracranial volume in MCA stroke predicted worse outcome (72). As in adult stroke, greater clinical stroke severity on the Pediatric NIH Stroke Scale in the acute setting is associated with worse neurologic outcome at 12 months (10).

Recurrent stroke risk has been evaluated with survival analysis in only three pediatric studies. A retrospective cohort of 181 neonates and children with AIS from Kaiser Permanente in California reported that the 5-year cumulative recurrence risk for neonatal AIS was 1.2%. The 5-year cumulative recurrence risk in older

children was 19% (95% CI, 12%–30%) (1). Similarly, a single-center study from the United Kingdom reported an 18% 5-year recurrence risk for childhood AIS, (95% CI, 11%–25%) (3). A German cohort reported recurrence in only 5%, but the CI was not provided (47).

■ CONCLUSIONS

Pediatric AIS is an underrecognized condition that carries a high degree of neurologic morbidity. Currently, management of pediatric stroke in the ICU is largely supportive, though antithrombotic therapy also plays an important role. The development of improved treatment strategies for pediatric AIS mandates collaborative trials to test acute therapies like thrombolytics as well as treatments for prevention of recurrent stroke.

■ REFERENCES

1. Fullerton HJ et al. Risk of recurrent childhood arterial ischemic stroke in a population-based cohort: the importance of cerebrovascular imaging. *Pediatrics*. 2007;119:495–501.
2. Fullerton HJ et al. Risk of stroke in children: ethnic and gender disparities. *Neurology*. 2003;61:189–194.

3. Ganesan V et al. Clinical and radiological recurrence after childhood arterial ischemic stroke. *Circulation*. 2006;114: 2170–2177.

4. Bernard TJ et al. Treatment of childhood arterial ischemic stroke. *Ann Neurol*. 2008;63:679–696.

5. Amlie-Lefond C et al. Predictors of cerebral arteriopathy in children with arterial ischemic stroke: results of the International Pediatric Stroke Study. *Circulation*. 2009;119: 1417–1423.

6. Monagle P et al. Antithrombotic therapy in neonates and children: antithrombotic therapy and prevention of thrombosis: American College of Chest Physicians evidence-based clinical practice guidelines (9th edition). *Chest*. 2012;141(2 Suppl):e737S-801S.

7. Roach ES et al. Management of stroke in infants and children: a scientific statement from a special writing group of the american heart association stroke council and the council on cardiovascular disease in the young. *Stroke*. 2008;39:2644–2691.

8. Srinivasan J et al. Delayed recognition of initial stroke in children: need for increased awareness. *Pediatrics*. 2009;124: e227–234.

9. Shellhaas RA et al. Mimics of childhood stroke: characteristics of a prospective cohort. *Pediatrics*. 2006;118:704–709.

10. Ichord R et al. Initial stroke severity measured by pediatric NIH stroke scale predicts 12-month outcome in children. Paper presented at: International Stroke Conference; February 2012, New Orleans, Louisiana

11. Ichord RN et al. Interrater reliability of the pediatric national institutes of health stroke scale (pednihss) in a multicenter study. *Stroke*. 2011;42:613–617.

12. Adams HP Jr et al. Guidelines for the early management of adults with ischemic stroke: a guideline from the american Heart Association/American Stroke Association Stroke Council, Clinical Cardiology Council, Cardiovascular Radiology and Intervention Council, and the Atherosclerotic Peripheral Vascular Disease and Quality of Care Outcomes in Research Interdisciplinary Working Groups: the American Academy of Neurology affirms the value of this guideline as an educational tool for neurologists. *Circulation*. 2007;115:e478–e534.

13. Sacco RL et al. Guidelines for prevention of stroke in patients with ischemic stroke or transient ischemic attack: a statement for healthcare professionals from the American Heart Association/American Stroke Association Council On Stroke: co-sponsored by the Council on Cardiovascular Radiology and Intervention: the American Academy of Neurology affirms the value of this guideline. *Circulation*. 2006;113:e409–e449.

14. Paediatric SWG. Stroke in childhood: clinical guidelines for diagnosis, management and rehabilitation. November 2004. http://bookshop.rcplondon.ac.uk/contents/f98c6540-a541-4bed-837d-ef293ac458bf.pdf. Accessed: September 10, 2012

15. Faustino EV, Apkon M. Persistent hyperglycemia in critically ill children. *J Pediatr*. 2005;146:30–34.

16. Hajat C, Hajat S, Sharma P. Effects of poststroke pyrexia on stroke outcome: a meta-analysis of studies in patients. *Stroke*. 2000;31:410–414.

17. Reith J et al. Body temperature in acute stroke: relation to stroke severity, infarct size, mortality, and outcome. *Lancet*. 1996;347:422–425.

18. Natale JE et al. Early hyperthermia after traumatic brain injury in children: risk factors, influence on length of stay, and effect on short-term neurologic status. *Crit Care Med*. 2000;28:2608–2615.

19. Abend NS et al. Seizures as a presenting symptom of acute arterial ischemic stroke in childhood. *J Pediatr*. 2011;159: 479–483.

20. Ruf B et al. Early decompressive craniectomy and duraplasty for refractory intracranial hypertension in children: results of a pilot study. *Crit Care*. 2003;7:R133–R138.

21. Vahedi K et al. Early decompressive surgery in malignant infarction of the middle cerebral artery: a pooled analysis of three randomised controlled trials. *Lancet Neurol*. 2007; 6:215–222.

22. Puetz V et al. Assessing the benefits of hemicraniectomy: what is a favourable outcome? *Lancet Neurol*. 2007;6:580; author reply 580–581.

23. Smith SE et al. Outcome following decompressive craniectomy for malignant middle cerebral artery infarction in children. *Dev Med Child Neurol*. 2011;53:29–33.

24. Mackay MT et al. Arterial ischemic stroke risk factors: the International Pediatric Stroke Study. *Ann Neurol*. 2011;69:130–140.

25. Amlie-Lefond C, Sebire G, Fullerton HJ. Recent developments in childhood arterial ischaemic stroke. *Lancet Neurol*. 2008;7:425–435.

26. Furlan AJ et al. Closure or medical therapy for cryptogenic stroke with patent foramen ovale. N Engl J Med. 2012;366:991-999.

27. Ganesan V et al. Investigation of risk factors in children with arterial ischemic stroke. *Ann Neurol*. 2003;53:167–173.

28. Goldenberg NA et al. Antithrombotic treatments, outcomes, and prognostic factors in acute childhood-onset arterial ischaemic stroke: a multicentre, observational, cohort study. *Lancet Neurol*. 2009;8:1120–1127.

29. Sebire G et al. Toward the definition of cerebral arteriopathies of childhood. *Curr Opin Pediatr*. 2004;16:617–622.

30. Askalan R et al. Chickenpox and stroke in childhood: a study of frequency and causation. *Stroke*. 2001;32:1257–1262.

31. Scott RM, Smith ER. Moyamoya disease and moyamoya syndrome. *N Engl J Med*. 2009;360:1226–1237.

32. Ozgur BM, Aryan HE, Levy ML. Indirect revascularisation for paediatric moyamoya disease: the EDAMS technique. *J Clin Neurosci*. 2006;13:105–108.

33. Robertson RL et al. Angiographic changes after pial synangiosis in childhood moyamoya disease. *AJNR Am J Neuroradiol*. 1997;18:837–845.

34. Khan N et al. Moyamoya disease and moyamoya syndrome: experience in europe; choice of revascularisation procedures. *Acta Neurochir (Wien)*. 2003;145:1061–1071; discussion 1071.

35. Earley CJ et al. Stroke in children and sickle-cell disease: Baltimore-Washington Cooperative Young Stroke Study. *Neurology*. 1998;51:169–176.

36. Ohene-Frempong K et al. Cerebrovascular accidents in sickle cell disease: rates and risk factors. *Blood*. 1998;91:288–294.

37. Switzer JA et al. Pathophysiology and treatment of stroke in sickle-cell disease: present and future. *Lancet Neurol*. 2006;5:501–512.

38. Preul MC et al. Intracranial aneurysms and sickle cell anemia: multiplicity and propensity for the vertebrobasilar territory. *Neurosurgery*. 1998;42:971–977; discussion 977–978.

39. Adams RJ et al. Stroke prevention trial in sickle cell anemia. *Control Clin Trials*. 1998;19:110–129.

40. Adams RJ et al. Prevention of a first stroke by transfusions in children with sickle cell anemia and abnormal results on transcranial doppler ultrasonography. *N Engl J Med*. 1998;339:5–11.

41. Kirkham FJ, DeBaun MR. Stroke in children with sickle cell disease. *Curr Treat Options Neurol*. 2004;6:357–375.

42. Fullerton HJ, Johnston SC, Smith WS. Arterial dissection and stroke in children. *Neurology*. 2001;57:1155–1160.

43. Rafay MF et al. Craniocervical arterial dissection in children: clinical and radiographic presentation and outcome. *J Child Neurol*. 2006;21:8–16.

44. Georgiadis D et al. Aspirin vs anticoagulation in carotid artery dissection: a study of 298 patients. *Neurology*. 2009;72: 1810–1815.

45. Benseler SM et al. Primary central nervous system vasculitis in children. *Arthritis Rheum*. 2006;54:1291–1297.

46. Kenet G et al. Impact of thrombophilia on risk of arterial ischemic stroke or cerebral sinovenous thrombosis in neonates and children: a systematic review and meta-analysis of observational studies. *Circulation*.121:1838–1847.

47. Strater R et al. Prospective assessment of risk factors for recurrent stroke during childhood—a 5-year follow-up study. *Lancet*. 2002;360:1540–1545.

48. Koga Y et al. Endothelial dysfunction in melas improved by l-arginine supplementation. *Neurology*. 2006;66:1766–1769.

49. Razvi SS, Bone I. Single gene disorders causing ischaemic stroke. *J Neurol*. 2006;253:685–700.

50. Rolfs A et al. Prevalence of fabry disease in patients with cryptogenic stroke: a prospective study. *Lancet*.2005;366:1794–1796.

51. Joutel A et al. Strong clustering and stereotyped nature of notch3 mutations in CADASIL patients. *Lancet*. 1997;350: 1511–1515.

52. Tissue plasminogen activator for acute ischemic stroke. The National Institute of Neurological Disorders and Stroke rt-PA Stroke Study Group. *N Engl J Med*. 1995;333:1581–1587.

53. Hacke W et al. Thrombolysis with alteplase 3 to 4.5 hours after acute ischemic stroke. *N Engl J Med*. 2008;359:1317–1329.

54. Del Zoppo GJ et al. Expansion of the time window for treatment of acute ischemic stroke with intravenous tissue plasminogen activator: a science advisory from the American Heart Association/American Stroke Association. *Stroke*. 2009; 40:2945–2948.

55. Furlan A et al. Intra-arterial prourokinase for acute ischemic stroke. The PROACT II Study: a randomized controlled trial. Prolyse in acute cerebral thromboembolism. *JAMA*. 1999;282:2003–2011.

56. Amlie-Lefond C et al. Thrombolysis in acute childhood stroke: design and challenges of the thrombolysis in pediatric stroke clinical trial. *Neuroepidemiology*. 2009;32:279–286.

57. Janjua N et al. Thrombolysis for ischemic stroke in children: data from the nationwide inpatient sample. *Stroke*. 2007;38:1850–1854.

58. Amlie-Lefond C et al. Use of alteplase in childhood arterial ischaemic stroke: a multicentre, observational, cohort study. *Lancet Neurol*. 2009;8:530–536.

59. Whelan HT et al. Practical model-based dose finding in early-phase clinical trials: optimizing tissue plasminogen activator dose for treatment of ischemic stroke in children. *Stroke*. 2008;39:2627–2636.

60. The international stroke trial (IST): a randomised trial of aspirin, subcutaneous heparin, both, or neither among 19435 patients with acute ischaemic stroke. International Stroke Trial Collaborative Group. *Lancet*. 1997;349:1569–1581.

61. CAST: randomised placebo-controlled trial of early aspirin use in 20,000 patients with acute ischaemic stroke. CAST (Chinese Acute Stroke Trial) Collaborative Group. *Lancet*. 1997;349:1641–1649.

62. Low molecular weight heparinoid, ORG 10172 (danaparoid), and outcome after acute ischemic stroke: a randomized controlled trial. The Publications Committee for the Trial of ORG 10172 in Acute Stroke Treatment (Toast) Investigators. *JAMA*. 1998;279:1265–1272.

63. Berge E et al. Low molecular-weight heparin versus aspirin in patients with acute ischaemic stroke and atrial fibrillation: a double-blind randomised study. HAEST Study Group. Heparin in Acute Embolic Stroke Trial. *Lancet*. 2000;355:1205–1210.

64. Bernard TJ et al. Anticoagulation in childhood-onset arterial ischemic stroke with non-moyamoya arteriopathy: findings from the colorado and german (coag) collaboration. *Stroke*. 2009;40:2869–2871.

65. Dix D et al. The use of low molecular weight heparin in pediatric patients: a prospective cohort study. *J Pediatr*. 2000;136:439–445.

66. Beslow LA et al. Hemorrhagic transformation of childhood arterial ischemic stroke. *Stroke*. 2011;42:941–946.

67. Lanthier S et al. Stroke in children: the coexistence of multiple risk factors predicts poor outcome. *Neurology*. 2000;54:371–378.

68. Fullerton HJ et al. Deaths from stroke in us children, 1979 to 1998. *Neurology*. 2002;59:34–39.

69. Ganesan V et al. Outcome after ischaemic stroke in childhood. *Dev Med Child Neurol*. 2000;42:455–461.

70. Hogan AM, Kirkham FJ, Isaacs EB. Intelligence after stroke in childhood: review of the literature and suggestions for future research. *J Child Neurol*. 2000;15:325–332.

71. deVeber GA et al. Neurologic outcome in survivors of childhood arterial ischemic stroke and sinovenous thrombosis. *J Child Neurol*. 2000;15:316–324.

72. Ganesan V et al. Lesion volume, lesion location, and outcome after middle cerebral artery territory stroke. *Arch Dis Child*. 1999;81:295–300.

73. Lo W et al. The cost of pediatric stroke care and rehabilitation. *Stroke*. 2008;39:161–165.

11 Cerebral Venous Sinus Thrombosis

SALLY M. SULTAN, REBECCA N. ICHORD, and LAUREN A. BESLOW

■ INTRODUCTION

Cerebral venous sinus thrombosis (CVST) refers to thrombotic occlusion of the cerebral dural venous sinuses. CVST occurs in healthy and chronically ill children of all ages. The diagnosis can be suspected based on clinical symptoms but requires appropriate imaging to confirm. The presentation of CVST can be dramatic with rapid progression to coma or insidious with mild or no symptoms. Identifying and managing risk factors are important. Existing published cohort studies, mostly retrospective, suggest that anticoagulation may be beneficial and carries little risk. However there are no pediatric randomized controlled trials to support any treatment recommendations. Outcome ranges from a full recovery to death.

■ EPIDEMIOLOGY

The incidence of pediatric CVST from population-based registries ranges from 0.34 to 0.67 per 100,000 per year (1–4). Reported incidence values are likely an underestimate since literature suggests that CVST is underdiagnosed. In a retrospective review of 131 children and adults referred to neuroophthalmology centers with a diagnosis of papilledema and presumed idiopathic intracranial hypertension, 9.4% were found to have CVST (5). In another cohort of 46 adults diagnosed with idiopathic intracranial hypertension, 26% were found to have CVST (6). Diagnosis of CVST may be more difficult in the pediatric population since symptoms are often nonspecific and nonlocalizing. Some children may even be asymptomatic.

The mean age of presentation in children has been estimated between 5.6 and 8.6 years (2,3,7). The age distribution is bimodal with a large peak in the neonatal period and a smaller peak during adolescence that is thought to be related to hormonal changes and downregulation of the fibrinolytic system (8). Male predominance for childhood CVST has been reported in several studies (9–11). The reason for this male predominance, seen also in childhood arterial ischemic stroke, is not completely understood.

■ PHYSIOLOGY OF CEREBRAL VENOUS DRAINAGE

Cerebral veins are thin-walled, without smooth muscle or valves. Deep veins within the parenchyma of the brain converge on internal cerebral veins that emerge from the brain and lie in the subarachnoid space. Cerebral veins enter the meningeal layer of the dura mater where they drain into cerebral dural venous sinuses which are formed from pockets in the dura mater. Outflow of blood follows deep veins to superficial sinuses and eventually to the internal jugular vein and extrajugular collaterals, the venous vertebral plexus, and emissary veins. In the supine position, the internal jugular vein is the major drainage pathway, and in the upright position, the venous vertebral system is the preferred drainage pathway. Cerebrospinal fluid reabsorption occurs though arachnoid villi which protrude into the cerebral dural venous sinuses and are most concentrated in the superior sagittal sinus.

■ VENOUS AND CEREBRAL DURAL VENOUS SINUS ANATOMY

Descriptions of the anatomy of the cerebral venous structures is provided below and in Figure 11.1.

Superficial system: The *superior sagittal sinus* (SSS) is confined by the attached borders of the falx cerebri. Blood from the medial and lateral surfaces of the frontal, parietal, and occipital lobes as well as from the scalp drains into the SSS. Cutaneous infections or contusions may cause SSS thrombosis. An anatomical variant exists in which the anterior portion of the SSS may be replaced by two superior cerebral veins that join behind the coronal suture. The SSS terminates at the junction of the *straight and transverse sinus* which is referred to as the confluence of the sinuses or torcula herophili. One transverse sinus, more often the right, may be dominant with mild or greatly diminished flow in the contralateral sinus (12–14). This is thought to be related to the more linear course from the right internal jugular vein to the superior vena cava and right atrium. Isolated lack or diminution of flow-related signal in one transverse sinus on time-of-flight magnetic resonance venogram (MRV) is typical in individuals with unilateral hypoplasia of the transverse sinus and should not be mistaken for a diagnosis of CVST. The *inferior sagittal sinus* lies in the falx cerebri free edge and drains into the straight sinus.

Deep system: The *straight sinus* is formed by the tentorium cerebelli and drains the vein of Galen and inferior sagittal sinus. It joins the torcula at the occipital protuberance. The *transverse sinuses* are formed from the attached borders of the tentorium cerebelli and drain blood from the posterior cerebral hemispheres, cerebellum, and brainstem into the sigmoid sinuses. The *sigmoid sinuses* drain the transverse sinuses into the internal jugular veins. The position of the sigmoid sinus over the inner aspect of the mastoid bone predisposes it to thrombosis with inner ear or mastoid infection (15).

Other: The *cavernous sinuses* are two large channels on either side of the sella turcica. The abducens nerve and internal carotid artery (carotid siphon) are located within the center of each cavernous sinus, and the oculomotor nerve, trochlear nerve, and ophthalmic and maxillary portions of the trigeminal nerve run along the lateral wall of each cavernous sinus. The cavernous sinuses drain the

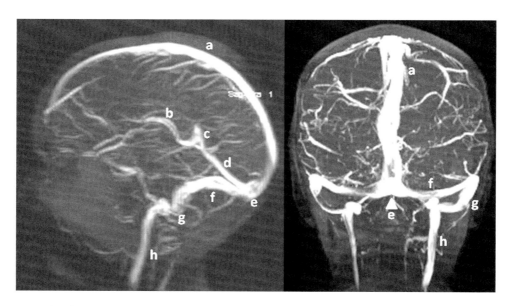

FIGURE 11.1 Sagittal (left panel) and coronal (right panel) magnetic resonance venograms demonstrating normal venous sinuses. (a) Superior sagittal sinus. (b) Internal cerebral veins. (c) Great vein of Galen. (d) Straight sinus. (e) Confluence of sinuses (torcula). (f) Left transverse sinus. (g) Left sigmoid sinus. (h) Left internal jugular vein. Note that the Inferior sagittal sinus is not visible in this figure.

ophthalmic veins and the anterior base of the brain via the middle cerebral vein. Infection of the face or sphenoid sinus predisposes to thrombosis of the cavernous sinuses. The *superior and inferior petrosal sinuses* drain the cavernous sinuses into the transverse and sigmoid sinuses, respectively. The *thalamostriate veins* drain the posterior frontal and anterior parietal lobes, the caudate nucleus, and the internal capsule. Deep structures of the frontal lobe drain into the *basal vein of Rosenthal*. The internal cerebral veins and basal vein of Rosenthal join to form the *vein of Galen* which drains into the straight sinus. Malformation of the vein of Galen results in arteriovenous shunting of blood and aneurysmal dilation of the vein and can be associated with thrombosis.

Anastomoses: The *vein of Trolard* connects the middle cerebral vein to the SSS. The *vein of Labbé* connects the middle cerebral veins to the transverse sinus. Anastomoses explain the absence of well-defined venous territories, and hence, well-defined clinical syndromes associated with thrombosis of a particular sinus or vein.

Sinuses most commonly involved: The most commonly involved sinuses with CVST are the SSS in 23% to 72% of cases (4,9,10,16–22), the transverse sinus in 6% to 74% of cases (4,9,10,16–22), the straight sinus in 13% to 33% of cases (9,17,18,20,21), and the internal veins in 1% to 8% of cases (4,9,17,20,21). Head computed tomography (HCT) is less sensitive for deep vein thrombosis, and thrombosis of deep veins may therefore be underrecognized (18,21). Involvement of multiple sinuses is common and is seen in 14% to 70% of cases (1,4,9–11,18,20–23).

■ PATHOPHYSIOLOGY

Many acute and chronic conditions are risk factors for CVST (Table 11.1). The cerebral veins and dural sinuses are common sites for thrombosis when one or multiple risk factors are present since blood flow is slow and follows a tortuous route. The presence of thrombosis causes venous outflow obstruction and creates a high pressure venous system that rivals the pressure in the arterial system. Capillary hydrostatic pressure increases as a result. Arterial perfusion may be inadequate when venous pressure exceeds arterial pressure, and ischemia may result. A high capillary hydrostatic pressure drives plasma filtrate into the interstitium leading to parenchymal edema. Thrombus in the dural sinuses, especially the SSS, may impair cerebrospinal fluid absorption through arachnoid villi and granulations (pacchionian bodies)

that protrude into these sinuses, resulting in communicating hydrocephalus. Parenchymal findings reflect the pathophysiology and include edema, hemorrhage, and ischemia.

■ CLINICAL MANIFESTATIONS

The clinical manifestations of CVST are nonspecific and variable. The classical presentation of CVST is a triad of headache, vomiting, and depressed level of consciousness. CVST can present suddenly with acute severe headache and rapid deterioration of consciousness or may develop insidiously over days to weeks.

In the largest multinational prospective observational study of CVST in adults, the evolution of clinical symptoms was acute in 37%, subacute in 56%, and chronic in 7% (24). Reflecting this variable course of symptom evolution, the time of symptom onset to hospital presentation in children ranges from 0 to 120 days. The median time to hospital presentation in children is 4 to 5 days (11,25), and the majority of children present within the first week (11,28). Delay in diagnosis often occurs, perhaps due to symptoms that are both nonspecific and often subtle.

Symptoms and signs associated with CVST are also associated with many other diagnoses that include arterial ischemic stroke, intracerebral hemorrhage, mass lesions such as brain tumor or abscess, meningitis, hydrocephalus, and idiopathic intracranial hypertension. The range of symptoms reported in children is broad (1–4,7,10,11,16,17,21,25–27). They include headache (21%–95%), nausea or emesis (21%–67%), visual symptoms (11%–38%), papilledema (22%–76%), cranial nerve abnormalities (10%–35%) often involving the sixth nerve (abducens nerve), hemiparesis (3%–33%), ataxia (6%–7%), aphasia (13%), and hemisensory loss. Fever is a common finding, seen in 29%–58% and may reflect the high association of CVST with infection. Seizures are reported in 20% to 48% of children, depressed consciousness or lethargy in 11% to 55%, and coma in 4% to 28% (1–4,7,10,11,16,17,21,25–27). Finally, CVST can be completely asymptomatic, found only when imaging is performed for another reason or because the patient has a known risk factor for CVST such as mastoiditis.

The involved sinuses cannot usually be distinguished by clinical features alone, but certain observations have been made. A review of 52 children with CVST found that depressed consciousness was common when the

■ Table 11.1 Risk Factors for Cerebral Venous Sinus Thrombosis

Chronic Conditions
Inflammatory bowel disease
Systemic lupus erythematosus
Behçet's disease
Cyanotic congenital heart disease
Nephrotic syndrome
Celiac disease
Liver disease
Multiple sclerosis

Head and Neck Infections
Otitis
Mastoiditis
Tonsillitis
Sinusitis
Meningitis

Prothrombotic Conditions
Protein C deficiency
Protein S deficiency
Antithrombin III deficiency
Factor V Leiden mutation
Prothrombin gene mutation
Anticardiolipin antibodies
Lupus anticoagulant
Hyperhomocysteinemia
Elevated lipoprotein (a)
Elevated factor VIII level

Anemia
Iron deficiency
Sickle cell
Thalassemia
Hemolytic

Head Injury

Malignancy
Brain tumors
Leukemia and lymphoma

Hydrocephalus (with or without shunt)

Pregnancy

Inherited Conditions
Homocystinuria
Trisomy 21

Acute Systemic Illness or Procedures
Dehydration
Hypoxia
Thyrotoxicosis
Postoperative
Postcatheterization

Medications
L-asparaginase
Oral contraceptives
Corticosteroids
Epoetin alfa

straight sinus was involved. Involvement of the SSS was observed with depressed consciousness, seizures, and focal signs. Papilledema with sixth nerve palsy occurred with thrombosis associated with mastoiditis (21).

■ RISK FACTORS

A risk factor for CVST is identified in 74% to 95% of children, and at least half of children affected by CVST have multiple risk factors (10,11,17,21,25). Table 11.1 lists risk factors for CVST.

Infections, particularly of the head and neck, are among the most common predisposing conditions, reported in 50% to 57% of children (2,3,7,10,11,21,

22,23,25,26). These include otitis media or mastoiditis in 9% to 62% and sinusitis in 2% to 36% (Figure 11.2). An intracranial infection, such as meningitis or intracranial abscess, is reported in 11% to 44%, and an extracranial infection in 24% to 33% of children. Sepsis is found more frequently in association with neonatal thrombosis but can also be a risk factor in childhood.

Dehydration and anemia are consistently described in children with CVST (11,17,23–25). Dehydration increases blood viscosity and is reported in 5% to 28%. The pathophysiology of the association between anemia and cerebral venous sinus thrombosis is not well understood and yet is reported in 10% to 19% of children. In one series, thrombocytosis was reported as a risk factor (25); however, thrombocytosis is a well-established physiologic response to anemia. It is not clear whether

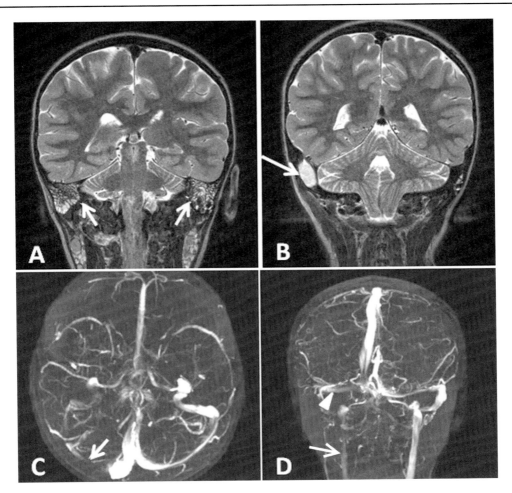

FIGURE 11.2 (A) Coronal T2-weighted magnetic resonance imaging (MRI) with bilateral mastoiditis (arrows). (B) Coronal T2-weighted MRI also demonstrates a right sided epidural abscess as a complication (arrow). (C) Axial time-of-flight MRV with decreased flow in the right transverse sinus (arrow) due to thrombus. (D) Coronal MRV again demonstrating decreased flow in the right transverse sinus (arrowhead) and merely a trickle of flow in the right internal jugular vein (arrow).

thrombocytosis is an independent risk factor for CVST in the absence of anemia.

The postsurgical state, in particular recent cranial surgery, is reported in 6% to 9% of children in two series (2,11). Recent head trauma is described in 4% to 6% (2,11,17). Closed head injury without skull fracture has also been reported as a risk factor (29).

Pregnancy and the puerperium are times of increased risk for CVST, seen in 14% and 6% of adults with CVST (24). Several medications have been associated with CVST. Oral contraceptive use is a well-established risk factor for thrombosis in adults and is reported as a risk factor in children (1,25). Corticosteroids have also been associated with CVST (30).

Certain chronic diseases have been implicated as risk factors for CVST and are present in 34% to 60% of affected children (1,3,7,11,17,21). Reported underlying conditions include hematologic malignancy, nephrotic syndrome, cardiac disease, and inflammatory conditions such as inflammatory bowel disease, celiac disease, systemic lupus erythematosus, and Behçet's disease.

Leukemia or lymphoma is reported in 5% to 18% of childhood CVST (3,7,17). The high blood viscosity conferred by hematologic malignancy may be important, and treatment with L-asparaginase increases risk (Figure 11.3). L-asparaginase, a chemotherapeutic often used to treat acute lymphoblastic leukemia (31), has been associated with CVST (31,32), possibly related

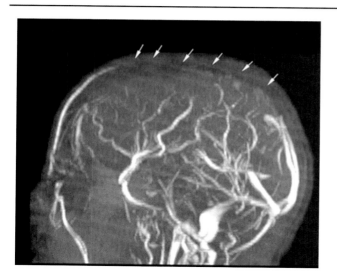

FIGURE 11.3 Sagittal MRV with decreased flow in the superior sagittal sinus (arrows) representing thrombus in a 17-year-old with acute lymphoblastic leukemia 10 days after receiving L-asparaginase.

to its effect on the synthesis of coagulation factors and inhibitors of coagulation such as proteins C and S. Nephrotic syndrome is rare in children but has been reported in 4% of children with CVST (11,21,23,25). Children with nephrotic syndrome have been found to have lower antithrombin III levels than healthy controls (33). Other potential contributors to a prothrombotic state in children with nephrotic syndrome are abnormal fibrinogen levels, abnormal lipid profiles, and reduced intravascular volume. A review of children with nephrotic syndrome found that when CVST was a complication, it was present with the first flare or within the first 6 months of diagnosis (34). Inflammatory conditions like systemic lupus erythematosus are seen in 4% to 7% of children with CVST (11,23). In systemic lupus erythematosus, secondary antiphospholipid syndrome characterized by anticardiolipin antibodies and/or lupus anticoagulant predisposes the child to venous and arterial thrombosis. A thrombotic event including CVST can herald the presentation of systemic lupus erythematosus (35). Behçet's disease is a vascular inflammatory disease with prominent venous involvement. The frequency of nervous system involvement was 13% among males and 6% among females in a 2-decade prospective cohort (36). In a series of children with Behçet's, 52% of thromboses were intracranial (37). In one series of children with CVST, 7% had Behçet's (3).

A prothrombotic risk factor has been reported in 40% to 76% of children with CVST (4,11,13,17,19,

21,23,38,39,40). In series that differentiate between children and neonates, a prothrombotic abnormality was found in 34% to 62% of children. The absence of standardized prothrombotic testing across institutions may account for these widely variable estimates of prevalence. In a large series of 149 children and neonates with CVST, univariate analysis showed a significantly higher prevalence of factor V G1691A mutation, elevated lipoprotein (a), protein C deficiency, and protein S deficiency in children with CVST compared to controls. However in multivariate analysis, only elevated lipoprotein (a), protein C deficiency, and a combination of a prothrombotic factor and another risk factor were independently associated with CVST (4). A recent large meta-analysis demonstrated significant associations between first CVST and prothrombotic risk factors. Prothrombotic factors with the highest association with CVST were antithrombin III deficiency, protein C deficiency, protein S deficiency, or the presence of > 2 prothrombotic traits. A significant though weaker association was present for factor V G1691A and factor II G20210A (41). In recent years, elevated factor VIII level has emerged as a possible risk factor for CVST (11), and both elevated factor VIII level and D-dimer levels have been reported in association with systemic thromboembolism (42,43).

■ DIAGNOSTIC STUDIES

Unenhanced HCT is routinely the first diagnostic test employed to screen for an acute intracranial process in children presenting with symptoms of CVST. In pediatric series, the sensitivity of unenhanced HCT for findings suggestive of CVST is 69% to 88% (2,22,25). Primary signs of CVST are the cord sign, the dense triangle sign, and the empty delta or empty triangle sign (Figure 11.4). The cord sign is visualized dense cortical veins or thrombosed sinuses. The dense triangle sign is a very early and transient sign. It is visualization of acutely congealed blood in the SSS. The delta or empty triangle sign is a late finding, requires contrast, and is the visualization of normally opacified collateral veins in the walls of the sinus, usually of the SSS, juxtaposed to nonopacified thrombus. In one series of 19 children, an empty delta sign was seen in 100%, a dense triangle sign in 42%, and a cord sign in only one subject (27).

On acute HCT, parenchymal effects of a CVST can sometimes be visualized. Early imaging findings may be

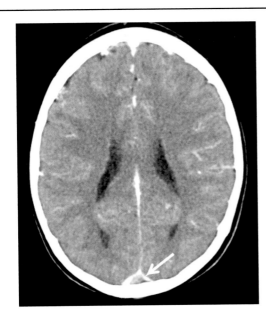

FIGURE 11.4 Contrast enhanced head computed tomography (HCT) demonstrating the empty delta or triangle sign (arrow) in a child with nephrotic syndrome and superior sagittal sinus thrombosis. There is low-attenuating thrombus within the superior sagittal sinus surrounded by a triangular area of enhancement.

restricted to vasogenic and cytotoxic edema. Isolated ischemic infarction was seen in 17% of children in one series (Figure 11.5) (16). Hemorrhage may be more common than isolated ischemia and has been reported in 16% to 23% of children (1,3,16,27). Hemorrhage can be parenchymal, intraventricular, or subarachnoid (16). Intraventricular hemorrhage is rare in children with CVST, reported in only 2% in two series (3,16). Hemorrhage on HCT along the transverse sinuses, in the biparietal region, or in the bithalamic region should prompt further evaluation for CVST, even if no clot is apparent because hemorrhage can obscure findings of the CVST itself (Figure 11.6). An absence of parenchymal findings has been reported in 14% to 26% of children (2,16). Children with polycythemia can have HCT findings that are difficult to differentiate from those present in CVST, so confirmatory vascular imaging should be performed quickly in most cases of suspected CVST so that appropriate treatment decisions can be made.

Confirmatory tests include magnetic resonance imaging (MRI) performed concomitantly with MRV, computed tomography venogram (CTV), and four-vessel conventional angiography with venous phase. An advantage of the combination of MRI and MRV is the absence of radiation and contrast exposure, a high sensitivity for

venous thrombosis, and the visualization of secondary parenchymal changes. Intraluminal thrombus is visualized on T2-weighted MRI as absence of a flow void or on T1-weighted MRI as hyperdense signal. The limitations of MRI are related to properties of blood flow and to the evolution of signal for thrombus over time. When blood flow is slow or the direction of blood flow is in the imaging plane, signal intensity is diminished and can be mistaken for thrombus. The appearance of thrombus changes with maturation of the clot. Within the first 5 days, deoxyhemoglobin is isointense on T1-weighted images and is hypointense on T2-weighted images. Deoxyhemoglobin can be mistaken for flowing blood. In the subacute phase, at 5 to 15 days, methemoglobin, which is easier to visualize, is hyperintense on both T1- and T2-weighted images (44). Therefore discussion with the neuroradiologist about the timing of the patient's presentation is helpful. Despite limitations, the combination of MRI and MRV has high sensitivity for CVST. In one study, 100% of children with CVST had a diagnostic MRI/MRV (25).

CTV has the advantage of rapid acquisition time, typically less than 1 minute, and can be used in children with medical devices that are not MRI compatible. However, drawbacks include radiation exposure and the risk of contrast nephropathy. Additionally, the quality of the study is related to appropriate timing between contrast administration and the image acquisition. At many centers the radiation dose for CTV (1–2.22 mSv) can be equivalent to or even lower than the radiation dose of unenhanced HCT (2.48 mSv) (45). On CTV, thrombosis is visualized as a filling defect, similar to the findings on conventional angiography with venous phase. When CVST is present, the time from administration of contrast to visualization of contrast in the cerebral veins and sinuses is delayed on the order of seconds (46). Many centers adjust their delay time for suspected CVST, but optimal delay time has not been established. In one study, the sensitivity and specificity of high resolution helical multidetector-row CT was found to be 100% (47).

When comparing MRI/MRV to CTV for the visualization of thrombosis, more than one study has demonstrated that both tests can establish the diagnosis well. CTV is superior to MRV for the visualization of smaller venous structures with low flow (48,49). MRI is superior to HCT for visualization of parenchymal changes secondary to cerebral venous thrombosis.

Four-vessel conventional angiography with venous phase is considered the gold standard test for CVST, but

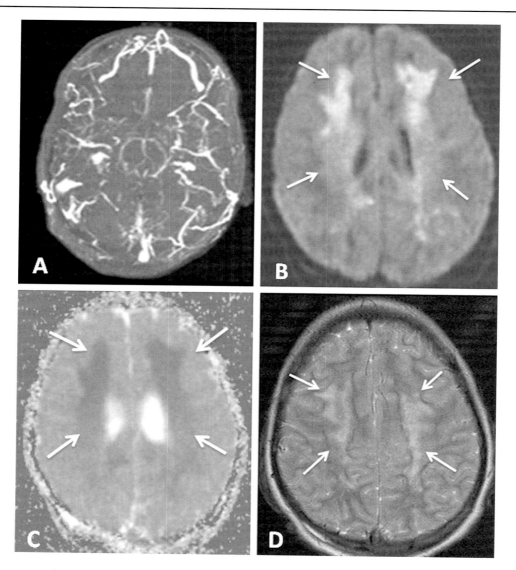

FIGURE 11.5 (A) Axial MRV with diffuse cerebral venous sinus thrombosis. (B) Axial diffusion weighted image with restricted diffusion representing ischemia in the white matter bilaterally (arrows). (C) Dark areas (arrows) on axial apparent diffusion coefficient map corresponding to areas of restriction on DWI confirm ischemia. (D) Axial T2-weighted image with hyperintensities (arrows) corresponding to the areas of abnormality on DWI and ADC.

with updated CT and MR techniques, conventional angiography is rarely needed to make the diagnosis.

■ LABORATORY EVALUATION

In the acute setting, a complete blood count (CBC) with differential and platelets, activated partial thromboplastin time (aPTT), prothrombin time (PT)/international normalized ratio, and basic metabolic panel (BMP)

should be sent. The CBC can help screen for infection, anemia, and thrombocytosis. Fibrinogen levels may be useful if the PTT or PT is abnormal. D-dimer is often but not always elevated in the setting of acute thrombus. The BMP can help assess for dehydration and electrolyte abnormalities such as hypernatremia.

A complete evaluation for thrombophilia is recommended in the American Heart Association (AHA) guidelines for the management of stroke in infants and children (50), but this recommendation has Class IIb/

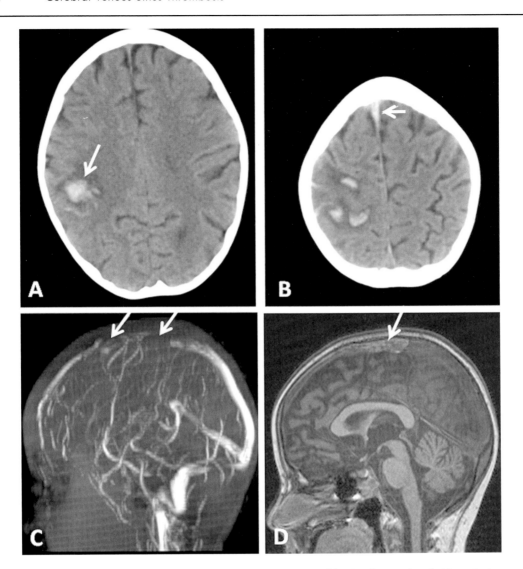

FIGURE 11.6 (A) HCT with hemorrhage in right frontal lobe (arrow) in a 6-year-old girl with acute lymphoblastic leukemia recently treated with L-asparaginase. (B) Higher on the same HCT, hyperdensity representing clot in the superior sagittal sinus is noted (arrow). (C) Sagittal MRV with flow void in anterior superior sagittal sinus representing thrombus (arrows). (D) Sagittal T1-weighted MRI with hyperintensity in area of anterior superior sagittal sinus representing thrombus (arrow).

Level B evidence. The combination of 2 prothrombotic factors or a prothrombotic factor plus another CVST risk factor is common (11), so evaluation for thrombophilia may be warranted even when another CVST risk factor is present. Thrombophilia evaluation typically includes protein C and protein S levels, antithrombin III level, homocysteine level, lipoprotein (a), antiphospholipid antibodies (immunoglobulin G and immunoglobulin M), dilute Russell venom viper time, and genetic testing for factor V G1691A mutation and factor II

G20210A variant. Some institutions also measure factor VIII levels. Prior to the initiation of anticoagulation, antithrombin III level must be sent since this level is altered once heparin is started. In the case of a prothrombotic abnormality, the laboratory test is often repeated weeks to months after the acute thrombus since the presence of thrombus itself can lower levels of certain factors such as proteins C and S. Consultation with a hematologist is strongly recommended to assist with interpretation of thrombophilia studies and with treatment. In children with anemia, a comprehensive diagnostic evaluation and treatment of the anemia are important.

If infection is suspected, a source should be investigated. Examination of the ears is part of the routine evaluation for all children. Sinus radiographs and blood cultures should be considered when there is suspicion for sinusitis and sepsis, respectively. Lumbar puncture with measurement of opening pressure and cerebrospinal fluid analysis should be considered in children who present with clinical signs of an intracranial infectious process. However, this may not be possible if there is evidence of mass effect or signs of greatly increased intracranial pressure. Even in CVST that is not associated with intracranial infection, cerebrospinal fluid analysis may be abnormal. In a series of 25 neonates and children with CVST, 19 underwent lumbar puncture. Elevated protein was present in 37% and subarachnoid hemorrhage was present in 79%. Opening pressure was measured in five and was elevated in four (26).

■ MANAGEMENT

Management of CVST focuses on providing supportive care, preventing and assessing for neurologic deterioration, and preventing propagation of thrombus.

Supportive Measures

It is crucial that patients with CVST be hydrated with isotonic fluids, and fluids are often administered at 1.5 times maintenance for at least 24 to 48 hours unless there is a contraindication. Very young infants may require hypotonic fluids, but this is usually not necessary after the neonatal period. Normoglycemia and normothermia are also goals. The head should be positioned at 30° or higher to promote venous outflow which may help to decrease intracranial pressure (ICP). If a bacterial etiology is suspected, broad spectrum intravenous antibiotics, with anaerobic coverage for possible sinus disease, should be initiated. For severe otitis media or mastoiditis, procedures including mastoidectomy, myringotomy, and/or tympanostomy may be indicated in addition to antibiotics. If an epidural abscess is present, neurosurgical drainage is often required.

Monitoring for and Treatment of Elevated ICP

In the acute phase, frequent neurologic examination is imperative. The clinician should pay particular attention to signs of elevated ICP including headache, emesis, hypertension, bradycardia, and deteriorating mental status including agitation and combativeness. Papilledema and changes in visual acuity, visual fields deficits, cranial nerve deficits (particularly nerves III and VI), and new motor deficits may also indicate elevated ICP or new parenchymal brain injury. In any child with an acute neurologic change, a noncontrast HCT should be obtained immediately.

Management of intracranial hypertension in children with CVST and cerebral edema or mass effect from hemorrhage is highly complex. The usual treatment strategies, including invasive ICP monitoring, hyperosmolar therapy, ventricular drainage, or decompressive surgery, must be used judiciously, balancing the risk of hemorrhagic complications and the need for suspending anticoagulation compared to the anticipated benefit.

Acetazolamide may be helpful in decreasing ICP since the medication is a carbonic anhydrase inhibitor and can decrease the production of cerebrospinal fluid; however, the medication will not acutely lower ICP in an emergency. There is limited literature on decompressive craniectomy for impending herniation in the setting of CVST. Case reports describe adult patients with large hemorrhagic infarcts accompanying CVST with signs of herniation that underwent successful decompressive craniectomy (51). A pediatric series also describes children who underwent decompression (22).

Monitoring for and Treatment of Seizures

There is concern that the metabolic demand of a seizure might worsen the extent of brain injury. If the child presents with a seizure, an antiepileptic medication should be considered. However, prophylactic anticonvulsants have not been studied in children with CVST. In patients who are comatose, sedated or paralyzed, or intubated, continuous electroencephalographic (EEG) monitoring should be strongly considered to screen for subclinical seizures (50). Other children may require continuous EEG monitoring including those with fluctuating mental status or who presented with seizures. In most cases even electrographic seizures without clinical manifestations are treated. In one series in which 8 of 15 children were monitored with EEG, it was abnormal in 75% due to diffuse slowing (26).

Anticoagulation

For many years the use of anticoagulation was considered counterintuitive in CVST because of the risk of concomitant hemorrhagic infarction. While there continues to be concern about the use of anticoagulation, especially in patients with large hemorrhages, treatment with anticoagulation is recommended in most cases of pediatric CVST (50,52). While there are no randomized controlled trials for anticoagulation in the pediatric population, recommendations supporting the use of anticoagulation in children are based on two randomized controlled trials in adult CVST (53,54) and experience from pediatric cohorts (9,16,23). The first adult trial comparing acute unfractionated heparin versus placebo was stopped early because complete clinical recovery at 3 months was seen in 80% of the heparin group compared with 10% of the placebo group (53). A larger blinded randomized controlled trial was conducted comparing acute treatment with low molecular weight heparin (LMWH) to placebo. A poor outcome (death or dependence) was seen in 13% of the anticoagulation group compared with 21% of the placebo group. These findings were not statistically significant despite a larger cohort (54). Both adult trials included patients with hemorrhage accompanying the CVST. In a Cochrane systematic review that pooled the results of the two adult randomized controlled trials, the relative risk of death in those treated with anticoagulation compared to placebo patients was 0.33 (95% confidence interval [CI] 0.08–1.21), and the relative risk of dependency was 0.46 (95% CI 0.16–1.31) (55). The pooled estimates did not reach statistical significance; however, no new symptomatic intracranial hemorrhages occurred in the patients treated with anticoagulation in either trial. The authors of the systemic review recognized that additional clinical trials would be difficult and concluded that anticoagulation in the setting of CVST seemed to be safe and had potential for reducing mortality and dependence (55).

Pediatric cohort studies also suggest that anticoagulation in the setting of CVST is safe. In one study of 30 children with CVST, 22 children without concomitant hemorrhage were treated with anticoagulation. Only one of these children had an intracranial hemorrhage after anticoagulation was initiated, and that hemorrhage was asymptomatic (23). In that same cohort, three deaths occurred among the 8 children who did not receive anticoagulation. In a larger cohort of children from the Canadian Stroke Registry, 66% of the children received antithrombotic therapy, most of which was anticoagulation. None of the children on anticoagulation died or experienced neurologic worsening due to hemorrhagic complications (1). In a more recent cohort study,

3 of 61 children treated with anticoagulation had major hemorrhages, but none with anticoagulation-related hemorrhage died. Two of these major hemorrhages occurred in children with intracranial hemorrhage prior to anticoagulation, and one occurred in a child without intracranial hemorrhage prior to anticoagulation. This study also demonstrated a statistically significant decrease in propagation of thrombus in children treated with anticoagulation compared to those who were not treated with anticoagulation. While not statistically significant in multivariate analysis, in univariate analysis anticoagulation was associated with favorable outcome compared to children who were not treated with anticoagulation (16). In another large multinational study with 396 patients from birth to age 18 years, only 6 of 22 children (27%) with recurrent thrombosis (systemic or cerebral) were receiving anticoagulation at the time of recurrence, a finding that suggests that anticoagulation might prevent recurrent thrombotic events in the setting of pediatric CVST (9).

Two practice guidelines for pediatric CVST have been published. The AHA guidelines for the management of pediatric stroke state that anticoagulation in children with CVST with either unfractionated heparin or LMWH, even in the presence of hemorrhage, is reasonable (50). The American College of Chest Physicians (CHEST) guidelines recommend that children with CVST without hemorrhage be anticoagulated with either unfractionated heparin or LMWH. For children with coexisting hemorrhage, the CHEST guidelines state that anticoagulation may be administered. Alternatively, the patient can be followed with neuroimaging at 5 to 7 days with anticoagulation started if there is evidence of thrombus progression (52).

Both unfractionated heparin and LMWH have been used to treat pediatric CVST (1,9,16,21,23). Oral vitamin K antagonists such as warfarin have also been used (1), although less frequently since vitamin K antagonists usually take several days to become therapeutic. In general, if unfractionated heparin is used, a bolus or loading dose is generally avoided to prevent supratherapeutic treatment which may increase the risk of intracranial hemorrhage in the setting of acute neurologic injury. However, a hematologist should be consulted to provide individualized recommendations. Some centers have set a goal for the aPTT of 60 to 85 seconds (16), but the goal aPTT for each patient should be considered individually and may change during the course of treatment. An advantage of unfractionated heparin is the ability to completely reverse the medication in the case of major bleeding or for a surgical procedure. In recent years, LMWH has been utilized with increasing frequency (16). LMWH has several advantages over unfractionated heparin. Pharmacokinetics are predictable with LMWH, monitoring is required less frequently, heparin-induced thrombocytopenia is rare, and administration does not require intravenous access. Disadvantages of LMWH include twice daily injections and less easily accomplished reversal of anticoagulation. The goal anti-Xa level for a child on LMWH is often considered 0.5 to 1.0 units/mL 4 to 6 hours after a dose (16,50), but the goal anti-Xa level may be individualized. Dosing for both unfractionated heparin and LMWH is dependent upon both age and weight, and is often guided by a pediatric hematologist. Monitoring should ensure adequate anticoagulation without supratherapeutic values. It is important to remember that no clinical trial comparing unfractionated heparin to LMWH in the setting of CVST exists (50). A child on anticoagulation with any acute neurologic alteration or any worrisome feature such as headache or new seizures should be imaged with a noncontrast HCT immediately to assess for intracranial hemorrhage. Surveillance imaging for hemorrhage is not usually required without new or concerning neurologic symptoms.

Some children with CVST may be postoperative from mastoidectomy or otolaryngology procedures, craniosynostosis repair, or other surgeries at the time of CVST presentation. The decision to use anticoagulation must be multidisciplinary in the postoperative scenario and sometimes is started cautiously at a lower dose or after several days.

While no studies evaluating the duration of anticoagulation have been performed in pediatric CVST, most treat for 3 to 6 months (50,52). At hospital discharge, children are often transitioned from unfractionated heparin or LMWH to oral warfarin with a goal international normalized ratio of 2.0 to 3.0 (16,21). A new oral direct thrombin inhibitor that does not require PT monitoring, dabigatran, has been introduced in the United States but has not been studied in pediatric CVST.

Thrombolysis and Thrombectomy

The first case of local urokinase used to treat SSS thrombosis was reported by J.A. Scott et al in 1988 (56). The literature on thrombolysis and thrombectomy is limited to observational studies in the setting of CVST (57,58). The subjects of these studies were assumed to have poor prognosis and were comatose or had continued deterioration despite systemic anticoagulation. Mechanical thrombectomy was conceived as a method of obtaining rapid recanalization without the use of local thrombolytics to reduce the risk of hemorrhage. Nevertheless, most reported cases of thrombectomy were also treated with chemical thrombolysis (57).

A review of the literature from 1988 through June 2009 described 161 adult CVST patients who underwent direct chemical thrombolysis and 34 patients who underwent a combination of chemical and mechanical thrombolysis/thrombectomy. Overall, 87% of the 161 subjects treated with direct thrombolysis had excellent or good outcomes, and 35% of the 34 patients treated with chemical and mechanical thrombolysis/thrombectomy achieved near-complete recovery (59). The largest retrospective study comparing local thrombolysis and systemic anticoagulation included 20 adults treated with local urokinase and 20 adults treated with systemic heparin. The patients who received thrombolysis had better outcomes at discharge, but two patients had hemorrhagic complications. The authors concluded that additional randomized studies are necessary (58). The Cochrane Collaboration reviewed thrombolysis for CVST and concluded that without data from randomized controlled trials there is insufficient information to recommend thrombolysis routinely; however, the group also recognized that thrombolysis is being used more frequently and that a randomized controlled trial for its use in the acute phase is warranted (60). Pediatric literature on thrombolysis is limited to case reports. In one report of a child with extensive thrombosis and early signs of herniation, there was improvement of anterograde venous flow and clinical symptoms (61). In another series of three children treated with local thrombolysis, there was one death (22).

Although mechanical thrombectomy has mostly been reserved for patients with poor mental status, coma, straight sinus thrombosis, or a large space-occupying lesion, 60% of patients in one series had minimal or no deficits. However, 10% had moderate or severe neurologic deficits, and 30% died. The deaths were mostly due to intracranial hemorrhage and resulting herniation (57).

The AHA guidelines state that thrombolysis may be used in certain pediatric patients (50), and the CHEST guidelines state that thrombolysis/thrombectomy may be used in children who do not respond to anticoagulation (52). Nevertheless, the optimal subject, thrombolytic, dosage of thrombolytic, and mechanical device approach are not known. Furthermore, thrombolysis may not be successful in recanalizing cortical veins.

Factor Replacement

Endogenous anticoagulant factor replacement with fresh frozen plasma can be considered in the setting of liver failure, nephrotic syndrome, or acquired deficiencies of antithrombin III, protein C, or protein S. However, no studies have demonstrated the efficacy of fresh frozen plasma in the setting of CVST.

Other Treatment Considerations

Children with iron deficiency anemia may require iron replacement or even transfusion of packed red blood cells if the anemia is severe. Children with sickle cell disease may require exchange transfusion or simple transfusion. In all cases of CVST in which an anemia is a risk factor, a hematologist should be consulted. In the case of young women on oral contraceptive pills, the medication should be discontinued immediately.

■ OUTCOME

Thrombus Propagation

One study of 79 children with CVST defined thrombus propagation as new thrombus in a venous sinus distal to or adjoining the initial thrombus within 14 days of the original diagnosis (16). Follow-up imaging was obtained within 14 days in 63 (80%) and showed clot propagation in 7 of 19 (37%) who were not treated with anticoagulation and in 3 of 44 (7%) children treated with anticoagulation (relative risk 3.1, 95% CI 1.6–5.8, P = .006). Propagation was symptomatic in 60% of the children and was accompanied by new venous infarction in 40%. Worse outcomes were associated with thrombus propagation (odds ratio 4.3, 95% CI 1.0–19.4, P = .053) (16).

Recanalization

The AHA guidelines state that repeated neuroimaging to assess for recanalization of the affected sinus(es) is sensible; however, the optimal timing of repeat imaging is not known. Many centers obtain follow-up imaging at 3 to 6 months when discontinuation of anticoagulation is typically considered (50). In mixed cohorts of neonates and children, the rates of recanalization are similar to those reported in adult series, with complete recanalization in 42% to 70%, partial recanalization in 23% to 42%, and persistent occlusion in 1% to 16%. (2,4,9,11,21,62). The presence of a prothrombotic risk factor was predictive of

failure to recanalize in one series (16) but was not associated with failure to recanalize in another study (4). Longer duration of symptoms has been associated with failure to recanalize (11,21). The administration of anticoagulation has not been found to be significantly associated with recanalization (4,11,16). Furthermore, propagation of thrombus within 2 weeks has not been associated with recanalization at 3 months. Both a pediatric and an adult series found that neither the number of vessels involved nor deep sinus thrombosis predicted recanalization (11,62). In a retrospective study of 16 children with CVST, 10 children had follow-up imaging. Neurologic deficits were present in all three subjects without recanalization compared to in 29% of children with complete or partial recanalization (2). In another retrospective series of 53 neonates and children, there was no significant correlation between recanalization and neurologic outcome (21).

Recurrence

The recurrence rate of CVST in pediatric cohort studies has been reported between 3% and 8%. The recurrence rate of systemic thrombosis after CVST has been reported between 3% and 7% (1,9,11,23). These estimates are similar to those in an adult study (24). From a multicenter mixed cohort of children and neonates from Europe and Israel with CVST, there were 22 recurrent venous thromboses of which 13 (59%) were cerebral. The recurrence rate for any venous thrombosis was 21.1 per 1000 person-years (95% CI 13.9–32.1 per 1000 person-years). Recurrent CVST was not seen in children < 2 years in this cohort, and the recurrence rate for any venous thrombosis in children older than 2 years was 29.1 per 1000 person-years (95% CI 18.9–44.7 person-years). Most recurrent CVST occurred within the first 6 months from initial diagnosis. Lack of treatment with anticoagulation, failure to recanalize, and heterozygosity for the G20210A mutation were all significantly associated with an increased risk of any recurrent venous thrombosis in a Cox proportional hazards model (9). Other smaller series report recurrences in children with underlying medical conditions such as nephrotic syndrome (11).

Neurologic Outcome

Neurologic outcomes in children with CVST range from normal to death. Normal follow-up examinations have been reported in 26% to 67% (1,11,23). Mortality estimates range from 3% to 13% (9,11,23). Death can be from the CVST itself or from underlying conditions. Neurologic deficits are present in 38% to 62% (1,11). In one cohort, deficits were motor in 80%, cognitive in 10%, developmental in 9%, speech in 6%, and visual in 6% (1). In a recent cohort, despite normal total scores on the Wechsler Intelligence Scale for Children, 14 of the 21 children given the scale had a cognitive abnormality in at least one subtest (3). In two other cohorts, 17% and 32% of children who survived had headache or other signs of elevated ICP (7,11). Epilepsy has been reported in 5% to 25% (7,11,63).

Since most cohorts are relatively small, predictors of neurologic outcome have not been elucidated fully. In one cohort, mortality was associated with coma at presentation and with seizures (22). In another study, younger children, seizures, and involvement of the straight sinus were predictors of severe sequelae while any combination of focal neurologic findings, seizures, and decreased consciousness were associated with any neurologic sequelae (21). In the cohort from the Canadian Pediatric Ischemic Stroke registry, seizures in nonneonates and infarction in neonates and nonneonates were associated with the composite outcome of neurologic deficits or death (1). Infarction has been associated with disability (3,18). In one study, good cognitive outcome was associated with older age at CVST presentation, involvement of the lateral and/or sigmoid sinuses, and anticoagulation (11). Another cohort demonstrated similar predictors of outcome in univariate analysis, although the findings were not significant in multivariate analysis (3). Other reported predictors of an unfavorable outcome are absence of recanalization or partial recanalization, thrombus propagation, presence of intraventricular hemorrhage, involvement of the straight sinus, and neurologic comorbidity (16).

■ CONCLUSIONS

CVST is an important cause of morbidity and mortality in children. The presenting symptoms and clinical course are variable. When there is suspicion for CVST, dedicated cerebral vascular studies, including MRI/MRV or CTV, should be performed. Treatment decisions often rely on a multidisciplinary approach among intensivists, neurologists, hematologists, and occasionally neurosurgeons and interventional radiologists. CVST

management includes supportive measures, identification and management of underlying risk factors, and in most cases anticoagulation. Systemic anticoagulation is generally safe, even in the presence of intracranial hemorrhage and may improve outcome, but further study is needed. Monitoring children with CVST demands close observation for neurologic deterioration. In the absence of randomized clinical trials, recommendations are based on data from cohort studies and from adult literature. The efficacy of any treatment, including anticoagulation, for the prevention of death or long-term neurologic sequelae requires adequately powered randomized controlled trials.

■ REFERENCES

1. deVeber G et al. Cerebral sinovenous thrombosis in children. *N Engl J Med.* 2001;345:417–423.
2. Barnes C et al. Cerebral sinus venous thrombosis in children. *J Paediatr Child Health.* 2004;40:53–55.
3. Grunt S et al. Cerebral sinus venous thrombosis in Swiss children. *Dev Med Child Neurol.* 2010;52:1145–1150.
4. Heller C et al. Cerebral venous thrombosis in children: a multifactorial origin. *Circulation.* 2003;108:1362–1367.
5. Lin A et al. Occurrence of cerebral venous sinus thrombosis in patients with presumed idiopathic intracranial hypertension. *Ophthalmology.* 2006;113:2281–2284.
6. Leker RR, Steiner I. Features of dural sinus thrombosis simulating pseudotumor cerebri. *Eur J Neurol.* 1999;6:601–604.
7. De Schryver EL et al. Long-term prognosis of cerebral venous sinus thrombosis in childhood. *Dev Med Child Neurol.* 2004;46:514–519.
8. Andrew M. Developmental hemostasis: relevance to thromboembolic complications in pediatric patients. *Thromb Haemost.* 1995;74:415–425.
9. Kenet G et al. Risk factors for recurrent venous thromboembolism in the European Collaborative Paediatric Database on Cerebral Venous Thrombosis: a multicentre cohort study. *Lancet Neurol.* 2007;6:595–603.
10. Carvalho KS et al. Cerebral venous thrombosis in children. *J Child Neurol.* 2001;16:574–580.
11. Sebire G et al. Cerebral venous sinus thrombosis in children: risk factors, presentation, diagnosis and outcome. *Brain.* 2005;128:477–489.
12. Widjaja E et al. 2D time-of-flight MR venography in neonates: anatomy and pitfalls. *AJNR Am J Neuroradiol.* 2006;27:1913–1918.
13. Rollins N et al. MR venography in the pediatric patient. *AJNR Am J Neuroradiol.* 2005;26:50–55.
14. Okudera T et al. Development of posterior fossa dural sinuses, emissary veins, and jugular bulb: morphological and radiologic study. *AJNR Am J Neuroradiol.* 1994;15:1871–1883.
15. Bales CB et al. Lateral sinus thrombosis as a complication of otitis media: 10-year experience at the children's hospital of Philadelphia. *Pediatrics.* 2009;123:709–713.

16. Moharir MD et al. Anticoagulants in pediatric cerebral sinovenous thrombosis: a safety and outcome study. *Ann Neurol.* 2010;67:590–599.

17. Bonduel M et al. Arterial ischemic stroke and cerebral venous thrombosis in children: a 12-year Argentinean registry. *Acta Haematol.* 2006;115:180–185.

18. Fitzgerald KC et al. Cerebral sinovenous thrombosis in the neonate. *Arch Neurol.* 2006;63:405–409.

19. Vielhaber H et al. Cerebral venous sinus thrombosis in infancy and childhood: role of genetic and acquired risk factors of thrombophilia. *Eur J Pediatr.* 1998;157:555–560.

20. Berfelo FJ et al. Neonatal cerebral sinovenous thrombosis from symptom to outcome. *Stroke.* 2010;41:1382–1388.

21. Vieira JP et al. Cerebral sinovenous thrombosis in children: clinical presentation and extension, localization and recanalization of thrombosis. *Eur J Paediatr Neurol.* 2010;14:80–85.

22. Wasay M et al. Cerebral venous sinus thrombosis in children: a multicenter cohort from the United States. *J Child Neurol.* 2008;23:26–31.

23. deVeber G et al. Anticoagulation therapy in pediatric patients with sinovenous thrombosis: a cohort study. *Arch Neurol.* 1998;55:1533–1537.

24. Ferro JM et al. Prognosis of cerebral vein and dural sinus thrombosis: results of the International Study on Cerebral Vein and Dural Sinus Thrombosis (ISCVT). *Stroke.* 2004;35:664–670.

25. Mallick AA et al. Cerebral venous sinus thrombosis: a case series including thrombolysis. *Arch Dis Child.* 2009;94:790–794.

26. Barron TF et al. Cerebral venous thrombosis in neonates and children. *Pediatr Neurol.* 1992;8:112–116.

27. Huisman TA et al. Cerebral venous thrombosis in childhood. *Eur Radiol.* 2001;11:1760–1765.

28. Shevell MI et al. Neonatal dural sinus thrombosis. *Pediatr Neurol.* 1989;5:161–165.

29. Matsushige T et al. Cerebral sinovenous thrombosis after closed head injury. *J Trauma.* 2009;66:1599–1604.

30. Shiozawa Z et al. Superior sagittal sinus thrombosis associated with Evans' syndrome of haemolytic anaemia. *J Neurol.* 1985;232:280–282.

31. Kieslich M et al. Cerebrovascular complications of L-asparaginase in the therapy of acute lymphoblastic leukemia. *J Pediatr Hematol Oncol.* 2003;25:484–487.

32. Ott N et al. Sequelae of thrombotic or hemorrhagic complications following L-asparaginase therapy for childhood lymphoblastic leukemia. *Am J Pediatr Hematol Oncol.* 1988;10:191–195.

33. Citak A et al. Hemostatic problems and thromboembolic complications in nephrotic children. *Pediatr Nephrol.* 2000;14:138–142.

34. Fluss J, Geary D, deVeber G. Cerebral sinovenous thrombosis and idiopathic nephrotic syndrome in childhood: report of four new cases and review of the literature. *Eur J Pediatr.* 2006;165:709–716.

35. Uziel Y et al. Cerebral vein thrombosis in childhood systemic lupus erythematosus. *J Pediatr.* 1995;126:722–727.

36. Kural-Seyahi E et al. The long-term mortality and morbidity of Behcet syndrome: a 2-decade outcome survey of 387 patients followed at a dedicated center. *Medicine (Baltimore).* 2003;82:60–76.

37. Krupa B et al. Pediatric Behçet's disease and thromboses. *J Rheumatol.* 2010;38:387–390.

38. deVeber G et al. Prothrombotic disorders in infants and children with cerebral thromboembolism. *Arch Neurol.* 1998;55:1539–1543.

39. Heller C et al. Prothrombotic risk factors in childhood stroke and venous thrombosis. *Eur J Pediatr.* 1999;158(suppl 3):S117–S121.

40. Kenet G et al. Paediatric cerebral sinus vein thrombosis. A multi-center, case-controlled study. *Thromb Haemost.* 2004;92:713–718.

41. Kenet G et al. Impact of thrombophilia on risk of arterial ischemic stroke or cerebral sinovenous thrombosis in neonates and children: a systematic review and meta-analysis of observational studies. *Circulation.* 2010;121:1838–1847.

42. Goldenberg NA, Knapp-Clevenger R, Manco-Johnson MJ. Elevated plasma factor VIII and D-dimer levels as predictors of poor outcomes of thrombosis in children. *N Engl J Med.* 2004;351:1081–1088.

43. Kreuz W et al. Familial elevated factor VIII in children with symptomatic venous thrombosis and post-thrombotic syndrome: results of a multicenter study. *Arterioscler Thromb Vasc Biol.* 2006;26:1901–1906.

44. Connor SE, Jarosz JM. Magnetic resonance imaging of patients with epilepsy. *Clin Radiol.* 2001;56:787–801.

45. Wetzel SG et al. Cerebral veins: comparative study of CT venography with intraarterial digital subtraction angiography. *AJNR Am J Neuroradiol.* 1999;20:249–255.

46. Gratama van Andel HA et al. Interobserver variability in the detection of cerebral venous thrombosis using CT venography with matched mask bone elimination. *Clin Neurol Neurosurg.* 2009;111:717–723.

47. Linn J et al. Diagnostic value of multidetector-row CT angiography in the evaluation of thrombosis of the cerebral venous sinuses. *AJNR Am J Neuroradiol.* 2007;28:946–952.

48. Ozsvath RR et al. Cerebral venography: comparison of CT and MR projection venography. *AJR Am J Roentgenol.* 1997;169:1699–1707.

49. Khandelwal N et al. Comparison of CT venography with MR venography in cerebral sinovenous thrombosis. *AJR Am J Roentgenol.* 2006;187:1637–1643.

50. Roach ES et al. Management of stroke in infants and children: a scientific statement from a Special Writing Group of the American Heart Association Stroke Council and the Council on Cardiovascular Disease in the Young. *Stroke.* 2008;39:2644–2691.

51. Stefini R et al. Emergent decompressive craniectomy in patients with fixed dilated pupils due to cerebral venous and dural sinus thrombosis: report of three cases. *Neurosurgery.* 1999;45:626-629; discussion 629–630.

52. Monagle P et al. Antithrombotic therapy in neonates and children: antithrombotic therapy and prevention of thrombosis: American College of Chest Physicians Evidence-Based Clinical Practice Guidelines (9th Edition). *Chest.* 2012;141(2 Suppl):e737S–801S.

53. Einhaupl KM et al. Heparin treatment in sinus venous thrombosis. *Lancet.* 1991;338:597–600.

54. de Bruijn SF, Stam J. Randomized, placebo-controlled trial of anticoagulant treatment with low-molecular-weight heparin for cerebral sinus thrombosis. *Stroke.* 1999;30:484–488.

55. Stam J, De Bruijn SF, DeVeber G. Anticoagulation for cerebral sinus thrombosis. *Cochrane Database Syst Rev.* 2002:CD002005.

56. Scott JA et al. Treatment of dural sinus thrombosis with local urokinase infusion. Case report. *J Neurosurg.* 1988;68:284–287.

57. Stam J et al. Endovascular thrombectomy and thrombolysis for severe cerebral sinus thrombosis: a prospective study. *Stroke.* 2008;39:1487–1490.

58. Wasay M et al. Nonrandomized comparison of local urokinase thrombolysis versus systemic heparin anticoagulation for superior sagittal sinus thrombosis. *Stroke.* 2001;32:2310–2317.

59. Rahman M et al. Direct thrombolysis for cerebral venous sinus thrombosis. *Neurosurg Focus.* 2009;27:E7.

60. Ciccone A et al. Thrombolysis for cerebral vein and dural sinus thrombosis. *Cochrane Database Syst Rev.* 2004:CD003693.

61. Griesemer DA et al. Local fibrinolysis in cerebral venous thrombosis. *Pediatr Neurol.* 1994;10:78–80.

62. Strupp M et al. Cerebral venous thrombosis: correlation between recanalization and clinical outcome—a long-term follow-up of 40 patients. *J Neurol.* 2002;249:1123–1124.

63. Hetherington R et al. Short-term intellectual outcome after arterial ischemic stroke and sinovenous thrombosis in childhood and infancy. *J Child Neurol.* 2005;20:553–559.

12 Nontraumatic Intracerebral Hemorrhage and Subarachnoid Hemorrhage

LAUREN A. BESLOW, GREGORY G. HEUER, and LORI C. JORDAN

■ INTRODUCTION

Intracerebral hemorrhage (ICH) refers to bleeding into the brain parenchyma (Figure 12.1) or ventricles (Figure 12.2). Subarachnoid hemorrhage (SAH) refers to bleeding into the subarachnoid space (Figure 12.3). Nontraumatic ICH accounts for about half of childhood stroke, but relatively little research has been devoted to its study. Childhood ICH most commonly occurs in previously healthy children with occult vascular malformations, although children with hematologic disorders, oncologic processes, and hypertension can be affected. SAH most commonly occurs in previously healthy children with occult aneurysms or other cerebral vascular malformations. Timely diagnosis, workup, and management are crucial, and a multidisciplinary team is usually required to manage these children.

■ EPIDEMIOLOGY

Estimates of the incidence of ICH in developed countries range from 1.1/100,000/year to 5.22/100,000/year (1,2). ICH is comprised of intraparenchymal hemorrhage (IPH) and intraventricular hemorrhage (IVH). SAH is generally discussed separately. A California population-based cohort estimated the incidence of SAH to be 0.4/100,000/year. ICH and SAH may occur in the context of traumatic brain injury, but this chapter will focus on nontraumatic causes.

Unlike adult ICH, in which hypertension and amyloid angiopathy are the most common etiologies, childhood

ICH is most commonly caused by ruptured vascular malformations including arteriovenous malformations (AVMs) (Figure 12.4), cavernomas (Figure 12.5), and aneurysms (Figure 12.6). Depending on the series, vascular malformations are responsible for 37.5% to 73.5% of pediatric ICH (3,4), with AVM the most common type of malformation. The prevalence of intracranial aneurysms in the pediatric population ranges from 0.5% to 4.6%, and the majority of these patients do not present with acute rupture (5–11).

Other common etiologies of ICH in children are hematologic abnormalities and coagulopathies, brain tumors, and cerebral infections (3,12). Although hypertension as a risk factor for ICH is less common than in adults, hypertension has also been associated with ICH in children (12,13). In recent cohorts, even after a thorough evaluation, between 9% and 23% of childhood ICH is considered idiopathic, although some of these cases may be due to vascular malformations that self-obliterate after the incident hemorrhage (12,14). Some children have underlying diseases that predispose them to ICH and/or to vascular malformations and are discussed in the section on special populations.

■ DIFFERENTIAL DIAGNOSIS AND PRESENTATION

The differential diagnosis for ICH is broad and is found in Table 12.1. Presentations of children with ICH can be rapid, occurring over minutes to hours, or insidious over several hours to days (13). In a recent cohort of children with IPH, the median time to hospital presentation was

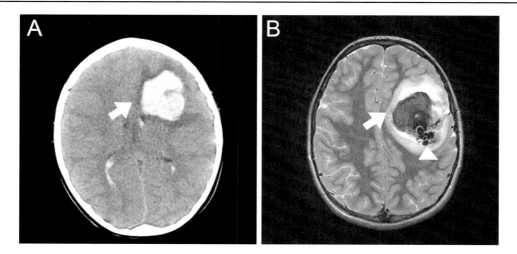

FIGURE 12.1 (A) Axial head computed tomography (HCT) with left frontal acute intraparenchymal hemorrhage (IPH, white arrow) and secondary intraventricular hemorrhage. (B) Axial fluid-attenuated inversion recovery sequence magnetic resonance imaging (MRI) from the same patient as in (A) at a different level with IPH (white arrow) and arteriovenous malformation at the posterior aspect of the hematoma (white arrowhead).

70 minutes, but 23% of children presented after 24 hours (14). Headache was the most common symptom in most series, affecting 45.6% to 77% of children (3,14). Altered level of consciousness was present in more than 50% of children in several series (3,12,14). Other common presenting symptoms include nausea and emesis, seizures (generalized or focal), neck pain, and focal neurologic deficits such as hemiparesis or aphasia (3,12,14). Common presenting symptoms for SAH also include severe headache, nausea, emesis, neck pain, meningismus, altermental status, and sometimes focal neurological deficits.

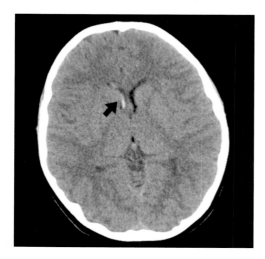

FIGURE 12.2 Axial HCT with intraventricular hemorrhage (black arrow) in the right lateral ventricle without hydrocephalus.

■ INITIAL EVALUATION AND MANAGEMENT

Acute studies in the emergency room or intensive care unit should be focused on rapid diagnosis of the hemorrhage, assessment for the presence of elevated intracranial pressure (ICP) and of herniation, and assessment of easily correctible risk factors such as thrombocytopenia or coagulopathy. In most cases, head computed tomography (HCT) is the initial imaging of choice. It is rapid, widely available, can be performed without sedation if the child has preserved airway reflexes and can protect his airway, and clearly diagnoses acute ICH.

In adult series, HCT can miss up to 5% of acute SAH (15–17). Therefore if SAH is suspected and a HCT does not demonstrate hemorrhage, a lumbar puncture should be performed in most cases. A spun down sample of cerebrospinal fluid (CSF) can be examined for the presence of xanthochromia (yellow discoloration of CSF secondary to bilirubin) to differentiate SAH from venous blood from a "traumatic tap." When sending a CSF sample for suspected SAH, it is important to indicate in the lab order that one wants to check for xanthochromia. A guideline for the analysis of lumbar puncture in adults with possible SAH from the United Kingdom states that if concern for SAH remains after a negative HCT, a lumbar puncture can be performed > 12 hours from symptom onset and the fourth tube sent

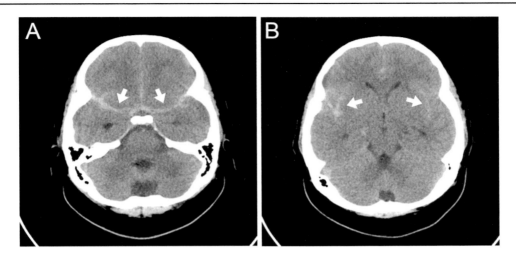

FIGURE 12.3 (A) Axial HCT with subarachnoid hemorrhage visible in bilateral basal cisterns (white arrows). (B) Axial HCT at a different level from the same patient as in A with SAH visible in the bilateral sylvian fissures (white arrows).

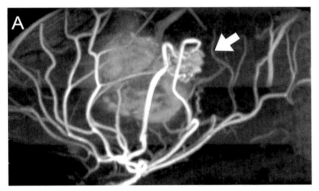

for spectrophotometry for bilirubin (18). An increase in CSF bilirubin supports the diagnosis of SAH although it is not specific for this diagnosis. Adjustment for elevated serum bilirubin may be necessary (19). Additionally, cell counts can be sent from the first and fourth tubes, since the red blood cell count should decrease between the first and fourth tubes in a traumatic tap whereas the red

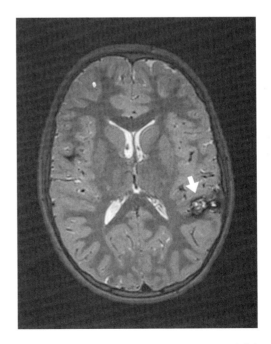

FIGURE 12.4 (A) Sagittal magnetic resonance angiography demonstrating arteriovenous malformation (AVM; white arrow). This AVM was the cause of the IPH shown in Figure 12.1. (B) Sagittal view of digital subtraction angiogram from the same patient demonstrating AVM supplied by distal branches of the left middle cerebral artery (black arrow).

FIGURE 12.5 Axial T2-weighted MRI sequence with left parieto-temporal cavernoma (white arrow).

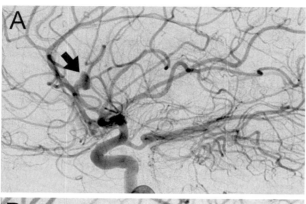

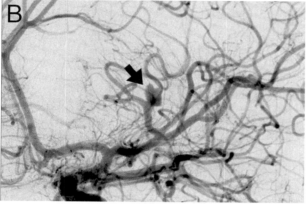

FIGURE 12.6 (A) Digital subtraction angiogram lateral view demonstrating left middle cerebral artery aneurysm (black arrow). (B) Digital subtraction angiogram posterior anterior view of the same patient demonstrating left middle cerebral artery aneurysm (black arrow).

blood cell count should not decrease between the first and fourth tubes in SAH. However, the magnitude of the decrease in red blood cells that can be used for this differentiation is controversial.

Acute laboratory studies include electrolytes, complete blood count with platelets, prothrombin time or international normalized ratio, activated partial thromboplastin time, and fibrinogen level. A type and screen should be sent as well.

The acute management of any child with ICH or SAH is focused on stabilization of the patient, detection and management of elevated ICP and herniation, and minimizing additional brain injury. No randomized trials exist for childhood ICH or SAH management, so most pediatric guidelines are adapted from those for adults (20–22) or are based on retrospective cohorts.

The patient should not be permitted to eat or drink, even when mental status is preserved since level of consciousness can deteriorate, and intubation or neurosurgical intervention may be required. Once ICH is diagnosed, a neurosurgeon should be contacted immediately. Consideration should be given to consultation with an interventional radiologist for diagnostic and/or therapeutic intervention. The head of the patient's bed should be elevated to at least 30° and the neck should be maintained in a midline position to promote venous drainage. Signs and symptoms of elevated ICP should be reassessed frequently (see section "Monitoring for Increased ICP"). For any neurologic deterioration, a repeat HCT should be obtained promptly to assess for worsening hemorrhage, hydrocephalus, edema, or herniation.

Isotonic fluids without glucose should be started immediately to maintain adequate hydration (20). Since temperature elevation > 37.5°C increases the likelihood of poor outcome in adult IPH (23), maintenance of normothermia with acetaminophen and cooling blankets is advised. Children who present with seizures should receive an anticonvulsant medication to reduce the likelihood of additional seizures.

Managing hypertension after ICH is challenging since no clear evidence exists in children. In adults

■ **Table 12.1** Differential Diagnosis for Intracerebral Hemorrhage
Arterial ischemic stroke with or without hemorrhagic transformation
Cerebral sinovenous thrombosis with or without venous infarction or hemorrhage
Brain tumor
Posterior reversible encephalopathy syndrome
Hypertensive urgency or emergency
Postictal Todd's paralysis
Migraine
Cerebral infections
Abscess
Encephalitis
Meningitis
White matter disease
Multiple sclerosis
Acute disseminated encephalomyelitis
Leukodystrophies
Metabolic derangements such as hypoglycemia
Organic or amino acidurias
Mitochondrial diseases such as mitochondrial encephalopathy with lactic acidosis and strokelike episodes
Cerebral autosomal dominant arteriopathy with subcortical infarcts and leukoencephalopathy

with ICH, treatment of elevated blood pressure may prevent expansion of the cerebral hematoma (24), and the adult ICH guidelines discuss management of hypertension (20). Logically, children with hypertension should be treated, and it is a reasonable goal to lower blood pressure to the 95th percentile for age and sex. However, this recommendation is not evidence-based. While lowering blood pressure may reduce the risk of hematoma expansion, it may reduce cerebral perfusion and thus exacerbate secondary brain injury if autoregulatory mechanisms are disturbed or if there is elevated ICP. If there is concern that hypertension is an autoregulatory response to maintain cerebral perfusion or that hypertension is refractory to initial management, ICP monitoring to allow management of ICP and cerebral perfusion should be considered. Antihypertensive medications should be chosen based on intracranial compliance. Vasodilators can reduce systemic blood pressure yet compromise cerebral perfusion pressure. Beta blockade may be helpful in maintaining cerebral perfusion pressure without the concomitant cerebral vasodilation.

For patients with hematologic abnormalities, a pediatric hematologist should be consulted. Patients with low platelet count or abnormal platelet function may require platelet transfusion. Patients with factor deficiencies such as factor XIII or IX deficiency usually require factor concentrate (25,26). Coagulopathy should be corrected for children with abnormal coagulation parameters secondary to liver failure or other medical causes. Children with ICH while on anticoagulation should have their anticoagulation reversed unless there is an overwhelming contraindication such as ongoing extracorporeal membrane oxygenation.

Recombinant activated factor VIIa (rFVIIa) was first used in patients with hemophilia who had developed inhibitors against coagulation factors. rFVIIa has been used in a variety of circumstances in neonates and children who do not have hemophilia, and the mechanism of action is induction of coagulation at sites in which tissue factor is present. However, its safety and efficacy in pediatric ICH has not been studied (27). In adults, a recent meta-analysis underscored that while rFVIIa reduces change in ICH volume, there has not been improvement in outcome or survival (28). Furthermore, there is an increase in thromboembolic events after rFVIIa. Adult studies of rFVIIa may have limited applicability in pediatric patients in whom vascular malformations are the most common cause of ICH since these patients were excluded from adult trials. Additionally, most pediatric patients lack the underlying cardiac and atherosclerotic risk factors that many adults with ICH possess. Other factor concentrates such as prothrombin complex concentrates have been studied in adult ICH in the setting of oral anticoagulation therapy to limit bleeding, but studies in children are lacking (29).

■ ACUTE MEDICAL AND SURGICAL MONITORING AND MANAGEMENT

Monitoring for Increased ICP

Declining mental status in a child with ischemic stroke or ICH is a worrisome sign and is a clear indication for ICP monitoring. Other symptoms and signs of increased ICP include positional headache (headache worse when supine, better when upright), vomiting, irritability or combativeness, sixth nerve palsies, and papilledema. Cushing's triad suggests elevated ICP and consists of hypertension, bradycardia, and irregular respirations. Cushing's triad is usually a late finding. With arterial ischemic stroke, increased ICP may develop several days after stroke onset as infarcted brain tissue becomes edematous. In ICH, increased ICP may occur acutely due to mass effect from a hemorrhage. Increased ICP may also occur acutely or subacutely if there is IVH accompanied by communicating hydrocephalus.

If monitoring is required, then an intraventricular catheter (IVC) is advantageous because it provides both a means to measure ICP and to manage ICP via drainage of CSF or blood in the case of IVH. IVC placement requires ventricular enlargement, so it is not an option for all ICH patients. In a recent series of children with IPH, 27% required a ventriculostomy (14). If an IVC cannot be placed due to size of the ventricles or other technical reasons, a subdural bolt can be placed for ICP monitoring. Brain tissue oxygen monitors can be placed to measure oxygen partial pressure, but experience using these types of monitors in pediatric ICH is limited.

Medical Management of Increased ICP

Nonsurgical methods for acutely lowering elevated ICP include keeping the head of the patient's bed at 30° to promote good cerebral venous drainage, hyperventilation to a Pco_2 of 25 to 30 mmHg, and hyperosmolar therapy to promote osmotic diuresis with either mannitol or hypertonic saline. Plasma osmoles and electrolytes must be monitored frequently when osmotic agents are used to avoid hypovolemia, hypotension, and renal failure. In some cases, sedation may be required to help manage elevated ICP. Hyperventilation and hyperosmolar therapy are generally temporizing measures. Corticosteroids should be avoided since adult randomized trials on ICH have not demonstrated efficacy (30,31). Hyperglycemia resulting from corticosteroids has been associated with worse outcome in adults (32,33). For ICH in the setting of a brain tumor, corticosteroids may be considered to limit edema surrounding the tumor.

Surgical Management of Increased ICP

Evacuation of Parenchymal Hemorrhage

While not studied in children, young adults with lobar hemorrhages with clinical deterioration due to mass effect have been reported to benefit from early surgical evacuation in a small retrospective series (34). The Surgical Trial in Intracerebral Hemorrhage (STICH) demonstrated that in adults with spontaneous supratentorial ICH, emergent surgical evacuation of hematoma within 72 hours of bleeding onset did not improve outcome beyond best medical management (35). However, few young patients were enrolled in this trial and children may require more urgent intervention to reduce ICP since they do not have cerebral atrophy that permits expansion of the hematoma. In adults, the revised 2010 guidelines for spontaneous ICH management state that patients with cerebellar hemorrhage, with clinical deterioration, with brainstem compression, or with obstructive hydrocephalus from compression of the ventricles should undergo surgical hemorrhage evacuation (20). Although this scenario has not been specifically studied in pediatric patients, children with cerebellar ICH may require evacuation to prevent herniation (36).

Hemicraniectomy

In adults, timely decompressive craniectomy may be both lifesaving and function-sparing when there is rapid deterioration in the setting of a large arterial ischemic stroke or ICH (37–39). A recent pooled analysis of the three European randomized controlled trials of hemicraniectomy for malignant middle cerebral artery (MCA) infarction demonstrated that hemicraniectomy

is a lifesaving procedure and can result in a favorable functional outcome when offered early in adults less than 60 years of age (39).

There are no formal studies of hemicraniectomy in children. In a recent case series of 10 children with malignant MCA infarction, seven underwent hemicraniectomy and all survived and had moderately good recovery (all had hemiparesis but were able to walk and had fluent speech despite left-sided infarcts) (40). The three children who died in this series did not have hemicraniectomy and died of elevated ICP. Time to surgery ranged from 18 to 291 hours, much longer than in adult studies where time to surgery was generally < 48 hours (39). The Glasgow Coma Scale score in children who survived ranged from 4 to 9 suggesting decompression may be beneficial even with deep coma. Although there is no class 1 evidence, some neurosurgeons will consider decompressive hemicraniectomy in patients with a large ICH and declining exam to reduce the likelihood of further deterioration. In a recent small series, 3 of 22 children with ICH had decompressive craniectomy, and all were functionally independent (14).

Monitoring for and Treatment of Seizures

Seizures are a common complication of stroke. Up to 20% of children with ICH will have a seizure (41). Prophylactic anticonvulsants are often used in the setting of ICH or SAH; however, the American Heart Association pediatric stroke guidelines recommend against prophylactic anticonvulsant use in ischemic stroke and do not make recommendations in ICH (22); there are no studies in children. A recent study analyzed data from the Cerebral Hematoma And NXY Treatment trial for neuroprotection in adults with ICH and found that prophylactic anticonvulsant use was associated with poor outcome. However, only 8% of study participants (n = 23) were placed on prophylactic medication (42). Similarly, in a prospective observational study of prophylactic anticonvulsant use in 98 adults with ICH, 12 (12%) received levetiracetam prophylaxis, 22 (22%) received phenytoin prophylaxis, 6 (6%) received both anticonvulsants, and 58 (59%) patients received neither anticonvulsant (43). In the seven patients with a clinical seizure, five occurred on the day of ICH. Phenytoin use was associated with a longer hospital stay and worse modified Rankin Scale at 14 days, 28 days, and 3 months. However, there was selection bias in these studies as patients with the largest ICH or who were sicker were most likely to receive prophylactic anticonvulsants.

Separate from the issue of preventing seizures with prophylactic anticonvulsants is the detection and management of convulsive or nonconvulsive seizures when seizures do occur. Continuous EEG monitoring is often utilized in the ICU but it is not of proven benefit to patients at this time. A recent study examined 100 children who had continuous EEG monitoring for a diverse array of clinical indications including some children with ICH and reported that EEG monitoring led to the initiation or escalation of antiseizure medications in 43 patients due to seizure detection (44). Many of these children had prolonged unresponsiveness after a seizure as the indication for EEG monitoring, so the application of these data to children with acute ICH is unclear. Continuous EEG monitoring should be strongly considered in children who have (1) persistently altered mental status that is not clearly explained by their ICH, or (2) movements or vital sign changes that are suggestive of seizure that cannot be captured on a routine EEG. In adult patients with SAH, EEG has been used to detect vasospasm (45) but this has not yet been studied in children.

■ DIAGNOSTIC STUDIES

If ICH or SAH is suspected, HCT is still considered the initial imaging study of choice by most authors (21). Magnetic resonance imaging (MRI) sequences such as gradient echo or susceptibility-weighted images clearly identify hemorrhage, but they are not universally available, may require sedation, show both old and new blood, and require some experience and training to correctly identify the hemorrhage (46). A child with ICH should have a thorough evaluation for vascular anomalies which account for 40% to 90% of pediatric ICH (3,13,14). Given this high rate of vascular malformations, high quality cerebrovascular imaging is critical. In one study of 116 children with hemorrhagic stroke between 1993 and 2003 only 65% had vascular imaging (47). A recent study documented vascular imaging in nearly 100% of nonneonates with IPH, perhaps leading to a higher percentage of confirmed ICH etiology (14). One study reported that a combination of MRI, magnetic resonance angiography (MRA), and magnetic resonance venography (MRV) images accurately identified the cause of ICH in 25 of 38 children (66%) (48). There were two MRIs that did not detect a vascular malformation that was in fact present: one patient had

a mycotic aneurysm, and the other had a peripherally located AVM identified on digital subtraction angiography or conventional cerebral angiography (CCA). In the same study, CCA alone had a diagnostic yield of 61% that was statistically equivalent to the yield from the combination of MRI, MRA, and MRV (48). However, in another series of children with nontraumatic ICH, the cause of bleeding was established in 97% of children who underwent CCA compared with 80% of children who did not have angiography (3). CCA can be relatively safe, although fewer than 50% of children with ICH undergo CCA (3,49,50). Even when a vascular malformation is detected on noninvasive imaging, neurosurgeons and interventional neuroradiologists might require CCA to characterize the malformation in more detail to determine the optimal management approach. CCA can also be used to administer treatment such as embolization of an AVM or coiling of an aneurysm prior to surgery. In a recent series of children who underwent surgical resection of AVM, intraoperative angiogram was useful for identifying residual lesion so that any remaining AVM could be resected prior to incision closure (51). Other methodologies including radiosurgery that are more commonly used in adults are being evaluated in children (52).

Recently, interest in CT angiography (CTA) has increased as it can be accomplished rapidly without sedation in some children. The disadvantages compared with MRI include the ionizing radiation exposure and iodinated contrast agent exposure. However, newer CTA protocols can reduce the amount of radiation to which the child is exposed. Another difficulty with CTA is the need to time the contrast bolus in a child with a small intravenous line (53). Some unsedated children move when contrast agent is injected, degrading the study. Advantages are that CTA is more widely available, and at many centers offers excellent and possibly superior visualization of vascular structures than MRA (54). Many neurosurgeons recommend that a CTA be obtained in any child in whom the initial HCT, lumbar puncture, or clinical history suggests the presence of an aneurysmal source since it can generally be performed quickly and is noninvasive. An undiagnosed ruptured aneurysm left untreated can have significant consequences for the patient including early rebleeding (55). CTA has a sensitivity of 95% and specificity of 83% in detecting aneurysms to about 2 mm in size in the adult population (56). However, CCA remains the gold standard (57). The American Heart Association guidelines for pediatric stroke state that when no cause for ICH is found via noninvasive vascular imaging, CCA should be strongly considered (22). Additionally, if an aneurysm is suggested by noninvasive imaging, a four vessel CCA should be performed to guide treatment.

Sometimes vascular malformations are not evident, even for months after the acute hemorrhage. Therefore, when vascular imaging is normal or inconclusive in the acute setting, studies should be repeated once the clot has been reabsorbed; this often takes 2 to 8 weeks. If no vascular cause of the ICH or SAH is identified at that point, additional vascular imaging may be required even later. The timing and frequency of additional studies has not been studied, so follow-up imaging is highly individualized.

Coagulation studies and other basic laboratory tests are recommended in the American Heart Association guidelines for management of ICH (20). No studies have been done to examine the yield of an extensive evaluation for a bleeding diathesis in children with ICH. Therefore, the guidelines for the evaluation and management of stroke in infants and children simply note that an evaluation for hematologic disorders, coagulation defects, and other risk factors may be appropriate (22). However, in children in whom a primary bleeding diathesis is suspected or in children in whom vascular imaging and MRI do not identify a cause of the ICH, hematology should be consulted, and a more detailed bleeding diathesis workup may be considered (58) (Table 12.2).

■ TREATMENT OF VASCULAR MALFORMATIONS

Treatments for vascular malformations include surgery, endovascular procedures, gamma knife radiosurgery, and proton beam therapy. The appropriate treatment for each patient is determined by the location and vascular anatomy of the lesion. A team of neurovascular specialists including neurology, neurosurgery, neuroradiology, interventional radiology, and radiation oncology is often needed to provide optimal care. As a generalization, vascular malformations other than aneurysm have a low acute risk of rehemorrhage although they may rehemorrhage later (59,60,61). Therefore many centers allow the hematoma to resolve prior to definitive treatment so that the full extent of the vascular malformation is evident and is not obscured by clot. However, some AVMs

---

■ Table 12.2 Laboratory Studies for Bleeding Diathesis

Initial Studies[a]

Complete blood count with platelets
Prothrombin time (PT) and international normalized ratio
Partial thromboplastin time (PTT)
Thrombin time
Fibrinogen

Advanced Studies[b]

Factor XIII (13) (deficiency does not prolong the PT and PTT)
Factor VIII (8) level
Factor IX (9) level
Von Willebrand disease (VW) studies: VW antigen, VW activity (previously ristocetin), factor VIII (8), platelet aggregation/secretion studies
Alpha-2-antiplasmin
Plasminogen activator inhibitor type 1 activity

---

[a] Should be performed as initial screen. If normal and suspicion for bleeding diathesis, consider the advanced level of testing. If any abnormalities on initial screen, proceed with additional testing based on abnormalities.
[b] Consider advanced studies in consultation with a hematologist.

---

have an aneurismal component that may cause rehemorrhage more acutely, underscoring the importance of high quality vascular images. Since aneurysms have a higher rate of acute rehemorrhage (55), aneurysm repair usually occurs in the acute setting. Recently, several groups have published their institutional case series on the surgical and endovascular treatment of children with cerebral aneurysms (62–65).

■ SPECIAL POPULATIONS

Sickle Cell Disease

Two (22,67) of three sets of pediatric stroke guidelines (22,66,67) recommend acute exchange transfusion for children with sickle cell disease (SCD) and acute arterial ischemic stroke; the goal is hemoglobin S < 30%. Ongoing chronic or periodic transfusions are also recommended by an evidence-based guideline for primary and secondary prevention of ischemic stroke (22,66,67). The American Heart Association guidelines mention that periodic transfusions have not been studied for primary or secondary prevention of ICH in children with SCD (22). There is no consensus that children with SCD and an acute hemorrhage should be treated acutely with simple or exchange transfusion (68), but management should be discussed with a pediatric hematologist in all cases. SCD can be associated with a large vessel arteriopathy that resembles moyamoya vessels which is generally located in the anterior circulation, but aneurysms can form as well, usually in the vertebrobasilar system. Therefore, children with SCD and ICH also required cerebrovascular imaging to identify possible vascular malformations (69).

Moyamoya Disease and Syndrome

Moyamoya is an arteriopathy characterized by progressive occlusion of the distal internal carotid arteries, but the posterior circulation can also be affected (22). Moyamoya disease is used when the arteriopathy is idiopathic, while moyamoya syndrome is used when the arteriopathy is secondary to an associated condition like cranial radiation or genetic syndromes like neurofibromatosis type 1 or trisomy 21 (70). Children with idiopathic moyamoya disease or moyamoya syndrome are most at risk for arterial ischemic stroke but may also present with ICH or SAH. The management of these children is not clear and must be highly individualized since lowering blood pressure in moyamoya patients who are often perfusion dependent may precipitate ischemia.

Other

Several genetic, connective tissue and rheumatologic, and systemic conditions can predispose children to ICH or SAH by causing vascular anomalies such as AVM or aneurysms or by causing vascular fragility (Table 12.3).

■ OUTCOME AFTER CHILDHOOD ICH

One study pooled data from non–population-based studies and reported an average mortality of 25% in children with ICH (71), but individual study estimates range from 7% to 54% (72). A more modern and population-based study found a case fatality rate for ICH of 5.2% (73). Several studies in children specifically addressed features that predict poor neurologic outcome after ICH. One study found that infratentorial location, Glasgow Coma Score (GCS) ≤ 7 at admission, aneurysm, age < 3 years at the time of ICH, and underlying hematologic disorder all predicted more severe

■ **Table 12.3** Rare Diseases Predisposing to Intracerebral Hemorrhage

Genetic
Autosomal dominant polycystic kidney disease (aneurysm)
Hereditary hemorrhagic telangiectasia (arteriovenous malformation [AVM], aneurysm)
Von Hippel-Lindau disease (cerebellar AVM)
Multiple cavernoma genes (CCM1, CCM2, CCM3)
Sickle cell disease

Connective tissue disorders
Fibromuscular dysplasia (aneurysm)
Ehlers-Danlos type IV (aneurysm)
Pseudoxanthoma elasticum (aneurysm)
Marfan syndrome

Rheumatologic
Takayasu arteritis (aneurysm)
Polyarteritis nodosa (aneurysm)
Behçet disease (aneurysm)
Kawasaki disease (aneurysm)
Primary central nervous system vasculitis

Other
Moyamoya disease and syndrome
Aortic coarctation (aneurysm)
Tuberculosis meningitis
Bacterial meningitis
Mycotic aneurysm

outcome (13). A recent retrospective study showed that ICH volume predicts poor outcome in children (12). This finding was confirmed in a prospective cohort, and altered mental status within 6 hours of hospital presentation was an added risk factor for short-term functional disability (14). This is consistent with adult literature that reports that larger ICH volume and GCS < 9 at the time of presentation are strong predictors of 30-day mortality (74). Bedside methods to estimate hemorrhage volume and therefore aid in clinical outcome prediction have recently been developed (75,76).

Little information exists on cognitive outcomes after ICH in children. One retrospective cohort study of 56 Dutch children < 16 years of age at onset of ICH who received care at a single medical center between 1978 and 1998 had long-term follow up (mean 10.3 years) on all 36 surviving patients; 10-year survival after ICH was 64% (77). In 31 subjects who reported for neuropsychological testing, 28 completed intelligence quotient (IQ) testing and mean full scale IQ was not below average (IQ 106, standard deviation 20) or left-shifted, but the standard deviation was large, indicating a range of IQs. Furthermore, 15 of 31 patients (48%) had signs of cognitive deficits when their performance was compared to their premorbid academic abilities or to those of their parents. Moderate to severe cognitive deficits were present in seven patients (23%).

■ RECURRENT ICH

Few studies comment on the incidence of rehemorrhage. In one retrospective cohort from Switzerland comprised of 34 children presenting between 1990 and 2000, recurrent ICH occurred in three children (9%) (13). All three recurrences occurred within the first year after the incident ICH and were in children with unknown cause of hemorrhage (one subject) or in children with unrepaired vascular anomalies (two subjects). In a population-based cohort of 116 children in Northern California presenting between January 1993 to December 2004, 11 (9.5%) had recurrent ICH (73). The recurrences occurred at a median of 3.1 months from the incident hemorrhage. Over 60% occurred within 6 months and over 90% occurred within 3 years. Of the children with recurrent ICH, none had idiopathic ICH and nine had vascular anomalies, six of which were never treated. The two children with medical etiologies of ICH recurred within 1 week of the incident hemorrhage. Therefore, children with an ICH must be discharged with clear follow-up plans so that appropriate decisions can be made for treatment of vascular anomalies and for follow-up of children with anomalies that are treated during the initial hospitalization.

As discussed above, aneurysmal hemorrhage carries an increased risk of rebleed immediately after a hemorrhage and therefore should be treated with prompt surgical and/or endovascular treatment. In adults, 4% of patients rebleed on day 1, and the highest risk occurs in the first 6 hours (55,78). In the first 2 weeks after the initial bleed, 15% to 20% of adult patients have rebleeding, and 50% have rebleeding within 6 months (55).

■ ARTERIAL ISCHEMIC STROKE AFTER ICH

In the population-based California cohort of pediatric ICH, four children (3.4%) had subsequent ischemic stroke, of which three occurred in the acute period (73). Arterial ischemic stroke after ICH can occur due to vasospasm after SAH, vasculopathy that predisposes to hemorrhage or ischemia like moyamoya vessels, mechanical compression of arteries from mass effect from the hemorrhage, or rarely as a complication of catheter angiogram. If an arterial ischemic stroke should occur its treatment depends on timing in relation to the ICH and to the severity and cause of the ICH. Multidisciplinary discussion and management are often required since the opposing processes of hemorrhage and ischemia are challenging.

The incidence of angiographic vasospasm in pediatric patients with aneurysmal SAH can be high, but it is not known if angiographic vasospasm is always clinically significant since some patients do not have clinical signs or symptoms (6,8,64,65,79–81). However, since the possibility exists for significant clinical decline associated with vasospasm and subsequent ischemia, it is important to monitor aneurysmal SAH patients for vasospasm. Hypovolemia should be avoided (82). In adults, oral nimodipine has been found to improve outcome after SAH (83), although the mechanism may not be through reduction of vasospasm and may rather be through neuroprotection via decreased calcium-induced excitotoxicity (82). Although the medication has not been specifically studied in pediatric aneurysmal SAH, pediatric patients are often placed on nimodipine as is done in adult ICUs. If a patient is unable to be given parenteral nimodipine, a low-dose intravenous calcium channel blocker such as nicardipine can be administered although adult data have not demonstrated that intravenous calcium channel antagonists statistically improve outcome (82,84). In pediatric patients, monitoring for vasospasm is typically performed with serial transcranial Doppler ultrasound, CTA with CT perfusion, and occasionally CCA. When detected and clinically significant, vasospasm is then treated with induced moderate hypertension, or when severe with angiographic techniques such as direct infusion of arterial dilating medications or balloon angioplasty of the affected vessel.

■ CONCLUSIONS

ICH and SAH are important causes of neurologic morbidity and mortality in the pediatric population. Optimal care of the patient requires collaboration among intensivists, neurologists, neurosurgeons, interventional neuroradiologists, and hematologists. Evidence-based monitoring and management of the pediatric ICH and SAH patients requires additional study and research.

■ REFERENCES

1. Fullerton HJ et al. Risk of stroke in children: ethnic and gender disparities. *Neurology.* 2003;61:189–194.
2. Giroud M et al. Cerebrovascular disease in children under 16 years of age in the city of dijon, france: a study of incidence and clinical features from 1985 to 1993. *J Clin Epidemiol.* 1995;48:1343–1348.
3. Al-Jarallah A et al. Nontraumatic brain hemorrhage in children: etiology and presentation. *J Child Neurol.* 2000;15: 284–289.
4. Broderick J et al. Stroke in children within a major metropolitan area: the surprising importance of intracerebral hemorrhage. *J Child Neurol.* 1993;8:250–255.
5. Dell S. Asymptomatic cerebral aneurysm: assessment of its risk of rupture. *Neurosurgery.* 1982;10:162–166.
6. Meyer FB et al. Cerebral aneurysms in childhood and adolescence. *J Neurosurg.* 1989;70:420–425.
7. Gerosa M et al. Intracranial aneurysms of childhood. *Childs Brain.* 1980;6:295–302.
8. Ostergaard JR, Voldby B. Intracranial arterial aneurysms in children and adolescents. *J Neurosurg.* 1983;58:832–837.
9. Roche JL et al. Intracranial arterial aneurysm in children. A cooperative study. Apropos of 43 cases. *Neuro-Chirurgie.* 1988;34:243–251.
10. Patel AN, Richardson AE. Ruptured intracranial aneurysms in the first two decades of life. A study of 58 patients. *J Neurosurg.* 1971;35:571–576.
11. Sedzimir CB, Robinson J. Intracranial hemorrhage in children and adolescents. *J Neurosurg.* 1973;38:269–281.
12. Jordan LC, Kleinman JT, Hillis AE. Intracerebral hemorrhage volume predicts poor neurologic outcome in children. *Stroke.* 2009;40:1666–1671.
13. Meyer-Heim AD, Boltshauser E. Spontaneous intracranial haemorrhage in children: aetiology, presentation and outcome. *Brain Dev.* 2003;25:416–421.
14. Beslow LA et al. Predictors of outcome in childhood intracerebral hemorrhage: a prospective consecutive cohort study. *Stroke.* 41:313–318.
15. Adams HP Jr. et al. Ct and clinical correlations in recent aneurysmal subarachnoid hemorrhage: a preliminary report of the cooperative aneurysm study. *Neurology.* 1983;33: 981–988.
16. van der Wee N et al. Detection of subarachnoid haemorrhage on early CT: is lumbar puncture still needed after a negative scan? *J Neurol Neurosurg Psychiatry.* 1995;58:357–359.
17. Boesiger BM, Shiber JR. Subarachnoid hemorrhage diagnosis by computed tomography and lumbar puncture: are fifth generation CT scanners better at identifying subarachnoid hemorrhage? *J Emerg Med.* 2005;29:23–27.
18. National guidelines for analysis of cerebrospinal fluid for bilirubin in suspected subarachnoid haemorrhage. *Ann Clin Biochem.* 2003;40:481–488.
19. Griffiths MJ, Ford C, Gama R. Revised national guidelines for the analysis of cerebrospinal fluid for bilirubin in

suspected subarachnoid haemorrhage: Interpret with caution. *J Clin Pathol.* 2009;62:1052.
20. Morgenstern LB et al. Guidelines for the management of spontaneous intracerebral hemorrhage: a guideline for healthcare professionals from the American Heart Association/American Stroke Association. *Stroke.* 41:2108–2129.
21. Broderick J et al. Guidelines for the management of spontaneous intracerebral hemorrhage in adults: 2007 update: a guideline from the American Heart Association/American Stroke Association Stroke Council, High Blood Pressure Research Council, and the Quality of Care and Outcomes in Research Interdisciplinary Working Group. *Stroke.* 2007; 38:2001–2023.
22. Roach ES et al. Management of stroke in infants and children: a scientific statement from a special writing group of the American Heart Association Stroke Council and the Council on Cardiovascular Disease in the Young. *Stroke.* 2008;39:2644–2691.
23. Schwarz S et al. Incidence and prognostic significance of fever following intracerebral hemorrhage. *Neurology.* 2000;54:354–361.
24. Anderson CS et al. Intensive blood pressure reduction in acute cerebral haemorrhage trial (interact): a randomised pilot trial. *Lancet Neurol.* 2008;7:391–399.
25. Lee CA, Berntorp EE, Hoots WK. *Textbook of Hemophilia;* 2010.
26. Ljung RC. Intracranial haemorrhage in haemophilia A and B. *Br J Haematol.* 2008;140:378–384.
27. Brady KM, Easley RB, Tobias JD. Recombinant activated factor VII (RFVIIA) treatment in infants with hemorrhage. *Paediatr Anaesth.* 2006;16:1042–1046.
28. Yuan ZH et al. A meta-analysis of the efficacy and safety of recombinant activated factor VII for patients with acute intracerebral hemorrhage without hemophilia. *J Clin Neurosci.* 17:685–693.
29. Imberti D et al. Emergency reversal of anticoagulation with a three-factor prothrombin complex concentrate in patients with intracranial haemorrhage. *Blood Transfus.* 2011;9(2):148–155.
30. Poungvarin N et al. Effects of dexamethasone in primary supratentorial intracerebral hemorrhage. *N Engl J Med.* 1987; 316:1229–1233.
31. Tellez H, Bauer RB. Dexamethasone as treatment in cerebrovascular disease. 1. A controlled study in intracerebral hemorrhage. *Stroke.* 1973;4:541–546.
32. Passero S, Ciacci G, Ulivelli M. The influence of diabetes and hyperglycemia on clinical course after intracerebral hemorrhage. *Neurology.* 2003;61:1351–1356.
33. Weir CJ et al. Is hyperglycaemia an independent predictor of poor outcome after acute stroke? Results of a long-term follow up study. *BMJ.* 1997;314:1303–1306.
34. Rabinstein AA, Atkinson JL, Wijdicks EF. Emergency craniotomy in patients worsening due to expanded cerebral hematoma: to what purpose? *Neurology.* 2002;58:1367–1372.
35. Mendelow AD et al. Early surgery versus initial conservative treatment in patients with spontaneous supratentorial intracerebral haematomas in the international surgical trial in intracerebral haemorrhage (stich): a randomised trial. *Lancet.* 2005;365:387–397.
36. Kumar R, Shukla D, Mahapatra AK. Spontaneous intracranial hemorrhage in children. *Pediatr Neurosurg.* 2009;45: 37–45.

37. Robertson SC et al. Clinical course and surgical management of massive cerebral infarction. *Neurosurgery.* 2004;55:55–61; discussion 61–52.

38. Ruf B et al. Early decompressive craniectomy and duraplasty for refractory intracranial hypertension in children: results of a pilot study. *Crit Care.* 2003;7:R133–R138.

39. Vahedi K et al. Early decompressive surgery in malignant infarction of the middle cerebral artery: a pooled analysis of three randomised controlled trials. *Lancet Neurol.* 2007;6:215–222.

40. Smith SE et al. Outcome following decompressive craniectomy for malignant middle cerebral artery infarction in children. *Dev Med Child Neurol.* 2011;53:29–33.

41. Jordan LC, Hillis AE. Hemorrhagic stroke in children. *Pediatr Neurol.* 2007;36:73–80.

42. Messe SR et al. Prophylactic antiepileptic drug use is associated with poor outcome following ich. *Neurocrit Care.* 2009;11:38–44.

43. Naidech AM et al. Anticonvulsant use and outcomes after intracerebral hemorrhage. *Stroke.* 2009;40:3810–3815.

44. Abend NS et al. Impact of continuous eeg monitoring on clinical management in critically ill children. *Neurocrit Care.* 2011;15(1):70–75.

45. Claassen J et al. Quantitative continuous eeg for detecting delayed cerebral ischemia in patients with poor-grade subarachnoid hemorrhage. *Clin Neurophysiol.* 2004;115:2699–2710.

46. Kidwell CS et al. Comparison of MRI and CT for detection of acute intracerebral hemorrhage. *JAMA.* 2004;292:1823–1830.

47. Jordan LC et al. The importance of cerebral aneurysms in childhood hemorrhagic stroke: a population-based study. *Stroke.* 2009;40:400–405.

48. Liu AC et al. Is there a role for magnetic resonance imaging in the evaluation of non-traumatic intraparenchymal haemorrhage in children? *Pediatr Radiol.* 2006;36:940–946.

49. Burger IM et al. Safety of cerebral digital subtraction angiography in children: complication rate analysis in 241 consecutive diagnostic angiograms. *Stroke.* 2006;37:2535–2539.

50. Lin CL et al. Spontaneous intracerebral hemorrhage in children. *Kaohsiung J Med Sci.* 1999;15:146–151.

51. Lang S et al. Follow-up imaging to detect recurrence of surgically treated pediatric arteriovenous malformations. *J Neurosurg Pediatr.* 2012;9(5):497–504.

52. Zadeh G et al. Pediatric arteriovenous malformation: University of toronto experience using stereotactic radiosurgery. *Childs Nerv Syst.* 2007;23:195–199.

53. Bowen BC. Mr angiography versus ct angiography in the evaluation of neurovascular disease. *Radiology.* 2007;245: 357–360; discussion 360–351.

54. Truwit CL. Ct angiography versus mr angiography in the evaluation of acute neurovascular disease. *Radiology.* 2007; 245:362–366; discussion 366.

55. Winn HR, Richardson AE, Jane JA. The long-term prognosis in untreated cerebral aneurysms: I. The incidence of late hemorrhage in cerebral aneurysm: a 10-year evaluation of 364 patients. *Annals of Neurology.* 1977;1:358–370.

56. Hsiang JN et al. The role of computed tomographic angiography in the diagnosis of intracranial aneurysms and emergent aneurysm clipping. *Neurosurgery.* 1996;38:481–487; discussion 487.

57. Chappell ET, Moure FC, Good MC. Comparison of computed tomographic angiography with digital subtraction angiography in the diagnosis of cerebral aneurysms: a meta-analysis. *Neurosurgery.* 2003;52:624–631; discussion 630–621.

58. Khair K, Liesner R. Bruising and bleeding in infants and children—a practical approach. *Br J Haematol.* 2006;133: 221–231.

59. Kondziolka D, McLaughlin MR, Kestle JR. Simple risk predictions for arteriovenous malformation hemorrhage. *Neurosurgery.* 1995;37:851–855.

60. Graf CJ, Perret GE, Torner JC. Bleeding from cerebral arteriovenous malformations as part of their natural history. *J Neurosurg.* 1983;58:331–337.

61. Ondra SL et al. The natural history of symptomatic arteriovenous malformations of the brain: a 24-year follow-up assessment. *J Neurosurg.* 1990;73:387–391.

62. Agid R et al. The role of endovascular treatment for pediatric aneurysms. *Childs Nerv Syst.* 2005;21:1030–1036.

63. Sanai N et al. Pediatric intracranial aneurysms: durability of treatment following microsurgical and endovascular management. [See comment]. *J Neurosurg.* 2006;104:82–89.

64. Stiefel MF et al. Endovascular and surgical treatment of ruptured cerebral aneurysms in pediatric patients. *Neurosurgery.* 2008;63:859-865; discussion 865–856.

65. Huang J et al. Intracranial aneurysms in the pediatric population: case series and literature review. *Surg Neurol.* 2005;63:424-432; discussion 432–423.

66. Monagle P et al. Antithrombotic therapy in neonates and children: antithrombotic therapy and prevention of thrombosis: American College of Chest Physicians evidence-based clinical practice guidelines (9th edition). *Chest.* 2012;141(2 Suppl):e737S-801S.

67. Paediatric SWG. *Stroke in Childhood: Clinical Guidelines for Diagnosis, Management and Rehabilitation.* November 2004. http://bookshop.rcplondon.ac.uk/contents/f98c6540-a541-4bed-837d-ef293ac458bf.pdf. Accessed: September 10, 2012.

68. Strouse JJ et al. Primary hemorrhagic stroke in children with sickle cell disease is associated with recent transfusion and use of corticosteroids. *Pediatrics.* 2006;118:1916–1924.

69. Preul MC et al. Intracranial aneurysms and sickle cell anemia: multiplicity and propensity for the vertebrobasilar territory. *Neurosurgery.* 1998;42:971–977; discussion 977-978.

70. Scott RM, Smith ER. Moyamoya disease and moyamoya syndrome. *N Engl J Med.* 2009;360:1226–1237.

71. Lynch JK, Han CJ. Pediatric stroke: what do we know and what do we need to know? *Semin Neurol.* 2005;25:410–423.

72. Livingston JH, Brown JK. Intracerebral haemorrhage after the neonatal period. *Arch Dis Child.* 1986;61:538–544.

73. Fullerton HJ et al. Recurrent hemorrhagic stroke in children: a population-based cohort study. *Stroke.* 2007;38:2658–2662.

74. Broderick JP et al. Volume of intracerebral hemorrhage. A powerful and easy-to-use predictor of 30-day mortality. *Stroke.* 1993;24:987–993.

75. Beslow LA et al. ABC/XYZ estimates intracerebral hemorrhage volume as a percent of total brain volume in children. *Stroke.* 41:691–694.

76. Kleinman JT, Hillis AE, Jordan LC. Abc/2: Estimating intracerebral haemorrhage volume and total brain volume, and predicting outcome in children. *Dev Med Child Neurol.* 2011;53(3):281–284.

77. Blom I et al. Prognosis of haemorrhagic stroke in childhood: a long-term follow-up study. *Dev Med Child Neurol.* 2003;45:233–239.

78. Inagawa T et al. Rebleeding of ruptured intracranial aneurysms in the acute stage. *Surg Neurol.* 1987;28:93-99.

79. Heiskanen O, Vilkki J. Intracranial arterial aneurysms in children and adolescents. *Acta Neurochir (Wien).* 1981;59:55–63.

80. Proust F et al. Pediatric cerebral aneurysms. *J Neurosurg.* 2001;94:733–739.

81. Pasqualin AM et al. Intracranial aneurysms and subarachnoid hemorrhage in children and adolescents. *Childs Nerv Syst.* 1986;2:185–190.

82. Bederson JB et al. Guidelines for the management of aneurysmal subarachnoid hemorrhage: a statement for healthcare professionals from a special writing group of the Stroke Council, American Heart association. *Stroke.* 2009;40:994–1025.

83. Barker FG, 2nd, Ogilvy CS. Efficacy of prophylactic nimodipine for delayed ischemic deficit after subarachnoid hemorrhage: a metaanalysis. *J Neurosurg.* 1996;84:405–414.

84. Dorhout Mees SM et al. Calcium antagonists for aneurysmal subarachnoid haemorrhage. *Cochrane Database Syst Rev.* 2007:CD000277.

13 Diagnosis and Endovascular Management of Cerebrovascular Malformations

BRYAN PUKENAS and ROBERT HURST

■ INTRODUCTION

Congenital cerebrovascular malformations are an uncommon but important group of intracranial lesions in the pediatric population. Congenital cerebrovascular malformations are generally divided into four major categories: arteriovenous malformations (AVMs), cavernous malformations, venous angiomas, and telangiectasias. Although quite rare in the general population, an additional congenital cerebrovascular lesion, the aneurysmal malformation of the vein of Galen (AMVG), is of considerable importance in the pediatric population, particularly in the youngest age groups.

Differences in angioarchitecture and hemodynamic flow differentiate the various types of cerebrovascular malformations. These differences also accentuate the imaging characteristics and dictate clinical behavior of the various lesions. At the present time, only those lesions characterized by arteriovenous shunting, including the AVM and AMVG, are amenable to endovascular treatment.

■ ARTERIOVENOUS MALFORMATIONS

Epidemiology

AVMs are the most common clinically symptomatic type of cerebrovascular malformation. They represent approximately 10% of all cerebrovascular malformations in the general population and have a prevalence of approximately 15 /100,000 (1). Hemorrhage related to an AVM most commonly occurs in the third and fourth decades (2). The annual risk of hemorrhage from an AVM is 2.4% (3) and the annual risk of death is 1% with a 10% mortality rate associated with the first hemorrhage (4). The rebleeding rate among survivors approaches 6% in the first year and is approximately 2% to 3% per year after that (4).

Morphology

AVMs have a characteristic angioarchitecture that consists of three components: feeding arteries, the nidus, and the draining venous system. Feeding arteries to an AVM are often enlarged and tortuous as a result of high flow through the vessels. The *nidus* consists of a group of histologically abnormal vessels that replaces the normal capillary bed and is the site of arteriovenous shunting. The nidus allows high pressure, high flow blood to shunt directly into the draining venous system. The venous system draining the AVM is frequently enlarged, reflecting the increased pressure and flow through the nidus.

Clinical

Intracranial hemorrhage, the most common clinical presentation of AVM, most commonly occurs in the second through fourth decades of life and is the presentation in up to 40% to 50% of all AVMs (5–6). AVM is the most common cause of nontraumatic intracranial hemorrhage in teenagers (6). Less commonly, AVMs may present with seizures or nonhemorrhagic neurologic deficits as a result of a number of potential mechanisms including mass effect, venous hypertension, or hydrocephalus.

Headache is also a frequent symptom leading to the diagnosis of AVM (7–8).

A number of features of AVMs have been evaluated to predict risk of future hemorrhage. These include patient related features, such as presentation with hemorrhage, patient age (3), drug use (9–10), and hypertension (11). A number of features of the AVM itself have also been related to future hemorrhage risk. These include location of the AVM, specifically an infratentorial location (11); size of the nidus (3); drainage into the deep or superficial venous system (12); single versus multiple venous drainage (13); feeding pedicle aneurysms (14); venous stenosis or focal enlargement; and associated features including aneurysms (12).

Imaging

Imaging evaluation of AVM is aimed at obtaining all necessary information to successfully plan and carry out therapy. A major feature of importance includes

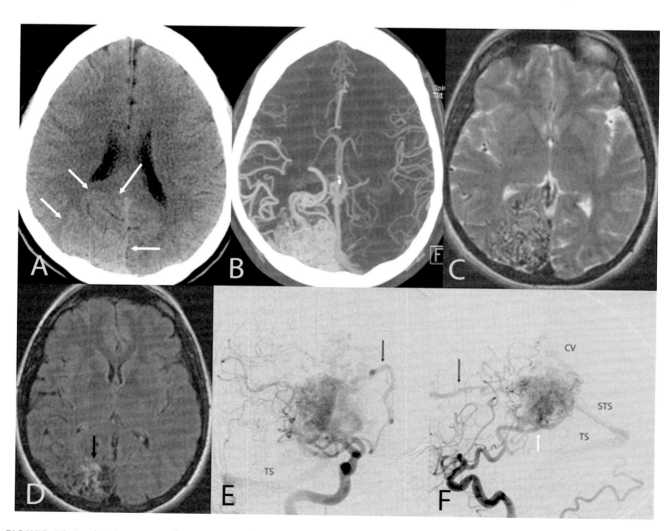

FIGURE 13.1 Arteriovenous malformation—axial unenhanced computed tomography (CT) (A), axial MIP CT angiography (CTA) (B), axial T2-weighted magnetic resonance imaging (MRI) (C), axial fluid-attenuated inversion recovery (FLAIR) MRI (D). Frontal oblique (E) and oblique lateral (F) angiograms (different patient). (A) Hyperdense area in the right occipital lobe is present (white arrows). (B) CTA demonstrating serpentine enhancing vessels supplying a large nidus. (C) Dilated feeding arteries and nidus appear as flow voids on the T2-weighted image. (D) Areas of increased signal within the nidus on FLAIR imaging, likely representing injury or gliosis (black arrow). (E) and (F) Enlarged right posterior cerebral (white arrow) and pericallosal (black arrow) arteries supplying a right medial temporoparietal nidus. There is rapid shunting into the straight (STS) and transverse sinus (TS) and superficially draining cortical vein (CV).

identification of the feeding arteries, specifically, to determine whether arteries solely provide supply to the AVM or also supply normal brain parenchyma. Evidence of AVM associated hemorrhage is also important to evaluate (15). This must include a determination of whether the hemorrhage is of recent or remote origin (16) and the relationship of the hemorrhage to the AVM components. The location and the size of the nidus also has significant implications for treatment (17). The venous drainage of the AVM must also be completely evaluated, including whether venous drainage is superficial or deep (17) and determining whether venous outflow restriction or mass effect exists (18–19). The brain parenchyma should also be evaluated to determine whether AVM related damage or evidence of prior treatment is present (20). Associated vascular lesions such as aneurysms and venous stenosis should also be sought. Multiple intracranial AVMs are extremely uncommon (21) but if present, the possibility of underlying conditions, including hereditary hemorrhagic telangiectasia, should be considered (22).

Selection of imaging modalities is extremely important, as each modality provides unique information regarding different features of the AVM (Figure 13.1). Generally AVMs are depicted on computed tomography (CT) as mildly hyperdense structures with minimal mass effect. CT should always be the first imaging study in patients with suspected intracranial hemorrhage as acute intracranial hemorrhage, including subarachnoid hemorrhage, is detected with very high reliability (23). Evaluation of brain parenchyma is also necessary to identify AVM associated injury (24) and hydrocephalus, if present, should also be identified. Calcification of AVM related structures also occurs with significant frequency and is readily detected with CT (25–26).

CT angiography (CTA) often provides valuable information regarding intracranial AVMs and exceeds CT in its ability to diagnose small AVMs (27–28). Feeding arteries, particularly if large, can be identified with considerable precision. In addition, the nidus, draining veins, and surrounding structures are well seen (29). Also, associated lesions including aneurysms are often well-characterized on CTA. The use of 4-dimensional CTA may become an important adjuvant for diagnosis of AVM (30). CTA is however limited in its ability to identify or characterize small aneurysms (less than 5 mm) or intranidal aneurysms (31).

Magnetic resonance imaging (MRI) and angiography (MRA) are most often the best screening techniques (32). Both are excellent for evaluating high flow structures

including the feeding arteries, nidus, and draining veins of the AVMs (33). Evidence of arteriovenous shunting is always present in AVMs and may not be optimally evaluated on static imaging modalities such as CT and MRI, but is easily identified with digital subtraction angiography (DSA). The characteristic MRI appearance of AVMs consists of groups of signal voids representing the high flow components of the lesion. Hemorrhage, with the exception of acute subarachnoid hemorrhage, is usually well evaluated on MRI. MRI also provides evaluation of the brain parenchyma for assessment of perilesional edema, gliosis, or infarction which may be associated with the AVM (34). Lastly, hydrocephalus is well evaluated on MRI.

Advanced MRI techniques including functional MRI and diffusion tract imaging have seen an increasing role in pretreatment evaluation of AVMs to determine the tracts (35–37). In addition, the use of arterial spin labeling has in some cases been able to demonstrate the temporal component of arteriovenous shunting necessary to confirm the diagnosis of AVM (38).

DSA remains necessary for complete evaluation of all AVMs. DSA gives the best depiction of arteriovenous shunting through the lesion, thereby confirming the diagnosis of AVM and permitting differentiation from other types of cerebrovascular malformations. In addition, DSA provides most accurate delineation of arterial supply, morphology of the nidus, and evaluation of the venous drainage. DSA is also excellent for identifying aneurysms associated with AVMs (39).

Evaluation of all arterial feeders to the lesion is necessary for complete characterization. This includes injecting all arterial circulations potentially providing contribution to the AVM and may include external carotid as well as internal carotid arteries and the vertebrobasilar system. Arteriovenous shunting with excessively rapid delivery of contrast into the venous system is essential to make a diagnosis of AVM. Consequently, immediate filling of the nidus and venous drainage is characteristic. Appropriate oblique views are necessary to determine the morphology of the nidus and its relationship to intracranial structures. An evaluation of drainage into the superficial and/or deep venous system is also necessary to fully characterize the lesion (40).

Management

Management options for AVMs include observation, surgical resection, radiosurgery, embolization, and combinations of the three latter techniques (41–42). The poorly characterized natural history of AVMs often makes management decisions difficult. At present, evidence from randomized trials comparing different treatments for brain AVMs which might guide the interventional treatment of brain AVMs is lacking (43). Currently an ongoing randomized controlled trial, A Randomized trial of Unruptured Brain Arteriovenous malformations (ARUBA), is comparing interventional treatment versus medical management for brain AVMs that have never bled (44).

Surgical Resection

For many years, surgical treatment was the only effective intervention for AVMs and remains the mainstay of treatment in many cases. The goal of surgical resection is the complete removal of the AVM, which probably reduces the risk of death, hemorrhage, and epilepsy (43). Surgical decision making is aided by various grading systems, the most widely utilized being the Spetzler-Martin grading system.

The Spetzler-Martin grading system is designed to determine the risk of surgery for AVM resection. The system evaluates three features of the AVM and assigns a score to each feature. The numerical value of each feature is added together to determine the surgical grade of the AVM. Features evaluated to grade an AVM using this system include the size of the nidus, whether or not there is drainage into the deep venous system, and whether or not eloquent brain is involved by the AVM. Eloquent brain is defined as primary sensorimotor, language, visual cortex, hypothalamus and thalamus, internal capsule, brainstem, cerebellar peduncles, and the deep cerebellar nuclei (17).

A number of studies have been published relating the estimated mortality and morbidity associated with surgical resection to the grade of the AVM (45–46). However, significant surgical issues remain unaddressed by grading systems. These include the timing of surgery and the combination of surgery with other AVM intervention techniques including radiosurgery and embolization (47–50). The vast majority of AVM resections are performed on an elective basis. This is almost always the case in nonhemorrhagic presentations. In addition, most authors advocate elective resection of AVMs following hemorrhage, usually weeks after a hemorrhage has occurred. Delayed resection permits liquification of acute clot, with formation of a discrete cavity in the region of prior hemorrhage, often minimizing brain retraction and

aiding resection. Nevertheless, early surgery may be required in patients with large hematomas to relieve mass effect and minimize progression of neurologic damage. The goal of early surgery may be complete resection of AVM and hematoma or may be restricted to removal of the acute hematoma.

Radiosurgery

Three radiosurgical techniques are commonly in use for treatment of AVMs. These include the Gamma knife (51), linear accelerator (52), and particle beam therapy (53). All three techniques deliver multiple radiation beams, consisting of gamma rays, high-energy photons, and charged particles respectively. The beams are targeted to converge on an isocenter, which is confined to the nidus of the AVM, thereby delivering a relatively high dose to that region with minimal dose to normal surrounding structures. The high isocenter dose damages the nidus vessels with subsequent smooth muscle proliferation, fibrosis, and obliteration of the nidus (54). Development of these changes requires a 2 to 5 year latent period for full effect. During the latent period, hemorrhage risk persists.

Obliteration rates following radiosurgical treatment are highly dependent on the size of the nidus treated and location (55). Radiosurgery obliterates 65% to 85% of AVMs under 3 centimeters and is best for treating AVMs with small, compact nidi (56). Lower obliteration rates are the rule for lesions exceeding 3 centimeters in diameter, limiting the use of radiosurgery for the treatment of large AVMs (57).

Embolization of AVMs

Embolization of AVMs involves selective endovascular catheterization of arterial feeders to the AVM with injection of embolic material into the nidus. The technique is designed to obstruct or obliterate flow within the vessels comprising the nidus and is generally performed to reduce the size and flow through the nidus prior to surgical resection or radiosurgical therapy, thereby making treatment safer or extending treatment options to lesions otherwise not amenable to therapy. It may also be performed to palliate or reverse progressive symptoms (58) or to selectively obliterate high risk features associated with the AVM (40).

In approximately 5% to 10% of cases, embolization alone may result in complete obliteration of an AVM.

The situation usually occurs in a setting of one or two direct feeders to a relatively small AVM (59). However, with the use of newer microcatheters, angiographic obliteration of the nidus after embolization may occur in up to 55% of cases (60).

Embolic materials utilized for AVM embolization include polyvinyl alcohol particles (PVAs) (61) and liquid embolic agents, including *n*-butyl cyanoacrylate (*n*-BCA) and Onyx (62). The liquid agents are most commonly used, and have the advantage of more permanent obliteration of the embolized components of the AVM. In addition, one study found a significantly higher rate of postembolization hemorrhage in patients embolized using PVA compared with *n*-BCA (63).

Complications of neuroendovascular AVM treatment consist primarily of ischemic and hemorrhagic events. Reported complication rates vary considerably, ranging from 4% to 14% for morbidity and 1% to 4% for mortality, likely reflecting differences in patient selection, embolization technique, and operator experience (64–65).

■ CAVERNOUS MALFORMATION

Epidemiology

Cavernous malformations represent from 5% to 15% of cerebrovascular malformations (66–68) with approximately one-fourth of cavernous malformations occurring in the pediatric population (69–70). Associated with an adjacent developmental venous anomaly (DVA) approximately 25% of the time (see below), cavernous malformations affect males and females with equal frequency, and are believed to have a prevalence of 0.02% to 0.9% in the general population (66,71–73). The incidence may be higher, however, as the increasing use of MRI has resulted in increased detection of asymptomatic lesions, with at least 40% detected incidentally in one study (68). Cavernous malformations may be single or multiple with multiplicity seen in up to 25% of sporadic cases. However, multiplicity also suggests a familial trait as 6% to 50% are associated with familial clustering with a higher prevalence noted in Mexican Americans (72,74). For unknown reasons, children with cavernous malformations tend to present in a bimodal pattern, at ages 0 to 2, and 13 to 16 years of age (75).

Morphology

Pathologically, cavernous malformations consist of unencapsulated collections of thin-walled sinusoidal channels separated by a collagenous stroma without mature vascular wall components (72). No normal brain parenchyma is found within cavernous malformations. Exceedingly slow blood flow and various stages of clot formation are found within the channels. Considerable fibrosis and collagen is present within the vessel walls and calcification may be present. Cavernous malformations are characterized by a complete rim of iron storage products surrounding the lesions and exert minimal mass effect in the absence of acute hemorrhage.

Cavernous malformations typically occur in subcortical locations of the cerebral hemispheres. The temporal and frontal lobes are most commonly involved, with approximately 10% of the lesions involving deep central regions of the brain. An infratentorial location is identified in approximately 20% of the lesions, with the majority of these affecting the brain stem, most commonly the pons. The spinal cord may be involved in up to 5% of cases and the lesions rarely may affect the third ventricle or be found extra axially.

Clinical

Cavernous malformations are most commonly asymptomatic, causing symptoms in approximately 15% of patients. When symptoms are present, they depend on the size and location of the lesion (76). Twenty-three percent to 79% of symptomatic supratentorial lesions give rise to seizures (74). Compared to other parenchymal lesions of similar volume and location, cavernous malformations are twice as likely to present with seizures (72). Focal neurologic deficits or gait ataxia are common presenting symptoms in patients with infratentorial lesions (74) and brain stem cavernous malformations may give rise to truncal ataxia, facial nerve paresis, dysphagia, diplopia, arm or leg weakness, numbness, dizziness, nausea, vomiting, or hiccups (77). Approximately half of symptomatic cases present with nonhemorrhagic neurologic deficits, and most patients present with multiple neurologic deficits (78). Hemorrhage is much less common when compared to AVMs, and is the presenting symptom in approximately 20% of cases, although some have reported a higher incidence of hemorrhage in the pediatric population (79–80).

Imaging

Cavernous malformations demonstrate characteristic features on MRI which most often permit confident noninvasive diagnosis (Figure 13.2). T2-weighted and gradient echo images demonstrate a complete rim of hypointense signal secondary to iron storage products (81–82). The central portion of the lesion is characterized by heterogeneous intensity, reflecting various stages of blood products. Minimal mass effect is present and no evidence of edema except in the setting of acute hemorrhage (83). Gradient echo images are most sensitive for detection of cavernous malformations and should be performed in every case as they can often identify lesions not appreciated on other sequences (84). Similar but less conspicuous features are identified on T1-weighted images (83). Minimal or no enhancement is present (85–86).

CT is much less sensitive than MRI in the detection of cavernous malformations. CT findings include areas of hyperdensity and occasional calcification (82). Mass effect and edema are most often absent on CT in the absence of hemorrhage (87).

Angiographic evaluation is rarely indicated in the evaluation of cavernous malformation. The study is generally performed to exclude an AVM in the setting of acute hemorrhage. The extremely slow flow through cavernous malformations accounts for them being angiographically occult.

Management

There is no role for endovascular management and cavernous malformations. Treatment, if indicated, is generally surgical resection.

■ DEVELOPMENTAL VENOUS ANOMALIES

Epidemiology

DVAs, also known as venous angiomas, are the most commonly identified incidental cerebrovascular malformation, with a prevalence of approximately 2% (88). They are believed to represent approximately 60% of cerebrovascular malformations detected at autopsy (89).

Morphology

DVAs represent anatomic variants of physiologically normal venous architecture. They consist of multiple dilated thin-walled vessels diffusely distributed in the normal white matter (90) that drain into an enlarged central trunk (91). The central trunk, in turn, drains into either the superficial or less often, into the deep venous system. DVAs occur in the subcortical white matter of the cerebrum, most often the frontal and parietal lobes (91).

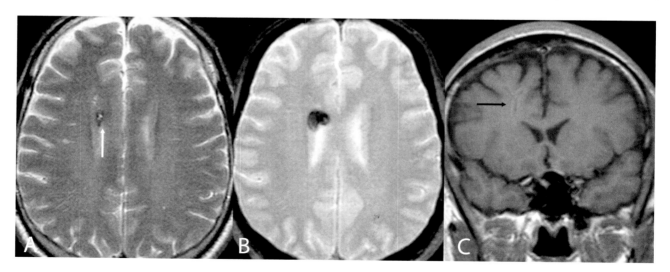

FIGURE 13.2 Cavernoma—axial T2-weighted (A), axial T2* gradient echo (B), and axial T1-weighted (C) images demonstrating a right frontal cavernoma with central heterogeneous signal completely surrounded by a hypointense rim (white arrow). Susceptibility artifact ("blooming") is present on the T2* gradient echo images. Post contrast coronal T1-weighted images demonstrate no enhancement. Notice the vertically oriented flow void characteristic of an associated developmental venous anomaly.

From 14% to 29% are located in the cerebellum (92). They are less often found in the basal ganglia (93) or brainstem (94). DVAs provide venous drainage to normal brain parenchyma within their distribution.

Imaging

DVAs have a characteristic MRI appearance, best evaluated on gadolinium enhanced T1-weighted images, as the dilated medullary venous system and enlarged central trunk are well seen (95). T2-weighted images may demonstrate small areas of the signal abnormality and signal void within the dilated central trunk secondary to flow related signal loss (96). No mass effect or edema is present (Figure 13.2C).

Angiographic evaluation of DVAs is rarely indicated. When MRI cannot differentiate DVA from AVM, angiography may be used to exclude AVM. Angiography shows filling of the DVA at the time of the normal venous drainage with no evidence of the characteristic arteriovenous shunting that characterizes an AVM (Figure 13.3).

Treatment

The vast majority of DVAs remain asymptomatic throughout life and require no treatment. Since they function as drainage pathways for normal brain, resection of DVAs may result in significant venous compromise or venous infarction (90).

■ CAPILLARY TELANGIECTASIA

Epidemiology

Capillary telangiectasias have an estimated prevalence of 0.4% at autopsy (97) and are believed to represent approximately 10% to 20% of cerebrovascular malformations (98–99).

Morphology

Telangiectasias are composed of numerous capillary-like vessels that lack smooth muscle or elastic fibers and are separated by normal parenchyma (99). There is little or no gliosis associated with the lesions. The vast majority occur in the pons, however they have been rarely reported in other locations throughout the brain and spinal cord (100–103).

Imaging

Telangiectasias are usually incidentally seen and are virtually always asymptomatic, almost never requiring treatment (Figure 13.4). They are generally occult on imaging except for MRI. Although variable signal characteristics have been described, capillary telangiectasias are generally isointense to hypointense on T1-weighted images and isointense to hyperintense on T2-weighted images most commonly in the midpons (104). Homogeneous or mildly heterogeneous enhancement is typically present and gradient echo images demonstrate

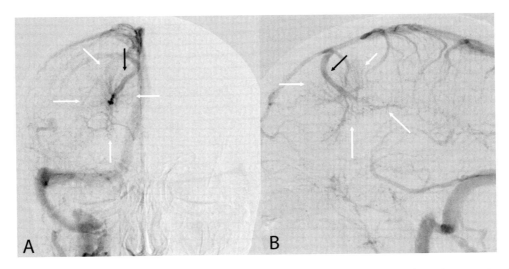

FIGURE 13.3 Developmental venous anomaly—Frontal (A) and lateral (B) angiograms in the venous phase demonstrating dilated medullary veins (white arrows) draining into enlarged central collecting vein (black arrow). The collecting vein then drains into the superior sagittal sinus. The dilated medullary veins appear simultaneously with normal venous structures, characteristic of a developmental venous anomaly.

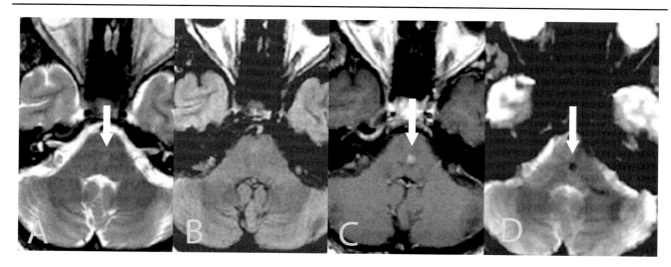

FIGURE 13.4 Capillary telangiectasia—axial T2-weighted (A), axial FLAIR (B), gadolinium enhanced axial T1-weighted (C), and axial T2* gradient echo (D) images demonstrating mild increase signal in the mid pons (white arrow) with no significant signal abnormality on FLAIR images. There is mild homogenous enhancement (white arrow) on the gadolinium enhanced post contrast images. Susceptibility artifact (blooming) is present on the T2* gradient echo images (white arrow).

focal hypointensity. Occasionally an enhancing adjacent vessel may be identified (100). There is no associated edema or mass effect. Rarely capillary telangiectasias can be seen as an area of focal enhancement on CT, sometimes with associated calcification (105).

■ ANEURYSMAL MALFORMATION OF THE VEIN OF GALEN

Epidemiology

Aneurysmal malformations of the vein of Galen consist of direct arteriovenous fistulas between an embryonic choroidal artery and an embryonic venous precursor to the vein of Galen. Aneurysmal malformations of the vein of Galen are rare, constituting less than 1% of all intracranial vascular malformations. They are however of significant importance in very young children, and represent nearly 30% of vascular malformations presenting in the neonatal and infant age groups (106). The lesions are congenital, but no convincing evidence of heritability has been demonstrated.

Anatomy

Aneurysmal malformations of the vein of Galen are located in the subarachnoid space within the cistern of the velum interpositum and quadrigeminal plate cistern

(107), thus differentiating them from pial AVMs and fistulas as well as from dural arteriovenous fistulas.

Two anatomic types of AMVG have been described (108–109). The *choroidal* type consists of numerous arteriovenous fistulas, often with extremely high blood flow through the shunts, which may represent the major portion of cardiac output. Choroidal AMVGs often present in the neonatal period. *Mural* type AMVGs consist of a few fistulas or even a single fistula, are characterized by lower arteriovenous shunt volumes, and usually present in infancy or even later in life (110).

Clinical

The volume of arteriovenous shunting through the AMVG is believed to be the major contributor to the clinical presentation of AMVG. Three age-specific clinical presentations have been described (111–112). Neonates, usually with choroidal type AMVG and large shunt volumes, experience high myocardial workload, often with decreased myocardial perfusion. Consequently, neonates usually present with high output heart failure. Infants and young children, usually with mural type AMVG, often present with macrocephaly, hydrocephalus, and developmental delay. Uncommonly, older children and even adults may present with headaches or subarachnoid hemorrhage due to AMVG.

A cranial bruit may frequently be auscultated, particularly in neonates with an open fontanelle. Intracranial hemorrhage associated with AMVG is uncommon in neonates and young infants. Intracranial hemorrhage in this age group may be due to an alternate diagnosis, including a pial AVM draining into the deep venous system (113–114).

Imaging

Unenhanced CT scans usually demonstrate the dilated venous drainage pathway as an isodense or hyperdense structure posterior to the third ventricle (115). Careful examination of the brain parenchyma is necessary to identify areas of gliosis or encephalomalacia which may contraindicate treatment. Evaluation for hydrocephalus, the most common associated imaging finding (116), should also be performed.

MRI combined with MRA sequences are usually the most important preangiographic evaluation in children with AMVG (115). Areas of signal void depict both the enlarged feeding arteries and dilated venous drainage that comprises the lesion (Figure 13.5A, 13.5B and 13.5C). As with CT, careful examination of the brain parenchyma

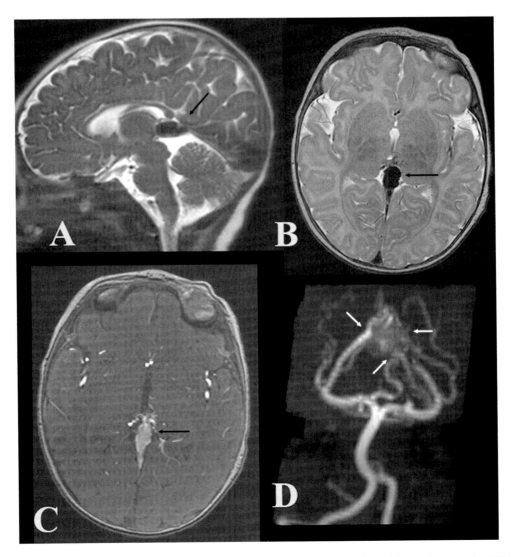

FIGURE 13.5 Aneurysmal malformation of the vein of Galen—midline sagittal T2-weighted (A), axial T2-weighted (B), axial magnetic resonance angiographic (MRA) source images (C), and coronal oblique MRA MIP images (D) demonstrate a large flow void in the cistern of the velum interpositum and quadrigeminal plate cistern (black arrows) fed by multiple branches of the posterior cerebral arteries (white arrows).

on MRI is necessary. MRA sequences, particularly with 3-dimensional reconstruction, often provide the best imaging to outline the anatomy of the lesion (Figure 13.5D). This information is most often useful to plan angiographic evaluation at the time of endovascular treatment.

Treatment

Embolization of the arteriovenous fistulas using neuroendovascular techniques constitutes the currently accepted management for AMVG (110,116–122). Open surgical treatment generally plays little role in the management of patients with AMVG (123–124). Selective catheterization of the feeding arteries is followed by occlusion at the site of the arteriovenous communication. Devices used include coils, *n*-BCA, and Onyx. Closure of the venous side of the AMVG has also been reported. This technique is uncommonly used today and may carry significant risk for intracranial hemorrhage and venous infarction (121,125–126).

Outcome

Untreated, the outcome of symptomatic AMVG is poor in both neonates and infants (123–124). Surgical treatment in AMVG also conveys very limited benefit in either patient group (123–124). Small series have emphasized improved survival benefit with endovascular as compared with open surgical treatment (127).

A number of series have reported endovascular management of AMVG (110,116–122). Despite the advances represented by endovascular treatment, AMVG in neonates remains a serious disorder with normal neurologic outcomes reported in from 25% to 60% of patients. Mortality rates have been reported to range from 15% to 60% in this age group. Results in older patients indicate a better outcome with normal neurologic development in 60% to 80% and mortality rates generally under 10%.

■ SUMMARY

A thorough understanding of the uncommon but clinically important group of congenital cerebrovascular lesions is essential for both the general pediatrician and pediatric specialist. The clinical presentations and imaging findings will help formulate a reasonable differential diagnosis and guide treatment options.

■ REFERENCES

1. Al Shahi R, Stapf C. The prognosis and treatment of arteriovenous malformations of the brain. *Practical Neurol.* 2005;5(4):194–205.
2. Soderman M et al. Management of patients with brain arteriovenous malformations. *Eur J Radiol.* 2003;46(3):195–205.
3. Hernesniemi JA et al. Natural history of brain arteriovenous malformations: a long-term follow-up study of risk of hemorrhage in 238 patients. *Neurosurgery.* 2008;63(5):823–829.
4. Wilkins RH. Natural history of intracranial vascular malformations: a review. *Neurosurgery.* 1985;16(3):421–430.
5. Hartmann A et al. Morbidity of intracranial hemorrhage in patients with cerebral arteriovenous malformation. *Stroke.* 1998;29(5):931–934.
6. Giroud M et al. Stroke in children under 16 years of age. Clinical and etiological difference with adults. *Acta Neurol Scand.* 1997;96(6):401–406.
7. Hofmeister C et al. Demographic, morphological, and clinical characteristics of 1289 patients with brain arteriovenous malformation. *Stroke.* 2000;31(6):1307–1310.
8. Geibprasert S et al. Hydrocephalus in unruptured brain arteriovenous malformations: pathomechanical considerations, therapeutic implications, and clinical course. *J Neurosurg.* 2009;110(3):500–507.
9. Baker SK, Silva JE, Lam KK. Pseudoephedrine-induced hemorrhage associated with a cerebral vascular malformation. *Can J Neurol Sci.* 2005;32(2):248–252.
10. Selmi F et al. Intracerebral haemorrhage due to amphetamine abuse: report of two cases with underlying arteriovenous malformations. *Br J Neurosurg.* 1995;9(1):93–96.
11. Langer DJ et al. Hypertension, small size, and deep venous drainage are associated with risk of hemorrhagic presentation of cerebral arteriovenous malformations. *Neurosurgery.* 1998;42(3):481–486.
12. Geibprasert S et al. Radiologic assessment of brain arteriovenous malformations: what clinicians need to know. *Radiographics.* 2010;30(2):483–501.
13. Gutierrez-Gonzalez R et al. Intraventricular haemorrhage caused by the rupture of a dural arteriovenous malformation of the middle cranial fossa. *Acta Neurochir (Wien).* 2009;151(8):1009–1012.
14. da Costa L et al. The natural history and predictive features of hemorrhage from brain arteriovenous malformations. *Stroke.* 2009;40(1):100–105.
15. Tsui YK et al. Susceptibility-weighted imaging for differential diagnosis of cerebral vascular pathology: a pictorial review. *J Neurol Sci.* 2009;287(1–2):7–16.
16. Grossman RI et al. MR imaging of hemorrhagic conditions of the head and neck. *Radiographics.* 1988;8(3):441–454.
17. Spetzler RF, Martin NA. A proposed grading system for arteriovenous malformations. *J Neurosurg.* 1986;65(4):476–483.
18. Vinuela F et al. Stenotic and occlusive disease of the venous drainage system of deep brain AVM's. *J Neurosurg.* 1985;63(2):180–184.
19. Shimizu S et al. Pial arteriovenous malformation with massive perinidal edema. *Neurol Res.* 1998;20(3):249–252.

20. Izawa M et al. Long-term complications after gamma knife surgery for arteriovenous malformations. *J Neurosurg.* 2005;102(suppl):34–37.

21. Komatsu F et al. Ruptured tectal arteriovenous malformation demonstrated angiographically after removal of an unruptured occipital lobe arteriovenous malformation. *Neurol Med Chir (Tokyo).* 2009;49(1):30–32.

22. Sadick H et al. Hereditary hemorrhagic telangiectasia: an update on clinical manifestations and diagnostic measures. *Wien Klin Wochenschr.* 2006;118(3–4):72–80.

23. Chiewvit P et al. Computed tomographic findings in nontraumatic hemorrhagic stroke. *J Med Assoc Thai.* 2009;92(1):73–86.

24. Lawton MT et al. Effect of presenting hemorrhage on outcome after microsurgical resection of brain arteriovenous malformations. *Neurosurgery.* 2005;56(3):485–493.

25. Kojima Y, Kuwana N. Progressive diffuse arteriovenous malformation—case report. *Neurol Med Chir (Tokyo).* Apr 1993;33(4):242–245.

26. Yu YL, Chiu EK, Woo E et al. Dystrophic intracranial calcification: CT evidence of 'cerebral steal' from arteriovenous malformation. *Neuroradiology.* 1987;29(6):519–522.

27. Gazzola S et al. Vascular and nonvascular mimics of the CT angiography "spot sign" in patients with secondary intracerebral hemorrhage. *Stroke.* 2008;39(4):1177–1183.

28. Anzalone N et al. Intracranial vascular malformations. *Eur Radiol.* 1998;8(5):685–690.

29. Tanabe S et al. Diagnosis of cerebral arteriovenous malformations with three-dimensional CT angiography. *J Clin Neurosci.* 1998;5(suppl):33–38.

30. Willems PW et al. The use of 4D-CTA in the diagnostic workup of brain arteriovenous malformations. *Neuroradiology.* Apr 2011;123–131.

31. White PM et al. Intracranial aneurysms: CT angiography and MR angiography for detection prospective blinded comparison in a large patient cohort. *Radiology.* 2001;219(3):739–749.

32. Al-Saleh S et al. Screening for pulmonary and cerebral arteriovenous malformations in children with hereditary haemorrhagic telangiectasia. *Eur Respir J.* 2009;34(4):875–881.

33. Wilms G et al. MRI of non-ischemic vascular disease: aneurysms and vascular malformations. *Eur Radiol.* 1999;9(6):1055–1060.

34. Essig M et al. Arteriovenous malformations: assessment of gliotic and ischemic changes with fluid-attenuated inversion-recovery MRI. *Invest Radiol.* 2000;35(11):689–694.

35. Stancanello J et al. BOLD fMRI integration into radiosurgery treatment planning of cerebral vascular malformations. *Med Phys.* 2007;34(4):1176–1184.

36. Berube J et al. Diffusion tensor imaging analysis of long association bundles in the presence of an arteriovenous malformation. *J Neurosurg.* 2007;107(3):509–514.

37. Caramia F et al. Neurophysiological and functional MRI evidence of reorganization of cortical motor areas in cerebral arteriovenous malformation. *Magn Reson Imaging.* 2009;27(10):1360–1369.

38. Wolf RL et al. Arteriovenous shunt visualization in arteriovenous malformations with arterial spin-labeling MR imaging. *AJNR Am J Neuroradiol.* 2008;29(4):681–687.

39. Gailloud P et al. Three-dimensional digital angiography: new tool for simultaneous three-dimensional rendering of vascular and osseous information during rotational angiography. *AJNR Am J Neuroradiol.* 2004;25(4):571–573.

40. Valavanis A, Yasargil MG. The endovascular treatment of brain arteriovenous malformations. *Adv Tech Stand Neurosurg.* 1998;24:131–214.

41. Hoh BL et al. Results of multimodality treatment for 141 patients with brain arteriovenous malformations and seizures: factors associated with seizure incidence and seizure outcomes. *Neurosurgery.* 2002;51(2):303–309; discussion 309–311.

42. Asgari S et al. AVM resection after radiation therapy—clinico-morphological features and microsurgical results. *Neurosurg Rev.* 2010;33(1):53–61.

43. Ross J, Al-Shahi Salman R. Interventions for treating brain arteriovenous malformations in adults. *Cochrane Database Syst Rev.* 2010;(7):CD003436.

44. Mohr JP. A randomized trial of unruptured brain arteriovenous malformations (ARUBA). *Acta Neurochir Suppl.* 2008;103:3–4.

45. Davidson AS, Morgan MK. How safe is arteriovenous malformation surgery? A prospective, observational study of surgery as first-line treatment for brain arteriovenous malformations. *Neurosurgery.* 2010;66(3):498–504.

46. Hamilton MG, Spetzler RF. The prospective application of a grading system for arteriovenous malformations. *Neurosurgery.* 1994;34(1):2–6.

47. Yuki I et al. Treatment of brain arteriovenous malformations with high-flow arteriovenous fistulas: risk and complications associated with endovascular embolization in multimodality treatment. Clinical article. *J Neurosurg.* 2010;113(4):715–722.

48. Iwama T et al. Emergency craniotomy for intraparenchymal massive hematoma after embolization of supratentorial arteriovenous malformations. *Neurosurgery.* 2003;53(6):1251–1258.

49. Millar C, Bissonnette B, Humphreys RP. Cerebral arteriovenous malformations in children. *Can J Anaesth.* 994;41(4):321–331.

50. Elhammady MS, Baskaya MK, Heros RC. Early elective surgical exploration of spontaneous intracerebral hematomas of unknown origin. *J Neurosurg.* 2008;109(6):1005–1011.

51. Lunsford LD, Flickinger J, Coffey RJ. Stereotactic gamma knife radiosurgery. Initial North American experience in 207 patients. *Arch Neurol.* 1990;47(2):169–175.

52. Deinsberger R, Tidstrand J. Linac radiosurgery as a tool in neurosurgery. *Neurosurg Rev.* 2005;28(2):79–88.

53. Fabrikant JI et al. Charged-particle radiosurgery for intracranial vascular malformations. *Neurosurg Clin N Am.* 1992;3(1):99–139.

54. Yamamoto M et al. Gamma knife radiosurgery for cerebral arteriovenous malformations: an autopsy report focusing on irradiation-induced changes observed in nidus-unrelated arteries. *Surg Neurol.* 1995;44(5):421–427.

55. Pollock BE, Gorman DA, Brown PD. Radiosurgery for arteriovenous malformations of the basal ganglia, thalamus, and brainstem. *J Neurosurg.* 2004;100(2):210–214.

56. Mitchell P et al. Surgical options in ICH including decompressive craniectomy. *J Neurol Sci.* 2007;261(1–2):89–98.

57. Kim HY et al. Gamma knife surgery for large cerebral arteriovenous malformations. *J Neurosurg.* 2010;113(suppl): 2–8.

58. Simon SD et al. Resolution of trigeminal neuralgia after palliative embolization of a cerebellopontine angle arteriovenous malformation. *Cen Eur Neurosurg.* 2009;70(3):161–163.

59. Rivera R et al. Single hole cerebral arteriovenous fistula between the anterior choroidal artery and the basal vein of Rosenthal in a child. *Childs Nerv Syst.* N2009;25(11): 1521–1523.

60. Maimon S et al. Brain arteriovenous malformation treatment using a combination of Onyx and a new detachable tip microcatheter, SONIC: short-term results. *AJNR Am J Neuroradiol.* 2010;31(5):947–954.

61. Sorimachi T et al. Embolization of cerebral arteriovenous malformations achieved with polyvinyl alcohol particles: angiographic reappearance and complications. *AJNR Am J Neuroradiol.* 1999;20(7):1323–1328.

62. Loh Y, Duckwiler GR. A prospective, multicenter, randomized trial of the Onyx liquid embolic system and N-butyl cyanoacrylate embolization of cerebral arteriovenous malformations. Clinical article. *J Neurosurg.* 2010;113(4):733–741.

63. N-butyl cyanoacrylate embolization of cerebral arteriovenous malformations: results of a prospective, randomized, multicenter trial. *AJNR Am J Neuroradiol.* 2002;23(5):748–755.

64. Haw CS et al. Complications of embolization of arteriovenous malformations of the brain. *J Neurosurg.* 2006;104(2): 226–232.

65. Taylor CL et al. Complications of preoperative embolization of cerebral arteriovenous malformations. *J Neurosurg.* 2004;100(5):810–812.

66. Giombini S, Morello G. Cavernous angiomas of the brain. Account of fourteen personal cases and review of the literature. *Acta Neurochir (Wien).* 1978;40(1–2):61–82.

67. Lonjon M et al. Intracranial cavernoma. 30 cases. *Presse Med.* 1993;22(21):990–994.

68. Batra S, Lin D et al. Cavernous malformations: natural history, diagnosis and treatment. *Nat Rev Neurol.* 2009; 5(12):659–670.

69. Hsu FPK, Rigamonti D, Huhn SL. *Epidemiology of Cavernous Malformations.* Park Ridge, IL: AANS Publications Committee; 1993.

70. Herter T, Brandt M, Szuwart U. Cavernous hemangiomas in children. *Childs Nerv Syst.* 1988;4(3):123–127.

71. Berry R, Alpers B, White J. *The Site, Structure and Frequency of Intracranial Aneurysms, Angiomas and Arteriovenous Abnormalities.* Baltimore, MD: Williams & Wilkins; 1996.

72. Maraire JN, Awad IA. Intracranial cavernous malformations: lesion behavior and management strategies. *Neurosurgery.* 1995;37(4):591–605.

73. Sage MR et al. Cavernous haemangiomas (angiomas) of the brain: clinically significant lesions. *Australas Radiol.* 1993;37(2):147–155.

74. Washington CW, McCoy KE, Zipfel GJ. Update on the natural history of cavernous malformations and factors predicting aggressive clinical presentation. *Neurosurg Focus.* 2010;29(3):E7.

75. Mottolese C, Hermier M, Stan H et al. Central nervous system cavernomas in the pediatric age group. *Neurosurg Rev.* 2001;24(2–3):55–71.

76. Lee JW et al. Management of intracranial cavernous malformation in pediatric patients. *Childs Nerv Syst.* Mar 2008;24(3):321–327.

77. Mattana M, Mattana PR, Roxo MR. Intractable hiccup induced by cavernous angioma in the medulla oblongata: case report. *J Neurol Neurosurg Psychiatry.* 2010;81(3):353–354.

78. Huang AP et al. Brain stem cavernous malformations. *J Clin Neurosci.* 2010;17(1):74–79.

79. Di Rocco C, Iannelli A, Tamburrini G. Cavernomas of the central nervous system in children. A report of 22 cases. *Acta Neurochir (Wien).* 1996;138(11):1267–1274.

80. Fortuna A et al. Cerebral cavernous angioma in children. *Childs Nerv Syst.* 1989;5(4):201–207.

81. Hardy PA, Kucharczyk W, Henkelman RM. Cause of signal loss in MR images of old hemorrhagic lesions. *Radiology.* 1990;174(2):549–555.

82. Rigamonti D et al. The MRI appearance of cavernous malformations (angiomas). *J Neurosurg.* 1987;67(4):518–524.

83. Biondi A et al. Magnetic resonance imaging of cerebral cavernous angiomas. *Acta Radiol Suppl.* 1986;369:82–85.

84. Lehnhardt FG et al. Value of gradient-echo magnetic resonance imaging in the diagnosis of familial cerebral cavernous malformation. *Arch Neurol.* A2005;62(4):653–658.

85. Mizoi K, Yoshimoto T, Suzuki J. Clinical analysis of ten cases with surgically treated brain stem cavernous angiomas. *Tohoku J Exp Med.* 1992;166(2):259–267.

86. Zakaria MA et al. Third ventricular cavernous angioma. *Med J Malaysia.* 2006;61(2):229–232.

87. Savoiardo M, Strada L, Passerini A. Intracranial cavernous hemangiomas: neuroradiologic review of 36 operated cases. *AJNR Am J Neuroradiol.* 1983;4(4):945–950.

88. Garner TB et al. The natural history of intracranial venous angiomas. *J Neurosurg.* 1991;75(5):715–722.

89. Osborn AG. *Diagnostic Cerebral Angiography.* 2nd ed. Philadelphia, PA: Lippincott Williams & Wilkins; 1999.

90. Abe M et al. Histologically classified venous angiomas of the brain: a controversy. *Neurol Med Chir (Tokyo).* 2003;43(1): 1–10.

91. Saba PR. The caput medusae sign. *Radiology.* 1998;207(3): 599–600.

92. Pereira VM et al. Pathomechanisms of symptomatic developmental venous anomalies. *Stroke.* 2008;39(12):3201–3215.

93. Dehkharghani S et al. Unilateral calcification of the caudate and putamen: association with underlying developmental venous anomaly. *AJNR Am J Neuroradiol.* 2010;31(10): 1848–1852.

94. Clatterbuck RE, Elmac I, Rigamonti D. The juxtaposition of a capillary telangiectasia, cavernous malformation, and developmental venous anomaly in the brainstem of a single patient: case report. *Neurosurgery.* 2001;49(5):1246.

95. Ostertun B, Solymosi L. Magnetic resonance angiography of cerebral developmental venous anomalies: its role in differential diagnosis. *Neuroradiology.* 1993;35(2):97–104.

96. Ruiz DS, Yilmaz H, Gailloud P. Cerebral developmental venous anomalies: current concepts. *Ann Neurol.* 2009;66(3): 271–283.

97. Sarwar M, McCormick WF. Intracerebral venous angioma. Case report and review. *Arch Neurol.* 1978;35(5):323–325.

98. Castillo M. *Neuroradiology Companion.* 3rd ed. Philadelphia, PA: Lippincott Williams & Wilkins; 2006.

99. Chaloupka JC, Huddle DC. Classification of vascular malformations of the central nervous system. *Neuroimaging Clin N Am.* 1998;8(2):295–321.

100. Barr RM, Dillon WP, Wilson CB. Slow-flow vascular malformations of the pons: capillary telangiectasias? *AJNR Am J Neuroradiol.* 1996;17(1):71–78.

101. Castillo M et al. MR imaging and histologic features of capillary telangiectasia of the basal ganglia. *AJNR Am J Neuroradiol.* 2001;22(8):1553–1555.

102. Huddle DC, Chaloupka JC, Sehgal V. Clinically aggressive diffuse capillary telangiectasia of the brain stem: a clinical radiologic-pathologic case study. *AJNR Am J Neuroradiol.* 1999;20(9):1674–1677.

103. Lee RR et al. Brain capillary telangiectasia: MR imaging appearance and clinicohistopathologic findings. *Radiology.* 1997;205(3):797–805.

104. Saba L, Pascalis L, Mallarini G. Magnetic resonance imaging of pontine capillary telangiectasia. *Eur J Radiol.* 2011 Dec;80(3):771-5. Epub 2010 Oct 6.

105. Tang SC et al. Diffuse capillary telangiectasia of the brain manifested as a slowly progressive course. *Cerebrovasc Dis.* 2003;15(1–2):140–142.

106. Lasjaunias P et al. [Dilatation of the vein of Galen. Anatomoclinical forms and endovascular treatment apropos of 14 cases explored and/or treated between 1983 and 1986]. *Neurochirurgie.* 1987;33(4):315–333.

107. Gupta A, Varma D. Vein of Galen malformations: review. *Neurology India.* 2004;52(1):43.

108. Lasjaunias P. Vein of Galen malformations. *Neurosurgery.* 1989;25(4):666–667.

109. Raybaud CA, Strother CM, Hald JK. Aneurysms of the vein of Galen: embryonic considerations and anatomical features relating to the pathogenesis of the malformation. *Neuroradiology.* 1989;31(2):109–128.

110. Fullerton HJ et al. Neurodevelopmental outcome after endovascular treatment of vein of Galen malformations. *Neurology.* 2003;61(10):1386–1390.

111. Gold A, Ransohoff J, Carter S. Vein of Galen malformation. *Acta Neurol Scand.* 1964;40(suppl 11):11–31.

112. Silverman BK et al. Congestive failure in the newborn caused by cerebral A-V fistula; a clinical and pathological report of two cases. *AMA Am J Dis Child.* 1955;89(5):539–543.

113. Lasjaunias P et al. Cerebral arteriovenous malformations in children. Management of 179 consecutive cases and review of the literature. *Childs Nerv Syst.* 1995;11(2):66–79.

114. Meyers PM et al. Hemorrhagic complications in vein of Galen malformations. *Ann Neurol.* 2000;47(6):748–755.

115. Martelli A et al. Aneurysms of the vein of Galen in children: CT and angiographic correlations. *Neuroradiology.* 1980;20(3):123–133.

116. Gupta AK et al. Evaluation, management, and long-term follow up of vein of Galen malformations. *J Neurosurg.* 2006;105(1):26–33.

117. Frawley GP et al Loughnan P. Clinical course and medical management of neonates with severe cardiac failure related to vein of Galen malformation. *Arch Dis Child Fetal Neonatal Ed.* 2002;87(2):F144–149.

118. Heuer GG et al. Diagnosis and treatment of vein of Galen aneurysmal malformations. *Childs Nerv Syst.* 2010;26(7):879–887.

119. Jones BV et al. Vein of Galen aneurysmal malformation: diagnosis and treatment of 13 children with extended clinical follow-up. *AJNR Am J Neuroradiol.* 2002;23(10):1717–1724.

120. Lasjaunias P. *Vascular Diseases in Neonates, Infants, and Children.* Springer; 1997:67–202.

121. Lylyk P et al. Therapeutic alternatives for vein of Galen vascular malformations. *J Neurosurg.* 1993;78(3):438–445.

122. Mitchell PJ et al. Endovascular management of vein of Galen aneurysmal malformations presenting in the neonatal period. *AJNR Am J Neuroradiol.* 2001;22(7):1403–1409.

123. Hoffman HJ et al. Aneurysms of the vein of Galen. Experience at the Hospital for Sick Children, Toronto. *J Neurosurg.* 1982;57(3):316-322.

124. Johnston IH et al. Vein of Galen malformation: diagnosis and management. *Neurosurgery.* 1987;20(5):747–758.

125. Gailloud P et al. Confirmation of communication between deep venous drainage and the vein of galen after treatment of a vein of Galen aneurysmal malformation in an infant presenting with severe pulmonary hypertension. *AJNR Am J Neuroradiol.* 2006;27(2):317–320.

126. Levrier O et al. Normal galenic drainage of the deep cerebral venous system in two cases of vein of Galen aneurysmal malformation. *Childs Nerv Syst.* 2004;20(2):91–97.

127. Ciricillo SF et al. Interventional neuroradiological management of vein of Galen malformations in the neonate. *Neurosurgery.* 1990;27(1):22–27.

14 Acquired Demyelinating Syndromes of the Central Nervous System

AMY T. WALDMAN, MICHAEL J. SHUMSKI, and GIHAN I. TENNEKOON

■ INTRODUCTION

Acquired demyelinating syndromes constitute a group of acute or subacute autoimmune disorders of the central nervous system (CNS) and include acute disseminated encephalomyelitis (ADEM), clinically isolated syndromes such as optic neuritis and transverse myelitis, multiple sclerosis (MS), and neuromyelitis optica (NMO). These disorders share an underlying pathology of an abnormal immune response resulting in inflammatory destruction of myelin, in addition to primary or secondary axonal damage, in the CNS. Therefore, treatment of these disorders is centered on altering the immune response.

Diagnosis of these disorders is difficult due to the similarities in their neurologic symptoms and neuroimaging findings; therefore, each disease must be distinguished by certain clinical criteria with supportive evidence from laboratory results and magnetic resonance imaging (MRI) scans (Table 14.1). Subtypes may vary substantially with respect to the severity of clinical signs and symptoms, frequency of recurrence, and outcome. After a brief description of the different acquired demyelinating disorders, this chapter will focus on the evaluation, diagnosis, and treatment of these disorders in a critical care setting.

■ OVERVIEW OF ACUTE DEMYELINATING SYNDROMES

Acquired demyelinating syndromes may be isolated or recurrent events. If a child is presenting with their first neurologic event, the diagnosis is either ADEM or a clinically isolated syndrome. If the child is encephalopathic and polysymptomatic, he or she meets criteria for ADEM (Figure 14.1) (1). Otherwise, an individual's first episode is referred to as a clinically isolated syndrome. A clinically isolated syndrome must not involve encephalopathy, but may involve either monofocal symptoms and signs (related to dysfunction at one CNS location) or multifocal symptoms and signs (localizing to multiple CNS areas) (1). A clinically isolated syndrome may present as optic neuritis, transverse myelitis, or brainstem, cerebellar, or hemispheric dysfunction.

If a child has a history of a demyelinating event, the diagnosis may be MS, NMO, recurrent ADEM, multiphasic ADEM, recurrent optic neuritis, recurrent transverse myelitis, or chronic relapsing inflammatory optic neuropathy (CRION). These diagnoses will be reviewed later in this chapter.

All demyelinating diseases are diagnosed by clinical signs and symptoms. However, often laboratory tests and neuroimaging are used to further define the extent of the disease. It is not always possible during an acute episode to confirm the diagnosis or establish the prognosis, which may not be apparent until follow-up testing is performed or there is a recurrence.

ADEM, NMO, transverse myelitis, and fulminant demyelinating diseases (acute hemorrhagic leukoencephalitis, Marburg variant, Balo concentric sclerosis, and tumefactive MS) are more likely to present to the intensive care unit (ICU). MS flares rarely require ICU admission, and isolated optic neuritis flares do not require ICU treatment; however, these are common demyelinating diseases and will be covered as well.

(text continues on page 230)

Demyelinating Disorder	Diagnostic Criteria			Supportive Data and Common Features			
	Inclusion Criteria	Exclusion	Comment	Clinical Features	MRI Characteristics[b]	CSF[b]	References
ADEM	1. Polysymptomatic neurologic dysfunction of the brain and spinal cord 2. Encephalopathy		More common in prepubertal children.	1. Antecedent infection or vaccination 2. Prodromal phase 3. Common features: pyramidal signs, ataxia, cranial neuropathies (bilateral optic neuritis), seizures	Diffuse T2-weighted hyperintense lesions of brain and spinal cord that are large (> 1–2 cm) and asymmetric with poorly defined margins. Basal ganglia and thalamic involvement may occur, with or without other supratentorial or infratentorial lesions. Spinal cord involvement is also common. Enhancement is variable.	Lymphocytic pleocytosis (mean 51 cells/mm³, range 0–270) or elevated protein (mean 73.9 mg/dL, range 45–120) was seen in 70%–75% of patients. Oligoclonal bands are present in 4%–29% of children with ADEM.	1, 2, 4, 5, 7–9
Recurrent ADEM	1. Polysymptomatic neurologic dysfunction of the brain and spinal cord at the same sites (no new involvement by history, examination, or neuroimaging) occuring 3 or more months after the initial ADEM event. 2. Encephalopathy	1. Steroids administered within the past month	No new lesions are seen on MRI; however, original lesions may be enlarged.	Same as the initial ADEM presentation	Same as the initial ADEM presentation, although some lesions may be enlarged.	Same as above	1

Multiphasic ADEM	1. Polysymptomatic neurologic dysfunction of the brain and spinal cord at the same sites with new involvement by history, examination, and neuroimaging occuring 3 or more months after the initial ADEM presentation 2. Encephalopathy	1. Steroids administered within the past month	1. While there are new lesions on the MRI of the brain, prior lesions seen during the initial presentation must show complete or partial resolution. 2. A recurrence without encephalopathy does not meet criteria for multiphasic ADEM or MS.	Compared to the first event, new clinical symptoms, such as pyramidal signs, ataxia, cranial neuropathies, seizures, are present (with the exception of encephalopathy which may be the same as the initial presentation)	New lesions are seen on the MRI of the brain and the initial lesions must show improvement or resolution.	Same as above	1
Clinically isolated syndrome	Monofocal or polyfocal neurologic disease localizing to the brain or spinal cord	Prior history of demyelination	Encephalopathy typically suggests ADEM; however, brainstem involvement in CIS may cause encephalopathy.	Unilateral or bilateral optic neuritis, transverse myelitis, or brainstem/cerebellar syndromes	Variable T2/FLAIR hyperintensities and enhancement after the administration of gadolinium	A lymphocytic pleocytosis, elevated protein, or markers of inflammation (presence of oligoclonal bands, elevated IgG synthesis, IgG index, or myelin basic protein)	1

(continued)

■ Table 14.1 Diagnostic Criteria and Supportive Features for Acquired Demyelinating Syndromes in Children *(continued)*

Demyelinating Disorder	Diagnostic Criteria			Supportive Data and Common Features			References
	Inclusion Criteria	Exclusion	Comment	Clinical Features	MRI Characteristics[b]	CSF[b]	
Clinically isolated syndrome—optic neuritis	1. Decreased visual acuity 2. Pain with eye movements 3. Decreased color vision 4. Visual field deficits	Ischemic, infectious, and hereditary causes of vision loss should be excluded	Not all symptoms are required for the diagnosis. Similarly, a relative afferent pupil defect and disc swelling are not required for the diagnosis as these exam findings are dependent upon the location of the inflammation.	"Blurry vision" in one or both eyes and pain with eye movements are the most common presenting symptoms	MRI of the orbits reveals enlargement of the intraorbital and intracanalicular segments of the optic nerve on T1-weighted images as well as hyperintensity on FLAIR and T2-weighted sequences. Postgadolinium images may reveal contrast enhancement. The presence of one or more lesions on an MRI of the brain (outside the anterior visual pathway) is considered high risk for MS.	CSF profile may be normal in isolated optic neuritis. A lymphocytic pleocytosis has been reported in up to 50%, and an elevated protein is seen in approximately 10% of patients. The presence of oligoclonal bands, seen in 11%–17%, raises concern for MS.	13–16, 18, 19, 114

Clinically isolated syndrome— transverse myelitis	1. Sensory, motor, or autonomic dysfunction localizable to the spinal cord 2. Bilateral involvement by history, exam, or imaging (with or without symmetry) 3. Presence of a sensory level 4. Inflammation documented by CSF pleocytosis, elevated IgG index, or gadolinium enhancement on MRI 5. Maximum deficit reached 4 hours to 21 days after symptoms onset	1. History of prior radiation to cord 2. Deficits consistent with anterior spinal artery infarct 3. Imaging suggesting AVM 4. Presence of brain lesions (suggests MS rather than TM)	Consider an ischemic process in children with the rapid onset of symptoms, reaching a nadir within 4 hours.	Weakness, loss or altered sensation, pain, and bladder dysfunction	MRI of the C- and T-spine may reveal T2-weighted hyperintensities that are < 3 spinal segments in length, longitudinally extensive lesions (≥ 3 spinal segments), or a combination. Longitudinally extensive lesions are common in transverse myelitis as a clinically isolated syndrome. T1-weighted images may reveal expansion of the cord.	A CSF pleocytosis and elevated protein may be present although normal CSF profiles have been reported in children with acute transverse myelitis. Markedly elevated CSF WBC should raise suspicion for neuromyelitis optica. The presence of OCB should raise concern for a first presentation of MS.

(continued)

227

Demyelinating Disorder	Diagnostic Criteria			Supportive Data and Common Features			References
	Inclusion Criteria	Exclusion	Comment	Clinical Features	MRI Characteristics[b]	CSF[b]	
Pediatric MS	Recurrent demyelination of the brain and spinal cord separated in time and space		After ADEM as a first attack, the diagnosis of MS is fulfilled after 2 or more non-ADEM attacks or after 1 non-ADEM attack with accrual of clinically silent lesions. In a patient with a clinically isolated syndrome characteristic of MS[b], it is possible to confirm a diagnosis of MS by showing dissemination in space and time using MRI.	The presentation is variable. Patients have paresthesias, visual dysfunction, motor problems, cranial neuropathies, cerebellar symptoms, ataxia and other gait problems, bowel and bladder dysfunction.	Lesions in the periventricular white matter, corpus callosum, junctions of the gray-white matter, and the spinal cord appear hyperintense on T2-weighted or FLAIR imaging and hypointense on T1-weighted imaging. Black holes (T1-weighted hypointensities) are the strongest predictor of MS. The presence of one or more periventricular lesions is also predictive of MS. Discrete lesions (with well-defined borders) and lesions perpendicular to the corpus callosum are also highly suggestive of pediatric MS. Enhancing lesions are seen in 25%–70% of children at their initial presentation.	A lymphocytic pleocytosis may be seen but the mean is decreased compared to ADEM (median 8/μL, range 0–61/μL). Protein may also be elevated. The presence of oligoclonal bands is variable and has been estimated in 40%–90% of children with pediatric MS.	1, 7, 33, 45, 46, 56, 57

| Neuromyelitis optica | 1. Optic neuritis
2. Myelitis
3. 2 of the 3: LE spinal cord lesion, NMO IgG positive, brain MRI does not fulfill criteria for MS | 1. The IPMSSG requires optic neuritis and myelitis as major criteria, and either longitudinally extensive spinal cord lesions or NMO-IgG positivity.
2. Brain lesions may be seen in children with NMO, especially in deep gray matter. | A clinical prodrome of fever, flulike symptoms, nausea and vomiting, or meningismus may occur. Bilateral optic neuritis and weakness, due to optic neuritis and myelitis, respectively, are common. Other patients present with encephalopathy or seizures. | Longitudinally extensive lesions (≥ 3 vertebral segments are present in the spinal cord). There may be enlargement of the intraorbital and intracanalicular segments of the optic nerves on T1-weighted images and hyperintensity on FLAIR and T2-weighted sequences. The chiasm may also be affected. Postgadolinium images may reveal contrast enhancement. MRI of the brain reveals large hemispheric lesions; the hypothalamus, thalamus, periaqueductal gray matter, brainstem, and the cerebellum, may also be affected. | A lymphocytic or neutrophilic pleocytosis is seen in the CSF in 55% of children (median 17, range 5–600). An elevated protein is seen in about half of patients (median 74 mg/dL, range 50–245 mg/dL). Oligoclonal bands are present in approximately 6% of children with NMO. | 1, 81–83, 115 |

Abbreviations: ADEM, acute disseminated encephalomyelitis; AVM, arteriovenous malformation; CIS, clinically isolated syndrome; IPMSSG, International Pediatric Multiple Sclerosis Study Group; CSF, cerebrospinal fluid; FLAIR, fluid-attenuated inversion recovery; IgG, immunoglobulin G; LE, longitudinally extensive; MRI, magnetic resonance imaging; MS, multiple sclerosis; NMO, neuromyelitis optica; OCB, oligoclonal bands; TM, transverse myelitis; WBC, white blood cell.

a Criteria have been proposed for demyelinating disorders in children; however, none have been validated.

b The diagnosis of these disorders is based on clinical features. MRI, CSF, and laboratory tests are supportive.

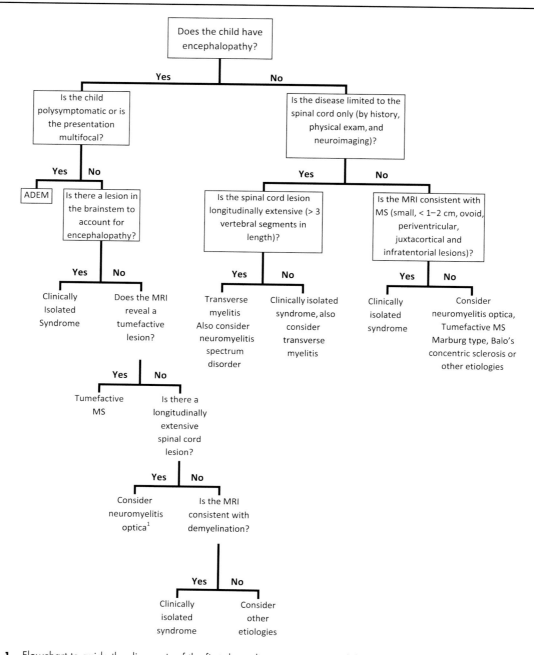

FIGURE 14.1 Flowchart to guide the diagnosis of the first demyelinating event in a child.
[1] While many children present with the classic findings of visual dysfunction or spinal cord symptoms, neuromyelitis optica may present with encephalopathy, seizures, or cranial nerve findings.

■ ACUTE DISSEMINATED ENCEPHALOMYELITIS

Introduction

ADEM has been considered the prototypic demyelinating disease in children as most first-time demyelinating events in children were labeled as ADEM. It is typically a monophasic disease, but relapses and even the subsequent development of MS have been reported. In an effort to better classify those with ADEM versus a suspected first presentation of MS (called a clinically isolated syndrome), consensus definitions were proposed by the International Pediatric Multiple Sclerosis Study Group in 2007 (1). The working definition of ADEM, not yet validated, requires a polysymptomatic presentation and encephalopathy. It is considered inaccurate to call all first demyelinating events ADEM if the event does not meet these two criteria.

Demographics

While ADEM can occur at any age, it is more common in children; especially prepubertal children (mean age 5–8 years). Males and females are equally affected, perhaps with a slight male predominance (2). There does not seem to be a racial or ethnic predominance.

Clinical Features

Children often have a prodrome of generalized malaise/fatigue, fever, headache, nausea, and vomiting prior to the onset of neurologic symptoms (3–6). Encephalopathy, manifested as fatigue or irritability to frank coma, is required for the diagnosis of ADEM according to the International Pediatric Multiple Sclerosis Study Group (1). Furthermore, the definition requires a polysymptomatic and multifocal presentation. Symptoms depend on the sites of inflammation; however, in general, motor symptoms are frequent, with 60% to 95% of children having unilateral or bilateral pyramidal signs (4). Ataxia, cranial neuropathies (including optic neuritis), and seizures are also common. If optic neuritis is present, there is often bilateral involvement. Sensory symptoms are less frequently reported. This may be due to pathophysiologic differences between ADEM and other demyelinating diseases (see Multiple Sclerosis, below) or simply because the severity of other neurologic symptoms and encephalopathy compromise the sensory examination.

Classically, ADEM has been diagnosed following an antecedent illness or vaccination in the month prior to the onset of neurologic symptoms. However, such an immune trigger is not always recognized, and a history of infection or vaccination is not required for the diagnosis of ADEM (2,4).

Imaging

A head computed tomography (CT) reveals multiple lesions in the white matter, but typically does not capture the extent of disease and may even be normal (5,7,8). The appearance of lesions on MRI is variable in ADEM. Most children present with diffuse fluid-attenuated inversion recovery (FLAIR) or T2-weighted hyperintense lesions of brain and spinal cord that are large (> 1–2 cm) and asymmetric with poorly defined margins. Basal ganglia and thalamic involvement may occur, with or without other supratentorial or infratentorial lesions. Spinal cord involvement is also common. Smaller lesions (< 5 mm) resembling MS are also possible.

Enhancement is variable. Some have proposed that all lesions should enhance indicating their acute nature since this would demonstrate a monophasic time course. In contrast, in MS there may be both enhancing and nonenhancing lesions suggesting prior episodes and a more chronic recurrent process. However, in some patients with ADEM both enhancing and nonenhancing lesions may occur, so the presence of some nonenhancing lesions should not alter the diagnosis. In addition, the development of lesions on MRI may lag behind the clinical symptoms in ADEM. Similarly, the MRI may reveal new or enlarging lesions within the first 3 months, even in the setting of clinical improvement.

Cerebrospinal Fluid

A lymphocytic pleocytosis (mean 51 cells/mm^3, range 0–270) or elevated protein (mean 73.9 mg/dL, range 45–120) was seen in 70% to 75% of patients who underwent a lumbar puncture (2,5,7). Other markers of CNS inflammation, such as the presence of oligoclonal bands, immunoglobulin G (IgG) synthesis, or myelin basic protein may be present in the cerebrospinal fluid (CSF), especially during the acute phase. According to some series, oligoclonal bands are present in 4% to 29% of children with ADEM (2,3,5,7), but they were not present in any patient with ADEM in another large study (9).

Prognosis, Recurrent ADEM, and Multiphasic ADEM

The prognosis is generally favorable, and most children with ADEM make a full recovery without sequelae. Residual deficits depend on the clinical sites involved, and the most common deficits are motor problems, visual impairment, cognitive impairment, behavioral problems, and seizures (4,7).

Relapse may occur after a first neurologic event consistent with ADEM. If symptoms recur within the first 3 months, this is considered part of the initial presentation and does not qualify as a relapse (Figure 14.2). Similarly,

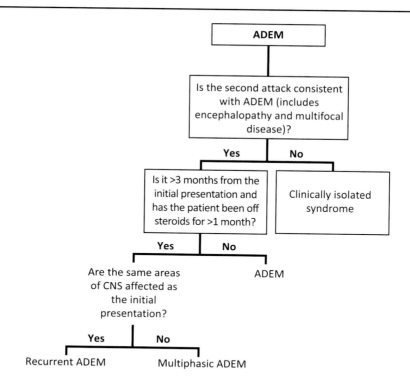

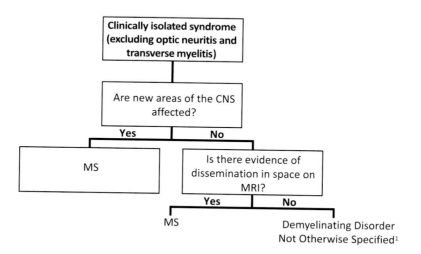

FIGURE 14.2 *Flowchart to guide the diagnosis of recurrent demyelinating diseases. The pathways depend on the initial diagnosis.*

[1] A relapse of a clinically isolated syndrome affecting the same area of the central nervous system fulfills dissemination in time; however, dissemination in space is required for a definition of pediatric multiple sclerosis.

[2] The diagnosis of neuromyelitis optica (NMO) requires the presence of both optic neuritis and spinal cord disease. In children who have one but not both criteria, especially in the setting of relapsing disease that is not consistent with multiple sclerosis, NMO immunoglobulin G (IgG) should be sent. If the serum NMO-IgG is positive the diagnosis is NMO spectrum disorder.

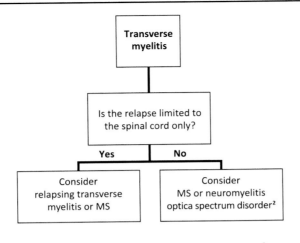

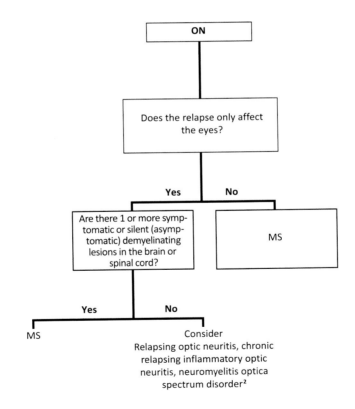

FIGURE 14.2 (*Continued*)

symptom recurrence within 1 month of discontinuing steroids is also considered part of the initial event, and is not considered a relapse. In contrast, neurologic symptoms occurring 3 months after the first episode and more than 1 month after discontinuing steroids may be due to recurrent ADEM, multiphasic ADEM, or MS. If the neurologic symptoms are exactly the same as the initial event (although there may be expansion of an existing lesion), the diagnosis is *recurrent ADEM*. If new symptoms or MRI lesions appear, the diagnosis is *multiphasic*

ADEM. For both recurrent and multiphasic ADEM, the presentation must include encephalopathy. If encephalopathy is not present, a clinically isolated syndrome is the likely diagnosis at the time of the relapse. MS requires 2 non-ADEM events; therefore, a single relapse after ADEM that does not fulfill criteria for ADEM currently does not meet MS criteria (1).

■ ACUTE HEMORRHAGIC LEUKOENCEPHALITIS

Introduction

Acute hemorrhagic leukoencephalitis or acute hemorrhagic encephalomyelitis (AHL or AHEM) is thought to be a fulminant form of ADEM. It may be distinguishable from typical ADEM on head CT or MRI by the presence of edema, mass effect, and hemorrhages (8).

Clinical Features

Similar to ADEM, AHL may follow a respiratory infection in some patients (2); however, a prior illness is not seen in all patients and is not required for the diagnosis. A prodrome of fever, headache, or vomiting may be present for 1 to 2 days prior to the onset of neurologic symptoms (10,11). Altered mental status is present, and various neurologic symptoms, such as weakness and seizures, occur depending on the location of the lesions. Pupillary asymmetry and vital sign instability occurs in the setting of herniation syndromes.

Imaging

Often, the lesions are large and confluent, and they may be unilateral or bilateral (8). A head CT may reveal cortical edema with midline shift or cerebellar involvement with brainstem compression and obstructive hydrocephalus. MRI of the brain may reveal hemorrhages using FLAIR or gradient echo techniques (8), although small, petechial hemorrhages may not appear on MRI.

Cerebrospinal Fluid

A granulocytic pleocytosis is seen in the CSF, and erythrocytes may be present (8). Compared to ADEM, the CSF white blood cell (WBC) and protein counts are often higher in AHL (median CSF WBC 145 and protein 115) compared to ADEM (median CSF WBC 15 and protein 32) (10). Elevations in the CSF IgG synthesis and myelin basic protein, or presence of oligoclonal bands, are also possible. The opening pressure is often elevated.

Prognosis

For AHL, death within 1 week has been reported (2) and 60% of pediatric cases are fatal (10). However, survival may be possible with aggressive treatment (10,11). Two surviving cases with pathologic confirmation were treated with decompressive craniotomies after failed medical management of elevated intracranial pressure (ICP) (10,11). Corticosteroids and other therapies, such as intravenous immunoglobulin (IVIg), have also been used.

■ CLINICALLY ISOLATED SYNDROMES

Introduction

A clinically isolated syndrome is a first demyelinating event in a child or adult that does not meet criteria for ADEM. This is an important distinction for 2 reasons. First, clinically isolated syndromes have a higher likelihood than ADEM of converting to MS. Second, disease modifying therapy is recommended for children and adults presenting with a clinically isolated syndrome who are "high-risk" for the conversion to MS since it delays the onset of MS; therefore, early recognition is essential.

Clinically isolated syndromes are a heterogeneous group of disorders, defined by the affected area within the CNS. The clinical presentation may be monofocal or multifocal. However, in contrast to ADEM, encephalopathy is not present (1), with one exception. If the brainstem is affected, encephalopathy may be present due involvement of the reticular activating syndrome. In this example, the patient may still meet criteria for a clinically isolated syndrome. The two most common clinically isolated syndromes are optic neuritis and transverse myelitis (12).

Optic Neuritis

Introduction

Optic neuritis is a common acquired demyelinating syndrome in children affecting the anterior visual pathway (optic nerve and chiasm). Optic neuritis can be an isolated clinical event without other neurologic signs and symptoms or associated with disseminated demyelination (as in ADEM, MS, or NMO). If isolated optic neuritis is present, the child would not be admitted to the ICU. However, optic neuritis could occur in the context of additional symptoms, and visual impairment may not be appreciated if encephalopathy is present. Optic neuritis may be unilateral or bilateral, and the distribution is defined by clinical history, physical examination, and neuroimaging.

Demographics

Bilateral optic neuritis is more common in younger children. Excluding children with ADEM, 72% of children < 10 years of age present with bilateral optic neuritis whereas 70% of children ≥ 10 years present with unilateral optic neuritis (13).

Clinical Features

The clinical presentation includes decreased visual acuity, contrast sensitivity, and color vision; visual field defects; and pain with extraocular movements in one or both eyes. There is considerable variation in the clinical features. For example, some children may have normal or slightly decreased visual acuity while others have no light perception (14,15). While subtle clinical features are possible, approximately two-thirds of children present with visual acuities of 20/200 or worse (16). The physical exam may reveal a relative afferent pupillary defect in unilateral cases. Fundoscopic exam may reveal disc edema when the inflammation occurs at the papilla (papillitis); however, swelling may not be present in retrobulbar optic neuritis and is therefore not required for a diagnosis. A formal neuroophthalmologic examination is often helpful in confirming the diagnosis and extent of inflammation.

Imaging

MRI of the orbits reveals enlargement of the intraorbital and intracanalicular segments of the optic nerve on T1-weighted images as well as hyperintensity on FLAIR and T2-weighted sequences. Postgadolinium images may reveal contrast enhancement. An MRI of the brain is also indicated, even in the absence of other neurologic signs or symptoms, as the presence of additional FLAIR and T2 hyperintensities outside the optic nerves and chiasm significantly increases the likelihood of developing further clinical attacks and a diagnosis of MS (see Prognosis and the section on Multiple Sclerosis, below) (13). In the United States, 54% of neurologists surveyed about practice patterns also obtain imaging of the cervical and thoracic spine (17). Similar to silent brain lesions, the presence of asymptomatic cord lesions would raise the possibility for MS or NMO, especially in cases of bilateral optic neuritis with longitudinally extensive cord lesions (see below), although such lesions are typically symptomatic.

Cerebrospinal Fluid

A lumbar puncture is not always performed in cases of isolated optic neuritis. In a study assessing practice patterns of U.S. neurologists, more than two-thirds of those surveyed routinely order CSF studies, such as oligoclonal bands or IgG index (17). A lymphocytic pleocytosis has been reported in about 43% to 50% of patients (15,18,19), and elevated protein has been reported in about 10%. In general, oligoclonal bands are seen in about 11% to 17%. The lumbar puncture is perhaps more helpful in patients with optic neuritis and normal MRI of the brain (excluding the optic nerves) as adults with oligoclonal bands in the CSF had an increased likelihood of developing MS (20).

Prognosis

The visual prognosis for children with optic neuritis is excellent. Despite often severe inflammation, most patients recover to a visual acuity of 20/40 or better with a short-course of intravenous (IV) steroids (14) (see treatment, below), although some recover without intervention. Optic neuritis may be a clinically isolated syndrome and never recur or may be the presenting symptom of MS or NMO. MRI scans (brain, C-, and T-spine) and laboratory studies (NMO IgG) can be helpful in identifying patients at risk for disease progression. Optic neuritis can also recur without brain or spine involvement, called sequential or recurrent optic neuritis depending on the affected eye and timing of relapse (in relation to the initial presentation and administration of an oral steroid taper).

CRION has been reported in adults and children (21,22). Initially described in adults, the optic neuritis in CRION is bilateral sequential (both eyes affected within days to weeks of each other) although relapses may occur years later in either eye. Clinically, there is severe pain and poor visual acuity, and MRI scans of the brain are typically normal, all of which help differentiate adult optic neuritis associated with CRION from optic neuritis typical of MS (21).

Transverse Myelitis

Introduction

Transverse myelitis is a demyelinating disease affecting the spinal cord. It is characterized by acute or subacute motor, sensory, and/or autonomic spinal cord dysfunction. Often, spinal cord inflammation occurs in the context of another demyelinating disease, such as ADEM, MS, or NMO, but may also occur as a clinically isolated syndrome. This section will cover transverse myelitis as a clinically isolated syndrome, and the differences between transverse myelitis as a clinically isolated syndrome and the other demyelinating diseases with spinal cord involvement will be highlighted. The terms complete and incomplete transverse myelitis have been used inconsistently; therefore, it is perhaps preferable to avoid such terms and rather describe the clinical and radiographic features.

Demographics

One study of 47 children with acute transverse myelitis at an academic center reported a bimodal incidence in toddlers (< 3 years of age, representing 38% of patients with transverse myelitis), and teenagers (> 11 years, 49%) (23). The remaining 13% were between ages 5 and 8 years. In this study, males and females were equally affected, and no correlation was seen between presentation and time of year. At another pediatric academic center where 38 patients were evaluated, only 5% of children were under the age of 3 years (24). In contrast to the prior study, more females were affected, especially over the age of 10 years. Similarly, when the cases were restricted to only transverse myelitis as a clinically isolated event (ie, without brain lesions or subsequent diagnosis of MS), more females were affected (all ages). In this study, 66% of children presented in colder months (November–April). The differences in demographics between these pediatric studies may be due to varying methodologies and inclusion criteria or referral practices for each academic institution.

Clinical Features

The presence of motor deficits, pain, bladder dysfunction, and sensory involvement should prompt consideration of acute transverse myelitis. A thoracic sensory level is often detected on examination, meaning sensory changes are seen below an identifiable level. However, all spinal levels (cervical through sacral) have been reported (23). Symptoms often progress over days (range 4 hours to 21 days). Symptom nadir typically occurs within 10 days for most patients (25). More rapid progression of symptoms (nadir in less than 4 hours) should raise concern for an ischemic process (26).

Acute transverse myelitis may be a clinically isolated syndrome in which only spinal cord symptoms and signs are present, or it may occur in the setting of MS (spinal cord and brain symptoms) or NMO (spinal cord and optic neuritis).

Imaging

On MRI axial and sagittal T2-weighted images the cord may reveal a single lesion or multiple lesions (< 3 spinal segments in length), longitudinally extensive lesions (≥ 3 spinal segments), or a combination (23,24). Longitudinally extensive lesions are common in ADEM, transverse myelitis (as a clinically isolated syndrome), and NMO, whereas smaller, asymmetric lesions with discrete borders are more common in MS (24). T1-weighted images may reveal expansion of the cord. While the clinical presentation often includes a thoracic sensory level, the MRI burden of disease is often more expansive than suggested by the clinical symptoms (23). Thus, a patient with a thoracic sensory level could have a lesion extending from the cervical cord to the conus. Normal MRI scans of the spinal cord have been reported in children with transverse myelitis (23,24). In such cases, localizable symptoms to the cord and inflammatory CSF profiles are used to establish the diagnosis of transverse myelitis (24).

MRI of the brain and orbits are helpful in assessing the extent of demyelination, especially in patients without referable brain symptomatology (ie, encephalopathy, cranial nerve deficits, seizures, etc), to determine risk for MS and NMO.

Cerebrospinal Fluid

A CSF pleocytosis and elevated protein may be present but are not required for the diagnosis. Normal CSF profiles have been reported in children with acute transverse myelitis (23,24). Markedly elevated CSF WBC should raise suspicion for NMO. The presence of oligoclonal bands is rare in acute transverse myelitis as a clinically isolated syndrome and may indicate that transverse myelitis is the first presentation of MS or a component of ADEM, and an MRI of the brain, if not previously performed, is warranted.

Prognosis

The recovery from neurologic deficits is influenced by associated demyelinating syndromes. Recovery is better if the spinal cord symptoms and signs occur in the setting of ADEM. In MS, spinal cord involvement may improve with time but could also result in persistent symptomatology, such as paresthesias. One pediatric study compared recovery when spinal cord demyelination occurred in the context of MS or as a clinically isolated syndrome. All MS patients were fully ambulatory with milder scores using the Expanded Disability Status Scale. Prognosis was not as favorable in acute transverse myelitis as a clinically isolated syndrome. Roughly 33% of patients recover without sequelae or minor neurologic symptoms, 33% have moderate deficits, and 33% have severe deficits. When part of a clinically isolated syndrome, children with motor and sensory deficits as well as bladder dysfunction were more likely to have permanent paralysis compared to children with partial syndromes (motor and/or sensory and/or bladder, but not all 3 symptoms) (24). In addition to motor symptoms, bladder dysfunction is a common long-term complication from acute transverse myelitis.

In adults with acute transverse myelitis, poor recovery was associated with rapid symptom progression, back pain, and spinal shock (26–30); however, rapid progression was not associated with poor outcome in a pediatric study (23). The same pediatric study reported that prompt diagnosis of acute transverse myelitis (< 7 days) resulted in improved outcomes (23); however,

time to treatment was not a factor in another pediatric study (24).

There have been a few pediatric deaths in children with acute transverse myelitis. High cervical cord lesions may result in respiratory failure (23). As many children are critically ill due to flaccid paralysis and respiratory difficulties, the acute treatment may be complicated by the failure of other systems. One death was reported during the acute hospitalization due to complications from a pulmonary embolus (24).

Approximately 70% to 90% of cases of acute transverse myelitis are truly isolated events that do not relapse or progress (25). There are a number of factors that help differentiate monophasic transverse myelitis from a first presentation of MS. The presence of one or more of the following is suggestive of a first presentation of MS: (1) predominantly sensory symptoms with motor preservation, (2) asymmetric examination, (3) discrete spinal cord lesions (less than two spinal segments), (4) positive oligoclonal bands in the CSF, and (5) an abnormal MRI of the brain (26). Longitudinally extensive MRI lesions, especially in the presence of optic neuritis or deep gray/brainstem lesions, should prompt consideration of NMO. Finally, transverse myelitis can relapse without brain MRI lesions or other features suggestive of MS or NMO (31).

■ MULTIPLE SCLEROSIS

Introduction

MS is the prototypical chronic demyelinating disease, and is one of the most common causes of neurologic disability in the world. Classically, MS has been diagnosed clinically by evidence of two CNS lesions "typical of MS" disseminated in time and space (32). More recently, criteria have been refined to include evidence from MRI (33,34). Acute, potentially devastating variants of MS include Marburg type, tumefactive MS, and to a lesser degree, Balo concentric sclerosis.

Demographics

In prepubertal children, MS affects males and females equally, or perhaps has a slight male predominance (35). However, postpuberty, there is a 2:1 female to male ratio. A higher proportion of African American and Hispanic children have been reported in pediatric MS compared to adult MS (36–38).

Clinical Features

The clinical symptoms of pediatric MS are quite variable depending on the areas of the brain and spinal cord affected. Pediatric MS most commonly presents with sensory symptoms (39,40) including numbness, tingling, or burning, present for more than 24 hours (and typically lasting 2–4 weeks), or optic neuritis (36). Such cases would not be admitted to the critical care unit. Other clinically isolated syndromes (such as some cases of transverse myelitis, as detailed above, or brainstem lesions) are more likely to require critical care observation and treatment. Children may also have motor problems, cranial neuropathies, cerebellar signs, vestibular disease, bowel and bladder involvement, cognitive problems, or fatigue.

Imaging

MS lesions classically appear hyperintense on T2-weighted or FLAIR imaging and hypointense on T1-weighted imaging. MS lesions are commonly found in the periventricular white matter, corpus callosum, junctions of the gray-white matter (called juxtacortical), and the spinal cord (41–44). The presence of one or more periventricular lesions is predictive of MS (45). Discrete lesions (with well-defined borders) and lesions perpendicular to the corpus callosum are also highly suggestive of pediatric MS (46) but may not be present on an initial MRI (45). Brainstem lesions (47,48) and large tumor-like lesions exhibiting mass effect (49,50) have been reported in fulminant cases (see below).

In general, the anatomic location and size of T2-weighted hyperintense lesions correlate well with histopathologic findings (51). Over time, the hypointensity of T1 lesions may increase or decrease, based on the permanence or reversibility of the process (52). Chronically, T1-hypointensity in MS lesions (called "black holes") are associated with severe white matter destruction, including axonal loss (53). T1-lesion load correlates well with changes in neurologic disability (54). Moreover, in children, the presence of T1 lesions, especially such lesions that are present on repeat imaging, are highly predictive of MS (45).

In adults, new lesions in MS typically enhance for an average of 3 weeks (range 1–13 weeks) (55). However, contrast-enhancement of lesions is not necessarily captured at the time of a first attack. At the time of the initial presentation, only 25% to 70% of children had enhancing lesions (45,46).

Cerebrospinal Fluid

A lymphocytic pleocytosis (median 8/μL, range 0–61/μL) is seen in about two-thirds of children with MS (56). Protein may also be elevated. The presence of oligoclonal bands is estimated between 40% to 90% of children with pediatric MS (57).

Prognosis

Recovery from MS flares is variable. Without treatment, symptoms may resolve within a few weeks. The use of corticosteroids may hasten recovery (58). While randomized controlled trials investigating the use of corticosteroids in adults with MS flares have confirmed their benefit in the treatment of acute symptoms, their long-term effect on disease progression or disability has not been proven (59,60).

Compared to adults, children experience more relapses, especially within the first few years of disease onset (38). This finding was confirmed when adjusted for sex, race, and disease modifying therapy. A natural history study revealed a median time to secondary progressive MS of 28.1 years in children versus 18.8 years in adults (61). While pediatric MS is more slowly progressive compared to adult-onset MS, children reach disability endpoints at earlier ages (41.4 years of age versus 52.1 years in adults). Frequent relapses and disability at younger ages were also seen in earlier studies (40,62).

Fulminant Disease—Marburg Type

Introduction

Marburg type of MS was originally described in 1906 as an MS variant with a fulminant course (63,64). The original cases were described as showing "hypercellular demyelinating plaques, with oedema, faint astroglial reaction, and presence of hypertrophic and giant astrocytes" (65). This fulminant demyelinating disease presents with acute lesions appearing to be of the same age in the context of a rapidly, progressive clinical course. Pathologically, there is extensive macrophage infiltration (47). Despite case reports detailing the pathology, imaging, and biochemical features of aggressive cases of demyelinating disease,

Marburg type remains best defined clinically by its rapidly progressive development and evolution of neurologic deficits. There has been one case of "acute multiple sclerosis" in a child, although this was likely Balo concentric sclerosis (see below) (66).

Clinical Presentation

Marburg type may present similarly to exacerbations or relapses of more typical forms of MS. Initial neurologic signs and symptoms may be focal or multifocal with variable severity. The rapid worsening of neurologic signs and the emergence of new deficits over the course of days to weeks is a hallmark of Marburg type. Neurologic signs may include gross motor and sensory disturbances, involvement of the anterior visual pathway, bulbar dysfunction, and areflexia (47). Respiratory failure may necessitate mechanical ventilation (67).

Imaging

Head CT may be normal (68) or may show a large hypodensity in the white matter or multiple hypodensities (63). Brain MRI reveals single or multiple hypointensities on T1-weighted images and hyperintensities on T2-weighted or FLAIR images, often with rim or diffuse enhancement (65,69).

Cerebrospinal Fluid

Similar to other demyelinating diseases, a pleocytosis, elevated protein, or markers of inflammation (the presence of oligoclonal bands, or elevated IgG synthesis or myelin basic protein) may be present.

Prognosis

Many patients die within a few months despite aggressive therapy (63,68,70). While survival has been reported, such cases may not truly reflect Marburg type (69,71).

Fulminant Disease—Balo Concentric Sclerosis

Introduction

Balo concentric sclerosis has long been considered a rare and acute variant of MS. In 1928, Balo originally described the condition in a 23 year-old law student presenting with aphasia and absent cremasteric reflexes, followed by diffuse neurologic signs, including facial weakness, hemiplegia, and incontinence, resulting in death (72,73). Autopsy revealed concentric lesions with alternating layers of normal and degenerated white matter, leading Balo to call the entity "encephalitis periaxialis concentric" (72).

Clinical Features

Many patients present with the acute onset of weakness, although a variety of neurologic symptoms, such as sensory symptoms, visual deficits, cognitive problems, and bulbar dysfunction, has been reported (74). The clinical manifestations are dependent on the regions of the brain affected.

Imaging

The MRI of the brain reveals a concentric pattern of hypodensities and hyperdensities in the white matter. After contrast administration, a thin border of enhancement is seen at the periphery of the lesion (8), and this is the key to differentiating Balo concentric sclerosis from other demyelinating disorders.

Cerebrospinal Fluid

Similar to other demyelinating diseases, a pleocytosis, elevated protein, or markers of inflammation (the presence of oligoclonal bands, or elevated IgG synthesis or myelin basic protein) may be present.

Prognosis

Early in the characterization of the disease, many adult cases were found to have resulted in death within weeks to months following onset. However, before the advent of MRI, when definitive diagnosis relied on postmortem pathologic study, patient selection for biopsy was based on the severity of the disease, allowing for the possibility of missing cases of Balo concentric sclerosis with a more benign course, thereby precluding diagnosis. Correlation of modern neuroimaging studies with pathologic findings has enabled antemortem diagnosis of Balo concentric sclerosis. This has lead to a trend in recent reports of Balo concentric sclerosis cases exhibiting prolonged survival, spontaneous remission, and an overall more benign disease course (74,75).

Pediatric Cases

Balo concentric sclerosis has been described in a 13-year-old female, who presented with hemianopsia and anomia (76). She had an elevated CSF WBC count (30 cell/μL) and large lesions with alternating hypointensities and hyperintensities on MRI in a concentric pattern with enhancement. She was also found to be positive for human herpesvirus 6. She was initially treated with IV methylprednisolone and foscarnet. Six months later, she deteriorated and was retreated with the same medications; however, she continued to progress and IVIg was initiated. She received IVIg monthly with clinical improvement and no further relapses.

There is one other reported case of a child with acute multiple sclerosis, published in 1965 in the case records of the Massachusetts General Hospital in the *New England Journal of Medicine* (66). A 6-year-old female presented 1 week after a brief respiratory illness and 3 days after a fall from a "horizontal bar" without loss of consciousness. Neurologic symptoms began hours after the fall, including blurry vision, and progressed over the next few days to include left hemiparesis, slurred speech, a right gaze preference, and she became unresponsive. Her temperature rose to 108°F. Her CSF did not reveal cells or an elevated protein, although the initial lumbar puncture revealed "a pressure of 100 mm." She was unresponsive to pain with fixed, unresponsive pupils, arm extension with increased tone, and flaccid paralysis of the lower extremities. For the increased pressure, neurosurgical intervention was required, and she had bilateral burr holes placed. She was treated with methylprednisolone, antibiotics, and phenytoin. She had multisystem organ failure requiring respiratory, cardiac, nutritional, and hematologic support. She developed seizures and further increases in ICP. Due to the poor prognosis, she was extubated. She died on hospital day 31. Pathology revealed diffuse perivascular lesions throughout the brain that varied in size and had clearly demarcated areas of demyelination. In addition, some of the "smaller lesions had a striking concentric pattern suggestive of altering zones of greater and lesser intensity of myelin." A dense cellular infiltrate consisting of macrophages was seen in larger lesions. She was diagnosed with acute multiple sclerosis.

Fulminant Disease—Tumefactive MS

Introduction

MS typically presents with small, discrete lesions in the periventricular, juxtacortical, or infratentorial brain. However, other patients have larger lesions in the brain with surrounding edema on head CT or brain MRI. Such lesions are called tumefactive and the imaging features

may raise concern for a malignancy, often resulting in a biopsy. However, clinical and radiographic characteristics suggestive of demyelination are described below to help distinguish a demyelinating disorder from a malignancy.

Clinical Features

Symptoms depend on the location of the tumefactive lesion. For example, acute weakness, cranial nerve involvement (including optic neuritis), and ataxia may be seen. Patients may present with headaches, seizures, nausea, and vomiting, which are uncommon in MS.

Imaging

Head CT may be normal or reveal hypodensities of the white matter. Patchy rim enhancement may be present on a postcontrast head CT. On T2-weighted or FLAIR MRI, lesions appear hyperintense in the periventricular white matter in older children. The lesions in younger children are present in the subcortical white matter. Rim enhancement of the lesion may be complete or incomplete. Greater enhancement may be seen on the side facing the ventricle (77). Spinal cord lesions may also be present.

Cerebrospinal Fluid

There are few reports of CSF findings in tumefactive MS in children. An elevated CSF WBC was seen (range 12–63 cells/μL), all had a normal CSF protein (77,78). In a single study, oligoclonal bands were present in one of the three children (78).

Prognosis

For some children, the disease is monophasic, without relapses, and the term "tumefactive MS" is a misnomer. However, for other children, tumefactive demyelination occurs during the course of MS. In other words, the initial presentation may be typical of MS; however, a relapse may include a tumefactive lesion.

■ NEUROMYELITIS OPTICA

Introduction

NMO (also known as Devic disease) is a demyelinating disease with predilection for the optic nerves and spinal cord. Initially thought to be a variant of MS, NMO is now believed to be a different demyelinating disease, largely due to the identification of a serum biomarker, IgG autoantibody (NMO-IgG), which may be present in the CSF as well (79,80). The clinical features of optic neuritis and spinal cord involvement are required for the diagnosis, which may be confirmed by the presence of the NMO-IgG antibody. Children who do not meet the clinical criteria, but are NMO-IgG positive, are often diagnosed with "NMO spectrum disorder."

Demographics

NMO spans the pediatric age spectrum, from 2–18 years (81). Females are predominantly affected (81,82). Two pediatric studies have noted a higher proportion of African-American children (34%–66%) compared to white children (27%–33%). Hispanic children are also affected (10%–33%) as well as Native American children (9%) (81,82). While NMO was previously thought to be more common in Asian adults, there were no Asian children in these cohorts.

Clinical Features

A prodrome of fever, viral illness, nausea, vomiting, hiccups, or meningeal signs may precede neurologic symptoms (81). Visual disturbance and weakness from optic neuritis and spinal cord disease, respectively, are the most common presenting symptoms (82). Vision loss is often bilateral and severe. Symptoms localizable to the brain, such encephalopathy, seizures, cranial nerve findings (other than optic neuritis), are common and should not preclude a diagnosis of NMO.

Diagnosis

While the evaluation is similar for most acquired demyelinating syndromes (see below), there are particularly important laboratory studies. First, there is an IgG autoantibody (NMO-IgG) that has been identified in the serum and CSF of pediatric and adult patients with NMO (79). The NMO-IgG antibody binds to an aquaporin-4 channel in the astrocytic foot processes in the blood-brain barrier. The presence of antibody in the serum (which is preferred) or CSF is not necessary for the diagnosis, which requires the presence of transverse myelitis and optic neuritis. Therefore, those with a negative NMO-IgG antibody may still be diagnosed with NMO (or NMO spectrum disorder if diagnostic criteria are not met). NMO-IgG positivity is dependent

upon treatment status, and may even appear later in the disease after an initial negative test (82).

NMO is associated with many other autoimmune diseases, such autoimmune rheumatologic, thyroid, and gastrointestinal diseases, and elevated antibodies (antinuclear antibodies and antiphospholipid antibodies) (83). Therefore, additional laboratory studies are required to further investigate these conditions.

Imaging

Spine MRI typically reveals longitudinally extensive lesions (≥ 3 vertebral segments); however, similar lesions are seen in ADEM, transverse myelitis, and, less frequently, MS (84). As described above, the optic nerves may reveal enlargement of the intraorbital and intracanalicular segments on T1-weighted images and hyperintensity on FLAIR and T2-weighted sequences. Postgadolinium images may reveal contrast enhancement. Children with NMO also have involvement of the optic chiasm. Brain MRI may reveal large hemispheric lesions or smaller lesions in the hypothalamus, thalamus, periaqueductal gray matter, brainstem, or cerebellum.

Cerebrospinal Fluid

A pleocytosis is seen in the CSF in 55% of children (median 17, range 5–600, with 50% lymphocytic and 50% neutrophilic) (81). While many patients have a low CSF WBC, others will have a markedly elevated CSF WBC, which should raise suspicion for NMO. Protein elevations are also seen in about half of patients (median 74 mg/dL, range 50–245 mg/dL). Oligoclonal bands are present in approximately 6% of children with NMO (81).

Prognosis

NMO is a relapsing disease, and recovery after an attack is often incomplete. Many children have residual weakness or visual impairment. NMO is associated with higher disability than MS in children. Death has been reported in adults with NMO (5-year survival of 68%) due to respiratory failure in the setting of brainstem disease (85,86). Fortunately, pediatric deaths due to NMO have not been reported.

Unique to NMO, there are comorbid or associated diagnoses that warrant further investigation. The hypothalamic-pituitary axis may be affected resulting in menstrual irregularities and the syndrome of inappropriate antidiuretic hormone. In addition, as noted above, patients with NMO often have symptoms or serologic evidence of other autoimmune diseases.

■ GENERAL APPROACH TO SUSPECTED DEMYELINATING DISEASE

History

The history of patients with demyelinating disease is markedly heterogeneous, even within the specific clinical entities. Nevertheless, a detailed history is critical to prompt disease recognition and the initiation of treatment. Isolated or multifocal neurologic signs and symptoms localizing to the CNS should give rise to increased clinical suspicion for these conditions. Symptoms may involve motor, sensory, cranial nerve, brainstem, cerebellar, cognitive, and/or autonomic deficits. Motor symptoms may localize to cerebral white matter, brainstem, or spinal cord. Deficits may result in weakness or paresis and may be focal or multifocal. Sensory deficits may include numbness or abnormal pain, temperature, or vibratory sensation. Lhermitte sign, which is an "electric-shock–like" sensation running down the spine or limbs associated with neck flexion or extension, may be present and is pathognomonic for cervical spinal cord disease. Bowel, bladder, and sexual dysfunction may be present in various forms and degrees of severity.

Seizures are more common in ADEM than MS. Isolated sensory symptoms, which are unlikely to require ICU care, are often present in MS whereas pyramidal involvement is more likely in ADEM, transverse myelitis, and NMO. Optic neuritis may be seen in ADEM, MS, NMO, infectious diseases, and other inflammatory or autoimmune disorders, or present as a clinically isolated syndrome.

Following a presentation suspicious for acute demyelination, the subsequent history should attempt to further support or refute specific etiologies and explore other potential diagnoses (Table 14.2). A history of prior demyelinating events is supportive of MS or NMO, or rarely, recurrent or multiphasic ADEM. Recent viral infection or vaccination is more commonly reported in ADEM and transverse myelitis than MS, although the exacerbation of MS symptoms can occur with an increase in body temperature (Uhthoff phenomenon). Such episodes may occur with a fever or illness or occur with exercise, hot showers, baths, or saunas, or hot weather.

Depending on the history, the differential diagnosis may still be broad, including rheumatologic/inflammatory, infectious, neoplastic, vascular, nutritional, toxic/metabolic, and traumatic causes (Table 14.2). Given the potentially large differential diagnosis, a thorough review of systems should be performed. Pertinent questions include fever, unintentional weight loss, abnormal skin changes or rashes, myalgias, arthralgias, hemoptysis, nosebleeds, hematuria, and abdominal pain. Neck stiffness and fever have been reported in acute transverse myelitis, making the distinction from meningitis/encephalitis difficult. Past medical history should address prior neurologic events, oncologic history, reasons for potential immunodeficiency, such as HIV, corticosteroid use, and transplant history, history of tuberculosis, sarcoidosis, fungal infections, glomerulonephritis, and sexually transmitted infections, most notably syphilis.

Social history should include questions regarding residence, pets (ie, cats), travel, diet, rigorous exercise, or trauma to identify risk factors for neuroborreliosis, toxoplasmosis, HTLV1 and 2, B_{12} deficiency, fibrocartilaginous embolic myelopathy, spinal cord compression, arterial dissection, etc. Additional questions regarding sexual activity, alcohol consumption, smoking habits, illicit drug use, and history of incarceration may be relevant depending on age to address risk factors for HIV, tuberculosis, and neurosyphilis. All of these conditions, many of which are rare, present with symptoms that mimic demyelinating disease. A family history of demyelinating disease, or a masquerading condition, may be supportive.

Physical Exam

Some aspects of the physical examination warrant particular attention. Mental status assessment, corroborated with baseline status and behavioral alterations, gathered from family and friends if necessary, should be used to discern encephalopathy, which is required for the diagnosis of ADEM, recurrent ADEM, and multiphasic ADEM, but may also be seen in NMO and rarely in MS.

Cranial nerve dysfunction, particularly involving the optic nerve and the ocular motor pathways, may be present. Signs of optic nerve dysfunction may include decreased visual acuity, color vision deficits, visual field defects, decreased contrast sensitivity, and pupillary

Table 14.2 Differential Diagnosis for Demyelinating Disorders in Children	
Rheumatologic disorders	PACNS
	Other vasculitis
	Sarcoidosis
	Sjögren syndrome
	Systemic lupus erythematosus
	Behçet syndrome
	Familial Mediterranean fever
	Anticardiolipin or antiphospholipid syndrome
	Scleroderma
Infectious diseases	Neuroborreliosis
	HIV
	Neurosyphilis
	HTLV
	Herpes viruses (HSV, VZV, HHV-6)
	Progressive multifocal leukoencephalopathy (JC virus)
	Mycoplasma
	Tuberculosis
	Neurocysticercosis
Neoplastic disorders	CNS lymphoma
	Glioma (especially low-grade gliomas or astrocytomas and optic pathway gliomas)
	Lymphoproliferative disorders
Vascular diseases	Watershed infarction
	CADASIL
Other neurologic conditions	Migraine
	Leukodystrophies
Nutritional	B$_{12}$ or folate deficiency
	Celiac disease
Toxic/metabolic	Mitochondrial disorders
	Congenital or hereditary optic neuropathy (such as Leber hereditary optic neuropathy, Kjer dominant optic neuropathy)
	Medications (infliximab, adalimumab, etanercept, amiodarone, cisplatin, digitalis, isoniazide, lead, methotrexate, organophosphates, tacrolimus, vincristine)
	PRES (also known as hypertensive encephalopathy or reversible posterior leukoencephalopathy syndrome)
	Thyroid disease (Hashimoto encephalopathy)
Trauma	Carotid dissection
	Concussion
	Fibrocartilaginous embolic myopathy
	Spinal cord compression

Abbreviations: CADASIL, cerebral autosomal dominant arteriopathy with subcortical infarcts and leukoencephalopathy; CNS, central nervous system; HHV-6, human herpes virus 6; HSV, herpes simplex virus; JC virus, John Cunningham virus; PACNS, primary angitis of the CNS; PRES, posterior reversible encephalopathy syndrome; VZV, varicella zoster virus.
Source: Adapted from Refs. 92, 116.

defects. Cranial nerves III, IV, and VI may be involved, impairing extraocular motility. Certain deficits of extraocular movements are characteristic of demyelinating diseases. Specific insult to the median longitudinal fasciculus (MLF) results in internuclear ophthalmoplegia (INO), clinically manifested as an adduction deficit on lateral conjugate gaze in the ipsilateral eye relative to the lesion. Such MLF lesions may be bilateral. If the brainstem lesion encompasses the abducens nucleus or the paramedian pontine reticular formation on the side ipsilateral to the MLF lesion, a "one and a half syndrome" may be apparent, in which only abduction in the eye contralateral to the lesion is preserved. Both INO and one and a half syndrome may be present in acute demyelinating disease, particularly MS; however, they are not specific to demyelinating diseases as other brainstem insults may result in their cause. Cranial nerves V, VII, and VIII may also be involved, resulting in trigeminal neuralgia or neuropathy, facial spasm or palsy, and vertigo, respectively.

Standard motor and sensory exams should attempt to localize lesions. Upper motor neuron signs localizing lesions to the CNS include hyperreflexia, spasticity, and a Babinski sign. Flaccid paralysis should raise suspicion for spinal cord or brainstem involvement. The sensory exam should pay attention to the sensory modalities (ie, pain, temperature, vibration) affected and the distribution of findings. While sensory symptoms may be due to lesions anywhere in the CNS, a sensory level may be helpful in differentiating between brain and spinal cord disease. The presence of a sensory level is not specific for transverse myelitis and may be seen in the other demyelinating diseases (ADEM, clinically isolated syndromes, MS, and NMO). The presence of encephalopathy or cranial nerve findings provides further evidence for brain involvement and helps differentiate these disorders.

Diagnosis

All demyelinating disorders are clinical diagnoses, and suggested diagnostic criteria for acquired demyelinating syndromes are presented in Table 14.1. However, there is considerable overlap between these diseases. Moreover, clinically silent lesions or CSF inflammation may be present thereby suggesting another disorder; therefore, additional tests are performed to improve diagnostic accuracy.

When considering certain diseases, such as malignancy in the setting of a large monofocal lesion on MRI, definitive diagnosis may be made by pathology; however, this is not always necessary as a detailed history, physical exam, and additional testing (MRI and CSF analysis) may provide further clues for demyelination. To assist in differentiating tumefactive lesions from CNS malignancies, Morin et al (78) have suggested that the following characteristics suggest demyelinating disease: (1) rapid evolution of clinical symptoms, typically within 1 week, (2) signs and symptoms of multifocal CNS involvement (especially if the MRI reveals only a single lesion), (3) recent viral infection by history, CSF, or laboratory evaluation, (4) MRI evidence of preferential white matter involvement, often with relative sparing of the cortex, (5) lesions exhibit little mass effect, and (6) treatment with corticosteroids results in rapid improvement in the MRI appearance.

Additional Considerations

The diagnosis of demyelinating disorders should not be dependent on age. While there is a higher prevalence of ADEM in prepubertal children compared to postpubertal children or adults, ADEM can occur at any age. MS is more common in older children but may be diagnosed in prepubertal children as well. Transverse myelitis can be seen in toddlers, and NMO has been reported across the pediatric age spectrum.

The latency in ADEM between antecedent illness and neurologic symptoms is approximately 2 weeks; however, this duration is much shorter in some patients (range 2–31 days) (7,9). The diagnosis of ADEM is often delayed in such patients, who are often diagnosed with infectious diseases, such as viral meningoencephalitis. Treatment with steroids is also delayed due to concern for the worsening of an infection, although the delay in initiating steroids due to this fear is often unwarranted (see below).

Optic neuritis may be associated with other demyelinating diseases or present as a clinically isolated syndrome. Younger children are more likely to present with bilateral optic neuritis or bilateral sequential optic neuritis (in which one eye is affected within a few weeks of the other eye), and children ≥ 10 years of age are more likely to present with unilateral optic neuritis. The presence of unilateral or bilateral disease does not influence the risk of MS (13). In children with unilateral or bilateral optic neuritis, the strongest predictor of MS is the presence of one or more lesion(s) in the brain (not including the optic nerves or chiasm). Accounting for such lesions, the risk of MS also increases with age in children presenting with optic neuritis.

Imaging

Head CT may be performed initially to explore other or emergent intracranial processes, such as aneurysm or subarachnoid hemorrhage, hemorrhagic infarct, or impending herniation from edema due to a variety of causes. However, MRI is the neuroimaging test of choice for demyelinating diseases. Depending upon the presenting symptoms, MRI of the brain, cervical, and/or thoracic spine may be required to define the extent of demyelination. Lesions in the conus and sacrum have been reported so imaging of the lower spine or conus should be considered if there are referable symptoms. Due to scheduling issues or patient instability, it may not be possible to obtain all of these images at one time, but acquisition should be attempted as early in the hospital course as possible. Even in a case of transverse myelitis, a brain MRI is indicated as radiographic disease without clinical signs or symptoms (silent lesions) are important in distinguishing transverse myelitis from MS.

While there are distinguishing characteristics which differentiate various demyelinating diseases from one another, these disorders share several common features. Conventional techniques used in the diagnosis include noncontrast T1-weighted, T2-weighted, and postcontrast (gadolinium) T1-weighted techniques (87). Generally, inflammatory demyelinating lesions share similar patterns of intensity and enhancement. Lesions on T2-weighted imaging appear hyperintense. T2-hyperintensity is nonspecific and may represent a range of underlying pathology such as inflammation, edema, demyelination, axonal loss, and Wallerian degeneration (41). Lesions on T1-weighted imaging appear hypointense, and have been referred to as black holes. Contrast-enhanced MRI with IV gadolinium is useful in identifying active demyelinating disease and assessing treatment effects. Gadolinium reaches areas of the CNS from the circulation via breaks in the blood-brain barrier, which may occur as the result of inflammation.

The size, number, location, distribution, and enhancement pattern of lesions suspicious for demyelination may help to further narrow the differential diagnosis. In children presenting with their first demyelinating event, the presence of T1 lesions on MRI is highly suggestive of MS (45). MS lesions are often discrete ovoid lesions affecting the periventricular white matter but are also seen in the white matter adjacent to the cortex (juxtacortical), brainstem, cerebellum, and spinal cord. While MS is a chronic relapsing disease, it is possible to confirm dissemination in space and dissemination in time in a child with a clinically isolated syndrome if MRI criteria are met (33). In a child with a clinically isolated syndrome, dissemination in space is confirmed by the presence of one or more T2-weighted lesions in at least two of the four following areas: periventricular, juxtacortical, infratentorial, and spinal cord. Dissemination in time is verified by the simultaneous presence of asymptomatic gadolinium-enhancing and nonenhancing lesions. Subsequent imaging revealing a new T2 or gadolinium-enhancing lesion can also be used to demonstrate dissemination in time.

Spinal cord lesions in MS are often focal (< 2 spinal segments) whereas longitudinally extensive lesions in the spinal cord are seen in ADEM, transverse myelitis, and NMO. There can be brain lesions, typically in the deep gray structures, thalamus, and brainstem, in NMO.

Similarly, the presence of large, ill-defined regions and thalamic or deep gray lesions are often seen in ADEM. In fact, the presence of thalamic lesions in ADEM may be a good prognostic sign and many of these children did not have a relapsing course (45). The presence of silent (asymptomatic) lesions in the brain or spinal cord in a patient with a clinically isolated syndrome is also suggestive of MS and such patients are considered high risk.

There is a clinicoradiologic paradox in demyelinating disorders (88). In other words, the clinical findings do not always localize to a CNS lesion, and silent lesions, for which there are no clinical symptoms, are frequently observed on neuroimaging.

Cerebrospinal Fluid

Table 14.1 provides a summary of the CSF findings for the demyelinating diseases. CSF analysis and culture is an important tool in the evaluation of CNS demyelinating diseases. CSF WBC and protein may be normal or elevated. Oligoclonal bands identified in the CSF that are not present in the serum indicate the presence of a local B-cell response in the CNS (89). To perform this test, CSF and serum samples must be sent at the same time for comparison. Therefore, a high index of concern for CNS demyelination is necessary for any patient presenting with neurologic signs and symptoms. The test for oligoclonal bands is considered positive if two or more IgG bands are present in the CSF and are not seen in the serum. The laboratory performing the test should use isoelectric focusing (90) and perform such studies regularly. The results must be interpreted with caution if such methods are not employed. Oligoclonal bands are seen in a variety of disorders and are not specific for MS (Table 14.3). Moreover, the presence of oligoclonal bands in the CSF is variable, even in MS, therefore, the presence of oligoclonal bands is not required for a diagnosis of demyelinating disease (91). The presence of oligoclonal bands in transverse myelitis raises concern for MS. Oligoclonal bands are infrequent in NMO. The utility of CSF myelin basic protein is unclear (17) but could be considered as another marker of myelin injury.

Normal Imaging and Cerebrospinal Fluid Studies

Some patients with suspected demyelinating diseases have both normal neuroimaging and CSF profiles at presentation. Such patients should undergo repeat

■ **Table 14.3** Differential Diagnosis for the Presence of Oligoclonal Bands in the Cerebrospinal Fluid

Demyelinating disease	Multiple sclerosis
	Acute disseminated encephalomyelitis (including recurrent ADEM and multiphasic ADEM)
	Clinically isolated syndromes (optic neuritis, transverse myelitis, brainstem and cerebellar syndromes, etc)
	Neuromyelitis optica
	Fulminant demyelinating disease (acute hemorrhagic leukoencephalitis, tumefactive MS, Marburg type, Balo concentric sclerosis)
Rheumatologic disorders	Primary angitis of the CNS (PACNS)
	Other vasculitis
	Sarcoidosis
	Sjögren syndrome
	Systemic lupus erythematosus
	Behçet syndrome
	Familial Mediterranean fever
	Anticardiolipin syndrome
Infectious diseases	Neuroborreliosis
	HIV
	Neurosyphilis
	Subacute sclerosis panencephalitis
	Herpes viruses (HSV, VZV, HHV-6)
	Viral meningoencephalitis
	Tuberculosis
Neoplastic disorders	CNS lymphoma
	Astrocytoma
	Germinoma
	Paraneoplastic syndromes
	Lymphoproliferative disorders
Vascular diseases	Infarction
	Cerebral hemorrhage
Other neurologic conditions	Creutzfeldt-Jakob disease
	Neuromyotonia
	Stiff person syndrome
	Inflammatory neuropathies
	Sydenham chorea
	Polyneuropathy
	Guillian-Barré syndrome (acute inflammatory demyelinating polyneuroapathy)
	CIDP
	Opsoclonus/myoclonus
	PLP1 mutations (gene associated with Pelizaeus-Merzbacher)
	Progressive myoclonic epilepsy
	Rasmussen encephalitis
	Limbic encephalitis
	Postinfectious encephalitis
	Paraneoplastic subacute cerebellar degeneration
Other	Vogt-Koyanagi-Harada syndrome

Abbreviation: CIDP, chronic inflammatory demyelinating polyneuropathy.
The presence of oligoclonal bands has been reported in patients with these disorders. The diagnosis of any disorder is dependent on the clinical history, physical examination, laboratory studies, and radiographic findings. See Table 14.2 for the differential diagnosis for demyelinating disorders.
Source: Adapted from Refs. 90, 117–124.

evaluations in approximately 1 to 2 weeks if the symptoms have not improved as the inflammation detected by these tests may lag behind the clinical symptoms.

Laboratory Studies

The broad differential diagnosis in a patient with suspected demyelinating disease necessitates several laboratory tests (Table 14.2). Rheumatologic, inflammatory, infectious, neoplastic, vascular, nutritional, toxic/metabolic, and traumatic disorders may be responsible for the presentation of focal or multifocal neurologic deficits localizing to the CNS. The determination of which tests are necessary in any given patient may be made on a case-by-case basis considering the clinical presentation of the patient in the context of prior medical history, laboratory findings, and imaging results. While some suggest that Lyme and HIV be excluded in every patient suspected of having MS (92), a study of U.S. neurologists did not reveal a consensus in the evaluation of a patient with suspected inflammatory demyelination (17).

Suggested blood tests include a complete blood count, erythrocyte sedimentation rate, NMO-IgG (serum), antinuclear antibody (ANA) profile (ANA, double-stranded DNA, or DNA biding, SS-A, SS-B, anti-SM, and anti-RNP), angiotensin-converting enzyme, antiphospholipid antibodies, B_{12}, and folate. Additional studies should be selected based on the history, examination, and imaging findings. Risk of MS may be influenced by the exposure to Epstein-Barr virus (EBV), vitamin D deficiency, or genetic susceptibility (31); therefore, EBV serologies, vitamin D 25-OH level, and HLA-DRB1*15 genotype are obtained, even though the results may not impact the acute care.

■ MANAGEMENT

Neurocritical Care

As with any significant or life-threatening illness, the patient's airway, breathing, and circulation should be assessed. Respiratory difficulties can occur in the setting of upper cervical cord lesions, and some patients may require intubation and respiratory support. Vital sign abnormalities may occur in patients with edema and mass effect. While midline shift and herniation syndromes are uncommon in MS, these may occur in fulminant demyelinating diseases with extensive inflammation (AHL, Marburg type, Balo concentric sclerosis, tumefactive MS).

If there are signs of elevated ICP, medical management should be initiated. If medical management is not successful, it may be necessary to place an ICP monitoring device and attempt to reduce the pressure. If elevated ICP remains refractory, and neuroimaging suggests mass effect or herniation, decompressive hemicraniectomy may be warranted (10,11,50). Decompressive hemicraniectomy has been used with success in pediatric patients with AHL (10,11). If the disease threatens life via maximum neurologic deficit, and not mass effect, hemicraniectomy would be unlikely to improve prognosis.

Corticosteroids

Treatment guidelines are based on suppressing the body's inflammatory response. Regardless of the demyelinating phenotype, initial treatment consists of high-dose, pulsed, IV corticosteroids. A typical treatment regimen consists of IV methylprednisolone, 15 to 30 mg/kg/day (maximum 1000 mg/day) for 3 to 5 days (17,93). While clinical trials have not been performed in pediatric demyelinating diseases, improved neurologic outcomes have been shown in multiple studies (9,94–96). Most neurologists recommend a steroid taper, although the length (ie, number of weeks) and dose have not been established (17). Some studies have concluded that relapses of disease are more common with short steroid tapers (mean of 3 weeks) compared to longer courses (mean of 6 weeks) (7,97); however, the side effects of steroids also need to be considered.

In children presenting with acute neurologic failure due to suspected demyelinating disease, the administration of corticosteroids should occur promptly. Often, corticosteroids are held due to concern for an underlying CNS infection, especially if the demyelinating disease presents with fever and meningismus (as can be seen in ADEM and NMO). However, current data support a benefit to the administration of steroids, even in the setting of bacterial meningitis (11). Furthermore, the delay in administering steroids cannot be justified in fulminant demyelinating disease. Payne et al (11) summarize recent studies refuting the belief that corticosteroids are harmful in CNS infections. Benefit from corticosteroids has been seen in herpes simplex encephalitis, *Haemophilus influenza* type B, and pneuomococcal meningitis.

For patients on high-dose corticosteroids, gastrointestinal prophylaxis is recommended for possible gastritis. One patient with ADEM treated with corticosteroids died after gastrointestinal bleeding (24). Other potential side effects include hypertension, insomnia, psychosis, hyperglycemia, hypokalemia, and avascular necrosis. Avascular necrosis has occurred in a patient on corticosteroids for less than 1 month (98,99).

Plasma Exchange

Plasma exchange has been used acutely in acquired demyelinating disorders. In adult randomized controlled trials (plasma exchange vs sham exchange), plasma exchange hastened recovery from acute symptoms (100,101). There are no randomized controlled trials in children; however, case reports and case series of children with various demyelinating disorders report benefit (102–105). In the critical care setting, aggressive treatment with plasma exchange (after failure to improve with corticosteroids) is warranted to hasten neurologic recovery. Patients with NMO at one academic center are treated with plasma exchange on day 7 if there has been no improvement after a 5 day course of IV methylprednisolone (30 mg/kg/day, with a maximum of 1 g/day, for 5 days) (82,83). A similar protocol has been proposed by other academic centers for acute demyelinating diseases with poor response to IV steroids (personal communication).

The optimal number and frequency of exchanges is not defined. Protocols using continuous flow centrifugation with 5 to 7 exchanges over 14 days (1.1 plasma volumes with 3.5% to 5% albumin) have been used. Common side effects include anemia and hypotension. Serious adverse events include infection (sepsis) from indwelling catheters. Rare complications that have been reported in adults include endotoxic shock, heparin-associated thrombocytopenia, pulmonary embolism, and death (100,101).

Intravenous Immunoglobulin

IVIg has been used in a number of autoimmune neurologic diseases. While randomized clinical trials have not been performed, benefit from IVIg has been demonstrated in pediatric demyelinating patients with diffuse cerebral and spinal cord involvement (106–108). Dramatic recovery has been seen in children, such as reversal of paralysis within days of receiving IVIg (109). In this patient, there was no response to corticosteroids, which were administered 2 weeks prior to the IVIg.

Similar severe cases of patients who were obtunded, quadriparetic, and required respiratory support showed dramatic improvement with IVIg, which was administered after a course of IV steroids (108). Publication bias may play a role in the reporting of severe encephalomyelitis responding to IVIg. Nevertheless, many experts believe that IVIg should be administered to those who have failed corticosteroids or those with contraindications to corticosteroids or plasma exchange (82,83,93,108).

An IVIg dose of 2 g/kg divided over 2 to 5 days is recommended. Common side effects include headache, nausea, vomiting, and aseptic meningitis. Pretreatment with acetaminophen and diphenhydramine are recommended. Prior to initiating treatment with IVIg, an IgA level may be checked as patients with IgA deficiency may develop anaphylaxis due to the presence of small amounts of IgA in pooled IVIg (110).

Cyclophosphamide

When other therapies fail, cyclophosphamide may be considered. In one study describing the use of cyclophosphamide in pediatric MS, various protocols were used: (1) induction therapy alone, (2) induction therapy followed by maintenance therapy, and (3) maintenance therapy alone (111). Many of the children in this cohort were receiving disease modifying therapy for MS or plasma exchange or steroids, or a combination of therapies. Overall, children treated with cyclophosphamide had a decrease in relapse rate and disability stabilized. Common side effects included nausea and vomiting, alopecia, and, as expected, pancytopenia. One patient developed bladder cancer and was successfully treated. Therefore, mesna is recommended for bladder prophylaxis.

Cyclophosphamide has also been used in the acute treatment of NMO (83). A one-time (induction) dose of 750 to 1000 mg/m^2 is recommended if there is no response to corticosteroids and plasma exchange.

Other Medications

Demyelinating diseases, especially transverse myelitis, NMO, and MS, may cause neuropathic pain, spasticity, fatigue, bladder dysfunction, or depression. Such symptoms require treatment; however, this may not be appropriate for the critical care setting as these symptoms may improve with the treatments listed above. Additional information on the symptomatic therapy can be found elsewhere (112,113).

Therapy

Physical, occupational, and/or speech therapy may be required depending upon the areas of the CNS affected. Many patients also require inpatient rehabilitation after their acute hospitalization. Otherwise, outpatient therapy may be arranged for children with residual deficits.

Disease Modifying Therapy

Patients fulfilling diagnostic criteria for MS or NMO and those identified as high risk for these disorders should be started on disease modifying therapy or immunosuppression (for NMO and NMO spectrum disorders). Such long-term therapy should be started by a neurologist and is often not appropriate for the ICU setting. The risks and benefits should be reviewed with the family with careful consideration of the age of the patient. Compliance with these therapies is improved if their benefits are clearly explained to the family; therefore, treatment is best recommended by a child neurologist with expertise in demyelinating diseases.

■ CONCLUSIONS

Acquired demyelinating syndromes, especially those affecting the brainstem and spinal cord, may require an admission to the ICU. Clinical symptoms may suggest a particular demyelinating disease; however, considerable overlap between the disorders exists. The evaluation of these disorders includes MRI scans of the brain, C-, and T-spine, a spinal tap, and blood work for mimics of demyelination. Treatment is also similar for acute demyelinating diseases. IV methylprednisolone is recommended; IVIg and plasma exchange are also commonly used. A pediatric neurologist with expertise in demyelinating diseases should be consulted for the long-term prognosis and management of these children.

■ REFERENCES

1. Krupp LB, Banwell B, Tenembaum S. Consensus definitions proposed for pediatric multiple sclerosis and related disorders. *Neurology.* 2007;68(16 suppl 2):S7–S12.
2. Hahn JS, Tenembaum S. Clinical and biological features of acute disseminated encephalomyelitis. In: Chabas D, Waubant E, eds. *Demyelinating Disorders of the Central Nervous System in Childhood.* New York, NY: Cambridge University Press; 2011:183–201.
3. Hynson JL et al. Clinical and neuroradiologic features of acute disseminated encephalomyelitis in children. *Neurology.* 2001;56(10):1308–1312.
4. Tenembaum S et al. Acute disseminated encephalomyelitis. *Neurology.* 2007;68(16 suppl 2):S23–S36.
5. Murthy SN et al. Acute disseminated encephalomyelitis in children. *Pediatrics.* 2002;110(2 pt 1):e21.
6. Brass SD et al. Multiple sclerosis vs acute disseminated encephalomyelitis in childhood. *Pediatric Neurology.* 2003;29(3):227–231.
7. Dale RC et al. Acute disseminated encephalomyelitis, multiphasic disseminated encephalomyelitis and multiple sclerosis in children. *Brain.* 2000;123(pt 12):2407–2422.
8. van der Knaap MS, Valk J. *Magnetic Resonance of Myelination and Myelin Disorders.* 3rd ed. New York, NY: Springer; 2005.
9. Tenembaum S, Chamoles N, Fejerman N. Acute disseminated encephalomyelitis: a long-term follow-up study of 84 pediatric patients. *Neurology.* 2002;59(8):1224–1231.
10. Leake JA et al. Pediatric acute hemorrhagic leukoencephalitis: report of a surviving patient and review. *Clin Infect Dis.* 2002;34(5):699–703.
11. Payne ET et al. Treatment leading to dramatic recovery in acute hemorrhagic leukoencephalitis. *J Child Neurol.* 2007;22(1):109–113.
12. Banwell B et al. Incidence of acquired demyelination of the CNS in Canadian children. *Neurology.* 2009;72(3): 232–239.
13. Waldman AT et al. Pediatric optic neuritis and risk of multiple sclerosis: meta-analysis of observational studies. *J AAPOS.* 2011;15(5):441–446.
14. Bonhomme GR et al. Pediatric optic neuritis: brain MRI abnormalities and risk of multiple sclerosis. *Neurology.* 2009;72(10):881–885.
15. Wilejto M et al. The clinical features, MRI findings, and outcome of optic neuritis in children. *Neurology.* 2006;67(2):258–262.
16. Waldman AT, Balcer LJ, Pediatric optic neuritis. In: Chabas D, Waubant E, eds. *Demyelinating Disorders of the Central Nervous System in Childhood.* New York, N: Cambridge University Press; 2011:223–233.
17. Waldman AT et al. Management of pediatric central nervous system demyelinating disorders: consensus of United States neurologists. *J Child Neurol.* 2011;26(6):675–682.
18. Alper G, Wang L. Demyelinating optic neuritis in children. *J Child Neurol.* 2009;24(1):45–48.
19. Brady KM et al. Optic neuritis in children: clinical features and visual outcome. *J AAPOS.* 1999;3(2):98–103.
20. Cole SR et al. The predictive value of CSF oligoclonal banding for MS 5 years after optic neuritis. Optic Neuritis Study Group. *Neurology.* 1998;51(3):885–887.
21. Kidd D et al. Chronic relapsing inflammatory optic neuropathy (CRION). *Brain.* 2003;126(pt 2):276–284.
22. Yeh EA et al. Retinal nerve fiber thickness in inflammatory demyelinating diseases of childhood onset. *Mult Scler.* 2009;15(7):802–810.
23. Pidcock FS et al. Acute transverse myelitis in childhood: center-based analysis of 47 cases. *Neurology.* 2007;68(18):1474–1480.
24. Thomas T et al. The demographic, clinical, and magnetic resonance imaging (MRI) features of transverse myelitis in children. *J Child Neurol.* 2012;27(1):11–21.

25. Pidcock FS, Sebire G. What is acute transverse myelitis in children? In: Chabas D, Waubant E, eds. *Demyelinating Disorders of the Central Nervous System in Childhood*. New York, NY: Cambridge University Press; 2011:243–254.

26. Proposed diagnostic criteria and nosology of acute transverse myelitis. *Neurology*. 2002;59(4):499–505.

27. Ford B, Tampieri D, Francis G, Long-term follow-up of acute partial transverse myelopathy. *Neurology*. 1992;42(1): 250–252.

28. Kalita J, Misra UK, Mandal SK, Prognostic predictors of acute transverse myelitis. *Acta Neurol Scand*. 1998;98(1):60–63.

29. Lipton HL, Teasdall RD. Acute transverse myelopathy in adults. A follow-up study. *Arch Neurol*. 1973;28(4):252–257.

30. Ropper AH, Poskanzer DC, The prognosis of acute and subacute transverse myelopathy based on early signs and symptoms. *Ann Neurol*. 1978;4(1):51–59.

31. Banwell B et al. Clinical, environmental, and genetic determinants of multiple sclerosis in children with acute demyelination: a prospective national cohort study. *Lancet Neurol*. 2011;10(5):436–445.

32. Poser CM et al. New diagnostic criteria for multiple sclerosis: guidelines for research protocols. *Ann Neurol*. 1983;13(3):227–231.

33. Polman CH et al. Diagnostic criteria for multiple sclerosis: 2010 revisions to the McDonald criteria. *Ann Neurol*. 2011;69(2):292–302.

34. McDonald WI et al. Recommended diagnostic criteria for multiple sclerosis: guidelines from the International Panel on the diagnosis of multiple sclerosis. *Ann Neurol*. 2001;50(1):121–127.

35. Pohl D. Epidemiology, immunopathogenesis and management of pediatric central nervous system inflammatory demyelinating conditions. *Curr Opin Neurol*. 2008;21(3):366–372.

36. Chitnis T et al. Demographics of pediatric-onset multiple sclerosis in an MS center population from the Northeastern United States. *Mult Scler*. 2009;15(5):627–631.

37. Langer-Gould A et al. Incidence of acquired CNS demyelinating syndromes in a multiethnic cohort of children. *Neurology*. 2011;77(12):1143–1148.

38. Gorman MP et al. Increased relapse rate in pediatric-onset compared with adult-onset multiple sclerosis. *Arch Neurol*. 2009;66(1):54–59.

39. Duquette P et al. Multiple sclerosis in childhood: clinical profile in 125 patients. *J Pediatr*. 1987;111:359–363.

40. Boiko A et al. Early onset multiple sclerosis: a longitudinal study. *Neurology*. 2002;59(7):1006–1010.

41. Zivadinov R, Bakshi R, Role of MRI in multiple sclerosis I: inflammation and lesions. *Front Biosci*. 2004;9:665–683.

42. Bakshi R et al. Magnetic resonance imaging findings in 22 cases of myelitis: comparison between patients with and without multiple sclerosis. *Eur J Neurol*. 1998;5(1):35–48.

43. Grossman RI, Barkhof F, Filippi M. Assessment of spinal cord damage in MS using MRI. *J Neurol Sci*. 2000;172(suppl 1):S36–S39.

44. Bot JC et al. Spinal cord abnormalities in recently diagnosed MS patients: added value of spinal MRI examination. *Neurology*. 2004;62(2):226–233.

45. Verhey LH et al. MRI parameters for prediction of multiple sclerosis diagnosis in children with acute CNS demyelination: a prospective national cohort study. *Lancet Neurol*. 2011;10(12):1065–1073.

46. Mikaeloff Y et al. MRI prognostic factors for relapse after acute CNS inflammatory demyelination in childhood. *Brain*. 2004;127(pt 9):1942–1947.

47. Johnson MD, Lavin P, Whetsell WO Jr. Fulminant monophasic multiple sclerosis, Marburg's type. *J Neurol Neurosurg Psychiatry*. 1990;53(10):918–921.

48. Giubilei F et al. Four-year follow-up of a case of acute multiple sclerosis of the Marburg type. *Ital J Neurol Sci*. 1997;18(3):163–166.

49. Wood DD et al. Acute multiple sclerosis (Marburg type) is associated with developmentally immature myelin basic protein. *Ann Neurol*. 1996;40(1):18–24.

50. Gonzalez Sanchez JJ et al. A case of malignant monophasic multiple sclerosis (Marburg's disease type) successfully treated with decompressive hemicraniectomy. *J Neurol Neurosurg Psychiatry*. 2010;81(9):1056–1057.

51. Newcombe J et al. Histopathology of multiple sclerosis lesions detected by magnetic resonance imaging in unfixed postmortem central nervous system tissue. *Brain*. 1991;114(pt 2):1013–1023.

52. Bitsch A et al. A longitudinal MRI study of histopathologically defined hypointense multiple sclerosis lesions. *Ann Neurol*. 2001;49(6):793–796.

53. van Walderveen MA et al. Histopathologic correlate of hypointense lesions on T1-weighted spin-echo MRI in multiple sclerosis. *Neurology*. 1998;50(5):1282–1288.

54. Truyen L et al. Accumulation of hypointense lesions ("black holes") on T1 spin-echo MRI correlates with disease progression in multiple sclerosis. *Neurology*. 1996;47(6):1469–1476.

55. Cotton F et al. MRI contrast uptake in new lesions in relapsing-remitting MS followed at weekly intervals. *Neurology*. 2003; 60(4):640–646.

56. Pohl D et al. CSF characteristics in early-onset multiple sclerosis. *Neurology*. 2004;63(10):1966–1967.

57. Ness JM et al. Clinical features of children and adolescents with multiple sclerosis. *Neurology*. 2007;68(16 suppl 2):S37–S45.

58. Beck RW et al. A randomized, controlled trial of corticosteroids in the treatment of acute optic neuritis. The Optic Neuritis Study Group. *N Engl J Med*. 1992;326(9):581–588.

59. Filippini G, Brusaferri F, Sibley WA, Citterio A, Ciucci G, Midgard R, Candelise L. Corticosteroids or ACTH for acute exacerbations in multiple sclerosis. *Cochrane Database of Systematic Reviews* 2000(4):CD001331: 10.1002/14651858. CD001331

60. Ciccone A, Beretta S, Brusaferri F, Galea I, Protti A, Spreafico C. Corticosteroids for the long-term treatment in multiple sclerosis. *Cochrane Database of Systematic Reviews* 2008(1): CD006264: 10.1002/14651858.CD006264

61. Renoux C et al. Natural history of multiple sclerosis with childhood onset. *N Engl J Med*. 2007;356(25):2603–2613.

62. Simone IL et al. Course and prognosis in early-onset MS: comparison with adult-onset forms. *Neurology*. 2002;59(12):1922–1928.

63. Mendez MF, Pogacar S. Malignant monophasic multiple-sclerosis or Marburgs disease. *Neurology*. 1988;38(7): 1153–1155.

64. Marburg O. Die sogenannte "akute multiple Skerose." *Jhrb Psychiatr Neurol*. 1906(27):211–312.

65. Capello E, Mancardi GL, Marburg type and Balo's concentric sclerosis: rare and acute variants of multiple sclerosis. *Neurol Sci*. 2004;25(suppl 4):S361–S363.

66. Case records of the Massachusetts General Hospital. Case 43-1965. *N Engl J Med.* 1965;273(14):760–767.

67. Bitsch A et al. Lesion development in Marburg's type of acute multiple sclerosis: from inflammation to demyelination. *Mult Scler.* 1999;5(3):138–146.

68. Johnson MD, Lavin P, Whetsell WO Jr. Fulminant monophasic multiple sclerosis, Marburg's type. *J Neurol Neurosurg Psychiatry.* 1990;53(10):918–921.

69. Walid MS, Sanoufa M. The diagnosis of Marburg disease is course-dependent. *GMS Ger Med Sci.* 2010;8:Doc06. 10.3205/000095. urn:de:0183-0000958

70. Wood DD et al. Acute multiple sclerosis (Marburg type) is associated with developmentally immature myelin basic protein. *Ann Neurol.* 1996;40(1):18–24.

71. Jeffery DR, Lefkowitz DS, Crittenden JP, Treatment of Marburg variant multiple sclerosis with mitoxantrone. *J Neuroimag.* 2004;14(1):58–62.

72. Balo J. Encephalitis periaxialis concentrica. *Arch Neurol Psychiatry.* 1928;19:242–264.

73. Pearce JM. Balo's encephalitis periaxialis concentrica. *Eur Neurol.* 2007;57(1):59–61.

74. Karaarslan E et al. Balo's concentric sclerosis: clinical and radiologic features of five cases. *AJNR Am J Neuroradiol.* 2001;22(7):1362–1367.

75. Yao DL et al. Concentric sclerosis (Balo): morphometric and in situ hybridization study of lesions in six patients. *Ann Neurol.* 1994;35(1):18–30.

76. Pohl D et al. Balo's concentric sclerosis associated with primary human herpesvirus 6 infection. *J Neurol Neurosurg Psychiatry.* 2005;76(12):1723–1725.

77. McAdam LC, Blaser SI, Banwell BL, Pediatric tumefactive demyelination: case series and review of the literature. *Pediatr Neurol.* 2002;26(1):18–25.

78. Morin MP et al. Solitary tumefactive demyelinating lesions in children. *J Child Neurol.* 2011;26(8):995–999.

79. Lennon VA et al. IgG marker of optic-spinal multiple sclerosis binds to the aquaporin-4 water channel. *J Exp Med.* 2005;202(4):473–477.

80. Lennon VA et al. A serum autoantibody marker of neuromyelitis optica: distinction from multiple sclerosis. *Lancet.* 2004;364(9451):2106–2112.

81. McKeon A et al. CNS aquaporin-4 autoimmunity in children. *Neurology.* 2008;71(2):93–100.

82. Lotze TE et al. Spectrum of pediatric neuromyelitis optica. *Pediatrics.* 2008;122(5):e1039–e1047.

83. McKeon A, Lotze TE, Neuromyelitis optica in children. In: Chabas D, Waubant E, eds. *Demyelinating Disorders of the Central Nervous System in Childhood.* New York, NY: Cambridge University Press; 2011:255–271.

84. Banwell B et al. Neuromyelitis optica-IgG in childhood inflammatory demyelinating CNS disorders. *Neurology.* 2008;70(5):344–352.

85. Wingerchuk DM et al. The clinical course of neuromyelitis optica (Devic's syndrome). *Neurology.* 1999;53(5):1107–1114.

86. Wingerchuk DM, Weinshenker BG. Neuromyelitis optica: clinical predictors of a relapsing course and survival. *Neurology.* 2003;60(5):848–853.

87. Bakshi R et al. The use of magnetic resonance imaging in the diagnosis and long-term management of multiple sclerosis. *Neurology.* 2004;63(11 suppl 5):S3–S11.

88. Barkhof F. The clinico-radiological paradox in multiple sclerosis revisited. *Curr Opin Neurol.* 2002;15(3):239–245.

89. Link H, Huang YM. Oligoclonal bands in multiple sclerosis cerebrospinal fluid: an update on methodology and clinical usefulness. *J Neuroimmunol.* 2006;180(1–2):17–28.

90. Mygland A et al. Isoelectric focusing is superior to immunofixation electrophoresis in diagnosing CNS inflammation. *Acta Neurologica Scandinavica.* 2007;115(2):122–125.

91. Polman CH et al. Diagnostic criteria for multiple sclerosis: 2005 revisions to the "McDonald Criteria". *Ann Neurol.* 2005;58(6):840–846.

92. Hahn JS et al. Differential diagnosis and evaluation in pediatric multiple sclerosis. *Neurology.* 2007;68(16 suppl 2):S13–S22.

93. Waldman AT, Tardieu M. Treatment and prognosis of acute disseminated encephalomyelitis. In: Chabas D, Waubant E, eds. *Demyelinating Disorders of the Central Nervous System in Childhood.* New York, NY: Cambridge University Press; 2011:212–222.

94. Lahat E et al. Rapid recovery from transverse myelopathy in children treated with methylprednisolone. *Pediatr Neurol.* 1998;19(4):279–282.

95. Straub J, Chofflon M, Delavelle J. Early high-dose intravenous methylprednisolone in acute disseminated encephalomyelitis: a successful recovery. *Neurology.* 1997;49(4):1145–1147.

96. Sebire G et al. High dose methylprednisolone in severe acute transverse myelopathy. *Arch Dis Child.* 1997;76(2):167–168.

97. Anlar B et al. Acute disseminated encephalomyelitis in children: outcome and prognosis. *Neuropediatrics.* 2003;34(4):194–199.

98. Richards RN. Short-term corticosteroids and avascular necrosis: medical and legal realities. *Cutis.* 2007;80(4):343–348.

99. Richards RN. Side effects of short-term oral corticosteroids. *J Cutan Med Surg.* 2008;12(2):77–81.

100. Weiner HL et al. Double-blind study of true vs. sham plasma exchange in patients treated with immunosuppression for acute attacks of multiple sclerosis. *Neurology.* 1989;39(9):1143–1149.

101. Weinshenker BG et al. A randomized trial of plasma exchange in acute central nervous system inflammatory demyelinating disease. *Ann Neurol.* 1999;46(6):878–886.

102. Khurana DS et al. Acute disseminated encephalomyelitis in children: discordant neurologic and neuroimaging abnormalities and response to plasmapheresis. *Pediatrics.* 2005;116(2):431–436.

103. Balestri P et al. Plasmapheresis in a child affected by acute disseminated encephalomyelitis. *Brain Dev.* 2000;22(2):123–126.

104. Miyazawa R et al. Plasmapheresis in fulminant acute disseminated encephalomyelitis. *Brain Dev.* 2001; 23(6):424–426.

105. Takahashi I et al. Childhood multiple sclerosis treated with plasmapheresis. *Pediatr Neurol.* 1997;17(1):83–87.

106. Kleiman M, Brunquell P. Acute disseminated encephalomyelitis: response to intravenous immunoglobulin. *J Child Neurol.* 1995;10(6):481–483.

107. Nishikawa M et al. Intravenous immunoglobulin therapy in acute disseminated encephalomyelitis. *Pediatr Neurol.* 1999;21(2):583–586.

108. Pradhan S et al. Intravenous immunoglobulin therapy in acute disseminated encephalomyelitis. *J Neurol Sci.* 1999;165(1):56–61.

109. Shahar E et al. Outcome of severe encephalomyelitis in children: effect of high-dose methylprednisolone and immunoglobulins. *J Child Neurol.* 2002;17(11):810–814.
110. Bashir K. Plasma exchange and IV immunoglobulin for acute demyelinating relapses. In: Chabas D, Waubant E, eds. *Demyelinating Disorders of the Central Nervous System in Childhood.* New York: Cambridge University Press; 2011:87–91.
111. Makhani N et al. Cyclophosphamide therapy in pediatric multiple sclerosis. *Neurology.* 2009;72(24):2076–2082.
112. Pohl D et al. Treatment of pediatric multiple sclerosis and variants. *Neurology.* 2007;68(16 suppl 2):S54–S65.
113. Venkateswaran S, Bennett S, Ness J. Symptomatic therapy in pediatric multiple sclerosis. In: Chabas, D, Waubant E, eds. *Demyelinating Disorders of the Central Nervous System in Childhood.* New York: Cambridge University Press; 2011:112–133.
114. Alper G, Heyman R, Wang L, Multiple sclerosis and acute disseminated encephalomyelitis diagnosed in children after long-term follow-up: comparison of presenting features. *Dev Med Child Neurol.* 2009;51(6):480–486.
115. Wingerchuk DM et al. Revised diagnostic criteria for neuromyelitis optica. *Neurology.* 2006;66(10):1485–1489.
116. Kuntz NL, Strober JB, Differential diagnosis of multiple sclerosis and acquired central nervous system demyelinating disorders in children and adolescents. In: Chabas D, Waubant E, eds. *Demeylinating Disorders of the Central Nervous System in Childhood.* New York: Cambridge University Press; 2011:58–74.
117. Iivanainen M et al. Oligoclonal bands in myoclonus epilepsy—reply. *Arch Neurol.* 1982;1982(39):321.
118. Iivanainen M et al. CSF oligoclonal bands, immunoglobulins, and viral antibodies in progressive myoclonus epilepsy. *Arc Neurol.* 1981;38(4):206–208.
119. Akman-Demir G et al. Inflammatory/demyelinating central nervous system involvement in familial Mediterranean fever (FMF): coincidence or association? *J Neurol.* 2006;253:928–934.
120. Bien CG et al. Slowly progressive hemiparesis in childhood as a consequence of Rasmussen encephalitis without or with delayed-onset seizures. *Eur J Neurol.* 2007;14(4):387–390.
121. Mehling M, Kuhle J, Regeniter A, 10 most commonly asked questions about cerebrospinal fluid characteristics in demyelinating disorders of the central nervous system. *Neurologist.* 2008;14(1):60–65.
122. Keshgegian AA. Oligoclonal bands in myoclonus epilepsy. *Arch Neurol.* 1982;39(5):321.
123. Gorman MP et al. Steroid-responsive neurologic relapses in a child with a proteolipid protein-1 mutation. *Neurology.* 2007;68(16):1305–1307.
124. Bourahoui A et al. CSF isoelectrofocusing in a large cohort of MS and other neurological diseases. *Eur J Neurol.* 2004;11:525–529.

15 Spinal Cord Disease and Injury

SHIH-SHAN LANG and LAUREN A. BESLOW

■ INTRODUCTION

Spinal cord injury (SCI) in pediatric patients is fortunately an uncommon event, and it represents a distinct entity from the adult SCI population in incidence, complications, and injury patterns. Only approximately 5% of all traumatic SCI occurs in children; in children the number of head injuries greatly outweighs the number of spine injuries (1). Since children have a greater head-to-body ratio than adults, this leads to a set of problems unique to the pediatric population. Management may also be complex because of the potential difficulty in obtaining a thorough history and physical examination. Treatment and intervention for SCI in the pediatric population is usually extrapolated from adult protocols and algorithms. There has been a shortage of literature analyzing outcome measures of pediatric long-term neurologic functions and quality of life after SCI. The most up-to-date treatment for pediatric patients with SCI encompasses traditional and historical techniques of prevention of secondary injury and spine stabilization. SCI also encompasses some rarer causes such as infection, tumors, vascular malformations, arterial ischemia, and demyelination. Demyelinating SCI is described in Chapter 14.

■ ANATOMY

Clinical care must be adjusted to account for differences in anatomical landmarks and growth of the pediatric patient. In infants, the location of the conus medullaris is much lower than in the adult, ending near the sacrum. Therefore, injury to the lower lumbar spine in infants may result in damage to the spinal cord. The inherent elasticity of the spinal column in infants and young children results in the classic and historical entity of "spinal cord injury without radiographic abnormality," abbreviated in the literature as "SCIWORA." SCIWORA is common, usually recoverable injury, accounting for a third of SCI in children (2). The spinal cord can stretch only a quarter inch in infants but the rest of the spinal column can stretch 2 inches (3). This means the spinal cord sustains considerable injury, but the damage to the bony structures and ligaments is trivial (4). Before the advent of magnetic resonance imagine (MRI), plain x-rays were unable to identify fractures or malalignment of the spine. Since many cases of SCIWORA were described prior to MRI, it is likely that a subset of these patients actually suffered from arterial spinal cord infarction.

■ PRESENTATIONS

The clinical presentation of acute SCI or disease depends on the levels of the injury and also on the rapidity of the process. For example, a trauma may present with acute paralysis while compression from metastases or a vascular malformation may present with progressive back pain, possibly accompanied by worsening weakness, and sensory or bladder symptoms. Acute myelopathy can present with spinal shock, a disruption of all reflex arcs characterized by flaccid plegia, absent sensation, absent reflexes, absent bowel and bladder tone, and priapism. Even without complete disruption of the cord, some children will have a flaccid paralysis with absent reflexes for days while some children develop spasticity and hyperreflexia quickly, even in the acute setting. Weakness of the arms and legs indicates that the process is affecting the cervical level, and depending on the cervical level affected, certain muscle groups may be intact while others have severe deficits. Additionally, cervical injuries may be accompanied by sensory deficits, respiratory difficulties, and loss of bladder and bowel control. Thoracic injuries can present with leg weakness, sensory deficits with preserved arm strength, and bowel and bladder dysfunction. Any injury above the T6 level that disrupts normal sympathetic outflow from the T1-L2 levels can present with neurogenic shock, a triad of hypotension, bradycardia, and peripheral vasodilation. Lumbar cord disease may present with leg weakness, decreased sensation there, decreased rectal tone, and urinary retention. Conus medullaris syndrome is caused by a sacral cord injury. The lumbar nerve roots may or may not be affected. The symptoms include variable motor and sensory loss in the legs, areflexia of the bladder, and decreased rectal tone. Cauda equina syndrome is caused by injury to the lumbosacral nerve roots in the spinal canal. Symptoms include variable loss of motor and sensory function to the legs, decreased rectal tone, and areflexia of the bladder. The lower extremities are areflexic since the injury is to nerve roots rather than to the cord itself.

When examining the pediatric patient with an acute spinal cord process, a careful and complete examination is paramount. All elements of the examination including tone, motor strength, sensation (pain, light touch, vibration, proprioception), and reflexes (deep tendon, abdominal, cremasteric, anal, plantar response) should be tested. The muscle groups affected and a sensory level can help to establish the diseased level. A motor level is defined as the most caudal muscles that have muscle strength of at least 3/5 or higher while the segment above is normal strength (5/5). A sensory level is the most caudal dermatome with normal sensation to pinprick and light touch. In some cases, particularly when there is flaccid paralysis with absent reflexes, it can be difficult to differentiate processes such as Guillain-Barré syndrome from acute spinal cord processes, but the presence of a sensory level and severely affected rectal tone and bladder retention may help differentiate the

processes. Table 15.1 includes motor functions, sensation, and reflexes affected by injury at some levels.

■ ACUTE STABILIZATION

The acute management of the child with a suspected spinal cord emergency hinges on immobilization and stabilization of the spine in cases of trauma or suspected trauma and on monitoring of autonomic function. Careful examination must be done to evaluate for respiratory compromise needing intubation, blood pressure instability, arrhythmias, and bladder retention. The two major causes of death in SCI are shock and aspiration. Therefore it is crucial to monitor airway and respiratory status as well for blood pressure instability and arrhythmias by using continuous cardiorespiratory monitors. Patients should be constantly evaluated for adequate oxygenation (FiO_2) and adequate ventilation. For children who are not intubated, vital capacity and negative inspiratory force should be followed to assess for respiratory deterioration. Cautious intubation may be required if the C-spine is not yet cleared. A neurologic examination and general examination must be performed since other major injuries may be masked below the level of the SCI. Patients with SCI may have disruption of their bowel and bladder circuits, therefore a urinary catheter is usually required. A nasogastric tube (to low suction) may also be needed to prevent aspiration and to decompress a paralytic ileus that is common in this population.

■ ACUTE IMAGING

Emergent diagnostic neuroimaging, including spine MRI to examine the cord itself and ligaments should be performed so that the pathologic process can be identified and treated immediately. In most cases, sagittal "scout" films of the entire spine should be performed since the full extent of injury may not be evident on the clinical examination. If that is not possible, several levels above and below the clinical level of injury should at least be studied. In many cases, a 1.5 Tesla MRI scanner images the spinal cord with more clarity than the stronger 3 Tesla scanner. If a tumor, infection, demyelinating process, or vascular malformation is suspected, an MRI performed with and without gadolinium should be performed.

■ **Table 15.1**	Motor Functions, Sensation, and Reflexes by Injury Level			
Level	Motor Function	Sensation	Deep Tendon Reflex	Other Reflexes
C5	Elbow flexors and scapula movement	Lateral arm	Biceps	
C6	Wrist extensors and humerus rotation	Lateral forearm, thumb, index finger	Brachioradialis	
C7	Elbow extensors	Index finger and middle finger	Triceps	
C8	Finger flexors	Fourth and fifth finger		
T1	Finger abductors and adductors	Fifth finger and medial arm		
T4		Nipple level		
T10		Navel		Upper abdominal T7-10, lower abdominal T10-L1[a]
T12		Midpoint of inguinal ligament		Cremasteric[b]
L2	Hip flexors	Lateral and midanterior thigh		
L3	Knee extensors	Anterior and medial thigh		
L4	Ankle dorsiflexors	Calf and medial malleolus	Patellar	
L5	First toe dorsiflexor	Lateral calf and dorsum foot		
S1	Ankle plantar flexors	Lateral heel	Achilles	
S2-4		Perianal and posterior thigh		Anal[c]

[a] Abdominal reflexes are elicited by stroking each section of the abdomen and noting whether the umbilicus moves toward the area stroked. Absence of this movement indicates pathology. (Beevor sign is seen in patients with damage to the spinal cord between T6-10. Patients have intact upper abdominal muscles but nonfunctioning lower abdominal muscles. When the patient sits up from a supine position, only the functioning upper abdominal muscles contract, thus the umbilicus is pulled caudally.)
[b] Stroke the inner aspect of the upper thigh. The scrotum pulls upward as the cremasteric muscle contracts.
[c] Gently touch the perianal skin. The external anal sphincter muscle contracts in response.

■ TRAUMA

Traumatic SCI in pediatric patients is an uncommon event, but can be devastating when it occurs. Fortunately, the incidence of traumatic SCI is less than 10% of all patients who have an SCI. Over 60% of SCIs in children occur in the cervical spine and less than 30% occur in the thoracolumbar spine (5). Children have a high head-to-body ratio, a sizeable amount of ligamentous laxity, and underdeveloped paraspinal muscles due to age. Due to these differences in anatomy and physiology, the pediatric population is predisposed to injury of the cervical spine in contrast to adults (6). More specifically, younger children (≤ 8 years) have the tendency for injuries of the upper cervical spine, and older children and adolescents have a predilection for injuries of the lower cervical spine (7). Injuries to the thoracolumbar spine occur more commonly in older children and adolescents and are often accompanied by thoracoabdominal injuries (5,8). The majority of children with cervical spine trauma can be managed nonoperatively with a hard collar or halo with good outcomes. However, it is not always the best quality of life option for a child to wear a hard collar or halo for many weeks. Surgical management such as anterior or posterior fusion and instrumentation may be necessary in severe unstable injuries, or for those patients who have a high likelihood of nonfusion secondary to anatomical or environmental influences (9). Fractures in the pediatric population are uncommon and tend to resemble fractures seen in adults

(Figures 15.1A and B). Fractures in the pediatric population are most often due to trauma.

Atlantooccipital Dislocation

Atlantooccipital dislocation (AOD) is a devastating condition that often ends in cardiorespiratory arrest prior to hospitalization. Historically, AOD had been considered almost always fatal and associated with devastating neurologic injury. The injuries are highly unstable and the mechanism of injury is almost always a hyperextension injury caused by a high velocity injury such as a motor vehicle accident (1). A large force is necessary to disrupt the ligaments that connect the cranium from the rest of the cervical spine. AOD is five times more common in the pediatric population versus the adult population (10). Additionally, children with trisomy 21 have atlantoaxial instability and are at particular risk for AOD with or without subluxation (11). Likely due to a variety of factors including improved prehospital resuscitation, diagnostic imaging, and a higher index of suspicion, there has been an increase in posttraumatic AOD survival rates (12).

Diagnosis can be made with plain cervical radiographs (Figure 15.2A) and is aided with computed tomographic (CT) scans and MRI (Figure 15.2B). For children who survive AOD with an incomplete SCI, the literature supports surgical intervention (occipital-cervical fusion) for older children (Figure 15.2C) and immobilization for infants (10,13,14). The signs of AOD are often subtle, and the possibility of this diagnosis must be kept high on the differential, especially in the pediatric population where ligamentous injury without bony fractures may not be apparent on x-rays or CT. Even in the absence of neurologic signs, a methodical approach to evaluating plain x-rays with subsequent use of CT scans and MRI is essential to identifying AOD.

Pseudosubluxation

Pediatric pseudosubluxation refers to the anterior displacement of C2 (axis) on C3. In children up to 10 years of age, the normal flexion mobility of C2 on C3 of 2 to 3 mm may be misinterpreted for pathologic motion (13). Especially in the presence of cervical muscle spasm, when the head is flexed, there may be an exacerbation of anterior displacement. This anatomical difference occurs because of the increased laxity in ligaments in children and also because of the increase

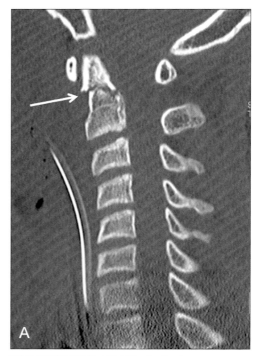

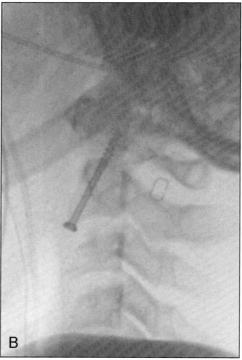

FIGURE 15.1 A 16-year-old male involved in a motor vehicle accident. Lateral C-spine x-ray showed an abnormality, thus a sagittal computed tomographic scan (A) was obtained which showed a type II odontoid fracture (arrow). The patient underwent an anterior instrumented fusion with an odontoid screw (B).

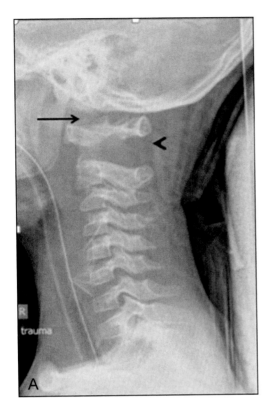
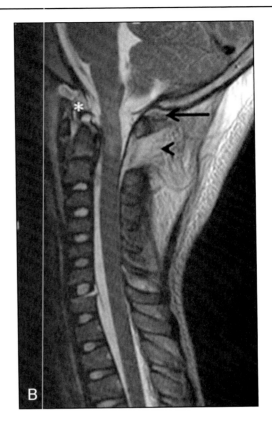
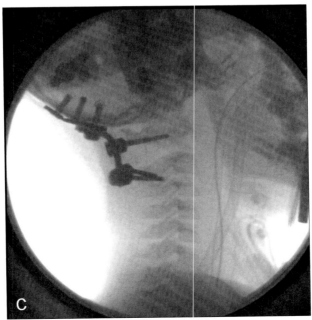

FIGURE 15.2 A 5-year-old boy unrestrained passenger in a motor vehicle accident was found to be quadriplegic but with Glasgow Coma Score of 15. Lateral radiographs (A) and magnetic resonance imaging (MRI) (B) revealed an atlantooccipital (arrow) as well as an atlantoaxial dissociation (arrowhead) with disruption of the cruciate and alar ligaments (asterisk). The patient underwent an occipital to cervical (C2) fusion (C).

in horizontal anatomical alignment of the facet joint than in adults (14).

Pharmacologic Treatment

A recent meta-analysis examined eight adult randomized controlled trials in which steroids were administered in the setting of acute spinal cord injury. Seven of the eight studies used high-dose methylprednisolone. A common regimen was a bolus of 30mg/kg followed by a 24 hour infusion at 5.4mg/kg/hour. The study concluded that steroids improved neurologic outcome at up to one year if started within 8 hours of the injury. One of the trials extended the infusion to 48 hours after injury and demonstrated that additional motor and functional improvement was gained by extending the length of the infusion. This was particularly true in patients in whom the treatment was not begun between 3 and 8 hours of the injury (50). There are no randomized clinical trials for high-dose steroids in the setting of acute pediatric spinal injury, but steroids may be considered in this setting. They are used routinely to decrease edema in other pediatric spine diseases like tumors and vascular malformations. However, in the settings of tumors and vascular malformations, dexamethasone given every 4 to 6 hours may be more commonly used than methylprednisolone.

■ INFECTIONS

Prompt diagnosis of spine infections is crucial since early treatment can decrease morbidity and mortality (15). Spine infections may be divided into a handful of major categories: vertebral osteomyelitis, discitis, epidural abscess, subdural abscess/empyema, meningitis, and cord abscess. We will discuss the two more common infections that affect the pediatric population.

Discitis and Vertebral Osteomyelitis

Discitis and vertebral osteomyelitis are interrelated and describe different aspects of the same clinical spectrum. Children rarely present to clinic with back pain, so the diagnosis of this disease can be challenging, leading to a delay in diagnosis or unnecessary and futile tests and treatments. Children of less than 3 years of age tend to be the age group most affected (16). Usually, children with discitis are younger than those with vertebral

osteomyelitis, and discitis most commonly affects the lumbar spine (17,18). The typical presentation is an older child who refuses to walk or to stand due to back pain or a toddler who refuses to sit. The underlying pathologic cause may be infectious, inflammatory, or traumatic. Discitis in younger children may be more common than in adults and older children because of the presence of abundant intraosseous arterial anastomoses that nourish the nucleus pulposus that disappear by adulthood (1). Since the cartilaginous disc has an abundant blood supply in children, the treatment of choice is long-term antibiotics. Surgery is a last resort, reserved for cases that progress despite antibiotic treatment or that develop spinal instability (19, 20).

Spinal Epidural Abscess

Epidural abscesses are uncommon in the adult population and even less frequent in the pediatric population; however, they are seen not uncommonly in the tertiary care setting. Because of the rare nature of this disease process in children, management is controversial with no consistent surgical and nonsurgical treatment approaches. In a study examining pediatric spinal epidural abscesses over 15 years (21), the incidence of epidural abscesses was stated as 0.6 per 10,000 hospital admissions, a figure comparable to an estimate in adults of 0.2 to 1.2 per 10,000 hospitalizations (22). Especially in the pediatric population, epidural abscess is often undiagnosed until the progression of neurologic deficits because of the rarity of the disease process (23). The common presenting symptoms are similar to those in adults, including fever, general malaise, pain, and gait difficulties. Some reports suggest that children may present with pain in the hip, leg, or abdomen, presumably from referred pain or radiculopathy rather than midline back pain (23,24). However because there is a broad range of nonspecific symptoms, the time from symptom onset to diagnosis and treatment can be prolonged, which increases the likelihood of developing neurologic deficits including weakness, paresthesias, and even paraplegia.

In contrast to adults, only a third of children have an underlying medical condition that predisposes them to spinal epidural abscesses (21). The most common disorders include sickle cell disease or immunosuppression from chemotherapy for malignancy (21). The lower thoracolumbar areas of the spine are more prone to epidural infections because the epidural space is wider and the

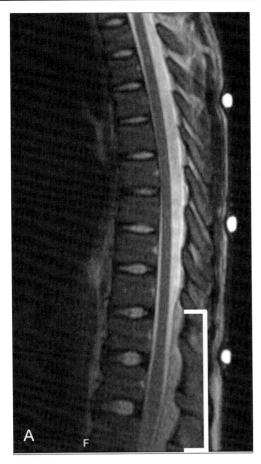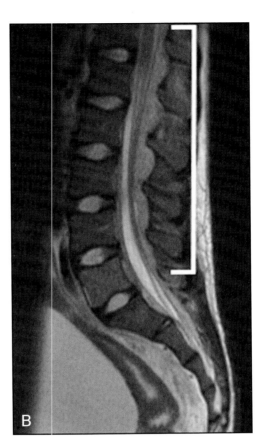

FIGURE 15.3 A 12-year-old male with sepsis from a urinary tract infection was found to have decreased motor strength (2/5) in his lower extremities with the inability to walk. Sagittal MRI of the thoracic (A) and lumbar (B) levels was obtained which showed an extensive thoraco-lumbar posterior epidural abscess without spinal cord infarction or compression (brackets). The patient's parents elected not to undergo any surgical intervention, and the patient was placed on antibiotics. One week later, the patient was walking unassisted with major improvement in his motor strength (4+/5).

spinal cord is narrower in this area. This epidural space is septated and contains larger amounts of adipose and vascular tissue which is the reason it has the potential to harbor infections. However, the septations are also potentially responsible for limiting extension of infection in adults. In children, the epidural space and vasculature are not as well developed and are still in the maturation phase with less adipose tissue. The anatomical differences between adults and children partially explain the age-related differences in abscess formation. Children, therefore, have the potential of multisegmented and very extensive epidural abscesses (Figure 15.3A and B). The most common mechanism of epidural abscess is hypothesized to be hematogenous spread into the epidural space from another infection such as endocarditis and urinary tract infections. There is also the possibility of direct extension from vertebral osteomyelitis or superinfection of a hematoma as the result of a trauma (24). Most of the literature, including reviews, report that over 80% of adult and pediatric epidural abscesses are caused by a *Staphylococcus aureus* infection (24). Some less common bacteria include *Pseudomonas*, *Pneumococcus*, and *Escherichia coli* (21). Mechanical compression from epidural abscesses may cause SCI, but this is not always the underlying cause of injury. Vascular mechanisms including thrombophlebitis of epidural veins or venous thrombosis and subsequent infarction have been described (22).

The treatment of spinal epidural abscess remains controversial especially in the pediatric population. There have been many articles in the adult literature that illustrate using antibiotic therapy only without surgical intervention for the treatment of epidural abscesses with good neurologic outcome (25,26). The caveat in these case series was that the patients tended to present early in the course of the infection with no neurologic compromise. There has been very limited literature with only a couple of case reports on spinal epidural abscesses in neurologically intact children that were successfully treated with antibiotics alone without surgical intervention (21,27). The gold standard treatment for epidural abscess includes combined surgical drainage and extended antibiotic therapy in children (28). The goal of surgical intervention is to decompress the spinal cord or thecal sac by performing a laminectomy to remove the compressive purulent material or granulation tissue. This will enable systemic antibiotics to penetrate the region (29). Exceptions to this approach can be made if the child has no neurologic deficit with extensive infection, where multilevel laminectomy would be the only treatment (27). The complications and morbidity associated with multilevel laminectomy in children are considerable, as this operation can lead to kyphosis and spinal instability.

■ TUMORS

Spinal cord tumors are a relatively rare diagnosis in both pediatric and adult populations. In children, the incidence is even less common and accounts for 0.5% to 10% of all pediatric central nervous system tumors (30,31) depending on the region of the world. Spinal tumors can be classified into three groups: extradural, intradural extramedullary, and intradural intramedullary. Extradural tumors arise from vertebral bodies or epidural tissues external to the leptomeninges and spinal cord (Figure 15.4A). Metastatic tumors to the spinal cord usually fall within this category; however, common pediatric tumors such as medulloblastomas or ependymomas may have intradural "drop mets" (Figure 15.4B). Intradural extramedullary tumors arise from the leptomeninges or nerve roots but arise outside of the neuronal tissue of the spinal cord. This category includes common adult tumors such as meningiomas and peripheral nerve sheath tumors. Intramedullary tumors also arise within

the meninges but from cells within the spinal cord itself. They are invasive and destructive to spinal cord tracts and gray matter (32,33). The incidence of intramedullary tumors is higher in children than in adults with reports citing ranges from 44% to 63% (31,34); this is compared to an average of 5% in the adult literature (1).

Glial neoplasms like astrocytomas are the most frequent intramedullary tumor in children followed by ependymomas (35). Other extradural or intradural extramedullary tumors that are also frequently encountered include tumor extension of neuroblastomas that originate outside of the central nervous system, nerve sheath tumors, and meningiomas (31,36). Spinal cord tumors are more frequently encountered toward the end of the first decade of life with no tendency for a particular sex (37).

Most children with spinal tumors will be diagnosed with imaging by a nonpediatric neurosurgeon or neuro-oncologist. Diagnostic imaging is key if a spinal cord tumor is in the differential, and MRI is the only imaging technique that can provide the necessary elements to confirm or exclude a tumor (38). If a child is suspected of having a spinal cord tumor, MRI should be the initial imaging modality (Figure 15.4C).

It is vital that children with this diagnosis be referred immediately to a specialist in order to prevent SCI and permanent disability. Many patients with spinal tumors are given dexamethasone during the acute management of their tumors since it can help reduce edema and inflammation which often improves symptoms. The treatment and management of spinal cord tumors is intricate and complex and must involve a multidisciplinary team of physicians. Treatment algorithms for spinal tumors are largely based on the histological type rather than the tumor location and generally follow the same surgical plan as adults. Surgery should be performed in a very short time frame after diagnosis before the development of irreversible neurologic deficits; however, surgery is usually not an emergency. If a tumor is extradural or intradural extramedullary, such as a meningioma or peripheral nerve sheath tumor, the goal of surgery is usually gross total resection. Intramedullary tumors are difficult; the goal for ependymoma treatment, especially myxopapillary ependymomas found at the filum terminale (1), should be a gross total resection. For low-grade astrocytomas, if a plane can be found between the tumor and spinal cord, gross total resection should be attempted (39). For high-grade astrocytomas or low-grade astrocytomas without a definitive plane, biopsy

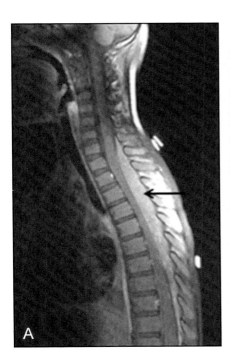 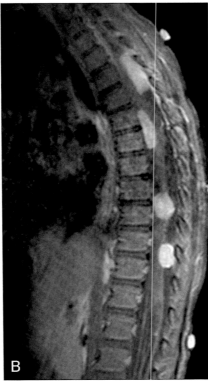 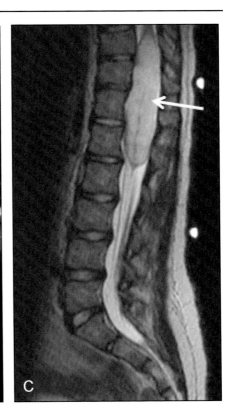

FIGURE 15.4 A 3-year-old male who presented with back pain and difficulty with ambulation (A). His neurologic deficit progressed to paraplegia and MRI showed a large cervicothoracic epidural lesion causing compression of the spinal cord (black arrow). He was taken to the operating room for gross total resection of the mass and pathology showed Burkitt's lymphoma. A 3-year-old female who was diagnosed with a large posterior fossa medulloblastoma (B). Surveillance spinal imaging showed multiple intradural extramedullary "drop mets" that enhanced with gadolinium on sagittal T2 MRI. She underwent surgical resection of her intracranial mass and went on to receive chemotherapy and radiation of her neuroaxis. At 5-year follow-up, she had no residual disease in her brain or spine. An 11-year-old female who started having abnormal gait around 18-months of age that was diagnosed as cerebral palsy (C). She had worsening paresthesias, wide-based gait, incontinence of urine and bowel, and motor strength of 3/5 in her left lower extremity. Sagittal T2 MRI shows a T10-L2 intradural intramedullary spinal cord tumor (white arrow). The patient underwent a moderate debulking, and pathology revealed a fibrillary astrocytoma. She underwent proton therapy and treatment with oral Temodar.

with limited resection is recommended (39). Depending on the age of the patient, tumor location, histological type and grade, and neurologic status after surgical intervention, adjuvant chemotherapy or radiation therapy may be warranted. Particular treatment protocols are beyond the scope of this chapter.

■ VASCULAR MALFORMATIONS

Vascular malformations of the spinal cord are rare lesions and account for only up to 4% of all primary spinal diseases (40,41). Most of these lesions are arteriovenous malformations (AVMs) or arteriovenous fistulae (AVFs).

Cavernomas and venous angiomas are rarely seen. There is limited literature regarding pediatric spinal vascular malformations, but the best estimates are that only 5% of all spinal vascular malformations occur in children (40). The majority of adult patients with any type of vascular malformation of the spine present as a progressive neurologic deficit, usually back pain with sensory loss, bladder or bowel dysfunction, and extremity weakness (41). However, it is more common in the pediatric population to see sudden onset of symptoms (40). Presentation with hemorrhage is more frequently encountered in children than in adults, except in very young toddlers and infants (42). In a minority of cases, vascular malformations can have a genetic association with hereditary hemorrhagic telangiectasia (43). The natural history of these lesions is usually a decline of neurologic status with no spontaneous improvement. It is crucial to diagnose and treat these lesions early since most patients will improve after appropriate treatment (40).

The most widely used classification of spinal vascular malformation categorizes these lesions into 4 types (41,44). Type I, termed dural AVF, is considered the most common type of malformation in adults (80%) but are extremely rare in children (45). Presenting symptoms such as cauda equina syndrome and motor deficits are due to the venous congestion of the cord (41). Type II AVM is labeled as glomus AVM and is a true intramedullary AVM of the spinal cord that can often present with hemorrhage (45). Type III, juvenile spinal AVM, is usually found in older children and is a large glomus AVM that usually encompasses the entire cord and possibly vertebral body, which may cause scoliosis (1). Type IV is a perimedullary AVM or AVF and can be found in children. These malformations can be very large direct fistulas and may also present with hemorrhage (Figure 15.5).

The gold standard evaluation of a suspected spinal vascular malformation is a diagnostic spinal angiogram. Angiography of the spinal arteries is not as routine as a typical cerebral angiogram and must be performed by an expert in the field at a center familiar with this procedure. Typically, type I AVFs are treated by open surgical removal of the malformation, and types II and IV malformations are most often treated by endovascular techniques. Type III AVM treatment is controversial since the natural history of the AVM may provide a better prognosis than surgical or endovascular treatment (41). Treatment options must be evaluated by a multidisciplinary team including interventional neuroradiologists, neurosurgeons, and stroke neurologists. Each vascular malformation requires an individualized approach with integration of endovascular and/or surgical techniques depending on the lesion's architecture and location and on the status of the patient.

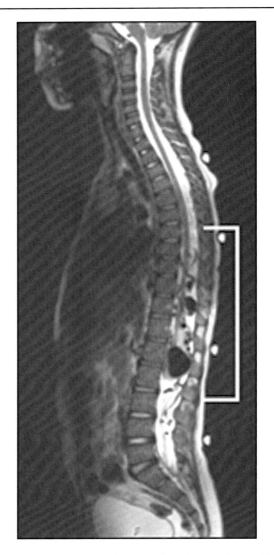

FIGURE 15.5 An 8-year-old boy with back pain, abnormally slow gait, and decreased flexibility. MRI/magnetic resonance angiography was obtained that showed type IV arteriovenous fistula of the spine (brackets). Based on the location, large size, and the significant risk of hemorrhage or enlargement of this lesion over time, the patient underwent embolization of the fistula.

■ ISCHEMIC SCI

Spinal cord infarction is extremely rare in children. In adults, anterior spinal cord infarction is most often seen in the setting of aortic surgery. Infarction can occur at any level but most often occurs in the T4-T8 watershed zone between the costocervical trunk that supplies the lower cervical to upper thoracic cord and the area supplied by the artery of Adamkiewicz (46). In children, spinal cord infarction has been related to minor trauma (47,48). Spinal cord infarction most often affects the anterior spinal artery which supplies the anterior two-thirds of the spinal cord including the anterior horn cells and the spinothalamic tract. This artery arises from paired branches of the vertebral arteries that combine to form the rostral origin. Intercostal arteries and lumbar segmental arteries develop a collateral supply as the artery runs caudally. A watershed area is in the mid-thoracic region (49).

A clue to anterior spinal artery infarction includes weakness with diminished pain and temperature sensation with preserved vibration sense and proprioception. Bladder and bowel dysfunction and priapism may also occur. Posterior spinal artery infarction is even less common. The paired posterior spinal arteries most frequently arise from the vertebral artery. These arteries supply the posterior one-third of the spinal cord including the dorsal columns that relay vibration sense and

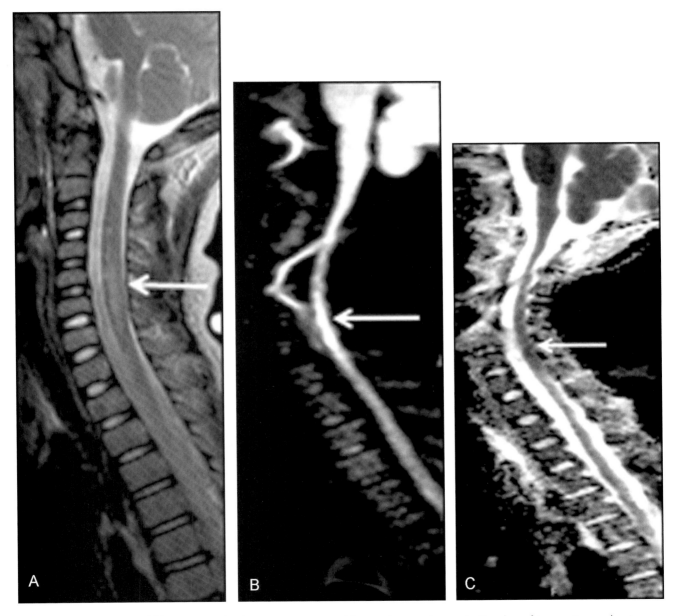

FIGURE 15.6 A 7-year-old boy presented with asymmetric arm and leg weakness, urinary retention, loss of temperature and pain sensations with preservation of vibration and proprioception. Sagittal T2-weighted MRI with hyperintensity from C3 through T2 (arrow) (A). Sagittal diffusion weighted imaging demonstrating restricted diffusion of water in the region of T2 hyperintensity seen in (A) (arrow) (B). Sagittal apparent diffusion coefficient map demonstrating a dark area corresponding to the region of restricted diffusion shown in (B) (arrow) (C).

proprioception. Therefore, infarction of the posterior spinal artery causes decreased vibration and proprioception with relative preservation of motor strength and temperature and pain sensation although motor function can be affected in some cases. Back pain often accompanies spinal cord infarction.

The mechanism for spinal cord infarction in children is not completely understood. Some postulated mechanisms include dissection, vasospasm, and fibrocartilaginous embolism, although none has been proven. When an ischemic cause of myelopathy is suspected, diffusion weighted imaging and apparent diffusion coefficient (ADC) maps on MRI should be obtained (Figure 15.6). Although these sequences can be difficult in the spinal cord, they have successfully been used in pediatric patients to help differentiate infarction from other causes of myelopathy (48). A spinal angiogram may be considered, but the risk of procedure-related infarction likely outweighs the benefit of additional diagnostic information, particularly given the ability to use diffusion weighted MRI with ADC mapping.

In any child with suspected anterior spinal artery infarction, aortic imaging should be considered to rule out an aneurysm or dissection, even though these diseases are rare in children. Blood pressure should be augmented with isotonic intravenous fluids, but the utility of pressors or a lumbar drain has not been established in the setting of pediatric ischemic cord injury. In many cases a complete hypercoagulable workup for children with ischemic cord injury is performed. (See Chapter 10 on arterial ischemic stroke for hypercoagulable testing.) Additionally, most patients were treated with aspirin for at least 1 year. If the diagnosis of spinal cord ischemia is not fully established, a lumbar puncture with testing for white matter disorders should be considered. However, it is important to recognize that myelin basic protein may be elevated in the setting of any SCI.

■ CONCLUSIONS

Acute myelopathy due to injury or other diseases is rare in children; however, spinal cord disease represents a true neurologic and often neurosurgical emergency. Thorough neurologic examination and timely definitive neuroimaging are crucial for diagnosis. Although some principles such as monitoring for respiratory compromise and autonomic instability are important for all

types of spinal cord disease, different underlying causes require tailored treatments. More research is needed for an evidence-based approach to management and treatment. It is important to refer to an expert in the field of pediatric neurosurgery and/or neurology if any of these acute spinal cord diseases is considered in the differential.

■ REFERENCES

1. Greenberg MS. *Handbook of Neurosurgery: Chapter 25.2 Pediatric Spine Injuries*. 7th ed; 2010. Thieme; New York, NY. p. 700
2. Reilly CW. Pediatric spine trauma. *J Bone Joint Surg Am*. 2007;89(suppl 1):98–107.
3. Leventhal HR. Birth injuries of the spinal cord. *J Pediatr*. 1960;56:447–453.
4. Pang D, Wilberger JE Jr. Spinal cord injury without radiographic abnormalities in children. *J Neurosurg*. 1982;57:114–129.
5. Muniz AE, Liner S. Lumbar vertebral fractures in children: four cases and review of the literature. *Pediatr Emerg Care*. 2011;27:1157–1162.
6. Jones TM, Anderson PA, Noonan KJ. Pediatric cervical spine trauma. *J Am Acad Orthop Surg*. 2011;19:600–611.
7. Platzer P et al. Cervical spine injuries in pediatric patients. *J Trauma*. 2007;62:389–396; discussion 94–96.
8. Dogan S et al. Thoracolumbar and sacral spinal injuries in children and adolescents: a review of 89 cases. *J Neurosurg*. 2007;106:426–433.
9. Oluigbo CO et al. Pattern, management and outcome of cervical spine injuries associated with head injuries in paediatric patients. *Childs Nerv Syst*. 2008;24:87–92.
10. Hosalkar HS et al. Traumatic atlanto-occipital dislocation in children. *J Bone Joint Surg Am*. 2005;87:2480–2488.
11. Taggard DA, Menezes AH, Ryken TC. Treatment of Down syndrome–associated craniovertebral junction abnormalities. *J Neurosurg*. 2000;93:205–213.
12. Gautschi OP, Woodland PR, Zellweger R. Complete medulla/cervical spinal cord transection after atlanto-occipital dislocation: an extraordinary case. *Spinal Cord*. 2007;45:387–393.
13. Goni Orayen C et al. Pseudosubluxation of C2-C3 in childhood: a frequent clinico-radiological diagnostic error. *An Esp Pediatr*. 1992;36:390–392.
14. Townsend EH Jr, Rowe ML. Mobility of the upper cervical spine in health and disease. *Pediatrics*. 1952;10:567–574.
15. Tehranzadeh J, Wang F, Mesgarzadeh M. Magnetic resonance imaging of osteomyelitis. *Crit Rev Diagn Imaging*. 1992;33:495–534.
16. Brown R et al. Discitis in young children. *J Bone Joint Surg Br*. 2001;83:106–111.
17. Fernandez M, Carrol CL, Baker CJ. Discitis and vertebral osteomyelitis in children: an 18-year review. *Pediatrics*. 2000;105:1299–1304.
18. Offiah AC. Acute osteomyelitis, septic arthritis and discitis: differences between neonates and older children. *Eur J Radiol*. 2006;60:221–232.

19. Cheung WY, Luk KD. Pyogenic spondylitis. *Int Orthop.* 2012;36:397–404.
20. Cebrian Parra JL et al. Management of infectious discitis. Outcome in one hundred and eight patients in a University Hospital. *Int Orthop.* 2012;36:239–244.
21. Auletta JJ, John CC. Spinal epidural abscesses in children: a 15-year experience and review of the literature. *Clin Infect Dis.* 2001;32:9–16.
22. Baker AS et al. Spinal epidural abscess. *N Engl J Med.* 1975;293:463–468.
23. Rubin G et al. Spinal epidural abscess in the pediatric age group: case report and review of literature. *Pediatr Infect Dis J.* 1993;12:1007–1011.
24. Jacobsen FS, Sullivan B. Spinal epidural abscesses in children. *Orthopedics.* 1994;17:1131–1138.
25. Leys D et al. Decreased morbidity from acute bacterial spinal epidural abscesses using computed tomography and nonsurgical treatment in selected patients. *Ann Neurol.* 1985;17:350–355.
26. Mampalam TJ et al. Nonoperative treatment of spinal epidural infections. *J Neurosurg.* 1989;71:208–210.
27. Bair-Merritt MH, Chung C, Collier A. Spinal epidural abscess in a young child. *Pediatrics.* 2000;106:E39.
28. Enberg RN, Kaplan RJ. Spinal epidural abscess in children. Early diagnosis and immediate surgical drainage is essential to forestall paralysis. *Clin Pediatr (Phila).* 1974;13:247–248 passim.
29. Hulme A, Dott NM. Spinal epidural abscess. *Br Med J.* 1954;1:64–68.
30. Stiller CA, Nectoux J. International incidence of childhood brain and spinal tumours. *Int J Epidemiol.* 1994;23:458–464.
31. Rosemberg S, Fujiwara D. Epidemiology of pediatric tumors of the nervous system according to the WHO 2000 classification: a report of 1,195 cases from a single institution. *Childs Nerv Syst.* 2005;21:940–944.
32. Wilne S, Walker D. Spine and spinal cord tumours in children: a diagnostic and therapeutic challenge to healthcare systems. *Arch Dis Child Educ Pract Ed.* 2008;95:47–54.
33. Huisman TA. Pediatric tumors of the spine. *Cancer Imaging.* 2009;9(Spec No A):S45–S48.
34. Wilson PE, Oleszek JL, Clayton GH. Pediatric spinal cord tumors and masses. *J Spinal Cord Med.* 2007;30(suppl 1):S15–S20.
35. Binning M et al. Spinal tumors in children. *Neurosurg Clin N Am.* 2007;18:631–658.
36. Asirvatham JR et al. Pediatric tumors of the central nervous system: a retrospective study of 1,043 cases from a tertiary care center in South India. *Childs Nerv Syst* 2011;27:1257–1263.
37. Rossi A et al. Tumors of the spine in children. *Neuroimaging Clin N Am.* 2007;17:17–35.
38. Baleriaux DL. Spinal cord tumors. *Eur Radiol.* 1999;9:1252–1258.
39. Nadkarni TD, Rekate HL. Pediatric intramedullary spinal cord tumors. Critical review of the literature. *Childs Nerv Syst.* 1999;15:17–28.
40. Du J et al. Clinical characteristic of spinal vascular malformation in pediatric patients. *Childs Nerv Syst.* 2009;25:473–478.
41. Dashti SR Toledo M, Kim LJ, Spetzler RF. Classification of spinal arteriovenous lesions: arteriovenous fistulas and arteriovenous malformations. In: Winn HR, ed. *Youmans Neurological Surgery.* 6th ed. Philadelphia, PA: Elesevier; 2011;4146–4152.
42. Lorenzoni PJ et al. Spinal cord arteriovenous malformation: a pediatric presentation. *Arq Neuropsiquiatr.* 2009;67:527–529.
43. Cullen S et al. Spinal arteriovenous shunts presenting before 2 years of age: analysis of 13 cases. *Childs Nerv Syst.* 2006;22:1103–1110.
44. Riche MC et al. Classification of spinal cord vascular malformations. *Radiat Med.* 1985;3:17–24.
45. Chuang NA et al. Slow-flow spinal epidural AVF with venous ectasias: two pediatric case reports. *AJNR Am J Neuroradiol.* 2003;24:1901–1905.
46. Mullen M, McGarvey ML. Spinal cord infarction: vascular anatomy and etiologies. In: *UpToDate.* Waltham, MA: Wolters Kluwer; 2009.
47. Nance JR, Golomb MR. Ischemic spinal cord infarction in children without vertebral fracture. *Pediatr Neurol.* 2007;36:209–216.
48. Beslow LA et al. Role of diffusion MRI in diagnosis of spinal cord infarction in children. *Neuropediatrics.* 2008;39:188–191.
49. Mohr JP, Benavente O, Barnett HJM. Spiral cord ischema. In: Mohr JP, Choi DW, Grotta JC, Weir B, Wolf PA, eds. *Stroke: Pathophysiology, Diagnosis and Management,* 4th ed. Philadelphia, PA: Churchill Livingstone; 2004:423–436.
50. Bracken MB. Steroids for acute spinal injury. *Cochrane Database Syst Rev.* 2012:CD001046.

16 Central Nervous System Infections

JENNIFER L. McGUIRE and ABBY M. GREEN

■ INTRODUCTION

Infections of the pediatric central nervous system (CNS) are a heterogeneous group of disorders with very diverse presentations, clinical courses, and prognoses. Presentations range from dramatic and imminently fatal (such as bacterial meningitis), to subacute or subtle (such as slow virus infections). A detailed history focused on why a particular child acquired a specific infection at a particular time, in conjunction with examination of host factors affecting susceptibility to various infections (including age, immune status, travel, endemic exposures, and animal exposures) is therefore crucial in the diagnosis of a suspected CNS infection.

Many CNS infections will require intensive care monitoring and treatment at some time during their course. This chapter aims to guide clinicians in the pediatric intensive care setting when thinking about the diagnosis and management of a possible CNS infection, but is not meant to be an exhaustive list of every pathogen that may affect the brain and spinal cord.

■ DIAGNOSTIC PROCEDURES IN SUSPECTED CNS INFECTIONS

Performing and Interpreting the Lumbar Puncture

Evaluation of the cerebrospinal fluid (CSF) is an essential component in the evaluation of a child with a suspected meningeal infection, subarachnoid hemorrhage, parenchymal brain infection, CNS neoplasm, or demyelinating disease. A lumbar puncture (LP) is a fast and safe procedure performed at the bedside for the majority of children, but there are several contraindications based on safety concerns that should be considered. Increased intracranial pressure (ICP) is an absolute contraindication to LP, given the risk of cerebellar tonsillar herniation (1). To minimize this risk, the Infectious Disease Society of America (IDSA) recommends intracranial imaging prior to LP in select infants and children (2) (Table 16.1). However, normal imaging does not definitively rule out increased ICP, so clinical judgment must be incorporated. Severe coagulopathy is another absolute contraindication to LP (3–5). In general, a patient who is actively bleeding, has severe thrombocytopenia with a platelet count < 50,000/microliter, or an international normalized ratio (INR) > 1.4 should not undergo LP prior to correction of each of these conditions unless there are specific extenuating circumstances indicating the LP. Finally, cardiovascular instability limiting appropriate positioning to perform an LP, and soft tissue or epidural infection at the puncture site (6) are both relative contraindications.

Patient positioning is extremely important in preparation for an LP. Children may lie in the lateral recumbent position with their hips and knees flexed, or they may sit upright with their hips flexed. While the interspinous space may be maximized in the sitting position (7), either position may be used according to clinician preference to maximize the success of the procedure. Use of local anesthetic may improve the likelihood of success in the absence of sedation (8). The needle

■ **Table 16.1** Infectious Disease Society of America Guidelines for Intracranial Imaging Prior to LP in Children

Immunocompromise
Papilledema
History of select CNS disease, including:
    Mass lesion
    CSF shunt
    Hydrocephalus
    Trauma
    Recent neurosurgery
Focal neurologic deficit (excluding palsy of cranial nerves VI or VII)

Abbreviations: CNS, central nervous system; CSF, cerebrospinal fluid; LP, lumbar puncture.
Source: Adapted from Tunkel AR et al. Practice guidelines for the management of bacterial meningitis. *Clin Infect Dis.* 2004;39:1267–1284.

should be introduced in the L3-4, L4-5, or L5-S1 space (6,9), with the bevel parallel to the longitudinal fibers of the dura.

Once CSF flow is obtained, an opening pressure (OP) should be measured on all patients with a standard manometer. For an accurate measurement, children should lie in the lateral recumbent position with legs either flexed or extended (10); it is not helpful to measure an OP if the patient is sitting upright. Pressures may be elevated in certain infections (such as *Cryptococcus*) and low in others (such as a spinal epidural abscess [EA] with spinal block). The commonly accepted normal range of CSF OP in adults is 10 to 25 cm H_2O (11). Normal values in children are poorly established. A recent prospective study of 197 children between 1 and 18 years old suggests that a range of 11.5 to 28 is probably normal (12).

After measuring the OP, a minimum of 4 tubes of CSF should be collected: the first and last for cell count, and the others for chemistries and Gram stain/bacterial culture. Additional tubes may be sent for analysis according to the specific testing indicated for each case. It is imperative to obtain two tubes to measure cell counts so elevated red blood cell (RBC) count in a traumatic LP may be distinguished from an intracranial hemorrhage. Withdrawing the needle with the stylet in place may reduce the risk of CSF leak and headache later (13). Common but treatable transient side effects following LP include back pain in 40% (6,14) and spinal headache in up to 60% (3,6).

Interpretation of the LP varies by age (Table 16.2), but basic cell counts, chemistries, and OPs can help

significantly narrow a differential diagnosis (Table 16.3). Several general rules of thumb in interpreting LP results are as follows:

- *Color:* Normal CSF should be clear and colorless; turbidity may be due to high white blood cell (WBC) or RBC. CSF may be grossly bloody with just 6,000 RBC (15). Xanthochromia refers to a yellow/pink discoloration of the CSF, due to the presence of bilirubin (related to blood breakdown products), elevated protein, or systemic hyperbilirubinemia. The presence of xanthochromia with RBCs suggests blood has been present in the CSF for at least 2 hours. Xanthochromia due to hemorrhage may persist for 2 to 4 weeks (16).
- *WBCs:* In general, infants have a higher normal CSF WBC than older children, with a higher percentage of polymorphonuclear cells (17,18). A WBC differential composed primarily of lymphocytes or monocytes is suggestive of, but not specific for, a viral process.
- *RBCs:* For LPs with gross blood, the WBC count may be corrected by decreasing 1 for every 700 RBC (19), when RBCs are below 10,000. Above 10,000, this rule of thumb may not be reliable. Grossly hemorrhagic LPs may be seen with a traumatic LP or intracranial (subarachnoid or intraparenchymal) hemorrhage. Hemorrhagic LPs can cause falsely negative herpes simplex virus (HSV) polymerase chain reaction (PCR) or falsely posi-

■ **Table 16.2** CSF Normal Values by Age

WBC (cells/μmL)	
Infants 0–28 days	0–19
Infants 29–56 days	0–9
Child	0–7
Glucose (mg/dL)	
Infants 0–28 days	30–61
Infants 29–56 days	30–66
Child	40–80
Protein (mg/dL)	
Infants 0–28 days	< 115
Infants 29–56 days	< 89
Child	5–40

Source: Adapted from Refs. 17, 18, 25, 26.

■ **Table 16.3** Different CSF Characteristics of CNS Infections

	Opening Pressure	WBC (cell/μL)	Predominant Cell Type in Differential (in Early Diagnostic Period)	Protein (mg/dL)	Glucose (mg/dL)	Culture	Miscellaneous
Bacterial meningitis	↑	↑↑↑	PMN	↑	↓	+	
Viral meningitis	Normal	↑	Lymphocyte, monocyte	Slightly ↑	Normal	−	
—HSV meningitis	↑	↑	Lymphocyte	↑	Normal	−	PCR
TB meningitis	↑	Normal or ↑↑	Lymphocyte	↑	↓	AFB	
Sarcoid		↑↑	Lymphocyte	↑	Normal or ↓	−	ACE
Neurosyphilis		↑↑	Lymphocyte, monocyte	↑	Normal		+VDRL/FTA
Lyme	Normal	↑	Lymphocyte	↑	Normal	−	+OCB
Fungal meningitis	↑	↑↑↑	Lymphocyte	↑	Normal or ↓	+	Ag
HIV	Normal or ↑	Normal or ↑	Lymphocyte	Normal or ↑	Normal	−	
Malignancy	Normal or ↑	Normal or ↑	Lymphocyte	↑	↓	−	
Postinfectious		↑↑	Lymphocyte	Normal or ↑	Normal	−	

Abbreviations: ACE, angiotensin converting enzyme; AFB, acid-fast bacilli; Ag, antigen; FTA, fluorescent treponemal antibody; HSV, herpes simplex virus; OCB, oligoclonal band; PCR, polymerase chain reaction; PMN, polymorphonuclear cell; TB, tuberculosis; VDRL, venereal disease research laboratory; ↑, elevated; ↓, depressed.

Source: Adapted from Refs. 27–29.

tive venereal disease research laboratory (VDRL) test for syphilis or Epstein-Barr virus (EBV) PCR. In addition, breakdown of the blood brain barrier (BBB) with hemorrhage may result in organisms or antibodies causing a peripheral/non-CNS infection to be found in the CSF, or may introduce an infection into the CNS.

- *Protein:* Normal protein concentration varies with age (Table 16.2), and may increase by 1 mg/dL per 1,000 RBC in older children and 2 mg/dL per 1,000 RBC in neonates in a hemorrhagic LP (20). Protein levels that are depressed are rarely pathologic, but proteins that are elevated may be due to anything that disrupts the BBB (21). For proteins over 100 to 200 mg/dL, spinal block should be considered and diagnostic spinal cord imaging should be performed. One may see elevated protein with a normal WBC (albuminocytologic dissociation) in acute inflammatory demyelinating polyneuropathies, such as Guillain-Barré syndrome (GBS).

- *Glucose:* Normal concentration ranges for CSF glucose are based on serum glucose measured within 1 hour prior to LP. A ratio of 0.6 CSF to serum or greater is normal (22,23). Hypoglycorrhachia may be seen with bacterial meningitis, tuberculous meningitis, some fungal meningitides, neurosarcoidosis, or tumors (21), but CSF glucose concentrations less than 18 mg/dL are strongly suggestive of bacterial meningitis (24). Glucose concentration in lymphocytic pleocytosis can greatly help narrow a differential diagnosis (Table 16.3)

- *Specific organism testing:* varies by pathogen. Please reference the Encephalitis/Myelitis and Immunocompromised Hosts sections of this chapter for specific recommendations.

Neuroimaging

CNS imaging is typically obtained in the child with focal neurologic deficits, obtundation, or seizures. A variety of imaging modalities exist, each with different advantages and disadvantages. Neuroimaging for specific disorders will be discussed in the following sections.

Computed tomography (CT) is a fast and effective study to help exclude acute problems that require interventional measures such as hemorrhage, large mass, obstructive hydrocephalus, or large vascular territory ischemic stroke. CT of the head is frequently used prior to the decision to perform an LP when there is concern for possible elevated ICP. Spinal CT with contrast is superior to a plain x-ray for detection of a paraspinal infection, but is not sensitive enough to exclude the presence of an early discitis or epidural abscess (EA), and does not assess the integrity of the spinal cord itself. Disadvantages of performing a CT include radiation exposure, the possibility of an acute allergic reaction to the radiodense, iodinating contrast agents, and the risk for acute kidney injury in subjects with underlying renal disease.

Magnetic resonance imaging (MRI) is more sensitive than CT for small structural lesions and inflammation. Diffusion-weighted imaging (DWI) is particularly sensitive to ischemia, and may also be helpful distinguishing an abscess or empyema from a necrotic tumor. Susceptibility-weighted imaging can be used to identify very small areas of hemorrhage which may not otherwise be seen on CT. MRI of the brain is also more likely than CT to show meningeal enhancement in uncomplicated meningitis. MRI with DWI is superior to CT in identification of ischemia, cerebritis, abscess, empyema, and ventriculitis. MRI does not involve radiation. However, the lengthy image acquisition time necessitates sedation for many children. In addition, any ferromagnetic materials in the imaging suite are incompatible with the strong magnetic field of the MRI. Therefore, children with myringotomy tubes, braces, metallic pacemakers, orthopedic implants, or metallic neurostimulators may be unable to safely undergo an MRI exam. Finally, gadolinium enhancement may be contraindicated in patients with renal disease given the small risk of nephrogenic systemic fibrosis or nephrogenic fibrosing dermopathy.

■ MENINGITIS

Meningitis refers to inflammation of the tissues surrounding the brain and spinal cord, usually caused by an infection of the CSF. Presentations range from acute and imminently life-threatening with acute bacterial meningitis, to chronic and smoldering with recurrent types of meningitis.

Acute Bacterial Meningitis

Epidemiology and Pathophysiology

Acute bacterial meningitis is one of the top 10 causes of infection-related death worldwide (30), with an annual incidence of about 2,000 pediatric cases in the United States per year (31), and accounting for about 5% of all cases of meningitis in developed countries (32). Bacterial meningitis is a medical emergency. Mortality in treated cases ranges from 3% to 40% (27,31,33), and approaches 100% without appropriate treatment. Even following optimal treatment, neurologic sequelae including hydrocephalus, visual and hearing loss, developmental delays, and cognitive deficits are common among survivors, given the rapid progression of infection and subsequent parenchymal damage.

Bacterial meningitis occurs when invading pathogens overcome host defenses to reach the subarachnoid space. In neonates, pathogens are typically acquired from maternal genital secretions. In children who suffer head trauma leading to skull defects causing CNS leaks, or with congenital dural defects, the CNS may be directly inoculated with an environmental pathogen (27). In most infants and children though, the route of pathogen entry is through the nasopharynx. In individuals with immature humoral immunity, or in the context of organisms with a particularly virulent capsule, colonizing bacteria may invade the nasopharyngeal epithelium (34). During subsequent bacteremia, a robust bacterial capsule again resists normal host defenses of complement mediated bactericidal activity, neutrophil phagocytosis, and circulating antibodies (35), allowing the organism to invade the CNS via one of several routes of entry: through the choroid plexus epithelium, through the dural venous sinus system, or through the cribriform plate. The CNS physiologically stocks lower concentrations of immunoglobulins and fewer complement factors than the systemic circulation, so once a pathogen reaches the subarachnoid space, bacterial seeding of the meninges proceeds relatively unhindered. Bacterial replication and autolysis then induces the release of proinflammatory cytokines, chemokines, and cellular toxins, causing inflammation and leukocyte recruitment into the subarachnoid space. This inflammatory response results in increased BBB permeability, increased CSF outflow resistance, and loss of autoregulation with changes in cerebral blood flow. Vasogenic edema, hydrocephalus with interstitial edema, and cytotoxic edema may ensue, all of which may culminate in increased ICP. Ventriculitis may also lead to pial vein, cortical arteriole, and venous sinus thrombosis, and subdural effusions (34).

Causative organisms vary depending on the route of pathogen entry and host factors affecting the pathophysiology of infection. Before 2000, *Haemophilus influenzae* type b (Hib) was the major cause of bacterial meningitis in children. However, following the introduction of a Hib vaccine to the infant vaccine schedule in the early 1990s, the overall incidence of bacterial meningitis in children less than 5 years of age was significantly reduced. The introduction of the *Streptococcus pneumoniae* (pneumococcus) conjugate vaccine to the infant vaccine schedule in 2000 reduced the incidence of pneumococcal meningitis in children

in the United States by 55% to 60%. However, *S pneumoniae* remains the most common cause of bacterial meningitis in children (31) because the standard pneumococcal vaccine includes only 13 of more than 90 serotypes. Host factors that may predispose a child to developing bacterial meningitis include lack of opsonizing antibodies, surgical or functional asplenia, complement deficiency, glucocorticoid excess, HIV infection, bacteremia, basilar skull fracture, or other traumatic or inflammatory breach of the BBB. Individuals with CSF shunts are particularly prone to staphylococcal infections with both coagulase-negative staphylococcal species and *Staphylococcus aureus*, in which the infection begins as ventriculitis but may spread to the meninges. Children in the early postneurosurgical period are particularly prone to *S aureus* meningitis, although this is rare. Finally, a child's age predisposes them to various infections, based on their environmental exposures and the maturation of their immune system (Tables 16.4 and 16.5).

■ Table 16.4   Acute Meningitis Etiologic Organisms Based on Age

Age	Bacterial Pathogen	Empiric Antibiotic Therapy
Neonate	Group B *Streptococcus* *Escherichia coli* *Listeria monocytogenes*	Ampicillin plus cefotaxime or gentamicin
Children ≥ 1 month and < 3 months	Group B *Streptococcus* Gram-negative bacilli[a] *Streptococcus pneumonia* *Neisseria meningitidis* *L monocytogenes*	Third or fourth generation cephalosporin plus vancomycin
Children ≥ 3 months and < 3 years	*S pneumoniae* *N meningitidis* Group B *Streptococcus* Gram-negative bacilli[a]	Third or fourth generation cephalosporin plus vancomycin
Children ≥ 3 years and < 10 years	*S pneumoniae* *N meningitidis* Other bacteria[b] Group B *Streptococcus*	Third or fourth generation cephalosporin plus vancomycin
Children ≥ 10 years and < 19 years	*N meningitidis* *S pneumoniae* Other bacteria[b] Group B *Streptococcus* Gram-negative bacilli[a]	Third or fourth generation cephalosporin plus vancomycin

[a] If there are Gram-negative bacilli on CSF Gram stain or there is a high level of suspicion for Gram-negative meningitis, empiric therapy should include a carbapenem plus gentamicin until the organism is identified and antibiotic susceptibilities are determined.

[b] Other bacteria = *L monocytogenes*, Group A *Streptococcus*.

Source: Adapted from Refs. 31, 36.

■ **Table 16.5** Acute Meningitis: Etiologic Organisms Based on Predisposing and Associated Conditions

Predisposing Conditions	Bacterial Pathogen	Empiric Antibiotic Therapy[a]

Otitis, mastoiditis, sinusitis	*Streptococci* spp
	Gram-negative anaerobes (*Bacteroides* spp,
	  Fusobacterium spp)
	Haemophilus spp
	Enterobacteriaceae
	Staphylococcus aureus
		Third or fourth generation
		  cephalosporin plus
		metronidazole +/– vancomycin

Surgical or functional asplenia	*Streptococci* spp	Third or fourth generation cephalosporin plus vancomycin
Lack of opsonizing antibodies	*Streptococci* spp	Third or fourth generation cephalosporin plus vancomycin
Postneurosurgical	Staphylococci spp Gram-negative bacilli	Vancomycin plus meropenem or third or fourth generation cephalosporin
Intraventricular device	Staphylococci spp Gram-negative bacilli	Vancomycin +/– third or fourth generation cephalosporin

[a] Antibiotic therapy should be tailored and specifically directed once the specific organism is identified and susceptibilities are determined.
Source: Adapted from Refs. 31, 36.

Clinical Presentation

Acute bacterial meningitis may present progressively over several days, or fulminantly over several hours, in which case it is more likely to be associated with significant brain edema. Signs and symptoms of meningitis may be preceded by an upper respiratory infection or otitis media. Most children initially present with fever and signs of meningeal inflammation (meningismus), including altered mental status (irritability or lethargy), headache, nuchal rigidity, emesis, and/or photophobia (36); however not all children have a classic presentation. For example, 6% to 20% of children may be afebrile (37,38) and up to 16% may not have meningeal signs. Nuchal rigidity is observed in less than 50% of children with meningitis (27,36) and may be absent in early infection (38). Nuchal rigidity is commonly assessed using Kernig and Brudzinski signs. A Kernig sign is present if the supine patient, with hips and knees flexed at 90°, has significant pain with extension of the knee less than 135°. A Brudzinski sign is present if the supine patient flexes the lower extremities during attempted passive flexion of the neck. Infants typically have a more nondescript presentation of bacterial meningitis, involving fever or hypothermia, altered mental status (irritability, restlessness, lethargy), poor feeding, respiratory distress, emesis or diarrhea, and/or a bulging fontanel. In all children, petechiae and purpura may be a sign of *Neisseria meningitidis* (meningococcal)

infection. The current immunization for meningococcus does not include serogroup B, which predominantly affects younger children and is responsible for one-third of the cases of meningococcal meningitis in the United States (27).

Neurologic findings in acute bacterial meningitis are variable. Altered level of consciousness, manifested primarily by irritability or lethargy is common, and children who are less responsive have a poorer prognosis. Increased ICP may result in a headache, bulging fontanel, or palsies of the third, fourth, or sixth cranial nerve (sixth nerve palsy is most common). Papilledema typically takes several days to develop, making it less helpful in the acute diagnostic setting. Up to 16% of patients, and 34% of those with pneumococcal meningitis, may have focal neurologic findings related to parenchymal extension of their meningitis (meningoencephalitis), increased ICP, or stroke, commonly related to an inflammatory vasculitis. Focal neurologic signs also correlate with increased morbidity and mortality. Finally, 20% to 30% of children with bacterial meningitis may have seizures, typically at the time of presentation. While most seizures are generalized and within the first 48 hours of admission, focal seizures may occur later in the course, and typically indicate a focal parenchymal injury. It is extremely unusual for bacterial meningitis to present with fever and a single brief generalized seizure alone. A study of 506 children aged 2 months to 15 years at two hospitals over a 20-year period found no cases of acute bacterial meningitis presenting solely with a simple febrile seizure (39). Another recent study examined 704 children aged 6 to 18 months presenting to a large tertiary care emergency department with a first time simple febrile seizure: none of these children had bacterial meningitis (40).

Diagnosis

As with all neurologic infections, a thorough history should be taken in all children with suspected bacterial meningitis, with particular attention to the course of illness, presence of predisposing immunologic factors, concurrent infections or head trauma, recent travel to areas with endemic meningococcal disease, and exposure to an individual with bacterial meningitis. Special attention should be given to immunization history. Complete physical and neurologic examinations should be performed. The constellation of systemic hypertension, bradycardia, and respiratory depression (Cushing triad) is a late sign of increased ICP. Children with bacterial meningitis may have concomitant bacterial infections at other sites (e.g., arthritis with *N meningitidis*, pneumonia or endocarditis with *S pneumoniae*).

Initial blood tests should include a complete blood count with differential, serum electrolytes, blood urea nitrogen, creatinine, glucose, and aerobic blood cultures. Blood cultures are positive in up to 80% of patients with previously untreated bacterial meningitis (41). Coagulation studies should be included if petechial or purpuric lesions are present. An LP should be performed in any child with suspected bacterial meningitis, unless specific contraindications are present (see above). Evaluation should include cell counts from two tubes, glucose, protein, Gram stain, and culture. Cell counts should be examined within 90 minutes of the LP to avoid WBC disintegration (41). Although several theoretical methods exist to differentiate between a traumatic LP versus a hemorrhagic LP, none have been validated (42), and clinicians should err on the side of treating conservatively while awaiting confirmatory results. In bacterial meningitis, CSF-to-serum glucose ratios are typically decreased to ≤ 0.6 in neonates, and ≤ 0.4 in children over 2 months of age (27). Specific organism testing may be performed as indicated (see Encephalitis and Myelitis section of this chapter, Table 16.21). Early in the course of disease, a

culture may be positive in the absence of a pleocytosis (43), and about 10% of cases with bacterial infection will have an initial lymphocytic predominance (44), making clinical differential diagnosis slightly more challenging. However, a high OP, pleocytosis with neutrophil predominance, elevated protein, and depressed glucose are more commonly observed (Table 16.3). Bacterial culture results in the definitive diagnosis, however growth from culture typically takes at least 24 hours (45). The sensitivity of CSF Gram stain exceeds 70%. Despite a high specificity of 80% to 92%, the positive predictive value of a Gram stain without culture is low (approximately 50%) given the very low prevalence of bacterial meningitis in the population at large (45–47). Reasons for falsely positive CSF Gram stains include observer misinterpretation, reagent contamination, and use of an occluded spinal needle, the latter of which leads to skin contamination. If CSF parameters are consistent with bacterial meningitis but culture does not yield bacterial growth, an empiric course of antibiotics should be considered.

Neuroimaging is typically normal in the early stages of bacterial meningitis, and is not necessary in uncomplicated disease. Neuroimaging in bacterial meningitis is appropriate when focal neurologic signs are present (raising concern for the presence of other pathologic conditions), if there is concern for a parameningeal infection focus (which is rare, and mostly seen in partially treated disease) or other anatomic condition predisposing a patient to the infection, or to look for obvious radiographic signs of elevated ICP prior to LP. Within several days of symptom onset, leptomeningeal enhancement and widened basal cisterns may be observed on CT. Occasionally, subdural effusions may be present later in the disease process, and less commonly, diffuse cerebral edema or abscess formation. Head ultrasound may be used for the examination of infants.

Complications

Acute and late neurologic complications of bacterial meningitis occur in 16% to 50% of survivors (48,49), and are related to the age and baseline health of the patient, causative organism, and the severity and duration of illness.

Early neurologic complications in children are varied. Increased ICP may occur within the first 48 hours in up to 50% of children who require intensive care monitoring (44). This elevation is typically associated with Cushing triad and progressive obtundation. Cranial nerve palsies (particularly third, fourth, sixth, and eighth) may occur secondary to elevated ICP, or as primary complications. Seizures occur in about 30% of children with bacterial meningitis early in the course of illness and often before presentation to medical care (2). In some cases seizures may be due to parenchymal spread of infection, in others they are thought to be due to cortical irritation resulting from associated inflammation, fever, and electrolyte changes. The majority of seizures resolve without directed intervention over several days. However, seizures that are prolonged or difficult to control may be associated with later neurologic sequelae (43,50). Subdural effusions occur in up to 50% of Hib meningitis, and in up to 30% with other infectious etiologies (27). They are typically sterile and self-resolve, however, if a child has protracted or focal symptoms, or partially treated meningitis with a prolonged course, subdural effusions may become superinfected and subdural drainage should be considered. Ventriculitis occurs most commonly in infants and presents with persistent fever. This complication requires prolonged antibiotics. Cerebritis and infarction result from direct spread of infection to the parenchyma of the brain, or due to inflammatory changes of the blood vessels related to the inflammatory cytokine milieu. Both are associated with abscess formation and poor prognosis.

Transient or permanent sensorineural deafness can result from inflammatory or bacterial damage to the eighth cranial nerve, cochlea, or labyrinth, or from the use of ototoxic antibiotics. Permanent hearing loss may occur in up to 11% of cases, and is more likely in children with a longer duration of symptoms, lack of petechiae (in the case of meningococcal disease), a low CSF glucose, and ataxia. In addition, it is significantly more common in Hib and pneumococcal infections than in meningococcal infections (51). All patients with bacterial meningitis need a hearing test prior to hospital discharge, and should be followed closely as outpatients.

Later neurologic complications include cognitive and behavioral deficits, seizures, and motor deficits. Less common complications of bacterial meningitis include transverse myelitis, infarction, permanent hydrocephalus, aneurysm formation of intracranial vessels, and cortical visual impairment.

Treatment

Treatment of bacterial meningitis is meant to inhibit bacterial replication, prevent cerebral edema, and prevent the secondary effects of proinflammatory cytokines in the subarachnoid space. Suspected meningitis should be treated immediately with empiric intravenous antibiotics; treatment must not be delayed if there is a contraindication to or a delay in ability to perform LP (36). In such situations, blood cultures should be obtained, and empiric antibiotics administered as soon as possible. Antibiotics typically sterilize a CSF culture and Gram stain within 2 to 48 hours, depending on the organism (52); earlier sterilization appears to occur with N meningitidis compared with other pathogens. CSF glucose begins to normalize over 12 hours following treatment (53). However, the CSF WBC and protein elevations frequently persist for up to 7 days (44). Once organism identification is made, and antibiotic susceptibilities are available, antibiotic selection can be appropriately directed. A repeat LP for test-of-cure in neonates with Gram-negative meningitis is recommended and may alter the duration of therapy, but is not routine for other clinical scenarios in which a child is recovering within the expected time course (2).

Choice of empiric antibiotics varies with age, and care must be taken to use antibiotics with appropriate CNS penetration. However in general, coverage should include a third generation cephalosporin, in addition to further coverage based on specific risk factors (Tables 16.4 and 16.5). In most cases of bacterial meningitis, a 10- to 14-day course of treatment is necessary, although some require longer durations of treatment. General recommendations for organism-specific antibiotics and duration of treatment are listed in Table 16.6, but individual treatment should always be discussed with an infectious disease specialist. Acyclovir should be added to an empiric regimen until HSV meningitis is definitively excluded.

Use of adjunctive corticosteroid therapy has been closely examined in bacterial meningitis with both prospective and retrospective randomized trials and meta-analyses in infants and children. When antibiotics are administered, the resultant bacterial lytic products, including endotoxin, increase the host inflammatory response in the subarachnoid space, resulting in further cellular damage. In general, glucocorticoids are thought to suppress proinflammatory

Table 16.6	Antibiotic Dosing and Schedules for Selected Organisms Causing Meningitis in Infants and Children[a]	
Organism	First-Line Therapy Choices and Doses	Treatment Duration
Listeria monocytogenes	Ampicillin 300 mg/kg/day divided q8h OR Penicillin G 0.3 mU/kg/day divided q4–6h	> 21 days
Aerobic Gram-negative bacilli	If susceptible: ceftriaxone 80–100 mg/kg/day divided q12–24h Other: meropenem 120 mg/kg/day divided q8h	~21 days

Streptococcus pneumonia	Based on penicillin minimum inhibitory concentration (MIC):
	  < 0.1 µg/mL:
	    Penicillin G 0.3 mU/kg/day divided q4–6h or
	    Ampicillin 300 mg/kg/day divided q8h
	  0.1–1.0 µg/mL:
	    Ceftriaxone 80–100 mg/kg/day divided q12–24h
	  ≥ 2 µg/mL:
	    Vancomycin 60 mg/kg/day divided q6h
	    Ceftriaxone 80–100 mg/kg/day divided q12–24h
		10–14 days

Streptococcus agalactiae	Ampicillin 300 mg/kg/day divided q8h OR Penicillin G 0.3 mU/kg/day divided q4–6h	14–21 days

Neisseria meningitidis	Based on penicillin MIC:
	  < 0.1 µg/mL:
	    Penicillin G 0.3 mU/kg/day divided q4–6h OR
	    Ampicillin 300 mg/kg/day divided q8h
	  0.1–1.0 µg/mL: third generation cephalosporin
	    Ceftriaxone 80–100 mg/kg/day divided q12–24h
		7 days

Haemophilus spp	β-lactamase negative: ampicillin 300 mg/kg/day divided q8h β-lactamase positive: ceftriaxone 80–100 mg/kg/day divided q12–24h	7 days

[a] Note: table does not include neonatal dosing.
Source: Adapted from Tunkel AR et al. Practice guidelines for the management of bacterial meningitis. *Clin Infect Dis.* 2004;39:1267–1284.

cytokines in the subarachnoid space, and therefore decrease eighth cranial nerve damage and subsequent hearing loss, the clinical duration of fever, parenchymal damage and later neurologic deficits, and perhaps mortality (54). In animal studies, it has also reduced cerebral edema, elevated ICP, and CSF outflow obstruction (27). However, it does not appear to reverse existing CNS damage.

The only proven indication for adjunctive glucocorticoid treatment of meningitis is in the setting of Hib infection. In this case, dexamethasone 0.4 mg/kg IV every 12 hours for 2 days is recommended. It is most beneficial when administered with, or just before parenteral antibiotics (33). The American Academy of Pediatrics recommends using dexamethasone only if it can be given within 1 hour of the first dose of antimicrobial therapy. Use in pneumococcal infections or as empiric therapy is more controversial. Several recent studies suggest no benefit to children for mortality (55) or hearing loss (56). The role for dexamethasone in the treatment of neonates is less clear (27).

Acute complications of meningitis require intensive care. Subdural empyemas (SDEs), intraparenchymal abscesses, and communicating hydrocephalus must be addressed surgically. The syndrome of inappropriate antidiuretic hormone (SIADH) may be treated with fluid restriction if the patient is hemodynamically stable; this frequently self-resolves with meningitis recovery. Patients who are stuporous or comatose may require ICP monitoring. Treatment for increased ICP include head of the bed elevation to 30°, hyperventilation to maintain Pco_2 at 25 to 30 cm H_2O, use of hyperosmolar agents such as hypertonic saline or mannitol, or neurosurgical decompression. Seizures are managed routinely, depending on frequency and type.

Chemoprophylaxis is recommended for close contacts or in outbreak situations for meningococcal disease and Hib. High-risk contacts include household members, incompletely immunized or immunocompromised contacts, and, in the case of meningococcal disease, those who had direct exposure to the index patient's respiratory secretions at any time within 7 days prior to onset of illness. Contact of patients with Hib meningitis should receive rifampin, and contacts of patients with meningococcal meningitis should receive rifampin, ceftriaxone, ciprofloxacin, or azithromycin. Chemoprophylaxis should be addressed for all contacts immediately following diagnosis.

Acute Viral Meningitis

Viral meningitis and encephalitis have similar epidemiologies, causative organisms, pathophysiologies, and treatments. For a complete review, please see Encephalitis and Myelitis section of this chapter. Briefly, the most common causes of viral meningitis are enteroviruses (EVs), followed by parechoviruses, herpesviruses, arboviruses, and influenza. The clinical presentation of viral meningitis is similar to acute bacterial meningitis, although symptoms are typically less severe and more indolent. However, anyone presenting with acute meningitis should be treated empirically as acute bacterial meningitis with immediate antibiotics until an alternate diagnosis becomes clear (32). LP is the diagnostic procedure of choice. Viral meningitides classically demonstrate a mildly elevated WBC, elevated protein, and normal glucose (Table 16.3). The pleocytosis is typically lymphocytic, although may be neutrophil predominant in the early stages of infection. In general, viral meningitis is much more common than acute bacterial meningitis; 95% of all children with pleocytosis are ultimately diagnosed with viral meningitis (47).

Subacute and Chronic Meningitis

Epidemiology and Pathophysiology

Subacute and chronic meningitis account for about 10% of all cases of meningitis (57), with an increased prevalence in the immunocompromised population (58). The pathophysiology is similar to acute bacterial meningitis, however subacute meningitis evolves over days to weeks, and chronic meningitis persists for over 4 weeks (2,58,59). Clinically, the distinction between subacute and chronic meningitis is not important

because both conditions are similar in presentation and etiology. In addition, patients rarely present after 4 weeks of meningeal symptoms, making the distinction unhelpful at the bedside. Therefore, subacute and chronic meningitis will be discussed here together. In broad terms, etiologies can be broken down into infectious versus noninfectious causes, however no etiology is found in 15% to 25% of cases (60). Noninfectious causes include autoimmune inflammatory disorders (Behçet, systemic lupus erythematosis, Wegener granulomatosis, or Vogt-Koyanagi-Harada syndrome), collagen vascular diseases, leptomeningeal neoplastic metastases, chronic subarachnoid bleeding, and chemical meningitides.

Infectious causes of subacute and chronic meningitis are diverse. Tuberculous (TB) meningitis (see Tuberculosis and Other Granulomatous CNS Infections section) and fungal meningitides (particularly cryptococcal disease; see Immunocompromised Hosts section) are the most common infectious causes. Other infectious etiologies include neurosyphilis (see Tuberculosis and Other Granulomatous CNS Infections section), neuroborreliosis, neurobrucellosis, rickettsial infections, *Listeria monocytogenes*, HIV (see Encephalitis and Myelitis and Immunocompromised Hosts sections), and parasitic diseases (see Protozoal and Helminthic infection section). Chronic viral meningitides outside of immunocompromised patients are rare.

Clinical Presentation

Most chronic meningitides present similarly, though more subacutely, to acute bacterial meningitis. Meningeal signs including headache and neck stiffness, lethargy, confusion, weight loss, and intermittent emesis predominate (58). If present, low-grade fevers are usually below 39°C (61). Less commonly, patients describe focal neurologic deficits, cranial nerve palsies, seizures, and radicular pain or paresthesias (58). Specific presentations of several etiologic organisms are as follows:

- *Borrelia burgdorferi* meningitis typically presents approximately 4 weeks after the erythema migrans rash of Lyme disease appears (57), and may be associated with persistent erythema migrans and/or arthritis. The course is subtle and fluctuant (61) and may be accompanied by a facial palsy or painful neuritis (58), most commonly optic neuritis.

- Systemic brucellosis presents with undulant fever, lymphadenopathy, and hepatosplenomegaly (61) following exposure to unpasteurized milk products or farm animals (60). Neurologic brucellosis occurs in less than 5% of cases of systemic disease (57). In the early septicemic phase an isolated leptomeningitis may occur, however patients may also develop a meningoencephalitis 2 months to 2 years following the initial episode (60), which may include cranial nerve palsies (61), radiculopathy, and peripheral neuropathy (57).
- Rickettsial chronic meningitis (particularly *Ehrlichia chaffeensis, Anaplasma phagocytophilum,* and *Babesia* spp) occurs in about 10% of rickettsial infections, and is frequently not identified due to low diagnostic baseline suspicion and lack of specific testing.
- *Listeria* causes basilar meningitis mimicking tubercular meningitis.
- Other etiologic considerations for clinical presentation of chronic meningitis include syphilis and neurocysticercosis (see Tuberculosis and Other Granulomatous CNS Infections section, and Protozoal and Helminthic infection section).

Diagnosis

Because several of the causes of chronic meninigitis are zoonoses, thorough travel and animal exposure histories are important in diagnosis, as is a thorough physical exam to investigate noninfectious etiologies. LP is the diagnostic test of choice for chronic meningitis, following a good examination and history. However, isolation of a causative organism from the CSF is often difficult because the pathogen load in chronic meningitis tends to be much lower than in acute bacterial meningitis (58). In addition, many pathologic organisms are fastidious and difficult to isolate in standard culture (such as *B burgdorferi, Rickettsia,* and *Ehrlichia*), or quickly degenerate without proper CSF handling (such as *Naegleria fowleri*). Blood and CSF serologies, PCR, pathogen-specific antigen tests, and other serum markers of systemic inflammation may be helpful (see Encephalitis and Myelitis section Table 16.21).

Most cases of chronic meningitis have nonspecific CSF findings. Typically, there is a moderate lymphocytic pleocytosis (< 500 WBC/mL), mildly elevated protein, and normal glucose (57). Persistent neutrophilic meningitides are rare, but can be associated with fungal infections, TB, or brucellosis. Noninfectious cases of chronic neutrophilic meningitis may be due to neoplasm, systemic lupus erythematosus, or chemical meningitis (58).

Neuroimaging may be helpful in determining an etiology of chronic meningitis; MRI with gadolinium enhancement is the best modality to do so. Table 16.7 reviews MRI findings suggestive of specific pathogens and processes. Vascular imaging by conventional angiography or magnetic resonance (MR) angiography may be helpful to look for evidence of vasculitis or aneurysm; however, vascular imaging is not 100% sensitive. Meningeal biopsy may be considered for focal areas of meningeal enhancement if the etiology is unclear; meningeal biopsy has the highest yield if underlying brain parenchyma is examined in tandem (58).

Treatment

Treatment for chronic meningitis is dependent on the etiologic agent (please see Acute Bacterial Meningitis

---

■ **Table 16.7** MRI Findings Associated With Specific Chronic Infections

MRI Finding	Possible Causative Infections
Basal meningeal enhancement	Tubercular, fungal, or *Listeria* infection
Focal meningeal enhancement	Granulomatous disease or leptomeningeal metastasis
Obstructive hydrocephalus	Tumor or ventricular neurocysticercosis
Parenchymal masses	Tuberculoma, abscess, neurocysticercosis, neoplasm
Subarachnoid or intraparenchymal hemorrhage	Vasculitic process, angioinvasive fungal infection, ruptured mycotic aneurysm

Abbreviation: MRI, magnetic resonance imaging.
Source: Adapted from Davis LE. Subacute and chronic meningitis. *CONTINUUM Lifelong Learning Neurol.* 2006;12:27–57.

and Tuberculosis and Other Granulomatous CNS Infections sections for organism specific treatment); however, as discussed above, a causative organism is frequently not found.

Recurrent Meningitis

Recurrent meningitis is defined by repeated episodes of appropriately treated acute meningitis, followed by periods of absent meningeal signs and normal CSF parameters (57). Recurrent meningitis may be bacterial, fungal, or aseptic.

Recurrent bacterial meningitis in children occurs with 1.3% to 5% of community acquired bacterial meningitis episodes (62). Most cases of recurrent bacterial meningitis are due to traumatic or congenital skull-based anatomic defects, parameningeal infectious foci, or immunodeficiencies (59). Following skull fracture, recurrent cases of *S pneumoniae*, Hib, and meningococcal meningitis have been described. Parameningeal foci include brain abscess, chronic osteomyelitis of a skull bone, or mastoiditis. Acute diagnostic testing and treatment are similar for recurrent bacterial meningitis as for chronic meningitis. Neuroimaging should be used to look for an anatomic source. If possible, anatomic defects should be repaired (63), and immune reconstitution should be implemented. Prophylactic antibiotic use in cases of known skull base defects is controversial, and not routinely recommended (62).

Recurrent aseptic meningitis may be caused by waxing and waning chronic meningitis (particularly *Cryptococcus*), although in these cases the CSF is persistently abnormal between acute episodes. Mollaret meningitis is a specific syndrome of benign recurrent aseptic meningitis characterized by sudden short bouts of fever, meningismus, and CSF profiles suggestive of viral infection. Mollaret meningitis primarily affects young adults, but has been reported in children as young as 5 years old (63). Typical episodes last 1 to 5 days, occurring at weekly, monthly, or yearly intervals, and often persist over many years. While some cases of Mollaret meningitis have been associated with HSV-2 CNS infection (57,63), many cases remain idiopathic. Patients with known HSV-2 CNS infection should be treated with antiviral therapy, although no controlled trials have formally evaluated this recommendation. The typical course of Mollaret meningitis is benign (63).

Latent infections such as HSV, EBV, and toxoplasmosis (59), chronic inflammatory diseases, and chemical meningitides may also cause a recurrent aseptic meningitis. Recurrent chemical meningitides may be due to intermittent discharge from epidermoid cysts or craniopharyngiomas, and neuroimaging may again be helpful in identifying these structural etiologies. Drug-induced recurrent aseptic meningitis is rare, but has been reported with nonsteroidal antiinflammatory drugs (NSAIDs), sulfa based antibiotics, and intravenous immunoglobulin (IVIg) (63). Vascular inflammatory disorders that are typically classified as chronic meningitis (such as Behçet) may also present with more intermittent symptoms and be clinically classified as recurrent cases.

Noninfectious Causes of Meningitis

There are multiple noninfectious causes for meningitis (Table 16.8).

■ **Table 16.8**   Noninfectious Causes of Meningitis

Acute Meningitis	Chronic Meningitis	Meningoencephalitis
Behçet	Granulomatous angiitis	Behçet
Chemical meningitis[a]	Chemical meningitis	ADEM
Systemic lupus erythematosus	Lymphomatoid granulomatosis	AHLE
Serum sickness	Systemic lupus erythematosus	Systemic lupus erythematosus
Sarcoidosis	Meningeal malignancy	Serum sickness
Cyst rupture	Sarcoidosis	Acute toxic encephalopathy
Parameningeal infection		
Febrile seizure		

Abbreviations: ADEM, acute disseminated encephalomyelitis; AHLE, acute hemorrhagic leukoencephalopathy.
[a] Due to nonsteroidal antiinflammatory drugs, sulfa drugs, intravenous immunoglobulin.

■ FOCAL SUPPURATIVE INFECTIONS

Brain Abscess

One thousand five hundred to 2,500 brain abscesses are diagnosed annually in the United States, and the incidence appears to be decreasing (64). While previously uniformly fatal, the advent of new neurosurgical techniques, antimicrobial therapy, and CT scanning (65) has improved morbidity and mortality with early and aggressive diagnostic and therapeutic strategies. However, brain abscesses continue to be a serious and difficult to treat suppurative intracranial infection, with a mortality rate in children of 4% to 12% (66).

Epidemiology and Pathophysiology

Brain abscess is defined as a focal intracerebral collection of pus surrounded by a well-vascularized capsule (67). Abscesses develop over the course of 2 weeks or more, beginning with a cerebritis stage, which is an ill-defined inflammatory infiltrate. The lesion progresses to become more organized and ultimately an encapsulated collection of necrotic tissue surrounded by a thick-walled capsule. A brain abscess can be staged based on clinical, histologic, and radiographic findings (Table 16.9).

In general, the brain is well protected from microbial invasion by an impermeable BBB. The BBB is composed of CNS endothelial cells joined by tight junctions (67) surrounded by a basal lamina. Astrocyte foot processes then ensheath these vessels on the parenchymal side. Interactions between these cells and immune cells regulate the permeability of the BBB, therefore modulating the inflammatory and microorganism milieu allowed entrance to the brain parenchyma. States of inflammation such as meningitis or disrupted blood flow following embolic events increase the permeability of the BBB. Physical disruptions, such as penetration by a foreign body in the case of surgery or trauma also upset this baseline homeostasis.

Bacteria reach the brain parenchyma via several different routes including direct extension from a cranial source of infection, hematogenous dissemination from a nearby or distant organ infection, or exogenous introduction. Direct extension is most common, typically from a paranasal sinusitis or otitis media; these sources may also reach the brain parenchyma via a valveless venous drainage system in the crania mucosa that communicates with the venous plexus of the dura mater (66,68) (Figure 16.1). Dental infections may also extend into parenchymal space (Tables 16.10 and 16.11).

Several known predisposing factors lead to brain abscesses in children, although 15% to 30% of cases remain cryptogenic (66) (Table 16.11). Some

■ Table 16.9 Brain Abscess Stages

Stage	Time Period (Days)	Histopathologic Findings	CT Findings	MRI Findings
Early cerebritis	1–3	Ill-defined lesion, inflammatory infiltrate, peripheral edema	Normal or ill-defined hypodensity, early enhancement	Focal edema
Late cerebritis	4–9	Central necrosis surrounded by ring of macrophages and other inflammatory cells	Early patchy enhancement progressing to ring enhancement	Ring enhancement (visualized early on MRI)
Early capsule formation	10–14	Necrosis and liquefaction; early formation of collagenous capsule; peripheral gliosis/fibrosis	Distinct contrast enhancement of capsule	Hyperintense central pus surrounded by hypointense capsule and peripheral edema
Late capsule formation	> 14	Full formed thick capsule		

Abbreviation: CT, computed tomography.

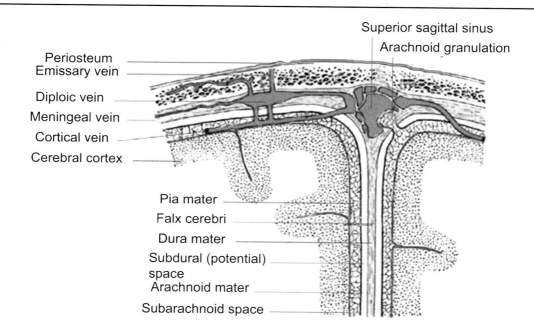

FIGURE 16.1 Anatomy of the meninges and vascular anatomy of sinuses. Adapted from *Gray's Anatomy of the Human Body,* 1918 (public domain).

organisms implicated in meningitis, specifically en-teric Gram-negative bacilli, are more likely to cause abscesses (64), and infants and toddlers are most sus-ceptible to parenchymal abscess formation following bacterial meningitis. Congenital heart disease, particu-larly with pronounced right-to-left shunting, is a risk factor for brain abscess: a patent foramen ovale or other atrioventricular septal defect may contribute to brain abscesses of unclear etiology (67). Intracranial trauma and surgery are risk factors for brain abscess with direct introduction of organisms to the sterile in-tracranial space. Trauma in which a foreign body or bone fragment is found in the brain parenchyma, or surgery which incorporates a foreign material into the intracranial space such as a ventriculoperitoneal shunt provide a nidus for infection. Children more frequently sustain penetrating orbital or otic trauma from sharp objects such as pencils, sticks, or lawn darts (66,69,70). Intracranial hemorrhage, ischemia, and tumors are additional risk factors for parenchymal abscess (67). These conditions affect certain pediatric populations, but occur more frequently in adults.

Epidemiologically, there is a male predominance among patients with brain abscesses and approximately 25% of brain abscesses occur in children (64,71). Brain abscesses are most common in children 4 to 7 years of age (66). Immunosuppressed patients and those with

congenital heart disease are at a higher risk of develop-ing brain abscess for the reasons discussed above.

Clinical Presentation

Headache is the most common reported presenting symptom of brain abscesses, occurring in up to 56% of patients (72), and is more often chronic and poorly characterized than acute (64,67). A sudden worsening of headache may be indicative of meningeal irritation due to rupture of abscess into the ventricular space. Fever occurs in approximately half of all cases. Papilledema is reported in 41% to 70% (66). Seizures, vomiting, nu-chal rigidity, focal neurologic deficits, and altered men-tal status are less common.

Prognosis is worse in patients who present with significantly altered mental status (65–67,72) and in those in whom abscess ruptures into the intraventricular space, in which case mortality is >80% (67). In pediatric populations, the rate of pervasive neurologic sequelae is approximately 15% with modern diagnostic and thera-peutic techniques (73).

Diagnosis

Early descriptions of brain abscesses report diagnoses made based on physical exam; however, prior to the late

■ **Table 16.10** Underlying Causes of Pediatric Brain Abscess

Otitis/mastoiditis	41%
Paranasal sinusitis	—
Dental	Up to 10%
Endocarditis	9%–10%
Bacteremia	8%
Pulmonary Infection	0.7%–9.8%
Folliculitis	1%–3%
Congenital heart disease	6%–51%
Meningitis	12%–36%
Penetrating injury	4.8%–16%
Neurosurgery	8%–10%
Hereditary hemorrhagic telangiectasia	—

Source: Adapted from Refs. 64, 66, 67, 71, 94.

■ **Table 16.11** Risk Factors for Poor Prognosis in Brain Abscess

Multiple abscesses
Deep-seated abscess
Intraventricular rupture
Congenital heart disease
Hydrocephalus
Poor neurologic status at presentation
Meningitis
Neonate
Initial error in diagnosis/delayed diagnosis
Unknown source of infection

Source: Adapted from Refs. 66, 72, 73.

19th century, brain abscess was 100% fatal and most diagnoses were made on postmortem examination. Perhaps the most influential factor in decreasing morbidity and mortality associated with brain abscess is the development of CT imaging in 1974. CT scanning allows for early diagnosis, localization for surgical procedures, and follow-up evaluation. Contrast-enhanced head CT is hypodense in the early cerebritis stage, reflecting focal edema. As the abscess organizes and encapsulates, CT will demonstrate a well-formed ring-enhancing lesion (64,67). Since the advent of CT neuroimaging, the rate of multifocal abscesses is recognized to be approximately 50%, which is significantly higher than previously suspected (64).

MRI with gadolinium is the preferred diagnostic study because it is more sensitive for detecting abscesses in the early cerebritis stage, with subtle edema demonstrated by T2 hyperintensity (66). Well-formed abscesses on MRI appear as T1 hypointense, T2 hyperintense, ring-enhancing lesions with surrounding edema. The necrotic core frequently diffusion restricts on DWI, as do some tumors and ischemic insults. MR spectroscopy can be helpful in the differential diagnosis of abscess and tumor based on different spectral profiles. Despite the advantages of modern brain imaging, brain abscess may be hard to distinguish from brain tumor. A surgical procedure is frequently necessary to make the definitive diagnosis.

LP is rarely helpful and potentially dangerous in patients with brain abscesses. If significant mass effect results from the abscess, there is a high risk of brainstem herniation during LP. The procedure is contraindicated in these cases. CSF examination is usually nonspecific, with pleocytosis and elevated protein, although may be normal and cultures are usually negative (67,72). Blood culture is often negative, but when positive, it may be helpful in identifying an organism.

Treatment

Treatment of brain abscess requires a combination of neurosurgical drainage, targeted antimicrobial therapy, and neurologic and intensive care supportive management. Initial stabilization measures are focused on decreasing ICP and controlling seizures. Seizures occur in 25% to 50% of brain abscesses (67) and are treated based on frequency and type. In cases of severe brain edema, mannitol and forced hyperventilation may be adjuncts to surgical care. Surgical stabilization, including decompressive craniotomy, is necessary for those patients with malignant ICP. An external ventricular drainage device may be warranted, especially in cases of intraventricular rupture of abscess (67).

Small lesions less than 2 centimeters may be managed successfully with only parenteral antibiotic therapy (64,67). Conservative therapy may also be appropriate for immature abscesses in the cerebritis stage or when multiple abscesses are present (68,72). However, early and aggressive surgical drainage should be performed for larger accessible lesions in appropriate patients. Several neurosurgical options exist: stereotactic biopsies may be done for deeper lesions, or complete excisions by craniotomy for multiloculated abscesses, those with resistant organisms, or lesions which have recurred despite prior drainage. Neither surgical option is associated with a more optimal outcome (66,72). Surgical management of paranasal sinusitis, otitis media, or other origin of infection must be undertaken in conjunction with abscess drainage.

Empiric antibiotic therapy is chosen based on the suspected origin of the infection. Brain abscesses are frequently polymicrobial due to the colonizing flora of the infection sources. The most common organisms are viridans group streptococci, *Streptococcus milleri*, and anaerobic bacteria (67,72). Abscesses of otic origin may include Gram-negative bacilli such as *Pseudomonas aeruginosa* and the Enterobacteriaceae (Table 16.12). Abscesses associated with trauma or surgical procedures are often caused by coagulase-negative staphylococci and *S aureus* (66,67).

Antibiotics must be both appropriate for the infecting organisms, and also the site of infection. In treating brain abscesses, antibiotics must have appropriate CNS penetration. First generation cephalosporins, clindamycin, and penicillins combined with beta-lactamase inhibitors have very poor CNS penetration. Quinolones and carbapenems have adequate CNS penetration, however, some drugs in these classes can lower seizure thresholds (67). A combination of antibiotics targeted at anaerobes, streptococci, and Gram-negative organisms should be employed for treatment of all brain abscesses. A late generation cephalosporin combined with metronidazole is appropriate empiric therapy. Vancomycin may be added in the case of trauma, postsurgical infection, or other cases in which *S aureus* is a suspected pathogen. Intraventricular antibiotics may be considered when there is intraventricular rupture of an abscess (66).

The yield of abscess material culture is reported to be 80% to 95% (66,72), and antibiotics may be narrowed to target those organisms identified; however, even with early and fastidious culturing of abscess material, strict anaerobes may be difficult to identify so all regimens should include anaerobic antibiotic therapy.

Corticosteroids have not been shown to cause appreciable difference in outcomes for patients with brain abscess (72) and should be reserved for those situations in which severe brain edema exists. Steroids may inhibit antimicrobial penetration into the CNS and clearance of infection (74). Therefore, corticosteroids should be administered for only short courses, if at all (64,68).

Intravenous antibiotic therapy should be given for approximately 6 to 8 weeks depending on the extent of infection and the organisms involved. Imaging should be repeated every 2 to 3 weeks until resolution of all lesions, and should be repeated immediately in the setting of clinical deterioration (64). Lesions usually resolve after 12 to 16 weeks but complete resolution may not occur for up to 6 months in some cases (66).

Subdural Empyema

SDE is defined as a purulent collection between the dura and the arachnoid meninges. Children with SDE are at high risk of increasing ICP, and therefore rapid neurologic deterioration. Prior to the advent of penicillin in 1944, the mortality rate of SDE was 100%. Currently, the mortality rate for children with SDE is 10% to 20%.

Epidemiology and Pathophysiology

SDE is a life-threatening infection that is primarily associated with otorhinologic infections during the summer months (75). These infections are most common in boys over the age of 7 years, which may be related to rapid growth of paranasal sinuses and related vasculature (76–79). In addition, approximately 2% of infants with meningitis will develop SDE as a complication (77). Less common etiologies of SDE include dental abscesses, superinfection of traumatic hematoma, or infection introduced during neurosurgical manipulation (76). Infants and young children can rarely develop SDE following upper and lower respiratory tract infections (77).

The subdural space is connected to the sinuses and middle ear by valveless diploic veins. Microbiologic organisms may enter this space via transport along these veins, direct intracranial extension of sinus infections through the posterior wall of the sinuses and the epidural space, or by thrombophlebitis of the interconnected venous system (68,77,79). Direct extension occurs more commonly in middle ear infections with associated mastoiditis (68). In infants with meningitis or respiratory infections, SDE occurs after a bacteremic event with seeding of a preexisting subdural effusion or hematoma (77). An alternate form of SDE occurs in infants following superinfection of meningitis-associated subdural effusions. This is seen less frequently since the initiation of routine immunization for pneumococcus and Hib.

Once pus exists in the subdural space, it can spread widely and rapidly over the entire cerebral hemisphere, into the interhemispheric fissure, and to the contralateral hemisphere due to the lack of septations within this space. SDE in pediatric patients is bilateral in 70% to 80% of cases (80). Most cases of SDE are supratentorial; approximately 0.6% are infratentorial and most of these are of otic origin (75). Although subdural pus begins as

■ **Table 16.12** Unusual Organisms Causing Brain Abscess

Organism	Characteristics	Susceptible Pediatric Host	Management	Prognosis	Other
Nocardia (95,96)	Gram-positive branched bacillus, acid-fast, member of actinomycetes family	Exposure to soil, immunosuppressed	Trimethoprim (TMP)-sulfa second line: imipenem or third generation cephalosporin; surgical drainage if > 2 cm; Duration: 12 months or longer if immuno-suppression persists	33%–37% mortality and higher with immunosuppression or multiple abscesses. Overall, mortality is 3 times higher than brain abscesses of other etiology.	Inhaled or cutaneous inoculation, brain involvement may be asymptomatic; insidious onset
Pseudallescheria boydii (97)	Dematiaceous fungus	Near-drowning, trauma, immunosuppressed	Voriconazole or posaconazole (resistant to amphotericin); surgical resection; prolonged duration	High mortality (75%), long-term neurologic sequelae common in survivors	Often accompanies lung infiltrates—organism probably inhaled during near-drowning episode
Citrobacter spp (98)	Gram-negative bacillus Colonizes gastrointestinal/genitourinary tract	Neonates	Cefepime, carbapenem (despite in vitro susceptibility to third generation cephalosporins, inducible resistance should be expected and these antibiotics should not be used); surgical drainage; duration: 4–6 weeks	33% mortality, 50% of survivors have neurologic sequelae	Occurs secondary to meningitis; 75% of those with *Citrobacter* meningitis have brain abscess
Listeria monocytogenes (99)	Gram-positive bacillus	Neonates, immunosuppressed	Ampicillin + aminoglycoside second line: TMP-sulfa; surgical drainage if possible duration: ampicillin minimum of 4 weeks, gentamicin 2–4 weeks; in one series all survivors received 2–14 weeks of antibiotic treatment with no difference in neurologic outcomes attributable to differences in duration	33 of 39 survivors in largest series	10% of all CNS infections caused by *Listeria* are brain abscesses; most have concomitant bacteremia; 1/3 have positive CSF culture
Other fungi (67,71,100)	*Candida, Cryptococcus, Aspergillus,* mucormycosis, coccidiomycosis, histoplasmosis, blastomycosis	Immunocompromised hosts; neonates at risk for *Candida*	Depends on organism	Organism-dependent; 95% mortality with *Aspergillus*; 10%–30% mortality with *Candida*	

liquid, it may become organized as infection progresses, resulting in loculation of advanced infections.

As with brain abscesses, the primary site of infection lends clues to the microbiologic etiology. Polymicrobial infection is common in sinus and otic-derived infections. In general, the most common bacteria found in SDE are streptococci, typically of the microaerophilic or nutritionally-deficient variety. Anaerobes can be isolated in up to two-thirds of cases (68), but fastidious collection techniques necessary for isolating anaerobes is both difficult and uncommon so this is likely an underestimate of the true proportion of anaerobic bacteria involved in SDE (Table 16.13).

Clinical Presentation

When a microbiologic organism enters the subdural space, it creates an inflammatory response, generating meningeal irritation and purulent exudate, blocking CSF reabsorption at the choroid plexus, resulting in increased ICP. This inflammation and elevated ICP causes headache, emesis, altered level of consciousness, focal neurologic deficits, and may cause seizures (77). New symptoms in a child with a known sinus or ear infection should raise suspicion for intracranial infection. In addition, a relapse of fever, enlarging head circumference, or new neurologic finding in an infant with known bacterial meningitis should prompt evaluation for an SDE. Duration of symptoms preceding diagnosis varies based on primary site of infection. Patients with extension of sinusitis have an average of 14 days of symptoms prior to diagnosis, whereas infants with meningitis and SDE present very acutely (76). Symptoms of primary infection are absent in 25% of patients at time of diagnosis of SDE (81). There may be incisional drainage at the site of postoperative infection.

Diagnosis

Cultures of material collected during surgical intervention are essential in providing guidance for targeted antimicrobial therapy. Blood cultures rarely yield pathogens. LP is generally contraindicated in SDE as ICP is increased. Neuroimaging is imperative in the diagnosis and surgical treatment planning of SDE, and should not be delayed if this diagnosis is suspected. A noncontrast head CT is the most rapid and available form of imaging, and typically demonstrates a hypodense area over the hemisphere or falx; contrast enhancement may help define specific margins. However, CT scanning is reportedly

normal in 50% of SDE (76). Gadolinium-enhanced MRI of the brain is the imaging study of choice when available promptly. MRI provides greater morphologic detail and higher sensitivity for fluid collection than CT. For planning and treatment, imaging should include the site of primary infection (paranasal sinuses, mastoids) to aid in surgical planning and to guide empiric antibiotic therapy.

Complications

Complications of SDE include sinus venous thrombus, cerebral edema, herniation, recurrent neurologic deficits, reaccumulation of empyema, and catheter-related complications due to long-term intravenous antibiotics (76–78,80). A 65-case series found sinus venous thrombus as the only statistically significant risk factor for mortality (82). Another series of 38 pediatric patients with SDE reported neurologic deficit and cerebral herniation at presentation as significantly associated with poor outcome (83).

Treatment

SDE is a neurosurgical emergency. Nearly all patients with SDE require at least one neurosurgical procedure; only very rare cases are managed successfully without surgery, and only in cases of well-localized, small collections of pus in minimally symptomatic patients (76,78,83). There remains some controversy surrounding the appropriate initial neurosurgical procedure to drain SDE. Craniotomy appears to have more success and requires fewer repeat operations, although there is a slightly higher risk of intraoperative bleeding and infection (75,82). In patients with significant cerebral edema, decompressive craniectomy may be required. If skull bones are infected, a bone flap removal is necessary. Burr holes are appropriate for drainage of localized collections, early infection when pus is still very liquid, or for patients too unstable to be taken to the operating room. In several large series however, the use of burr holes as initial surgical technique was a risk factor for repeated operation (76,80). In one large series of pediatric patients with SDE, 26% required reoperation, 83% of whom had primary burr hole placement (82). Surgical intervention for the origin of infection should be performed simultaneously with drainage of subdural collections. Early sinus drainage and mastoidectomy contribute to lower mortality and decreased incidence of reoperation in cases of rhinosinogenic SDE (77,79).

Cultures of pus should be obtained during surgical intervention. Cultures are sterile in 7% to 53% of cases (77,78,82) likely due to exposure to antibiotics

■ **Table 16.13** Pathogens, Sites of Primary Infection, and Empiric Treatment of Brain Abscess

Pathogen	Origin of Infection	Empiric Antibiotic Treatment

Microaerophilic streptococci
Anaerobes
  Fusobacterium spp
  Prevotella spp
  Peptostreptococcus spp
  Bacteroides spp
  Clostridium diversus
Eikenella corrodens
Nontypeable Haemophilus influenzae
	Sinus, Gingiva	Third generation cephalosporin
		+
		Metronidazole

S. pneumoniae	Middle ear	Third generation cephalosporin + Metronidazole
S. aureus *Coagulase-negative Staphylococcus*	Post-operative	Vancomycin + Third generation cephalosporin +/– Metronidazole
H. influenzae type B *E. coli* *Group B Streptococcus*	Meningitis	Third generation cephalosporin +/– Vancomycin
Salmonella spp.	Other (Cryptogenic)	Vancomycin + Third generation cephalosporin +/– Metronidazole

Source: Adapted from Refs. 68, 76, 78, 79, 81, 83.

and difficulty isolating anaerobic bacteria. Generally, empiric antibiotic therapy should be broad and include Gram-positive, Gram-negative, and anaerobic bacteria. Empiric therapy may be tailored to the site of originating infection if it is known at diagnosis. *S aureus* is a rare pathogen in sinusitis-related intracranial infection, occurring in only 4% to 8% of cases (77), so vancomycin need not be included in empiric therapy unless there are specific concerns for *S aureus* infection (Table 16.13).

Antibiotics should be tailored to pathogens grown in cultures of subdural pus. Although no randomized studies exist regarding the duration of antibiotics, few treatment failures are observed when intravenous antibiotics are given for 3 weeks following operative drainage (80). Patients with SDE who are managed conservatively without surgical intervention should receive approximately 6 to 8 weeks of intravenous antibiotics (78). Metronidazole is enterally bioavailable and adequately penetrates the BBB, so may be given orally.

Intensive care management should include anticonvulsant therapy either to treat or prevent seizures in cases of severe SDE. Any patient with severe neurologic compromise (Glasgow Coma Score < 8) should be mechanically ventilated for airway protection and monitored with continuous electroencephalogram (EEG) to detect subclinical seizures. Management of intracranial hypertension may require hyperventilation, mannitol, and external ventricular device placement. Corticosteroids should be reserved for only the most refractory cases of increased ICP, as the immunosuppressive effects of steroids are deleterious in treating intracranial infections.

Epidural Abscess

EA is a collection of pus in the potential space between the calvarium and the dura mater. Its origin is similar to those of SDE, however EA-related mortality is low and good neurologic outcomes are expected. EA is an uncommon entity in the developed world due to the early recognition and treatment of otorhinologic infection.

Epidemiology and Pathophysiology

EA is the most common complication of acute bacterial sinusitis. Sixty percent to 90% of epidural space infections occurring in children are a secondary complication of sinusitis or middle ear infections (84). Like SDE, EA occurs more frequently in males, and in patients 7 to 20 years of age (85), probably for similar reasons. Pathophysiologically, a network of valveless bidirectional veins passes from sinuses and mastoid air cells through the epidural space and into the subdural space, thereby creating a passageway for bacteria to travel from extracranial to intracranial structures (Figure 16.1) (84). Less frequently, sinus and mastoid infections extend directly through the skull wall into the epidural space.

The dura mater is tightly adhered to the skull and forms a space only when penetrated. This precludes epidural infections from spreading rapidly and protects the patient from focal neurologic symptoms in most cases. Because of the proximity of this space to the skull, osteomyelitis may be comorbid in EA. Pott puffy tumor is a specific predisposing factor for EA in children and adolescents. Described by Percival Pott in 1760 (76), the "tumor" describes localized swelling of the forehead indicating osteomyelitis of the frontal bone with subperiosteal abscess secondary to frontal sinusitis. Although not always included in this constellation of findings, EA is a common comorbidity.

Children may also develop EA following superinfection of a traumatic head injury. Blood is excellent culture media, so patients with traumatic epidural effusions may develop superinfection of the hematoma therefore creating EA. In cases of superinfected epidural effusions, the hematomas are likely seeded by bacteremic events, which may be transient and asymptomatic, or pathologic. In these patients, staphylococci, streptococci, and Gram-negative bacilli must be considered. Most commonly, EAs are polymicrobial infections. Streptococci are found in a disproportionately high number of cases, and anaerobes are often present in cases of sinogenic origin (Table 16.13) (86).

Clinical Presentation

EA presents more subtly than SDE, often with several days of fever, headache, and neck pain. Mental status change and focal neurologic deficits occur less frequently than in SDE, although seizures may occur (84,85). Extension of sinus disease into the epidural space usually occurs in the frontal region, so frontal headaches may be present. Patients with prior trauma or surgery may suddenly develop fever or erythema and dehiscence at the skin incision.

Diagnosis

The diagnostic evaluation of EA is very similar to that of SDE. Blood cultures should be obtained, as well as abscess culture if surgical intervention occurs. CT scanning is often the first imaging modality used in acute bacterial sinusitis, and may detect a low-attenuation extraaxial collection consistent with EA. MRI with gadolinium is the imaging modality of choice, with 90% to 95% sensitivity and at least 90% specificity in detection. It is better able to clearly delineate abscess from normal tissue, and effectively shows thickening of the dura, which differentiates a purulent collection from a benign effusion (84).

Treatment

Although EA does not pose the same neurosurgical emergency as SDE, surgical management in combination with intravenous antibiotic therapy ensures the best outcomes (80). Craniotomy is preferred as burr holes are associated with abscess recurrence. Small EA less than 2 cm in patients without neurologic compromise may be treated successfully with antibiotics alone (84). Surgical management of osteomyelitis, sinusitis, and mastoiditis should occur concurrently with drainage of EA.

Empiric therapy should include coverage of streptococci, Gram-negative bacilli, and anaerobic bacteria. Staphylococci are infrequently found in EA originating from otorhinologic infection, although should be considered in posttraumatic or postoperative cases of EA. Empiric antibiotics should include a third-generation cephalosporin and metronidazole, and vancomycin if staphylococci are suspected pathogens. In EA originating in the sinuses, narrowing antibiotic coverage based on culture data is not recommended because anaerobic bacteria are difficult to grow in culture and may not be recovered in microbiology specimens (85).

A 3-week course of intravenous antibiotics is appropriate following surgical drainage of EA. In patients managed medically without surgical intervention or those with comorbid osteomyelitis, a 6- to 8-week course of antibiotics is necessary (80,84).

Spinal EA

Spinal location accounts for a small proportion of all epidural infections; in one large pediatric series only 8.6% of 70 patients with extraaxial CNS infections occurred in the spine (76). When present, spinal EA may threaten the spinal cord or cauda equina by either compression, or vascular supply compromise. Spinal EA may occur secondary to spinal manipulation, hematogenous spread from distant sites of infection, superinfected traumatic hematoma, or local extension of vertebral osteomyelitis. Patients typically present with backache and lower-limb weakness (76). Spinal SDE is exceedingly rare.

Spinal EA is often medically managed with success. Surgical intervention is high-risk and reserved for those patients with progressive or concerning neurologic deficits indicative of spinal cord compression (87). Empiric antibiotic treatment is aimed at the organisms responsible for the primary site of infection; because spinal EA is often associated with bacteremic events, *S aureus* is the most common pathogen, occurring in 60% to 90% of infections, and anaerobes are rarely found. Gram-negative bacilli must be considered (76,86). Vancomycin and a third or fourth generation cephalosporin are appropriate empiric coverage.

Suppurative Jugular Thrombophlebitis

Also known as Lemierre syndrome, suppurative jugular thrombophlebitis describes a well-known syndrome of pharyngitis with septic thrombosis of the internal jugular veins, bacteremia, and possible distant septic metastasis. This entity was first described by Dr Andre Lemierre (88) in 1936 and is commonly caused by *Fusobacterium necrophorum*, an anaerobic resident of the oral flora.

Epidemiology and Pathophysiology

Oral bacteria cause pharyngitis in superinfection of a viral upper respiratory infection. This pharyngitis rarely extends to the carotid sheath, which encloses both the carotid artery and the internal jugular vein. However when it does, infection and inflammation of those vessels may create a local thrombophlebitis, which can extend both intracranially (to cause cavernous sinus

thrombophlebitis), and to distant sites as septic thromboemboli. Metastatic disease most frequently affects the lungs and causes cavitary pneumonia but also may affect musculoskeletal sites, and other distant organs (89).

Lemierre syndrome is rare in the antibiotic era, especially with attention paid by primary care providers to prompt treatment of bacterial pharyngitis in an effort to prevent rheumatic heart disease. One Scandinavian retrospective review estimated a current incidence of 0.8 cases per million people (90). Lemierre is seen most frequently in adolescents and young adults, and has a male-to-female incidence of 2:1 (91). The mortality rate has been reported as 0% to 8% in the postpenicillin era (89,91).

F necrophorum, a Gram-negative anaerobe and oral commensal organism causes 80% of Lemierre syndrome cases (92). However, many other organisms have been described in association with this syndrome including *S aureus*, Pneumococcus, *Streptococcus pyogenes* and other streptococcal species, and other Gram-negative bacilli such as *Proteus mirabilis* (91,93). These organisms enter the pharyngeal space from odontogenic sites via erosions or breaks in the pharyngeal mucosa.

Clinical Presentation

Lemierre syndrome classically presents acutely with fever, chills, shock, and cardiovascular instability in the context of a recent history of resolved pharyngitis. Patients may have pain at the mandibular angle or the sternocleidomastoid muscle, and may have concurrent focal edema. Patients with intracranial extension of septic thrombophlebitis may have cranial nerve palsies.

Diagnosis

Lemierre syndrome is diagnosed based on clinical symptomatology as well as the presence of bacteremia. A thorough history and physical exam, with focus on the head and neck, as well as blood and pharyngeal cultures should be done. In children without a clear source, a thrombophilia evaluation should be considered.

All children with Lemierre syndrome should be evaluated radiographically. Ultrasound is a safe, sensitive, available, and noninvasive modality to visualize a thrombus of the internal jugular vein, however, it is limited in elucidating intracranial extension. The diagnosis of intracranial venous thrombosis is best established with more advanced imaging. Sinus venous thrombosis is best seen on MRI with MR venography, but contrast-enhanced CT is also very sensitive and specific, and is often more readily available. Contrast-enhanced CT typically demonstrates a low density intraluminal thrombus, a sharply defined bright vessel wall, soft tissue swelling surrounding the internal jugular (IJ) vein, and a distended IJ vein proximal to the thrombus. In addition, CT provides information regarding parameningeal foci of infection such as subdural or epidural collections (93).

Treatment

The mainstay of therapy for jugular thrombophlebitis is antibiotic treatment. Most patients do not require ligation of the vessel or other surgical intervention if prompt and appropriate antibiotic therapy is initiated at diagnosis. Empiric antibiotic therapy should include coverage for *Fusobacterium* spp, as well as other anaerobes (*Bacteroides*, *Peptostreptococcus*), all streptococcal species, and *S aureus*. Metronidazole plus a third or fourth generation cephalosporin plus vancomycin should be initiated upon diagnosis. Antibiotic therapy can be narrowed based on blood culture results, but clinicians should remember that up to one-third of Lemierre syndrome cases are caused by polymicrobial infections (91). Antibiotics should be continued for a minimal duration of 3 to 6 weeks, and patients with intracranial thrombophlebitis and multiple distant metastatic sites should receive longer courses (93).

Patients with Lemierre syndrome often present with septic shock and may require cardiorespiratory support with mechanical ventilation and vasopressors. Given this risk, patients with a clear diagnosis of jugular thrombophlebitis who are not yet in extremis should be admitted to an intensive care unit (ICU) for close observation during the initiation of treatment.

The role of anticoagulation in jugular thrombophlebitis is controversial and is reserved for patients with a large intracranial clot burden, progressive thrombosis despite adequate antibiotic therapy, and no clear contraindications (93).

■ TUBERCULOUS AND OTHER GRANULOMATOUS CNS INFECTIONS

Tuberculous Meningitis

Mycobacterium tuberculosis represents a complex of seven nearly genetically identical species which are slow-growing, fastidious, aerobic bacteria most notable for causing granulomatous disease of the lungs. *M tuberculosis* also causes an array CNS diseases including meningitis, tuberculoma, and spondylitis.

Epidemiology and Pathophysiology

The most devastating CNS disease caused by *M tuberculosis* is meningitis. The pathogenesis of tuberculous meningitis begins during primary infection, which is most often transmitted by inhaling organism into the pulmonary tree. From there, the bacillus is hematogenously disseminated and may form small granulomas throughout multiple organs, including the meninges. In time, CNS granulomas, called "rich foci," form central caseation and eventually rupture, spilling organism into the CSF and causing meningeal inflammation and exudates. The time course of this rupture depends on the host's immune status, but often occurs 2 to 6 months after initial infection (101).

Three processes lead to the intracranial destruction incurred by *M tuberculosis*. First, *M tuberculosis* has a propensity to form gelatinous exudates within the CSF, particularly in the basal portion of the brain including the sylvian fissures, basal cisterns, brainstem, and cerebellum (102). This exudate can coat cranial nerves resulting in focal cranial neuropathy, and/or often creates a significant obstruction to CSF flow resulting in hydrocephalus. The degree of hydrocephalus present at initial diagnosis portends important prognostic factors. Second, obstruction and inflammation of meningeal blood vessels causes vasculitis and infarcts. This may be an early finding or may occur after treatment has been initiated. Third, small tuberculomas may coalesce or expand to form larger lesions that cause mass effect on surrounding tissue.

General epidemiologic risk factors for TB include poverty, crowded living spaces, and living in endemic areas. The highest disease burden of TB exists in Southeast Asia and Africa. In 2008, the five countries with the highest incidence of TB reported were Nigeria, India, China, South Africa, and Indonesia (103).

Tuberculous meningitis is three times more common in children than adults, and children often have more severe disease manifestations than adults (104). Approximately 4% of children with TB develop tuberculous meningitis (105). Children are thought to be at risk due to relative immunologic immaturity. In addition, patients who are immunosuppressed by HIV/AIDS, malnutrition, or immunosuppressive therapy are at a high risk for severe disease caused by TB including tuberculous meningitis.

Clinical Presentation

Patients with tuberculous meningitis present with a spectrum of clinical manifestations, most commonly irritability and focal neurologic deficits. In 1947, the British Medical Research Council described three disease stages of increasing severity (Table 16.14); more severe disease at presentation is directly related to poorer outcomes (106). Stage I involves nonspecific and often subtle neurologic signs without focal deficits. This stage lasts for several weeks and the diagnosis of tuberculous meningitis is usually not made during this time. Stage II is more acute and typical of bacterial meningitis. The hallmark of this stage is focal neurologic findings. Stage III represents late and severe disease, including stupor and coma.

Diagnosis

The differential diagnosis of tuberculous meningitis includes typical bacterial meningitis, viral meningoencephalitis, and other CNS vasculitides such as Behçet disease and sarcoidosis.

The diagnosis of tuberculous meningitis is made difficult by the slow growth rate of *M tuberculosis* and therefore long time period required for culture positivity of CSF samples. A high level of suspicion must be maintained in order to not delay treatment. Several clinical findings help to distinguish tuberculous meningitis from other causes of CNS infection: (1) illness greater than 7 days at presentation, (2) optic atrophy on fundoscopic exam, (3) focal neurologic deficit, (4) movement disorders, and (5) lymphocyte predominance of CSF WBC (107).

An LP is required for diagnosis, although because patients are at significant risk for cerebral edema,

imaging prior to LP should be considered (see Diagnostic Procedures section). OP is usually elevated. CSF sampling yields a lymphocyte-predominant pleocytosis, although neutrophils may be the predominant cell early in the disease process. WBC is generally elevated, but may be normal. Low or normal WBC count is associated with poor prognosis (102). An elevated protein level in the CSF and hypoglycorrhachia are consistent findings (Table 16.3). CT and MRI findings include hydrocephalus, infarcts, and basal meningeal enhancement.

Additional supportive laboratory findings include hyponatremia secondary to metabolic derangement such as cerebral salt wasting or SIADH, and central diabetes insipidus (107). Chest radiography may be normal, or may show signs of active or resolved pulmonary TB including hilar lymphadenopathy, pleural effusion, or calcification. Less than half of patients diagnosed with tuberculous meningitis have an abnormal chest x-ray (105), although this number may be somewhat higher in pediatric patients (104). Tuberculin skin testing is unreliable in diagnosing tuberculous meningitis, especially in early stages of disease. Even in later stage disease, tuberculin skin testing is positive in only approximately half of patients (108,109). Again, this number may be greater in children though, where tuberculin skin testing has been reported to be positive in up to 85% to 90% of children with tuberculous meningitis. Children who are vaccinated with bacilli Calmette-Guerin will have positive tuberculin skin testing transiently following vaccination. The tuberculin reactivity rapidly wanes at 6 to 12 months following vaccination, and reactivity to tuberculin skin testing thereafter is no different between vaccine recipients and those who are unvaccinated (110,111).

Microbiologic diagnosis is traditionally made by large volume CSF culture. A large amount is required due to the paucity of organisms in CSF. Acid-fast stains of CSF are positive in only 5% to 30% of samples (112), but *M tuberculosis* can be expected to grow in culture within 3 to 4 weeks, and occasionally sooner if a large burden of organisms exists. Alternate body fluid sources such as sputum or gastric aspirate may be positive in cases of suspected tuberculous meningitis and should be examined both to support the diagnosis and for infection control purposes. Nucleic acid amplification testing is now routinely used in the United States and assays are available for CSF. Nucleic acid amplification testing is > 95% specific, but depending on the burden of organisms, may have sensitivity ranging from 44% to 95%

■ **Table 16.14** Tuberculous Meningitis: Stages of Severity at Presentation

Stage I	Fever, irritability, lethargy, headache Regression of developmental milestones
Stage II	Nuchal rigidity, seizures, focal neurologic deficits, vomiting Movement disorders, cranial nerve palsies (predilection of *Mycobacterium tuberculosis* for basilar portion of brain) Cerebral edema, infarction
Stage III	Paraplegia, cardiovascular instability Posturing, eventual death

Source: Adapted from Council MR. Streptomycin treatment of tuberculous meningitis: report of the committee on Streptomycin in Tuberculosis Trials. *Lancet*. 1948;1:582–597.

(113). Nucleic acid amplification testing is not superior to bacteriologic diagnosis, but may remain positive following empiric treatment for a longer period of time than traditional culture (102).

Complications

Approximately 80% of children diagnosed with tuberculous meningitis will either die or be significantly neurologically impaired (112). However, prognosis is largely determined by stage of disease at presentation. In one retrospective description, all patients who presented in stage I disease had a normal outcome (114). Patients who present in stage II or III disease have a high incidence of mortality, and those who survive suffer significant neurologic sequelae. Permanent neurologic impairment includes movement disorders, vision and hearing impairment, mental retardation, and cranial nerve palsies (105).

Treatment

Any patient with suspected tuberculous meningitis should be immediately empirically treated to prevent disease progression and worsened outcome; treatment should not be delayed until diagnosis is confirmed if a high clinical suspicion for TB meningitis exists. Empiric therapy for tuberculous meningitis in the United States consists of a four-drug regimen of isoniazid (INH), rifampin, ethambutol, and pyrazinamide, given for at least the first 2 months of therapy. Thereafter, patient-specific mycobacterial isolates and accompanying drug susceptibility testing may help narrow the chemotherapeutic regimen. In pan-sensitive isolates, chemotherapy would be narrowed to INH and rifampin. Because *M tuberculosis* grows slowly in culture, an isolate from the source case to which a child was exposed is frequently identified prior to the growth of that child's culture, and may be used to guide the child's therapy until testing of their own isolate is available. Antituberculous therapy should be given for a total of 12 months (107). Multidrug resistant TB may be suspected based on the source case exposure history, or travel to regions with high prevalence of multidrug resistant TB. In this case, empiric therapy may be adjusted to account for the probability of INH or other drug-resistant TB and therapy may be extended for up to 24 months (107).

Adjunctive corticosteroids are recommended in all cases of tuberculous meningitis because they decrease the risk of serious neurologic morbidity and mortality.

Dexamethasone or prednisone is typically given for 2 to 8 weeks including dosage taper. If neurologic disability remains significant, duration of corticosteroid treatment may be extended.

If hydrocephalus is significant, patients may require external ventriculostomy or ventriculoperitoneal shunting. Shunts are frequently complicated by obstruction, which is often due to elevated protein and subsequent increased viscosity of CSF in tuberculous meningitis.

Following initiation of treatment, patients are often noted to have worsening hydrocephalus, and new or larger ring-enhancing lesions on brain imaging. Patients may also have increased CSF pleocytosis. This represents a "paradoxic expansion" of disease, which does not require a change in antituberculous therapy or further neurosurgical intervention (104) although some experts recommend continuation of steroid treatment should this occur (112).

TB and HIV Coinfection

Coinfection with HIV and TB is common in the third world. HIV infection increases the risk of the development of TB. Patients with HIV have a high incidence of abnormal chest radiographs and CT scans of the brain, and are prone to falsely negative tuberculin skin testing, making the diagnosis of TB in such patients quite difficult (115). However, small studies have shown that the clinical presentation of TB meningitis is not different in patients with and without HIV infection (116). Treatment for patients with HIV and TB meningitis remains the same as for those without HIV. Immune reconstitution should be instituted when possible, although care must be taken to monitor closely for immune reconstitution inflammatory syndrome (IRIS), which can be fatal in patients with HIV undergoing treatment for TB.

Infection Control

An investigation into the source case should be undertaken for all children with tuberculous meningitis both to identify an isolate for drug susceptibility testing, as well as for infection control purposes. Fifty-one percent to 69% of children diagnosed with tuberculous meningitis have an identifiable close contact with active TB (114). Family members and close contact should undergo tuberculin skin testing and chest radiography as indicated. If any patient contact has active pulmonary TB, he or she should be excluded from visiting the hospitalized child and should obtain an appropriate medical evaluation. Children with tuberculous meningitis who do not have active pulmonary disease are considered noninfectious and do not need to be isolated or placed in a negative pressure environment.

Tuberculoma

Intracranial tuberculomas are rare, large, caseating granulomas that present as mass lesions. The most common clinical manifestation is focal seizures (105), occurring in around 44% of patients (117). Focal neurologic deficits may also be present, depending on the size and location of individual lesions. Tuberculomas may be single or multiple (113).

Contrast-enhanced CT or MRI of the brain reveal ring-enhancing lesions with surrounding edema. The differential diagnosis includes malignancy, brain abscess, sarcoidosis, neurocysticercosis, and toxoplasmosis. Antituberculous therapy should be initiated for any presumed diagnosis of tuberculoma. Surgical biopsy for pathologic examination is often required for definitive diagnosis, although excision of the tuberculoma is not required for successful treatment. The neurosurgical staff should be alerted to the presumed diagnosis of TB because this will require specific preparation of the operating room and sterilization procedures. Chemotherapeutic regimens for tuberculoma are the same as those for tuberculous meningitis (118). Although no trials involving corticosteroid treatment for tuberculoma without meningitis have been done, most experts extrapolate from data regarding treatment of tuberculous meningitis and use corticosteroids in the initial treatment of tuberculoma.

Tuberculous Spondylitis

Vertebral TB, first described by Percival Pott in 1779 who coined the eponym Pott disease, is a primary bone infection affecting vertebral bodies and intervertebral joints. Pott disease is frequently complicated by neurologic symptoms due to close proximity to CNS structures. It represents one-third to one-half of all cases of skeletal TB (113,119). The clinical presentation of vertebral TB is typically more indolent and less severe than primary CNS TB. Vertebral TB, an infection which begins in the bone, must be distinguished from spinal tuberculoma, which arises within the spinal cord, sometimes causing symptoms similar to that of bony disease (102).

Pathophysiology/Epidemiology

The thoracic spine is the most common spinal region to be affected by tuberculous spondylitis due to the spread of mycobacteria from the pulmonary lymphatic system to spinal lymphatics. Other routes of spread include hematogenous dissemination during initial infection and bacteremia, or contiguous spread from other tissue sites.

TB begins at the anteroinferior part of the vertebral body, the destruction of which develops a "wedge" deformity. Vertebral bodies are preferentially affected due to their significant vascularity. Once in the vertebral body, mycobacterial spread occurs along the anterior spinal ligament and may involve contiguous discs and vertebral bodies (119). The posterior portion of the spine is often spared. Paraspinal abscesses occur in approximately 50% of cases and may dissect along tissue planes for a great distance, occasionally affecting distant vertebral bodies (113). Other contiguous sites of abscess reported include epidural, psoas, retropharynx, and gluteal muscles depending on the vertebral level affected (120–122). Intradural manifestations are caused by compression of the cord or nerve roots by edema or abscess.

The development of TB of the spine indicates a prolonged infection with *M tuberculosis*. In underdeveloped parts of the world and endemic areas, spinal TB is predominantly a disease of adolescents and young adults (113). In the United States and other developed countries, spinal TB affects older patients.

Clinical Presentation

Nonspecific back pain and limb weakness are the most common presenting symptoms. Spinal TB is not often accompanied by systemic symptoms such as fever, night sweats, and weight loss. Focal neurologic deficits such as urinary/fecal incontinence, paraplegia, and sensory loss indicate advanced disease (119).

On physical exam, spinal tenderness and edema may be present. Kyphoscoliosis and other spinal deformities are common in children and may persist or progress despite appropriate antituberculous treatment.

Diagnosis

The diagnosis of tuberculous spondylitis is frequently delayed due to vague, nonspecific symptoms; delay in diagnosis from time of initial presentation may range from 3 weeks to several years (123). Spinal radiographs are typically normal in early stages of the disease; plain radiographs of advanced disease show destruction and collapse of anterior vertebrae and resulting wedge-shape. CT and MRI are more sensitive and reveal abnormalities earlier in the disease course.

When possible, a biopsy of vertebral lesion should be examined for histologic changes and microbiologic evidence of TB including acid-fast smear and culture, and antibiotic susceptibility profile. Pathology specimens will show granuloma formation.

Tuberculin skin test may be positive in spinal TB, but is not diagnostic. Chest x-ray and sputum culture should be examined if the patient has symptoms consistent with pulmonary TB.

Treatment

Treatment for vertebral TB begins with the same 8-week regimen as described for tuberculous meningitis. This should be followed by a period of INH and rifampin, with a total treatment duration of 6 to 9 months. Corticosteroids are not recommended for the treatment of tubercular spondylitis unless is occurs concurrent with tuberculous meningitis.

The role of surgery in the treatment of vertebral TB is largely supportive and probably not required for successful treatment, although a paucity of appropriate trials exists regarding this matter. Surgical management is indicated for spinal stabilization, abscess drainage, and decompression of neurologic structures (119).

Syphilis

Syphilis, one of medicine's "great masqueraders," is caused by the spirochete *Treponema pallidum*. In the pre-penicillin era, syphilis was on nearly every neurologic differential diagnosis because the population prevalence was very high, and it was known to cause a vast spectrum of neurologic disease. However, since the advent of penicillin and more sophisticated diagnostic tools, the incidence and prevalence of syphilis has markedly decreased. Due to these epidemiologic shifts, and the fact that neurologic effects of syphilis occur only after many years or decades of infection, neurosyphilis is rare among children. The important manifestations, diagnostic, and therapeutic tools are described in this section.

Pathophysiology/Epidemiology

As of 2007, 12 million new cases of syphilis were diagnosed each year, 100,000 of which were in North America

(124). Children may be infected by syphilis via vertical transmission (congenital syphilis) or as an acquired sexually transmitted infection. The prevalence of congenitally acquired syphilis mirrors the pattern of prevalence of infected women (125). The incidence and prevalence of syphilis dramatically decreased with the availability of penicillin in 1942, although both have again been increasing in the United States over the last 11 years (126), particularly in men who have sex with men (127). Reasons for this are not entirely clear, although it may be related to an increase in unprotected sex among HIV positive individuals (who are now surviving longer with HIV infection, and less afraid of transmitting HIV infection through unprotected sex), and trading drugs for sex.

Spirochetes invade many organs, including the CNS, early in the course of infection when a high burden of spirochetemia exists (128). Seventy percent to 80% of patients clear spirochetes from the CNS early in disease, regardless of treatment, or after a brief meningitis (125,126). However, those who do not clear their initial CNS infection progress to persistent meningitis, and further CNS manifestations. Neurosyphilis may be divided into 2 categories based on time to manifestation. Early neurosyphilis is a meningitis caused by obliterative endarteritis and infarction of small vessels of the CNS, known as meningovascular syphilis (127). This is the primary manifestation seen in pediatrics. Late neurosyphilis irreversibly affects the CNS parenchyma in the form of atrophy, gummas, and progressive vascular disease, and manifests decades after primary infection occurs (125).

Clinical Presentation

Syphilitic meningitis may be symptomatic or asymptomatic. Given the variability in clinical presentation, CSF evaluation should be done when a high index of suspicion exists. Typical symptoms include fever, headache, photophobia, and neck stiffness. Meningovascular syphilis presents with focal neurologic deficits dependent on the specific location of ischemia. Cranial nerve palsies, seizures, and altered mental status are common (129). Additionally, patients may have independent otic or ophthalmologic involvement.

Neurologic manifestations of congenitally acquired syphilis occur either early in life as aseptic meningitis or, more commonly, at age 2 to 3 years as deafness, cranial neuropathies, seizures, or other symptoms consistent with meningovascular syphilis.

Diagnosis

Systemic syphilis is diagnosed by a sensitive but non-specific screening serologic test (Venereal Disease Research Laboratory [VDRL] or rapid plasma reagin [RPR]); followed by a confirmatory treponemal test such as fluorescent treponemal antibody-absorption. CSF examination is indicated for any patient with a serologic diagnosis of syphilis and neurologic symptoms or for patients who do not respond with an appropriate decrease in RPR titer after treatment (fourfold or greater decline 6 to 12 months after therapy) regardless of neurologic symptoms. CSF testing often demonstrates lymphocytic pleocytosis ranging from 5 to 2,000 cells/mL depending on the stage of infection (Table 16.3), but in general, CSF testing is insensitive. CSF may be normal early in the course of infection, and CSF VDRL is negative in up to 70% of patients with neurosyphilis (130). Centers for Disease Control (CDC) diagnostic criteria are shown in Table 16.15 (126). CSF should be reexamined every 6 months until abnormalities have resolved (126).

All infants being evaluated for congenital syphilis based on clinical suspicion or maternal history should undergo LP (125). CSF findings are similar to those of older children and adults including pleocytosis and elevated protein, although these abnormalities may not be present if LP is done early in the course of infection (128).

Treatment

Penicillin is the standard of care for patients with neurosyphilis, however small studies have suggested that intravenous ceftriaxone 2 grams daily may be equally efficacious (130). Benzathene penicillin, recommended for nonneurologic syphilis, does not provide spirocheticidal levels of antibiotic in the CSF (129), so the recommended agent to treat neurosyphilis is aqueous crystalline penicillin G 2 to 4 million units every 4 hours intravenously for 10 to 14 days. An alternate regimen of penicillin G procaine 2.4 million units per day intramuscularly for 10 to 14 days is approved and should be given with oral probenecid 500 mg 4 times daily. The treatment for congenital syphilis is aqueous crystalline penicillin G 50,000 units/kg every 12 hours for 1 week, then every 8 hours for 3 weeks, then every 4 to 6 hours for 10 to 14 days (128).

■ ENCEPHALITIS AND MYELITIS

Inflammation of the brain or spinal cord parenchyma on histopathologic examination associated with clinical neurologic dysfunction formally defines encephalitis or myelitis, respectively. However the diagnosis of these entities in practice rests primarily on clinical presentation and history, since tissue is rarely obtained for pathologic examination. For the purposes of this section, encephalitis will be defined as acute CNS dysfunction (seizure, focal neurologic deficits, or altered mental status) in the context of laboratory or radiographic evidence of brain parenchymal inflammation. Myelitis will be similarly defined with respect to the spinal cord. Both encephalitis and myelitis may be caused by a host of inflammatory etiologies, including infectious, neoplastic, toxic/metabolic, vascular, or autoimmune disorders.

There is some inherent overlap in the clinical presentation of primary encephalitis and myelitis with meningitis, since inflammation of the brain or spinal cord frequently involves the meninges, and primary inflammation of the meninges frequently spreads to involve adjacent brain parenchyma (131). However, in this section, we will consider these separate entities, and aim to broadly discuss the epidemiology, diagnosis, and treatment of primary infectious encephalitis and myelitis based on various clinical

■ **Table 16.15** Centers for Disease Control Diagnostic Criteria for Neurosyphilis	
Confirmed Neurosyphilis[a]	**Presumptive**[a]
Any stage of syphilis	Any stage of syphilis
	Nonreactive CSF VDRL
Reactive CSF VDRL	CSF pleocytosis or elevated protein
	Clinical signs or symptoms consistent with syphilis
	without an alternate diagnosis to account for these

[a] Must fulfill all criteria in one column for diagnosis. Adapted from Ref. 126.

presentations. Finally, a brief discussion of non-infection-related primary encephalitis and myelitis will follow.

Primary Infectious Encephalitis

There are at least two different forms of infection-related encephalitis/myelitis: primary infectious encephalitis/myelitis, and postinfectious (or immunologically mediated) encephalitis/myelitis (i.e., acute disseminated encephalomyelitis [ADEM]) (132). While the clinical presentation of these two entities may be similar, the distinction in pathogenesis is important because clinical course, treatment, and prognosis may differ significantly (133). Primary encephalitis results from direct parenchymal invasion of the offending pathogen and largely affects the gray matter, whereas postinfectious encephalitis is immunologically mediated and more prominently affects the white matter (132). This section will discuss primary infectious encephalitis and myelitis only. For a discussion of immunologically mediated encephalitis, please see the chapter on "Acquired Demyelinating Syndromes of the Central Nervous System."

Epidemiology and Pathophysiology

Primary infectious encephalitis causes an estimated 7.3 hospitalizations per 100,000 people in the United States annually, leading to about 1,400 deaths per year, predominantly in children and the elderly (132,133). The true incidence of encephalitis in the United States population in unknown, but probably ranges between 2.6 and 27.7 cases per 100,000 child-years (134,135); the highest rates occur in children less than 1 year of age. Among cohorts of children 1 to 18 years of age, the mean incident age of encephalitis is 6 years (135).

The pathogenesis of primary infectious encephalitis varies broadly by the etiologic organism, but overall is poorly understood. Some organisms enter the CNS from the bloodstream following systemic viremia via infected cells allowed across the BBB (HIV), or via infection of capillary endothelial cells (arboviruses). Other organisms enter the CNS via retrograde transport in infected axons (rabies). Finally, others may enter directly via the olfactory mucosa (*N fowleri*) or following trauma. Once in the CNS, different organisms have different tissue tropisms, and thus clinical manifestations vary based on the site of significant tissue invasion (132).

More than 100 different pathogens have been associated with primary infectious encephalitis (134,136), and common culprits have evolved over time as vaccine-preventable etiologies diminish (measles, mumps, rubella), newer pathogens emerge (West Nile virus, Nipah virus), and new laboratory methods are developed for pathogen detection (132). In general, viruses, particularly herpesviruses and arthopod-borne viruses (arboviruses), are the most common identified etiologies of encephalitis. However, bacteria (*M tuberculosis, L monocytogenes*), fungi, parasites, and other noninfectious agents may also be responsible (Table 16.16) (132). The frequency and distribution of etiologic agents varies with geographic region and climate, epidemics, arthropod presence, and variations in immunization programs (136). In a prospective study of 1,570 cases referred over 7 years to the California Encephalitis Project (CEP), only 16% of encephalitis cases had a confirmed or probable infectious etiology (69% viral, 20% bacterial, 7% prion, 2% parasitic, 1% fungal); 13% had a possible infectious etiology, and 8% had a noninfectious etiology (such as neoplasm, vasculitis, metabolic disorders, etc.) (137). Perhaps most striking however, is that no etiology was found in 63% of cases (137). Another prospectively observed cohort of 253 subjects in France (10% of whom were pediatric), who were hospitalized for at least 5 days, found an infectious etiology in only 52% (138). Of these, 69% were viral, and 30% were bacterial (10% *Listeria*, 15% *M tuberculosis*). An epidemiologic summary of encephalitis is organized by infectious etiology in Table 16.16 by specific historical clues or exposure in Table 16.17.

Failure to determine a specific etiologic agent is common in clinically diagnosed primary infectious encephalitis for several reasons. First, given the wide geographic variation in etiology, each study period, setting, and particular clinical definition for primary infectious encephalitis is variable and nonspecific between studies. Second, diagnostic method practices (such as timing of serology acquisition, use of PCR, etc.) and sensitivities vary. Finally, the laboratory case definition of encephalitis is continuously evolving. As of 2010, cases were only considered confirmed if an organism was found in the CSF or if intrathecal antibody production was demonstrated (136).

Clinical Presentation

Clinical manifestations of primary infectious encephalitis vary significantly according to the etiologic pathogen, which portions of the CNS are affected, and specific host factors. Eighty percent to 100% of affected individuals demonstrate encephalopathy (149), 64% to 81% have

(text continues on page 298)

■ Table 16.16 Common Infectious Etiologies and Epidemiology of Encephalitis

Pathogen	Transmission, Vector, Reservoir	Age, Season, Geography, other Epidemiology	Incidence, Morbidity, and Mortality
Viruses			
Adenovirus	Droplet transmission	Sporadically affects children and immunocompromised hosts	
Arboviruses (arthropod-borne viruses)			Affect 150–3,000 persons per year
EEE	Mosquito vector Avian (N America), rodent, and marsupial (S America) reservoirs	Sporadically affects children < 15 years old east of the Mississippi river, and in gulf coastal regions in the summer and early fall.	U.S. incidence of ~5 cases/year Case fatality 50%–70%
WEE	Mosquito vector Avian reservoir	Affects children < 4 years old in the central United States between April and September. Endemic and epidemic (last in United States in 1994)	Case fatality 3%–4%, higher in infants
SLE virus	Mosquito vector Avian reservoir	Typically a low-level endemic disease in the elderly, most cases west of the Mississippi river. Sporadic large outbreaks every 10–15 years between August and October.	U.S. incidence ~35 cases/year Case fatality 2%–20%
California encephalitis group (LCV, California encephalitis virus)	Mosquito vector	Most common in children 5–9 years old in midwestern and southeastern United States between July and September	U.S. incidence ~70 cases/year. Most common cause of pediatric arboviral encephalitis in North America. Case fatality < 1%
WNV	Mosquito vector Avian reservoir Transmission also reported via transfusion, transplantation, breast-feeding	Endemic in the Middle East, Africa, and Asia, mostly in children. First occurred in the United States in 1999 on Atlantic seaboard, now seen throughout the United States in the summer, mostly in the elderly.	1/150 infections develop CNS disease. Most common arboviral infection in the United States. Case fatality of all CNS disease is 10%–15%. If subject has encephalitis and weakness, this increases to 30%.
JEV	Mosquito vector Avian reservoir, domestic pigs serve as amplifying host	Primarily found endemically in Asia; JEV is rare among travelers to endemic areas, but occasionally is found in military personnel, expatriates, and travelers in the United States between March and October.	1/300 infections develop encephalitis. Worldwide incidence ~50,000 cases/year. Most common cause of viral encephalitis worldwide. Case fatality ~30%, higher in younger children.

(continued)

■ **Table 16.16**   Common Infectious Etiologies and Epidemiology of Encephalitis (*continued*)

Pathogen	Transmission, Vector, Reservoir	Age, Season, Geography, other Epidemiology	Incidence, Morbidity, and Mortality
Tick-borne encephalitis TBE	Tick vector and reservoir Transmission also via unpasteurized milk	Typically epidemic and sporadic in Eastern Russia, central Europe, and Asia, primarily affecting the elderly from April to November.	2/3 of cases are asymptomatic. Case fatality ranges from < 2% to 40%, depending on the virus subtype
Colorado tick fever	Tick vector and reservoir	Western United States and Canada, mostly above elevations of 4,000 ft	Several hundred cases in United States annually. Second most common arboviral infection in the United States. Case fatality rare, but more common in children.
EV Coxsackievirus A and B Echovirus EV serotype 71 Parechovirus Poliovirus	Fecal-oral transmission	EVs affect all ages (but primarily children) between June and September worldwide. Poliovirus specifically affects unvaccinated individuals in developed countries, and infants in developing countries.	Mortality is low for most CNS EV infections, except for EV71.
Herpesviruses CMV	Blood product transfusion, solid organ and stem cell transplantation, placental, and breast milk transmission	Primarily affects immunocompromised individuals.	Nearly 100% fatality without immune reconstitution.
EBV	Respiratory/saliva transmission	Primarily affects immunocompromised individuals.	1%–5% of acute EBV cases are complicated by CNS involvement
HSV HSV-1	Unknown transmission	More common in adults, but affects all ages. 2/3 of cases are due to reactivation of HSV-1. Does not vary by season or geography.	Most common cause of sporadic fatal encephalitis. U.S. incidence ~2.2 cases/ million population per year.
HSV-2	Perinatal transmission	Most common in neonates, particularly with prolonged rupture of membranes, instrumentation during delivery, or if primary maternal infection occurred perinatally.	Case fatality 29%–85% in disseminated disease, 4%–50% in CNS disease, depending on use of antiviral therapy
HHV6	Unknown transmission Likely via saliva	Typically occurs in infants or the immunocompromised. No seasonal predilection.	Not fatal
VZV	Transmitted via direct contact, droplets	Affects all ages, during all seasons (possible increase in late winter and spring).	Case fatality ~100% in immunocompromised hosts, about 15% in immunocompetent hosts

(continued)

Pathogen	Transmission, Vector, Reservoir	Age, Season, Geography, other Epidemiology	Incidence, Morbidity, and Mortality
HIV	Blood product, sexual activity, needle sharing transmission	All ages, all seasons, worldwide.	
Influenza	Transmitted via direct contact, droplets	Most common in children < 5 years old, with seasonal peaks in the winter.	5% of North American pediatric encephalitis cases. Case fatality is unknown.
LCMV	Transmitted by rodents	Peaks in autumn.	Case fatality is < 1%
MV	Transmitted via direct contact, droplets	Unvaccinated children and adults at higher risk.	Case fatality about 10%. May progress to measles body inclusion encephalitis, or SSPE (100% fatal)
Mumps	Transmitted via direct contact, droplets	Unvaccinated children and adults at higher risk.	Case fatality is low
Nipah virus	Transmitted via exposure to infected pigs, bats, or humans	South Asia	Case fatality ~40%
Rabies virus	Transmitted by bite of infected animal, or organ donation	Rare and sporadic in the United States	Worldwide: 50,000–100,000 deaths annually. Case fatality 100%.
Bacteria			
Bartonella henselae	Transmitted by cat bite or scratch, or by rodent, dogs, fleas	Primarily affects children and young adults, during all seasons.	1%–7% of *Bartonella* infections develop encephalopathy
Listeria monocytogenes	Food-borne or transplacental transmission	Neonates, pregnant patients, and immunocompromised (especially cell-mediated) patients are at higher risk of *Listeria* infection.	Case fatality for all *Listeria* infections is 20%–30%
Mycobacterium tuberculosis	Droplet transmission	See Granulomatous Disease section	
Rickettsial and ehrlichial Infections			
Rickettsia rickettsii (Rocky Mountain spotted fever)	Tick vector, dogs can carry ticks. 51% of pediatric cases do not remember a bite	Typically affects children on the east coast of the United States between April and September.	U.S. incidence ~2,000 cases/year Case fatality 2%–10% with early treatment, 25%–30% in untreated patients
Coxiella burnetii (Q fever)	Tick vector. Cattle, sheep, and goat reservoirs Transmission also via contaminated dairy	Primarily affects adults worldwide throughout the year.	Case fatality is rare
Ehrlichia chaffeensis (ehrlichiosis)	Tick vector. White-tailed deer reservoir, lone star tick is vector. 72% remember the tick exposure	Affects mostly adults in the southeastern United States and Atlantic seaboard from April to September.	U.S. incidence at least 0.7 cases/million population Case fatality ~3%

(continued)

■ Table 16.16 Common Infectious Etiologies and Epidemiology of Encephalitis (*continued*)

Pathogen	Transmission, Vector, Reservoir	Age, Season, Geography, other Epidemiology	Incidence, Morbidity, and Mortality
Spirochetes			
Borrelia burgdorferi	Tick vector	Endemic in North America, Europe, and Asia, occurring in all age groups between May and November.	Fatality rare
Treponema pallidum	Transmitted perinatally and via sexual contact	Affects all ages worldwide.	Fatality rare with antimicrobial treatment
Fungi			
Coccidioides spp *Cryptococcus neoformans* *Histoplasma* spp	Discussed in Immunocompromised section		
Protozoa			
Acanthamoeba spp	Transmitted via exposure to contaminated water	Typically affects chronically ill or immunocompromised individuals worldwide, any time of year	Case fatality ~100%
Balamuthia mandrillaris	Transmitted via exposure to contaminated soil, or via solid organ transplantation	Affects all ages, in warmer regions of the globe throughout the year. Higher incidence in subjects with Hispanic ethnicity.	~60 cases over 35 years in the United States, mostly fatal
Naegleria fowleri	Transmitted via exposure to contaminated fresh, warm water	Typically affects children and young adults in warmer regions throughout the world in the spring and summer	0–8 cases per year in the United States Case fatality > 95%
Plasmodium falciparum *Toxoplasma gondii* *Trypanosoma* spp	See Tropical medicine section See Immunocompromised Host section See Tropical medicine section		

Abbreviations: CMV, cytomegalovirus; EBV, Epstein-Barr virus; EEE, Eastern equine encephalitis virus; EV, enterovirus; HHV, human herpesvirus; JEV, Japanese encephalitis virus; LCMV, lymphocytic choriomeningitis virus; LCV, La Crosse virus; MV, measles virus; SLE, St Louis encephalitis; SSPE, subacute sclerosing panencephalitis; TBE, tick-borne encephalitis; U.S. United States; VZV, varicella-zoster virus; WEE, Western equine encephalitis virus; WNV, West Nile virus.
Source: Adapted from Refs. 131–133, 137, 139–148.

fever (134,149,150), many have headache, 14% to 78% have seizures (134,137,149,150), and 44% to 78% (149,150) have focal neurologic signs. However, all of these symptoms are noted in older children (149). Infant presentation can be very nonspecific, but should be considered in the context of seizure, temperature alteration (fever or hypothermia), poor feeding, irritability, or lethargy.

The CEP has attempted to group primary infectious encephalitides into groups based on characteristics of clinical presentation (137). For example, HSV-1 is the most common cause of temporal lobe symptoms, however, varicella-zoster virus and EVs may also cause temporal lobe specific findings. Table 16.18 provides a summary of infectious agents frequently associated with specific clinical findings.

■ **Table 16.17** Epidemiologic and Historical Clues to the Etiology of Encephalitis	
Risk Factor	**Possible Etiologies**
Age < 28 days	CMV, HSV-1 or HSV-2, rubella, *Listeria monocytogenes, Toxoplasma gondii, Treponema pallidum*
Blood transfusion or transplant (bone marrow or solid organ transplantation)	CMV, EBV, HIV, rabies, TBE, WNV, *T pallidum, Rickettsia rickettsii, Cryptococcus neoformans, Coccidioides* spp, *Histoplasma capsulatum, T gondii*
Immunodeficiency	CMV, EV, HHV6, HSV, VZV, WNV, *T gondii*, HIV, *Listeria, Mycobacterium tuberculosis, C neoformans, Coccidioides* spp, *H capsulatum*
Animal exposures	
Mosquito bite	Arboviruses, *Plasmodium falciparum*
Tick bite	*Borrelia burgdorferi, R rickettsii, Ehrlichia chaffeensis, Anaplasma phagocytophilum,* TBE, Colorado tick fever, Powassan
Bats	Rabies virus, Nipah virus
Pigs	Nipah virus, JEV
Cats/dogs	*Bartonella* spp, *Toxocara* spp, rabies virus, *T gondii*
Sheep/goats	*Coxiella burnetii*
Raccoons	Rabies virus
Rodents	LCMV, EEE, TBE, LCV
Horses	EEE, WEE
Birds	WNV, EEE, WEE, SLE, JEV, *Cryptococcus* (bird droppings)
Season	
Summer	EV, TBE, arboviruses
Late summer/fall	Arbovirus, agents transmitted by tics (see above)
Winter	Influenza
Unpasteurized dairy exposure	*Brucella*, TBE, *L monocytogenes, C burnetii*
Rural exposure	*Francisella tularensis, Rickettsia typhi*
Recreational activities	
Swimming	EV, *Naegleria, Acanthamoeba* spp
Spelunking	Rabies virus, *H capsulatum*
Sexual activity	HSV, HIV, *T pallidum*
Travel	
Asia	JEV, Nipah virus
Africa	Lassa fever, malaria
Europe	TBE
Immunization preventable	Measles, mumps, rubella, VZV, JEV

Abbreviation: SLE, St Louis encephalitis virus.
Source: Adapted from Refs. 132, 133, 136, 137, 149.

Diagnosis

Diagnosis of primary infectious encephalitis is based upon a combination of historical information and clinical findings (Tables 16.16 and 16.18), and is supported by blood and CSF analysis, EEG, and neuroimaging. Supportive evaluation is directed by a specific child's exposures and presenting symptoms (133,149). Because an etiologic agent is not found in up to 65% of cases of encephalitis (137,149), and because proving causality between a microbe found in the periphery and clinical encephalitis is difficult (136,137), clinical criteria are most helpful in diagnosing encephalitis. For example, the CEP defines encephalitis as encephalopathy (depressed or altered level of consciousness for ≥24 hours, lethargy, or change in personality) requiring hospitalization, plus at least one of the following: fever, seizure, focal neurologic findings, CSF pleocytosis, or EEG or neuroimaging findings consistent with encephalitis (137). Identification of a specific organism as causative of clinical encephalitis is then based on specific

■ **Table 16.18**   Clinical and Laboratory Findings: Possible Etiologic Agents

Clinical Finding	Possible Etiologies
General Findings	
Parotitis	Mumps
Rash	
Vesicular	HSV, VZV (although 44% of subjects will lack skin findings)
Hand, foot, mouth	EV
Erythematous macules and papules with cephalocaudad spread	Measles virus
Beginning on extremities	*Rickettsia rickettsii*
Respiratory findings	Nipah virus, Influenza, adenovirus, *Mycoplasma pneumoniae*, *Coxiella burnetii*, *Mycobacterium tuberculosis*, *Histoplasma capsulatum*
Retinitis	CMV, *Toxoplasma gondii*, WNV, *Bartonella henselae*, *Treponema pallidum*
Urinary symptoms (dysuria, urgency, incontinence)	SLE virus (during prodrome)
Neurologic Findings	
Cerebellar ataxia	VZV, EBV, mumps, SLE virus, JEV, WNV
Cranial nerve palsies	HSV, EBV, mumps, *Listeria monocytogenes*, *M tuberculosis*, *T pallidum*, *Borrelia burgdorferi*, *Cryptococcus neoformans*, *H capsulatum*, JEV
Dementia	HIV, *T pallidum*, *Tropheryma whipplei*
Cognitive and language impairments	JEV (30%)
Parkinsonism	JEV, SLE virus, WNV, Nipah, *T gondii*
Tremor	WNV
Poliomyelitislike flaccid paralysis	JEV, WNV, TBE, EV71, Coxsackievirus, poliovirus
Rhomboencephalitis	EV71, HSV, WNV, *L monocytogenes*
Laboratory Findings	
Neutropenia	Colorado tick fever, ehrlichiosis, HSV, measles virus, rickettsial infections, rubella
Thrombocytopenia	Rickettsial infections (especially ehrlichiosis)
Hyponatremia	Rickettsial infections, EEE
SIADH	SLE virus, HSV
Hypoglycemia, acidosis, hyperammonemia	Uncommon in primary infectious encephalitis, consider alternative diagnosis such as metabolic encephalopathy or toxic exposure

Abbreviations: SIADH, syndrome of inappropriate antidiuretic hormone; SLE, St Louis encephalitis.
Source: Adapted from Refs. 133, 137, 148.

microbial criteria (136). Typically, each potential etiologic pathogen is classified as confirmed, probable, possible, or excluded, depending on the types of specimens available, strength of previously established associations, clinical characteristics, and epidemiologic profiles of each agent (136,137). Many cases remain probable when clinicians are unable to obtain specific evidence of CNS disease to establish causality, or when convalescent serologies are not available.

Peripheral blood work, including a complete blood count, electrolytes, liver function testing, and coagulation studies, should be obtained in all children with suspected infectious encephalitis, both to aid in the differential diagnosis, and to assess for possible multiorgan complications (Table 16.18). Serologic evaluation, serum PCR, antigen detection, and cultures should be obtained based on clinical suspicion for particular pathogens, and the time course of illness. Specifically, serologies may be negative very early in the course of illness, and culture or molecular techniques may be negative depending on the time course of infection and presentation (146). Serologies in general should be obtained at presentation, and 21 days later. An acute infection will result in a $\geq 4\times$ increase in titers on paired acute/convalescent sera. Table 16.19 summarizes screening blood and body fluid testing for all individuals with suspected infectious encephalitis.

Spinal fluid analysis in all cases of suspected encephalitis (unless specifically contraindicated) should routinely include OP, cell counts, glucose, protein, Gram stain, bacterial and acid-fast bacilli (AFB) culture with smear, and HSV and EV PCR. If the WBC is elevated, a differential should be obtained (146). Forty-five percent to 55% of all children with viral encephalitis will demonstrate a CSF lymphocytic pleocytosis, although within the first 24 to 48 hours this may be neutrophil predominant (149,150). In general, RBCs in the CSF outside of a traumatic LP are rare, and suggest HSV, California encephalitis group, Eastern equine encephalitis, or amoebic encephalitis if present. CSF protein in most viral encephalitis is slightly elevated, and glucose is typically normal or slightly low in HSV or mumps. Viral cultures are not routinely recommended due to low sensitivity (133). Other specific CSF serologies and assays should be dictated by the individual's specific history and presentation. CSF immunoglobulin M (IgM) should be measured in conjunction with serum IgM: when IgM is found in the CSF out of proportion to serum levels, this is likely representative of true disease, because IgM does not cross an intact BBB. CSF PCRs in general are very specific, but not 100% sensitive, and negative results should be interpreted with caution. Specifically, if an HSV PCR is negative but a clinical suspicion remains, this should be retested in 3 to 7 days following initial LP. EBV PCR may generate false positive results related to latently infected

mononuclear cells in the CSF from prior infection. In addition, sensitivities of CSF PCR vary with specific viral strains. For example, EV71, a particularly neurotropic strain of EV, is rarely detected by CSF PCR, and diagnosis relies on conventional skin and rectal swabs instead. Table 16.20 summarizes recommended screening CSF labs for individuals with suspected infectious encephalitis.

MRI is the most sensitive imaging modality to detect inflammation associated with encephalitis, and should be performed in all patients with suspected infectious encephalitis to aid in diagnosis, and to rule out mimics of infectious etiologies requiring different treatments (133). Initial MRI findings are abnormal in up to 60% of subjects with infectious encephalitis (137), 30% with patterns suggesting specific etiologies (149). The remainder reveal nonspecific findings such as diffuse edema, focal edema or ischemia, multifocal edema, or infarct (150).

EEG should be performed in all subjects with suspected encephalitis to diagnose clinical or subclinical seizures associated with altered mental status (133). However, while EEG is abnormal in 43% to 96% of encephalitis cases (134,149), it is rarely helpful in establishing a specific etiologic organism. Electrographic abnormalities observed include diffuse slowing, focal or lateralized slow wave abnormalities, focal seizures, periodic lateralized epileptiform discharges, and frontal or occipital intermittent rhythmic delta activity (150).

■ Table 16.19 Screening Blood and Body Fluid (Non-CNS) Labs in Suspected Infectious Encephalitis

CBC with differential
Electrolytes and liver function testing
Coagulation studies
Respiratory pathogen screen
Bacterial blood cultures
Screening serologies for most common infectious encephalitis pathogens:
  —HSV and varicella-zoster virus PCR, HIV testing, arbovirus panel (including St Louis encephalitis virus, California encephalitis group, Eastern equine encephalitis virus, Western equine encephalitis virus, West Nile virus) of serologies, lymphocytic choriomeningitis virus serologies
Consider:
  —Rheumatologic screen with atypical presentation: ANA, ANCA, ACE, RF, ESR, CRP
  —Hashimoto encephalitis testing if prominent seizures: antithyroid peroxidase antibody, antithyroglobulin antibody
  —Other acute and convalescent serologies, depending on clinical suspicion and exposures
  —Culture or PCR of skin lesions if present for HSV, varicella-zoster virus, and/or rickettsial infection
  —Viral cultures and analysis (antigen detection, PCR) of other potentially affected body fluids (tracheal aspiration, urine, stool) or mucosal sites (throat, nasopharynx, rectum)

Abbreviations: ANA, antinuclear antibody; ANCA, anti-neutrophil cytoplasmic antibodies; CBC, complete blood count; CRP, C-reactive protein; ESR, erythrocyte sedimentation rate; RF, rheumatoid factor.

■ **Table 16.20** Screening CSF Labs in Suspected Infectious Encephalitis

Opening pressure
Cell counts, tubes 1 and 4
Chemistries (glucose, protein)
Gram stain, bacterial culture, AFB smear and culture
HSV and enterovirus PCR
Varicella-zoster virus, HIV, lymphocytic choriomeningitis virus, arbovirus (St Louis encephalitis virus, California encephalitis group, Easter equine encephalitis virus, Western equine encephalitis virus, West Nile virus) serologic testing
Consider:
—Virus-specific IgM, other PCR depending on clinical suspicion, exposures or travel history, and time of year
—Repeat HSV testing 3–7 days after initial test if clinical suspicion remains
—Brain biopsy in subjects with a progressive deterioration despite empiric therapy.
—Fungal cultures (immunocompromised hosts)

Abbreviation: IgM, immunoglobulin M.

A brain biopsy may be obtained to attempt a tissue diagnosis depending on the area of brain involved and its surgical accessibility. However, such studies are high risk and typically low-yield in the case of encephalitis, and therefore rarely pursued.

Table 16.21 summarizes specific clinical presentations, diagnostic testing, imaging and EEG characteristics, and recommended treatment by etiologic agent.

Complications

Fluid and electrolyte disturbances, SIADH, seizures or status epilepticus, cerebral infarction, cerebral sinus venous thrombosis, cardiorespiratory failure, aspiration pneumonitis, upper gastrointestinal bleeding, and disseminated intravascular coagulation are common complications of primary infectious encephalitis and must be managed expectantly. Cerebral edema or cerebellar inflammation may result in herniation.

Treatment

Initial treatment of viral encephalitis should focus on stabilizing airway, breathing, and circulation. Children should be admitted to the ICU for close monitoring, supportive care, and standard treatment of any associated complications. The following discussion will focus on immunologically competent children.

Empiric therapy (Table 16.22) should include acyclovir for all children with suspected primary infectious encephalitis, pending a negative HSV PCR. Empiric acyclovir should continue despite a negative HSV PCR if clinical suspicion is high, in which case LP should be repeated. Doxycycline should be initiated empirically during

rickettsial season in patients with an appropriate history, endemic region, or clinical suspicion. Empiric antibiotic therapy should be given if bacterial meningitis is suspected and supported by initial CSF studies until CSF bacterial cultures are negative. Other empirical antimicrobial agents may be started based on specific etiologic suspicions (133).

Adjunctive corticosteroids may be helpful in HSV (152) and varicella-zoster virus infections (151), and have been suggested in small case series to be effective in early stages of other viral encephalitis with progressive alteration in consciousness (153). However, corticosteroids may halt the immune clearance of infectious organism, so the use of corticosteroids in the context of active infectious encephalitis is controversial.

Surgical decompression is indicated for impending herniation or medically-refractory elevated ICP (151). Seizures are managed with anticonvulsants. SIADH should be managed symptomatically with frequent evaluation of fluid balance and serum sodium levels.

Isolation is not required for community acquired acute infective encephalitis, but should be considered for severely immunocompromised patients, those with rabies, those with exanthematous encephalitis, and those with a contagious hemorrhagic fever (151). Infection control specialists should be consulted for proper precautions.

Prognosis

Prognosis in primary infectious encephalitis varies according to pathogen, severity of CNS symptoms, and time course prior to treatment. In general, those presenting with diffuse cerebral edema, intractable seizures, or movement disorders have a poor neurologic recovery

(*text continues on page 308*)

■ Table 16.21 Acute Infectious Encephalitis Presentation, Diagnostic Testing, Imaging, and EEG Characteristics by Organism

Pathogen	Unique Clinical Features	Diagnostic Testing	Imaging and EEG	Treatment
Viruses				
Adenovirus	Associated respiratory symptoms	• Acute and convalescent serology • PCR of CSF • PCR of respiratory specimen and blood	No specific findings	Supportive
Arboviruses EEE	Abrupt onset with fulminant course	• Acute and convalescent serology • WBC > 300 cell/mm^3	MRI with nonenhancing focal lesions in thalami, BG, and midbrain, diffuse edema	Supportive
WEE	Headache, seizures, relatively mild course	• Acute and convalescent serology • CSF IgG, Ag	No specific findings	Supportive
SLE	Causes meningoencephalitis in young people Urinary symptoms are early features. SIADH in 1/3	• Acute and convalescent serology (may cross-react with other flaviviruses) • CSF IgM	MRI demonstrates T2 hyperintense lesions in thalami, BG, and substantia nigra	Supportive Consider IFN-2α (experimental)
California encephalitis group (LCV, California encephalitis virus)	Mild meningoencephalitis that may progress Seizures (50% of children), paralysis.	• Acute and convalescent serology • CSF IgM, elevated RBC	No specific findings. EEG may be focal	Supportive
WNV	Movement disorders, poliomyelitislike flaccid paralysis, CN dysfunction, ataxia Fine maculopapular rash	• Acute and convalescent serology (may cross-react with other flaviviruses) • CSF IgM (after 4 days of symptoms, WNV PCR (insensitive)	MRI shows T2 hyperintense lesions in the substantia nigra, BG, and thalami. Meningeal and periventricular enhancement	Supportive Ribavirin is not recommended
JEV	Seizures and movement disorders common Poliomyelitislike flaccid paralysis	• Acute and convalescent serology • CSF IgM	MRI demonstrates T2 hyperintense and T1 hypodense lesions in thalami, BG, brainstem, and cerebellum	Supportive IFN-α is not recommended
TBE	Poliomyelitislike paralysis	• Acute and convalescent serology • CSF IgM, PCR (before day 4)	No specific findings	Supportive
Colorado tick fever	Nonspecific encephalitis	• Acute and convalescent serology	No specific findings	Supportive

(continued)

■ **Table 16.21** Acute Infectious Encephalitis Presentation, Diagnostic Testing, Imaging, and EEG Characteristics by Organism (*continued*)

Pathogen	Unique Clinical Features	Diagnostic Testing	Imaging and EEG	Treatment
EV Coxsackievirus A and B Echovirus EV71 Parechovirus Polio virus Herpesviruses	Rash or exanthem common in all EV EV71 may cause a rhomboencephalitis with myoclonus, tremors, ataxia, and CN deficits	• Acute and convalescent serology • CSF EV PCR • Enteroviral PCR from a mucosal surface supports, but does not confirm diagnosis	MRI shows T2 hyperintensity in the midbrain, pons, medulla and/or anterior horn of the spinal cord	Supportive
CMV	Retinitis, pneumonitis, myelitis, encephalitis, polyradiculopathy	• Acute and convalescent serology • CSF CMV PCR	MRI demonstrates diffuse nonspecific white matter T2 hyperintensities and subependymal enhancement	Ganciclovir or foscarnet Immune reconstitution
EBV	Patients often lack symptoms associated with mononucleosis (fever, pharyngitis, lymphadenopathy Focal deficits, cerebellar ataxia, psychosis, and cranial nerve palsies	• Acute and convalescent serology (EBV VCA, EBNA) • Elevated EBV VCA titer in CSF • CSF EBV PCR • CSF viral loads < 1,000 copies/mL have unclear significance—may represent incidental detection of latent virus. Viral loads ≥ 1,000 are probably significant. • Heterophile antibody test frequently negative in CNS disease	MRI may demonstrate T2 hyperintensity in the BG, thalami, and cortex	Supportive Acyclovir not recommended Corticosteroids may be helpful in protracted or severe disease
HSV-1 and HSV-2	Clinical presentation reflects temporal lobe involvement: seizures, autonomic dysfunction, language abnormalities, and personality change SIADH occurs less commonly	• CSF HSV PCR • CSF IgM may also be used to track therapy	MRI with temporal lobe, cingulate gyrus, insular involvement in HSV-1 Diffuse involvement including periventricular white matter, may spare medial temporal and inferior frontal lobes in HSV-2 EEG changes in 80%–94%, most commonly PLEDs	Acyclovir

(*continued*)

■ **Table 16.21** Acute Infectious Encephalitis Presentation, Diagnostic Testing, Imaging, and EEG Characteristics by Organism (*continued*)

Pathogen	Unique Clinical Features	Diagnostic Testing	Imaging and EEG	Treatment
HHV6	Exanthem, seizures, ~80% infected by age 2, rare in > 3 years of age	• Acute and convalescent serology • CSF HHV6 PCR	MRI may show T2 hyperintensity in frontal and parietal white matter, and/or edema in temporal lobes	Supportive Ganciclovir or foscarnet (only in severe disease, usually associated with immunocompromised hosts)
VZV	Vesicular rash Vasculopathy involving either large or small vessels Cerebellar deficits common	• Acute and convalescent serology • CSF VZV PCR • Culture of skin lesions	MRI may show large vessel arteritis, ischemic and/or hemorrhagic infarcts, demyelinating lesions MRA may demonstrate angiitis	Acyclovir Consider ganciclovir as alternate Use of adjunctive corticosteroids is controversial
HIV	Acute encephalopathy with seroconversion, or chronic progressive neurocognitive deficit/dementia	• Acute and convalescent serology • CSF HIV PCR • Quantitative serum HIV RNA viral load	MRI may show atrophy and nonspecific periventricular white matter changes. In later stages, may reveal opportunistic infections or malignancy	Initiate HAART
LCMV	Psychosis, cranial nerve deficits, hydrocephalus, acute aseptic meningitis	• CSF and serum serology	No specific findings	Supportive
Measles virus (rubeola)	Focal neurologic signs, obtundation SSPE: chronic, progressive	• Acute and convalescent serology • CSF serology • RT-PCR of nasopharynx and urine for MV RNA	No specific findings	Supportive Vaccine-preventable Vitamin A has been shown to improve symptoms SSPE: interferon and ribavirin are experimental
Mumps	Parotitis Sensorineural hearing loss	• Acute and convalescent serology • CSF mumps PCR • Saliva culture	No specific findings	Supportive
Nipah virus	Pneumonitis Myoclonus, dystonia, areflexia, hypotonia	• Acute and convalescent serology • CSF serology, cell culture	MRI may show discrete focal lesions on T2 imaging in subcortical and deep white matter	Supportive, consider ribavirin

(*continued*)

■ **Table 16.21** Acute Infectious Encephalitis Presentation, Diagnostic Testing, Imaging, and EEG Characteristics by Organism (*continued*)

Pathogen	Unique Clinical Features	Diagnostic Testing	Imaging and EEG	Treatment
Rabies virus	Paresthesias at or near inoculum site Symptoms may present days or years after exposure, depending on site of bite "Furious form": progressive encephalopathy, hydrophobia "Paralytic form": ascending paralysis	• Acute and convalescent serology • CSF IgG/IgM, CSF rabies PCR • Saliva culture and RT-PCR • Ag detection on histopathology (Negri bodies)	No specific findings	Postexposure prophylaxis with rabies Ig and vaccine prior to clinical symptom onset 100% fatal
Bacteria				
Bartonella henselae	Regional adenopathy days prior to CNS manifestations Neuroretinitis	• Acute and convalescent serology • Lymph node tissue PCR	No specific findings	No definitive evidence for use of antimicrobials Often treated with erythromycin or doxycycline (+/− rifampin) Alterative therapy includes quinolones, azithromycin, clarithromycin
Listeria monocytogenes	Rhomboencephalitis	• Blood culture • CSF culture	No specific findings	Ampicillin + gentamycin or bactrim
Mycobacterium tuberculosis	Rhomboencephalitis, lacunar infarcts, hydrocephalus	• CSF AFB smear and culture, PCR • PCR and culture of respiratory secretions	See Granulomatous Disease section	Isoniazid, rifampin, pyrazinamide, ethambutol + dexamethasone
Rickettsial and ehrlichial disease	Nearly all present with fever, headache, and rash appears in 85% by the fifth day of illness			
Rocky Mountain Spotted Fever (*Rickettsia rickettsii*)	Rash in 90% due to small vessel vasculitis Subarachnoid hemorrhage and other CNS complications in about 25%	• Acute and convalescent serology • PCR of any skin lesions (available through the CDC)	MRI shows T2 hyperintensity in perivascular spaces that resolves with clinical improvement	Doxycycline Seroconversion may be delayed, treat empirically if suspected infection
Q fever	Worst headache of life, encephalitis, dementia, peripheral neuropathy	• Acute and convalescent serology • PCR of any skin lesions	No specific findings	Doxycycline or tetracycline

■ **Table 16.21** Acute Infectious Encephalitis Presentation, Diagnostic Testing, Imaging, and EEG Characteristics by Organism (*continued*)

Pathogen	Unique Clinical Features	Diagnostic Testing	Imaging and EEG	Treatment
Ehrlichiosis	20% have CNS involvement Meningoencephalitis Rash (spares face, palms, and soles), fever, cytopenias	• Acute and convalescent serology • CSF *Ehrlichia* PCR	MRI may show leptomeningeal enhancement EEG demonstrates nonspecific slowing	Doxycycline
Spirochetes *Borrelia burgdorferi*	Facial nerve palsy, meningitis, and radiculitis	• Acute and convalescent serum • Acute CSF serology	No specific findings	Ceftriaxone, cefotaxime
Treponema pallidum (see Granulomatous Diseases section)	Meningoencephalitis, general paresis, tabes dorsalis	• Serum RPR and FTA-ABS • CSF VDRL and FTA-ABS	No specific findings	Penicillin G
Fungi				
Coccidioides spp *Cryptococcus neoformans* *Histoplasma*	See Immunocompromised section			
Protozoa and Helminths				
Acanthamoeba spp	Subacute presentation Skin nodules/ulcers	• Acute and convalescent serology • Saliva culture • Direct visualization on wet mount of fresh CSF, or Giemsa/Wright stained smears of CSF • Cysts and trophozoites on brain tissue	MRI may show enhancing space occupying lesions or hydrocephalus	Multidrug therapy: pentamidine + azole + sulfonamide +/−flucytosine Alternative options: rifampin, trimethoprim + sulfamethoxazole, surgical debulking
Balamuthia mandrillaris	Cranial nerve palsies, ataxia	• Acute and convalescent serology • Cysts and trophozoites on brain tissue • Wet mount of CSF	MRI may show enhancing space occupying lesions or hydrocephalus	Macrolide + pentamidine + flucytosine + fluconazole + sulfadiazine (combination used in 3 of 4 survivors reported in United States)

(*continued*)

■ **Table 16.21** Acute Infectious Encephalitis Presentation, Diagnostic Testing, Imaging, and EEG Characteristics by Organism (*continued*)

Pathogen	Unique Clinical Features	Diagnostic Testing	Imaging and EEG	Treatment
Naegleria fowleri	Change in taste or smell at onset Rapid progression Fatal	• Direct visualization on wet mount of fresh CSF	No specific findings	Amphotericin B (IV and IT) with optional addition of quinolones or rifampin Few survivors
Plasmodium falciparum	See Tropical medicine section			
Toxoplasma gondii	See Immunocompromised section			
Trypanosoma spp	See Tropical medicine section			

Abbreviations: BG, basal ganglia; CDC, Centers for Disease Control; CN, cranial nerve; EBNA, Ebstein-Barr nuclear antigen; EEG, electroencephalogram; FTA-Abs, fluorescent treponemal antibody-absorption; HAART, highly active antiretroviral therapy; IFN, interferon; IT, intrathecal; IV, intravenous; MRA, magnetic resonance angiography; PLED, periodic lateralized epileptiform discharge; RBC, red blood cell; RPR; RT-PCR, reverse transcriptase polymerase chain reaction; SLE, St Louis encephalitis virus; VCA, viral capsid antigen; WBC, white blood cell.
Source: Adapted from Refs. 131–133, 136–138, 146, 151.

and increased risk of mortality, whereas those with self-limited seizure activity tend to have a more rapid recovery (137). Mortality statistics by etiologic agent are given in Table 16.16; the overall mortality for all types of primary infectious encephalitis is between 0% to 7%. In general, fatality is associated with age, presence of malignancy, immune status at baseline, need for mechanical ventilation, etiologic agent, presence of coma after 5 days, and presence of sepsis after 5 days (138,147).

Morbidity in surviving children generally consists of persistent headache in 60% to 75%, as well as fatigue

■ **Table 16.22** Empiric Therapy Dosing Schedules for Viral Encephalitis

Acyclovir

≤ 28 days	20 mg/kg per dose IV 3 times daily × 21 days[a]
> 28 days to < 12 years	20 mg/kg per dose IV 3 times daily × 21 days[a]
≥ 12 years	10 mg/kg per dose IV 3 times daily × 21 days[a]

Doxycycline

2.2 mg/kg/dose twice daily (max dose 100 mg) by mouth (PO) or IV until 3 days after fever subsides and clinically improving (typically 5–7 days in rickettsial and ehrlichial infections)

[a] Consider repeat LP for the best of cure before discontinuation of therapy.

and cognitive problems for months following hospitalization (149,150); this may be higher with certain infections, such as HSV. Less common long-term problems include epilepsy, motor function disability, and moderate to severe learning disabilities. Younger children with abnormal EEG or imaging, a high degree of BBB damage, focal neurologic signs, or severe encephalopathy, all have poorer prognosis (149). Seizures at presentation are not predictive of persistent seizures at discharge.

Noninfectious Causes of Encephalitis

There are a variety of noninfectious diagnoses that may mimic primary infectious encephalitis. First and foremost, an immune-mediated postinfectious process may be present, and this may actually overlap with the active primary infection, in which case treatment and prognosis would be different than isolated primary infectious encephalitis. Please see the chapter on "Acquired Demyelinating Syndromes of the Central Nervous System" for more information on demyelinating disease. Other noninfectious, nonautoimmune processes that may mimic encephalitis and myelitis are reviewed in Table 16.23.

Acute Primary Infectious Myelitis

Epidemiology and Pathophysiology

Primary infection of the spinal cord is rare, with an incidence between 1 and 4.5 cases/million people a year

■ **Table 16.23** Common Mimics of Infectious Encephalitis	
Disorder	**Diagnosis**
Endocrinologic	
Hashimoto thyroiditis	Thyroid function tests, anti-thyroperoxidase Ab, anti-thyroglobulin Ab
Rheumatologic	
Systemic lupus erythematosus	ANA, anti-DS DNA
Other rheumatologic conditions	RF, anti-SSA, anti-SSB
Metabolic	
Hypoglycemia	Serum glucose
Uremic encephalopathy	Blood urea nitrogen and creatinine
Hepatic encephalopathy	Serum aminotransferases, ammonia
Inborn errors of metabolism	Serum amino acids, urine organic acids, acylcarnitine profile, lactate, pyruvate
Other	
Head trauma	History, neuroimaging
Nonconvulsive status epilepticus	EEG
Acute confusional migraine	Diagnosis of exclusion
Intracranial hemorrhage or thrombosis	Neuroimaging
Toxin	
Acute ingestion	Toxicology screen

Abbreviations: Ab, antibody; DS, double strand; SSA, Sjögren's syndrome A; SSB, Sjögren's syndrome B.

(154). Frequently, myelitis occurs in conjunction with meningitis, encephalitis, or radiculitis. While etiologic organisms are rarely found, some viruses are specifically neurotropic and tend to attack the spinal cord, including EVs, West Nile Virus, and HSV. Certain bacteria (syphilis, *B burgdorferi*), parasites (*Schistosoma*), and fungal infections (*Coccidioides, Aspergillus*) may also primarily affect the spinal cord. Organism-specific epidemiology is the same as in primary infectious encephalitis (Table 16.16).

Clinical Presentation

Viral infections of the spinal cord may result in one of two classic pathophysiologic courses and clinical presentations (155). First, the virus may specifically target the gray matter of the spinal cord resulting in an acute lower motor neuron disease, or acute flaccid paralysis (155,156). Viruses typically responsible for this syndrome include EVs (particularly EV71 and polio) (157) and flaviviruses (particularly West Nile virus) (139,155). These infections are frequently accompanied by other symptoms of acute viral infection, including fever, headache, and meningismus. Onset of anterior horn cell infection occurs within days, and may occur in a focal or segmental pattern. Clinically, this results in an asymmetric flaccid weakness with hyporeflexia. Sensory symptoms are uncommon given the specific tropism for anterior horn cells of these viruses.

The second common pathophysiology and clinical presentation of a primary viral infection of the spinal cord is quite similar to a postinfectious transverse myelitis. Certain viruses, including members of the herpesvirus family (HSV, cytomegalovirus [CMV], varicella-zoster virus, EBV) and hepatitis C more preferentially affect the white matter. These cases in general present with more diffuse white matter involvement, and thus may also include sensory symptoms and bladder dysfunction (155) in addition to the weakness, flaccid paralysis, and hyporeflexia seen in anterior horn cell syndromes.

Diagnosis

The primary differential diagnosis of acute infectious myelitis includes other causes of myelopathy (structural and compressive etiologies, vascular abnormalities, or metabolic disorders), and immune-mediated causes, such as acute disseminated encephalomyelitis (ADEM). Diagnostic testing is primarily aimed at exclusion of treatable causes of myelopathy, particularly compressive or extramedullary lesions (155). The mainstay in the radiographic diagnosis of acute infectious myelitis is MRI imaging. While MRI findings are variable in acute infectious myelitis, T2 hyperintensity in the anterior horns of the spinal cord across multiple vertebral body segments (157) in anterior horn cell specific disease may be demonstrated. Focal edema or hemorrhagic necrosis may also be present, and contrast enhancement may be present for several days (155).

CSF should also be examined in the diagnosis of acute infectious myelitis. A lymphocytic pleocytosis is present in about 83% of children with an acute viral myelitis, and an elevated protein is present in about 66% (154). An IgG index ([CSF IgG/CSF Albumin]/[Serum IgG/ Serum Albumin]) is typically normal, which may help distinguish infectious cases from those that are immune-mediated. Similar to encephalitis, CSF PCR is the gold standard for diagnosis of an etiologic organism (155).

Finally, electrodiagnostic testing may be helpful in the diagnosis of acute infectious myelitis by helping to objectively localize symptoms to the spinal cord, if imaging is normal. Typically, electromyography and nerve conduction studies demonstrate normal sensory nerve action potentials, mildly reduced compound motor action potentials, and positive sharp waves and fibrillations.

Treatment

Treatment of primary infectious myelitis is largely supportive, unless a strong clinical suspicion for a specific pathogen is present, or if there is evidence for a primary etiology. If HSV or varicella-zoster virus is suspected, acyclovir therapy is appropriate. If CMV is suspected, ganciclovir or foscarnet may be used. Finally, if there is any clinical suspicion of an immune-mediated component of disease, high dose methylprednisolone should be administered.

■ SLOW INFECTIONS OF THE NERVOUS SYSTEM

The phrase "slow virus infection" was coined by Dr Bjorn Sigurdsson (158) in 1954 to describe slowly progressive neurologic and pulmonary diseases in sheep (159). He defined slow infections as caused by organisms that continuously multiplied and produced progressive abnormality in a host over months and years, following a long incubation period, and often localized to a single organ (158,160). These infections are distinct from reactivation of latent viruses with respect to the time course of their slow accumulation of pathogen, followed by a slowly progressive

but unrelenting disease course (161). Slow infections of the nervous system are quite rare, however, most are devastating and require intensive care treatment and monitoring in later stages of disease, either related to progressive obtundation, brainstem dysfunction, or intractable seizures.

Progressive Multifocal Leukoencephalopathy

Progressive multifocal leukoencephalopathy (PML) was the first slow virus infection of the nervous system definitively linked to a virus (161). PML is caused by the DNA *Polyomavirus* JC (JCV), and results in widespread and frequently fatal CNS demyelination via lysis of oligodendrocytes and astrocytes. While latent JCV infection of the kidneys and lymphoid organs is reportedly present in 50% of children age 9 to 11 years and up to 80% of healthy adults (162), PML is rare, with an incidence of about 0.6 cases per million adults (163). The incidence is lower in children, and is mostly associated with HIV infection (164). Profound suppression of cellular immunity appears to play a role in the reactivation of JCV and progressive development of PML (165), although PML may also rarely occur in patients with minimal or occult immunosuppression (166).

Clinical signs and symptoms of PML are insidious, progressive, multifocal, and nonspecific, depending on what region of the brain is affected by the extensive demyelination caused by JCV. Diagnosis is based on clinical and radiographic guidelines in an at-risk individual, coupled with identification of the virus on CSF PCR or brain biopsy sample. CSF is typically acellular. The most effective treatment of PML is to reconstitute the immune system. There is no definitive effective pharmacologic therapy for JCV or PML. Highly active antiretroviral therapy (HAART) has improved survival in HIV-infected adults with PML, although no comparable data for pediatrics is available. Several specific therapeutics have been investigated, including intrathecal cytosine arabinoside and oral cidofovir, mefloquine, and mirtazapine, although none have been shown to be definitively effective. Thus, standard therapy consists of immune reconstitution and supportive care.

Subacute Sclerosing Panencephalitis

Subacute sclerosing panencephalitis (SSPE) was first described clinically in 1934 (167), and was shown to be caused by the measles virus in 1969 (168). Measles virus is thought to gain entry to the CNS during acute infection, where it enters neurons, alters cellular machinery to avoid immune surveillance, and slowly replicates intracellularly over many years, while undergoing hypermutations of its proteins to avoid recognition (169,170). Unlike systemic measles, release of infectious progeny is not routine (171). In fact, typical infectious measles virus has never been isolated either from the brain or the CSF of patients with SSPE, and histopathologic exams have consistently failed to reveal the typical morphologic changes associated with virus maturation (172). Instead, spread to neighboring neurons is thought to be very slow via direct cell-to-cell interaction (169).

SSPE typically presents 6 to 8 years (170,172) following an acute wild-type measles infection (171,173). In the United States, the incidence is about 0.01 cases per million people, or four to five cases per year. Worldwide, 1 to 11 cases of SSPE can be expected for every 100,000 cases of measles (170). SSPE typically presents between 8 and 13 years of age, although latencies of up to 30 years have been reported (172). Other clear risk factors include male gender, younger age at measles onset, living in a rural area, poverty, and overcrowding (171). SSPE has a variable clinical presentation, but progressive intellectual deterioration (poor school performance and attention span), personality changes, and behavioral abnormalities (emotional lability, forgetfulness, and trouble sleeping) are common (170,171). These nonspecific symptoms are followed by a steady motor decline in 100%, with myoclonus in 74%, seizures in 10%, cognitive decline in 86%, dyspraxia, visual disturbances in up to 50% (171), autonomic failure, and rigidity (170). SSPE ultimately leads to akinetic mutism and death (Table 16.24).

Diagnosis of SSPE rests on an appropriate clinical history, elevated CSF measles antibody titers, and either a specific EEG pattern, CSF profile, or molecular diagnostic tests to identify the measles virus mutated genome in brain tissue specimens (171,172). CSF typically reveals pleocytosis, elevated IgG and oligoclonal bands, normal glucose, elevated or normal protein, and anti-measles virus IgG titers ranging from 1:40 to 1:1280 (170,171), with a CSF-serum ratio ranging from 5:1 to 40:1 (170,171). Enzyme-linked immunosorbent assay (ELISA) for measles virus IgG in the CSF has a 100% positive predictive value in individuals with the appropriate clinical presentation, assuming CSF albumin is negative (implying no breakdown of the BBB, and therefore true intrathecal antibody production). EEG shows stereotyped, bilaterally synchronous, symmetric periodic complexes in 65% to 83% of individuals with SSPE, which may occur in sleep, and can be stimulus-induced in the early stages. These last approximately

■ **Table 16.24** Clinical Stages of SSPE

Stage	Clinical Manifestations
Stage 1	Personality, behavioral, and cognitive changes. Slurred or regressive speech.
Stage 2	Frequent myoclonus, dyskinesias, poor coordination, seizures
Stage 3	Pyramidal and extrapyramidal symptoms, disappearance of myoclonus, decreased level of consciousness, autonomic instability
Stage 4	Vegetative state, autonomic failure

Source: Adapted from Refs. 170, 171, 174.

1 to 3 seconds each, with 2- to 20-second intervals between complexes. Lateralization or regionalization is less common (170). MRI is not particularly helpful in diagnosis because findings do not correlate with clinical stages, and sometimes progress despite clinical stabilization. In general, posterior cortical and subcortical asymmetric T2 hyperintensities mark the early stages, which progress to periventricular white matter lesions, progressive cortical and deep gray matter atrophy, accompanied by enhancement and restricted diffusion (170–172). Pathologic findings are variable, depending on when during the course of the disease, and where in the brain they are sampled. Edema is prominent early, and an acute inflammatory phase is demonstrated later, with perivascular inflammation (with relative sparing of the cerebellum), spongiosis, demyelination, and neuronal loss as the disease progresses.

Most SSPE is relentlessly progressive and the disease is almost always fatal. The mean survival in children ranges from 21 to 36 months (170), and less than 7% of individuals are alive after 6 years (175). Up to 10% of cases progress even faster (death can occur within 6 months from symptom onset), and are labeled atypical and fulminant (171). At best, trials have shown that 30% to 35% of individuals benefit from therapy aimed at bolstering the immune system or slowing clinical progression (170). Clinical improvement is much less likely. Isoprinosine (inosiplex), interferons, ribavirin, and various combinations of these medications have been attempted through several delivery mechanisms (oral, subcutaneous, intrathecal, intraventricular) in an attempt to improve the disease course. The most effective therapy reported to date has been a combination of weekly intrathecal interferon alfa and daily oral Isoprinosine, however, 50% of patients treated with this regimen do not achieve stabilization of symptoms and ultimately, regardless of treatment, nearly all progress to death (170).

Progressive Rubella Panencephalitis

Progressive rubella panencephalitis is a rare, insidiously progressive, and ultimately fatal neurologic disorder caused by latent infection with the rubella virus (159). Most commonly it is a late sequelae of congenital rubella syndrome presenting sometime in the second decade of life, although it has also been reported following postnatal childhood rubella infections (176–178). Clinically, it presents similarly to SSPE, except that marked cerebellar dysfunction and ataxia are dominant features (176), whereas in SSPE the cerebellar functions are largely notably spared. CSF demonstrates a mild mononuclear pleocytosis with elevated protein and increased CSF to serum rubella IgG ratio (159,176,178). Pathology shows a panencephalitis with diffuse destruction of white matter, neuronal loss, and gliosis similar to SSPE, but with the unique feature of amorphous vascular deposits in the white matter and diffuse cerebellar atrophy (159). Recovery of the rubella virus from brain biopsy or autopsy has been documented, but is rare. Therapeutically, there is no known treatment. Isoprinosine has not been shown to be helpful in small case series, despite its minor success in SSPE. Supportive care is the standard.

Retroviral Infections

HIV-1

As of 2009, the World Health Organization (WHO) estimated that of the 33.3 million HIV-infected individuals worldwide, 2.5 million were children. There were 370,000 new infections and 260,000 deaths worldwide in children less than 15 years old in 2009 (179). In the United States, by the end of 2008 approximately 30,000 adolescents and young adults 13 to 24 years of age were living with a diagnosis of HIV (Centers for Disease Control, United States).

HIV causes a variety of neurologic diseases in children and adults, some of which are a direct consequence of HIV itself, and some of which are related to the immunosuppression it induces and subsequent opportunistic infections (OI) (see Immunocompromised Hosts section). For the purpose of this section, we will address only acute neurologic complications caused directly by HIV infection that may require intensive care support; these complications typically occur around the time of seroconversion. In fact, up to 20% of persons with HIV may present initially with a neurologic disorder (180,181). HIV is thought to enter the CNS early in infection via infected monocytes and lymphocytes crossing a disrupted BBB.

Aseptic meningitis or meningoencephalitis may occur with seroconversion, either in isolation, or in association with a mononucleosis-like syndrome (181), in up to 50% of patients. The presentation and screening CSF testing is consistent with any viral meningitis, so care must be taken in the evaluation of these children to identify any risk factors that may indicate specific HIV testing. At the time of acute infection, serologic testing will typically be negative. However, in a suspicious clinical scenario, these may be positive upon repeat testing 2 to 3 months following the initial presentation. During the acute phase of infection, PCR is the test of choice for HIV-seroconversion syndromes. Neuroimaging is typically unrevealing in HIV seroconversion-associated meningoencephalitis (181). Symptoms typically resolve over the course of about 2 weeks with supportive therapy alone.

Acute inflammatory demyelinating polyneuropathy (Guillan Barre Syndrome [GBS]) has also been reported in the early stages of HIV infections. Again, the presentation of HIV-associated GBS is similar to that of uninfected subjects, primarily with progressive motor weakness, nonspecific sensory symptoms, autonomic dysfunction, and areflexia. However, in contrast to the classic cytoalbuminemic dissociation seen in GBS outside of HIV infection, HIV-infected subjects tend to demonstrate a lymphocytic pleocytosis (181). Thus, testing for HIV should be considered in these cases of GBS, and in general, attention should be paid to HIV risk factors in all GBS patients. Conventional therapy with corticosteroids, IVIg, or plasmapheresis is indicated, and prognosis is similar to uninfected subjects (181).

As HIV infection progresses into the chronic phase, vacuolar myelopathy, neurocognitive impairments, neuropathies, and myopathies may insidiously develop as a direct consequence of infection as well; however, given the chronicity of these symptoms, intensive care is rarely required.

Human T-Lymphotropic Virus 1–Associated Myelopathy/Tropic Spastic Paraparesis

HTLV (human T-lymphotropic virus) was the first retrovirus recovered from man and associated with human disease (161). From a neurologic standpoint it primarily causes HTLV-1–associated myelopathy/tropic spastic paraparesis (HAM/TSP), but has also been associated with uveitis, some facial nerve palsies (182), mild cognitive deficits, and peripheral neuropathy. From a nonneurologic standpoint, it is associated with adult T-lymphocyte leukemia/lymphoma and several rheumatologic disorders (182). HTLV affects 10 to 20 million people worldwide (183), with transmission occurring primarily through breast milk; 42% of breast fed infants in endemic areas will be infected (161,182,184). Transmission may also occur via exposure to blood products, needle sharing, and sexual intercourse. While the prevalence of infection in the United States and Europe is less than 1%, prevalence in endemic areas such as the Caribbean and Japan may be as high as 30%. The estimated lifetime risk of HAM/TSP for infected individuals is less than 2% (182,183), with onset of symptoms ranging from 4 months to 50 years after infection. Clinically, symptoms are largely localized to the thoracic spinal cord and include slowly progressive gait spasticity, incontinence, impotence, and ill-defined, nonlocalizable sensory symptoms. CSF may show a mild lymphocytic pleocytosis and elevated protein, or may be normal; blood and CSF should be tested for the presence of HTLV-1 antibodies or antigens. Pathology is necrotizing and demyelinating (161). There is no proven treatment for HTLV and no vaccine (182). However, typically HTLV-1 is not fatal, unlike the other slow virus infections (161). In one prospective study of 123 patients diagnosed with HAM/TSP, neurologic symptom progression from disease onset to wheelchair confinement occurred over a median of 21 years (183).

■ TRANSMISSIBLE SPONGIFORM ENCEPHALOPATHIES

Transmissible spongiform encephalopathies (TSEs), or prion ("proteinaceous infectious agents") diseases, are a group of uniformly fatal, slowly progressive neurodegenerative diseases in animals and humans (185). They are caused by misfolded isoforms of a normal host-encoded cell membrane glycoprotein, called prion protein (PrP) (186), encoded by the PRNP gene. The natural form of PrP (PrP^C) is expressed in many human tissues, but is most concentrated in the brain. When PrP^C misfolds into an abnormal isoform (PrP^{SC}) through unclear mechanisms, it progressively accumulates in the CNS (185), and propagates itself by imposing its conformation on the normal host cell protein (187).

TSEs may be sporadic, acquired, or heritable (186). Infection is acquired by ingestion or inoculation with infected CSF or neurologic tissues; brain tissue is thought to be 100,000 times more infectious than peripheral

tissues including blood (187). Agents that inactivate viruses and nucleic acid in biologic specimens or on medical equipment (such as heat, ionizing radiation, alcohol, formalin, proteases, and nucleases) do not effectively inactivate prions. Once infected, there is no host immune response to infection, and a noninflammatory pathologic process ensues. Incubation after infection with a prion is typically months to years; neurologic manifestations are then slowly progressive until death (185).

Diagnosis is established based on clinical and exposure history, CSF examination, EEG, neuroimaging, and postmortem histopathologic findings. Treatment is supportive. Prognosis is uniformly fatal. Specific epidemiology, clinical manifestations, and diagnostic tools for different human prion diseases are presented in Table 16.25.

■ PROTOZOAN AND HELMINTHIC INFECTIONS

The following section will discuss various clinical, diagnostic, and therapeutic aspects of common parasitic infections of the CNS. Parasitic infections specific to the immunocompromised host (including *Toxoplasma gondii*) will be discussed in the Immunocompromised Hosts section. Emphasis is again placed on parasitic infections causing illness severe enough to warrant critical care.

Protozoan Infections

Cerebral Malaria

In 2002, over 2 billion people worldwide were exposed to malaria, resulting in an estimated 515 million clinical cases of acute *Plasmodium falciparum* infection (189), and about a million deaths, mostly in children less than 5 years old (190). *Plasmodium falciparum* is the most aggressive form of malaria, and the most common parasite to infect the CNS in immunocompetent individuals (191). The pathogenesis of cerebral malaria (CM) is probably multifactorial (192). Infected erythrocytes are sequestered in multiple organs by adherence to venule endothelial cells, particularly in the brain (193). This cytoadherence is thought to promote parasite growth in a relatively hypoxic environment and to allow the infected erythrocytes to evade destruction in the spleen. Sequestration is also thought to reduce microvascular flow (193) and, aggravated by poor RBC deformity, results in vessel occlusion (194). This cerebrovascular obstruction, in combination with possible seizures, metabolic derangements, impaired

■ **Table 16.25** Transmissible Spongiform Encephalopathies in Humans

	Epidemiology	Clinical Presentation	Labs/Imaging/EEG	Pathology
CJD				
sCJD	Most common form of human prion disease, Comprises 85% of CJD, most common between 50–75 years old. Annual incidence 0.5–2 cases/million population. No seasonal or geographic predisposition. Possible genetic predisposition— Sephardic Jewish individuals have a 30× higher frequency than Ashkenazi Jewish individuals.	Rapid progressive dementia, spontaneous or induced myoclonus, cerebellar dysfunction with variable ataxia. Pyramidal and extrapyramidal dysfunction may also be present. Akinetic mutism typically prior to death.	*CSF:* mildly elevated or normal protein. Nonspecific 14-3-3 protein elevated in >50% of cases. *Neuroimaging:* brain atrophy on head CT. >50% have MRI with high T2, FLAIR, or DWI in basal ganglia or in cerebral or cerebellar cortex. *EEG:* initial slow wave activity, later with pseudoperiodic 1 hertz sharp wave complexes.	CNS amyloid plaques in 5–15%, spongiform changes universal.
iCJD	Acquired via corneal transplants, allografts of dura mater, electrocorticographic electrodes, neurosurgical equipment, and via administration of cadaver-derived gonadotropic hormones. Incubation time is < 2 years. Rare.	Similar to sCJD	Similar to sCJD	Similar to sCJD
fCJD	5–15% of CJD cases. Autosomal dominant inheritance, but with variable penetrance and poor phenotype/genotype correlation.	Similar to sCJD	Similar to sCJD	Similar to sCJD
nvCJD	Acquired via eating prion-infected beef or potentially via exposure to infected blood or plasma components. Reported age of onset ranges from 16–39 years (mean 29 years), with an average duration 18 months before death. By Feb 2012, 225 definite and probable cases in the world, 3 in the United States. Unknown number of asymptomatic infections.	Prominently psychiatric presentation (agitation, aggression, depression, anxiety, etc). Cerebellar ataxia and dysesthesias are also uniform, and not typical of sCJD. Later: urinary incontinence, progressive immobility, and akinetic mutism.	*CSF:* Nonspecific elevation of 14/3/3 protein. *Neuroimaging:* Bilateral increased thalamic densities on MRI *EEG:* generalized slowing, no periodic complexes.	Florid amyloid plaques surrounded by spongiform lesions ("florid plaques") in basal ganglia and thalamus, with widespread accumulation of abnormal PrP. Thalamic gliosis.

(continued)

■ **Table 16.25** Transmissible Spongiform Encephalopathies in Humans (*continued*)

	Epidemiology	Clinical Presentation	Labs/Imaging/EEG	Pathology
Kuru	Acquired via ritualistic cannibalism in the Fore linguistic group of Papua New Guinea. Likely started via consumption of a sCJD case	Cerebellar ataxia, movement disorder (tremor, choreiform and athetoid movements), cranial nerve abnormalities.		Amyloid plaques common. Spongiform changes, neuron loss, astrocytic microgliosis.
GSS syndrome	Autosomal dominant inheritance. Annual incidence is 1 in 100 million population. Disease onset between 30–60 years old, with progression over 3.5–9.5 years.	Cerebellar ataxia, gait abnormalities, dementia, cranial nerve disorders, rare myoclonus, spastic paraparesis, Parkinsonism. Altered sleep and temperature rhythms	EEG rarely helpful.	Amyloid plaques are universal. Wide range of spongiform changes, neuron loss, astrocytic microgliosis, and neurofibrillary tangles
FFI	Autosomal dominant inheritance; previously known as "thalamic dementia." Presents between 20–72 years old, at an average age of 49 y/o, with an average survival of 18.4 months.	Insomnia or disrupted sleep, dysautonomia, ataxia, myoclonus, dysarthria, dysphagia, pyramidal signs, late mild dementia	*Polysomnogram:* reduction in sleep type and disorderly transition b/t sleep stages *PET:* hypometabolism in thalamus and cingulate cortex	Predominantly affects the thalamus. No amyloid plaques, minimal vacuolation.
SFI	Sporadic, rare.	Same as FFI, but no family history.		Predominantly affects the cerebral cortex.

Abbreviations: CJD, Creutzfeldt-Jakob Disease; fCJD, familial CJD; FFI, fatal familial insomnia; GSS, Gerstmann-Sträussler-Scheinker; iCJD, Iatrogenic CJD; nvCJD, new variant CJD; sCJD, sporadic CJD; SFI, sporadic fatal insomnia.
Source: Adapted from Refs. 185–188.

perfusion, elevated ICP and cerebral edema, and infection-specific toxins all likely contribute to coma in CM (195).

The WHO defines CM as a clinical syndrome characterized by coma at least 1 hour after termination of a seizure or correction of hypoglycemia (Blantyre coma scale ≤ 2) (196,197), *P falciparum* parasitemia, and exclusion of other obvious causes of encephalopathy (195,198). Nearly all children with any type of malaria present with fever, rigors, and/or chills (193). Sixty percent to 80% of children with CM also present with seizures (193,199), which may be related to hypoxia and ischemia, sequestration of infected erythrocytes, or parasite-derived toxins. Brainstem signs are common and are frequently associated with increased ICP and cerebral edema (195), however, other focal neurologic findings are less common. Malarial retinopathy, manifested by retinal whitening, vessel changes, and hemorrhages is common. Papilledema may or may not be present (199). Systemically, metabolic aberrations including hypoglycemia, hyponatremia, and metabolic acidosis are common (195).

In general, children affected by CM are slightly older than those with uncomplicated malaria, have a shorter duration of illness, and have a higher parasite burden. There is no clear association between hemoglobin concentration and level of consciousness (200), although all children with malaria should be evaluated for anemia on an ongoing basis. Factors independently associated with neurologic involvement include past history of seizures, fever lasting at least 2 days, delayed capillary refill, acidosis, and hypoglycemia.

The diagnosis of CM is difficult to confirm in endemic areas where rates of asymptomatic parasitemia may be as high as 80%, and in the context of limited availability of diagnostic tools (199). Approximately 25% of children who qualify for a clinical diagnosis of CM may in fact have nonmalarial etiologies of coma and seizure (201). Therefore, LP must be performed to exclude other etiologic causes of encephalopathy. In isolated CM, CSF may be normal or may demonstrate a mild pleocytosis, elevated protein (195), depressed glucose, or CSF–serum adenosine deaminase ratio of < 0.38. A low CSF glucose appears to be the most helpful factor in discriminating CM from viral encephalitis (202). Parasites are not reliably found in the CSF on microscopic examination. EEG is nonspecific, and may be consistent with diffuse anoxia or hypoglycemia (197). CT of the brain may demonstrate cerebral edema. The presence of malarial retinopathy improves diagnostic accuracy, and has a 90% to 100% specificity and 95% sensitivity for identification of CM in fatal disease (199). Given the difficulty in diagnosis, CM should be considered in the differential diagnosis of anyone with the appropriate symptomatology who has recently traveled to an endemic region.

Quinine, quinidine, and artemisinin derivatives are the treatment of choice for CM. Mefloquine should be avoided due to a possible increased risk of neuropsychiatric toxic effects in CM. Erythrocytapheresis or exchange transfusion is indicated for patients with known CM or a peripheral parasite burden above 10% to 15% due to the probability of developing CM. Metabolic derangements and anemia must be corrected, with close monitoring and good supportive care. Steroids, aspirin, and heparin are harmful in patients with CM. Anti-tumor necrosis factor monoclonal antibodies are associated with a worsened neurologic outcome (195).

Untreated, CM is almost uniformly fatal. Following appropriate antimalarial therapy, the mortality rate of CM is between 18.6 and 22.2% (190), compared to 13.6% of malaria cases without neurologic involvement (200). Most deaths occur within 24 hours of admission (195), and occur due to a variety of mechanisms, including herniation and cardiopulmonary arrest related to metabolic acidosis. Another 6% to 29% of affected children have gross neurologic deficits at the time of hospital discharge (190,193), and it is estimated that about one-fourth of

children who survive CM have persistent neurologic or cognitive impairments or epilepsy (200), and particularly develop deficits in attention and working memory (203). Cerebellar ataxia is particularly common in CM. A "postmalaria neurologic syndrome" consisting of acute confusion, psychosis, generalized convulsions, and/or tremor is seen in about 0.1% of patients after severe malaria, and is associated with mefloquine use (193).

Trypanosomiasis

Human African trypanosomiasis (HAT), or "sleeping sickness" is caused by the trypanosome *Trypanosoma brucei*. There have been three major outbreaks over the last century, and HAT is now present in 36 sub-Saharan countries (204,205), with an estimated 300,000 to 500,000 individuals currently infected, resulting in about 100,000 deaths annually (206,207). In the United States, HAT is very uncommon, and seen only in immigrants, refugees, and individuals who have traveled to affected regions of Africa, most commonly game parks in East Africa (208). There are two morphologically similar strains of *T brucei* that cause human disease: *T b gambiense* is present more in Western and Central Africa, and causes endemic disease, whereas *T b rhodesiense* is seen primarily in East Africa, and causes an acute epidemic disease (207).

HAT is typically transmitted to humans through the bite of the tsetse fly, although there have also been case reports of vertical and blood-product transmission (209). Following a bite by an infected tsetse fly, a chancre frequently develops at the site of inoculation due to a local inflammatory response and parasitemia ensues, triggering B-lymphocyte activation, IgM production, immune complex formation, and reticuloendothelial hyperplasia. End-organ damage is caused by a combination of direct parasite invasion, immune complex deposition, inflammatory infiltrates, and vascular infiltration (210).

Clinically, both types of *T brucei* infection are characterized by an early hemolymphatic stage, and following CNS invasion, a late meningoencephalitis stage. In *T b gambiense*, the early phase may last months to years, whereas *T b rhodesiense* evolves more aggressively over weeks to months (208). Manifestations of the early stage include a chancre in 50% of *T b rhodesiense* infections and generalized lymphadenopathy, classically seen in posterior cervical nodes and called *Winterbottom sign* in *T b gambiense* (204,209). Successive waves of headache, fevers, malaise, and arthralgias ensue in both strains. Adenopathy, pruritis, rash, edema, anemia, cardiac disorders, and neuroendocrine disturbances may also develop over time. CNS involvement of the late stage is progressive with diffuse meningoencephalitis and parenchymal edema causing progressive sleep disturbance, headache, neuropsychiatric symptoms, weakness, tremor, and dyskinesias (208). Sleep disturbances, generating the moniker of "sleeping sickness," are related to a dysregulated circadian rhythm and fragmented sleep pattern. The end result is stupor and death (208).

Diagnosis requires demonstration of the parasite from the blood, lymph node aspirate, or CSF. A card agglutination test for trypanosome-specific antibodies is used on blood for endemic *T b gambiense* population screening (208,211). LP is recommended by the WHO for all suspected cases of HAT in order to define the stage of disease, and dictate treatment (212). Late stage disease is pathologically defined by the WHO as the presence of > 5 WBC, trypanosomes, or elevated protein > 370 mg/L in CSF (208). Lack of trypanosomes does not rule out neurologic involvement if trypanosomes have been demonstrated from other sampled sites, and the patient otherwise meets clinical criteria. EEG findings in late-stage HAT include sustained low-voltage background, paroxysmal waves, or various types of delta wave and rapid intermittent high-voltage delta bursts between periods of lower-voltage delta activity. MRI findings are typically nonspecific, but frequently include diffuse hyperintensities in the basal ganglia, internal and external capsules, asymmetric white matter abnormalities, and ventricular enlargement. Perhaps more importantly, MRI can help distinguish HAT from other CNS syndromes (204).

HAT is fatal if left untreated (208). Treatment regimens are different for *T b gambiense* and *T b rhodesiense*, and vary depending on whether or not there is known CNS involvement. Late-stage infections are treated with melarsoprol (a trivalent arsenical compound, available from the CDC on a compassionate use protocol), eflornithine, or nifurtimox. All treatment regimens are expensive and toxic, and between 2.5% and 10% of individuals with late infection are estimated to die from adverse effects of treatment alone (212). Overall, mortality with treatment is 10% to 20% (204). Following treatment, blood and CSF should be re-examined every 6 months over the subsequent 2 years to ensure no further trypanosomes are detected in blood, lymph, or CSF before a subject is considered cured (204,212).

Helminthic Infections

Neuroschistosomiasis

Schistosomiasis (also known as *Bilharzia*) infects up to 300 million people worldwide each year in 79 endemic countries throughout South America, the Middle East, and sub-Saharan Africa (213). Nearly all infections are transmitted transdermally following direct contact with fresh water that harbors the larval forms of the parasite known as *cercariae* (214) and the intermediary host, the freshwater snail (213). Transmission by organ transplantation has also been reported.

Acute hepatosplenic schistosomiasis (Katayama fever) presents with fever, urticaria, myalgias, eosinophilia, and bloody stools, which may last for weeks (211). Neuroschistosomiasis is rare, occurring in 4.3% of cases in one series (213,215), and typically developing weeks to months after initial infection (211). The larger *Schistosoma mansoni* tends to cause spinal cord disease (211), whereas the smaller *Schistosoma japonicum* causes most brain infections (213,215).

Myelopathy (including transverse myelitis) is the most common neurologic complication of schistosomiasis (213); the cauda equina or conus medullaris are the most common sites of involvement (211). Individuals with acute schistosomal myelopathy rarely have clinical evidence of systemic schistosomiasis (213). Other spinal manifestations include anterior spinal artery syndrome (211), bladder/rectal sphincter incontinence, painful radiculopathies, chronic asymmetric myeloradiculopathy, and extraaxial granulomas. Cerebral complications have been reported in 2.3% of travelers and other nonimmune subjects (213), and are characterized by cerebral edema, mass lesions (214), and hematomas, resulting in seizures, visual field impairment, altered mental status, cognitive difficulties, focal motor deficits, and cerebellar syndrome (213). A tumorlike syndrome may be seen with *S mansoni*, manifested as slowly increasing ICP resulting in headache, ataxia, nausea, emesis, and ataxia. Cases of acute encephalitis and cerebral vasculitis have also been reported during primary infection with *S mansoni*.

The diagnosis of CNS schistosomiasis is difficult, and requires the identification of an egg in a biopsy tissue specimen (211). Serologic testing is helpful only for those patients from nonendemic regions. CSF typically demonstrates a lymphocytic pleocytosis, elevated protein, presence of eosinophils, and elevated IgG index. Neuroimaging classically reveals one or more edematous cortical (213) or cerebellar (214) lesions with variable contrast enhancement. In addition, the brain may appear "arborized" on MRI, with linear enhancement surrounded by punctate enhancing nodules (211).

Praziquantel is curative of schistosomiasis in 60% to 90% of cases (211), however, feces and urine should be reexamined 1 month after treatment to ensure treatment efficacy (213). Oxamniquine is an alternative therapeutic option. Adjunctive steroids should be considered for subjects with rapid neurologic decline or significant edema, and large granulomas may need to be surgically removed (211). Complete recovery is only seen in 30% of S mansoni myeloradiculopathy patients and fewer transverse myelitis patients (213).

Neurocysticercosis

At least 50 million people worldwide are infected with Taenia solium, transmitted via ingestion of the larval stage of the pork tapeworm shed in the stool of a human tapeworm carrier (216). Cysticercosis is endemic in regions of Central and South America, sub-Saharan Africa, India, and Asia (217), but is also seen not uncommonly in the United States in immigrant populations, travelers to endemic countries, and their close contacts (218). Humans become tapeworm carriers (taeniasis) by ingesting undercooked pork containing larval cysts in muscle tissue. However, an individual must ingest an actual egg to develop cysticercosis; eggs are only present in the feces of a tapeworm-carrying human (216,217). About 5% to 40% of people infected by cysticercosis are tapeworm carriers, but most carriers do not develop symptomatic cysticercosis (219). Interestingly, pigs also acquire infection by ingesting contaminated human feces. The most common source of infective eggs is from asymptomatic household tapeworm carriers (216).

Several weeks or months following ingestion of tapeworm eggs, tissue cysticerci consisting of membranous walls filled with fluid and an invaginated scolex develop throughout the body including the brain as well as intraventricular, subarachnoid, intraocular, and spinal sites (216). Most cysts are asymptomatic for 3 to 5 years, and some may remain asymptomatic for up to 30 years (218). Cysts do not initially cause large local inflammatory reactions (220), and are not large enough to cause symptoms related to mass effect. Over time however, the cysts degenerate and attract an inflammatory response (217,220), and later form a calcified granuloma (220). Seizures are the primary manifestation of parenchymal neurocysticercosis and occur in 50% to 80% of patients with parenchymal disease (217). In fact,

neurocysticercosis is the most frequent cause of epilepsy in adults in the developing world (220). In children and adolescents, parenchymal neurocysticercosis may also generate an intense immune response with a high cyst burden, resulting in cerebral edema and a picture similar to encephalitis. Extraparenchymal neurocysticercosis may result in hydrocephalus, arachnoiditis, vasculitis, meningitis, and strokes. Spinal cysticercosis occurs in about 1% of cases. Ocular cysticercosis occurs in about 1% to 3% of cases (217).

The diagnosis of neurocysticercosis (NCC) is based primarily on clinical and radiographic criteria. Identification of a scolex (a round or elongated bright object) in a cystic lesion on CT, MRI, or fundoscopic examination is pathognomonic (218). In cases without an identified scolex, head CT typically demonstrates round, nonenhancing, hypodense lesions ranging from 0.5 to 2 cm in diameter at the gray-white junction of the cerebral cortex or within the brainstem. As a cyst degenerates, the wall increases in density and is surrounded by edema and contrast enhancement. Later, a calcified granuloma may be seen (217). Mass effect, diffuse edema, and infarction are significantly less common. Overall, HCT has a 95% sensitivity and specificity for the diagnosis of NCC (220). MRI may be helpful in detecting very small or degenerating lesions (216,220). Serologic testing as an adjunctive diagnostic test to neuroimaging can be helpful, however its negative predictive value is poor, as is it's specificity in endemic regions (216). LP is typically used to rule out other diagnoses, and must be used with caution with concern for elevated ICP. A fundoscopic examination should always be performed prior to treatment, but no other routine laboratory studies are necessary.

Treatment of NCC is primarily symptomatic, and centers on adequate seizure control with typical antiepileptic medications for focal seizures. Antiparasitic therapy using albendazole (doses vary depending on location of involvement) may hasten resolution of active cysts, decrease risk of seizures, and decrease recurrence of hydrocephalus, although it also risks increasing inflammation around a degenerating cyst (217), thereby worsening neurologic symptoms. As such, corticosteroids should be used as adjunctive therapy to antiparasitic medications. Of note, the same regions and groups at risk for NCC are typically at risk for TB and strongyloidiasis. Patients should be screened for both illnesses prior to initiating corticosteroid treatment. Antiparasitic drugs should not be used in cysticercal encephalitis, since enhanced killing can exacerbate host inflammatory response and lead to diffuse edema and potential herniation syndromes. Surgery for cyst excision is recommended for intraocular cysts to prevent vision loss associated with inflammation (221), in addition to antiparasitic therapy and corticosteroids. Ventriculostomy or ventriculoperitoneal shunt may be necessary for symptomatic hydrocephalus (216). Finally, open resection should be used for giant cysticerci and life-threatening mass effect.

■ RASMUSSEN ENCEPHALITIS

Rasmussen encephalitis (RE) is a rare progressive inflammatory disease of the brain involving one hemisphere (222), first described in 1958. It primarily affects children, although there are case reports of affected teenagers and adults. RE was originally thought to be viral in etiology (223), and connections with EVs, EBV, CMV, and HSV were described. However, no specific virus has been definitively linked to RE (224), and some now wonder if it is a postviral syndrome instead (225). Circulating autoantibodies have also been found in RE cases, supporting an autoimmune pathophysiology (222), and more recently, a cytotoxic T-lymphocyte reaction against neurons by the release of granzyme B has been proposed (222,224,226). Neuropathology is significant for T-lymphocyte dominant inflammation, microglial activation and nodule formation, neuronal loss, and astrocytic activation. However, there are no other known human or experimental autoimmune diseases that occur unilaterally, so the true etiology of RE is still in question (224).

Clinically, RE causes an acute onset of medically refractory focal epilepsy, particularly epilepsy partialis continua and progressive unilateral neurologic and functional deficits due to chronic localized encephalitis (226). The course of the disease can be conceptually broken down into three stages. The prodromal stage lasts a median of 7 months (longer in teens and adults), and involves relatively low seizure frequency and rare hemiparesis. The acute stage lasts a median of 8 months. During this time, RE progresses to manifest as frequent simple partial motor seizures. MRI abnormalities during this stage initially appear to be monofocal in the perisylvian area, but then spread across the ipsilateral hemisphere. Finally, a residual stage develops characterized by permanent and stable hemiparesis and decreased seizure frequency (222).

Diagnosis is primarily based on clinical presentation in conjunction with MRI evaluation and histopathology, when available (227). MRI of the brain initially demonstrates diffuse unilateral inflammation, and later a "burnout" atrophy that appears to correlate to a decreasing number of activated T-lymphocytes and reactive astrocytes on pathology (222).

The most effective treatment of RE is hemispherectomy (222,228). More recently, immunomodulatory therapy including corticosteroids, IVIg, and cyclophosphamide (228) has been attempted, but has not yet been studied in a randomized, objective fashion (222). Seizures are treated with standard antiepileptic drugs, which do not halt the progression (227). Prognosis overall is poor (222).

■ CNS INFECTIONS IN IMMUNOCOMPROMISED HOSTS

Immunodeficiency may involve any of the functional components of the immune system (B-lymphocytes, T-lymphocytes, complement, phagocytes, etc), and may be congenital or acquired. Congenital, or primary, immunodeficiencies (PIs) refer to genetic defects which cause abnormalities in one or more arms of the immune system; these typically present in childhood with recurrent or severe infections. In the developed world, secondary, or acquired, immunodeficiencies may be related to the treatment of cancer, stem cell or solid organ transplant, or immunosuppressive therapy for autoimmune diseases. In the developing world, secondary immunodeficiencies are more commonly associated with malnutrition and HIV infection.

A good understanding of the basic pathogenesis of each type of deficiency will aid the clinician in understanding the particular CNS infections to which an individual may be predisposed, forming a differential diagnosis and delivering appropriate empiric treatment rapidly. The following section outlines basics of the immune system, ways in which children are immune deficient, and particular opportunistic CNS pathogens.

Immunology Basics

The immune system is comprised of two arms: innate and adaptive, which complement each other in fighting different types of infections in different circumstances. The innate immune system is present from birth and does not vary significantly throughout one's lifetime. The adaptive immune system is comprised of cellular and antibody-mediated defenses supplied by lymphocytes, which are constantly changing to meet the needs of the host's immune challenges.

The Innate Immune System

The innate immune system is nonspecific and serves as the first line of defense against microbial invasion. It is comprised of the body's skin and mucosal barriers, toll-like receptors (TLRs), phagocytes and other inflammatory cells, and complement. There are many other proteins, molecules, and supportive cells involved in innate immunity, the details of which are beyond the scope of this chapter.

- *Skin and mucosa.* External barriers are made up of endothelial cells connected by tight junctions, which physically prevent invasion of most infectious organisms. The mucosa also contains many enzymes and protective proteins that can chemically neutralize any organisms attempting to invade the physical barrier.
- *TLR.* TLRs are transmembrane receptors expressed on cells of the innate immune system that inherently recognize a wide variety of pathogen-associated molecular patterns (PAMP) and are the first line of defense against invading pathogens. When TLRs recognize a specific PAMP, they initiate a cascade of cellular signals resulting in microbicidal activity. There are 10 distinct TLRs known in the human repertoire; a deficiency of one of these predisposes the host to specific pathogen invasion. For example, TLR4 recognizes and responds to lipopolysaccharide, a cell wall component of Gram-negative bacteria. Deficiency or defect of TLR4 predisposes to Gram-negative bacterial infection.
- *Phagocytes.* Neutrophils, monocytes, macrophages, and dendritic cells are phagocytic leukocytes present in blood and tissue; the word phagocyte is derived from the Greek word for *devour*. Neutrophils are the most common of these cells and are the first recruited to a site of infection. Neutrophils ingest and destroy pathogens by activating the complement system, which opsonizes, or kills, foreign invaders. Macrophages and monocytes serve a similar function and also act as antigen presenting cells (APCs) to activate the adaptive immune response. Decreased quantity or quality of phagocytic cells predisposes an individual to life threatening bacterial and fungal infections (229).
- *Other cells.* Other cells involved in innate immunity, pathogen clearance, and the inflammatory response include natural killer (NK) cells and mast cells. These cells target pathogens and pathogen-infected cells nonspecifically by initiating both cytokine release and apoptosis of a target foreign cell (230). While deficiencies of NK cell number or function may affect susceptibility to a variety of infections, overwhelming herpesvirus infections (HSV, CMV, EBV) are the most common clinical manifestation.
- *Complement.* The complement system is a destructive enzymatic cascade composed of more than 30 components that act in conjunction with the innate and adaptive immune responses in the defense against microbial pathogens. The complement cascade is first activated by recognition of cellular and pathogen components. It then opsonizes the surfaces of specific bacteria (labeling them for phagocytosis), creates bactericidal activity within serum though the membrane attack complex, and acts as a potent chemoattractant to bring other portions of the immune system to the site of infection (230). Complement deficiencies are rare and result in heterogeneous manifestations, depending on which complement protein and activation system is impaired. The most common complement deficiencies predispose affected individuals to recurrent encapsulated bacterial infections (particularly *Neisseria*).

The Adaptive Immune System

The adaptive immune system contains cell mediated and antibody mediated (humoral) components. It is activated to direct an antigen-specific response against a pathogen, and is comprised of T and B lymphocytes and antibody responses. The adaptive immune response may be further broken down into cell mediated and humoral immunity.

Cell Mediated Immunity

T-lymphocytes are the central orchestrators of the adaptive immune response and comprise about 75% of circulating lymphocytes. Naive T-lymphocytes circulate through lymphoid tissues to look for antigenic small peptide fragments presented by APCs that they recognize. Upon this discovery, the naive T-lymphocyte is activated and develops into a defense specific to that antigenic fragment. Activated T-lymphocytes become either effector cells, which are dispatched to contribute to the inflammatory milieu, or memory cells, which are quiescent and monitor for future invading pathogens.

APCs (usually comprised of dendritic cells and macrophages) express major histocompatibility complex (MHC) class II receptors on their surface and activate CD4+ T-lymphocytes. At the cellular level, CD4+ T-lymphocytes promote antibody formation by B-lymphocytes, initiate cytotoxic events by interaction with CD8+ cells, and activate macrophages. Deficiencies in CD4+ T-lymphocytes, such as in HIV infection, which specifically targets and destroys these cells, lead to OIs such as *Cryptococcus* and mycobacteria, as well as malignancies and autoimmune disorders.

CD8+ T-lymphocytes make up the cytotoxic arm of cell-mediated immunity. They are activated both by APCs expressing MHC I and CD4+ T-lymphocytes and function to initiate cytokine release as well as apoptosis of target cells (phagocytes). Deficiencies in cytotoxic T-lymphocytes lead to recurrent bacterial and viral infections. T-lymphocyte defects can also affect B-lymphocyte mediated antibody production, if the required T-lymphocyte costimulation is inadequate (229).

Antibody-Mediated (Humoral) Immunity

B-lymphocytes are critical for pathogen-specific immunity via their production of antibodies, and comprise about 10% to 15% of circulating lymphocytes. Naive B-lymphocytes are stimulated by a combination of antigen and CD4+ T-lymphocytes to mature and proliferate. They differentiate into memory B-lymphocytes or antibody-secreting plasma cells. During a new antigen (primary) exposure, a prolonged process of creating specific antibodies directed toward the antigenic challenge ensues; this process occurs during vaccination. When a previously primed memory B-lymphocyte is reexposed to an antigen, it is able to quickly produce specific antibodies (secondary response). As B-lymphocytes mature, the production of antibodies becomes increasingly sophisticated and higher affinity antibodies are created. Humoral immune deficiencies typically present with recurrent bacterial and viral respiratory infections, particularly those caused by encapsulated bacteria.

Combined B and T-lymphocyte deficiencies are particularly devastating, and predispose a host to all types of infections.

Mechanisms of Immunodeficiency

Children with prolonged profound neutropenia, as found in those receiving chemotherapy or those with aplastic anemia, are at high risk for invasive fungal infections. Children treated with chronic steroids are at risk for skin and mucosal barrier breakdown. Children with prolonged T-lymphocyte depletion as in solid organ transplant are at high risk for overwhelming viral infection. These examples of the varied risks posed to children with different immunodeficiencies illustrate the importance of understanding each model of immunosuppression in order to formulate a differential diagnosis and adequately target diagnostic and therapeutic efforts. Because of the morbidity and mortality associated with OIs, the fields of cancer therapy and transplant medicine are continuously evolving toward decreasing immunosuppressive therapy and providing appropriate antimicrobial prophylaxis either empirically or when indicated based on screening tests. The following sections present a brief overview of the common mechanisms of immune deficiency in children.

Pharmacologic Immunosuppression

Children with autoimmune disease, hematopoietic stem cell transplant, or solid-organ transplantation are frequently treated with immunosuppressive agents to reduce their immune response. Table 16.26 reviews the basic mechanisms of various immunosuppressive medications and the infection susceptibility they each confer. When evaluating the infectious risks of immunosuppressive therapy, special attention should be paid to the combination of agents and dosing. High-dose and multiagent therapy is associated with more frequent and severe infection. Of note, children with autoimmune diseases, even without iatrogenic immunosuppression, are at higher risk for infection (231).

Cancer/Neutropenia

Nearly all pediatric cancers are treated with myelosuppressive chemotherapy which constitutes a secondary immunodeficiency. Children undergoing treatment for leukemia and lymphoma undergo chemotherapy for up to 3 years with periods of profound, sometimes prolonged neutropenia and progressive lymphopenia as cumulative effects of bone marrow damage occur. Pediatric patients with solid tumors generally have less profound and prolonged neutropenia.

■ **Table 16.26**	Immunomodulatory and Immunosuppressive Medications, Mechanisms, and Susceptibility to Infection		
Class of Medication	**Immune Target**	**Example Drugs**	**Infection Susceptibility**
Steroids	⇓ Inflammatory cytokines/ chemokines ⇓ Circulating lymphocytes ⇓ Neutrophil trafficking ⇓ Immunoglobulin production Hyperglycemia	Hydrocortisone, dexamethasone, prednisone	Bacterial, mycobacterial, fungal (including PCP), *Nocardia*
Nucleotide inhibitors	Inhibition of DNA synthesis ⇓ Lymphocyte proliferation	Azathioprine 6-Mercaptopurine Mycophenolate mofetil	Herpesvirus (CMV)
Calcineurin inhibitors	⇓ T-lymphocyte activation ⇓ IL-2 and other cytokine production	Cyclosporine A Tacrolimus (FK506) Rapamycin (sirolimus, mTOR inhibitor)	Herpesvirus (CMV) Low rate of infection with cyclosporine
Alkylating agents	Cytotoxic ⇓ B and T-lymphocyte number/function	Cyclophosphamide (cytoxan)	Similar to steroids; herpesvirus, bacterial, fungal
Antimetabolite	Inhibits folic acid metabolism Cytotoxic ⇓ T-lymphocyte synthesis	Methotrexate	Fungal, herpesvirus, mycobacterial
Polyclonal antibody	Nonspecific T-lymphocyte depletion	Antilymphocyte globulin	Herpesvirus, *Polyomavirus*, fungal
Monoclonal antibody	Depletion of specific cell expressing antigenic target	Rituximab (anti-CD20) Alemtuzumab (anti-CD52) CD52 is present on most lymphocytes and some NK cells and neutrophils, immune depletion with anti-CD52 persists for months to years conferring a high risk of infection	Low risk of infection with rituximab; prolonged and high risk of opportunistic infection (herpesvirus, fungal, *Polyomavirus*, *Nocardia*, myco-bacteria) with alemtuzumab
Direct cytokine inhibitors		Anakinra (anti–IL-1 receptor) Etanercept, infliximab (anti–TNF-a)	Mycobacterial, bacterial (pneumococcal, *Listeria mono-cytogenes*)

Abbreviations: IL, interleukin; mTOR, mammalian target of rapamycin; NK, natural killer; PCP, *Pneumocystis carinii*; TNF-α, tumor necrosis factor α.
Source: Adapted from Refs. 231, 232, 233–235, 236, 237, 238.

Several other aspects of pediatric cancer care confer increased risk for invasive infection. Central venous catheters are frequently used for chemotherapy administration to protect against vesicant infusions and to enable easy vascular access for hydration, transfusion support, and frequent blood work. Central venous catheters have varying risks of infection: an implanted port that is unaccessed when not in use is a lower risk factor than a Hickman-Broviac tunneled line or a peripherally inserted central catheter (239,240). Disruption of the skin by central catheters predisposes the patient to infection with skin flora including coagulase-negative staphylococci and *S aureus*.

Chemotherapeutic agents have the unintended side effect of disrupting the gastrointestinal mucosa, allowing for translocation of mouth and intestinal flora into the blood stream. Even when controlling for neutropenia, mucositis is independently associated with a significantly increased incidence of infection. One large study reported documented infection in 58% of patients with mucositis (241). This pathophysiology accounts for many of the infections caused by *Candida* and Gram-negative bacteria in this population (242).

CNS infections occur in children with cancer when a bloodstream infection gains access to the intracranial space either by disruption of the BBB from inflammation or medical devices such as ventriculoperitoneal shunts. These shunts are placed temporarily and permanently in children with hydrocephalus caused by intracranial tumors.

Hematopoietic Stem Cell Transplant

Hematopoietic stem cell transplant (HSCT) refers to the process of eradicating a patient's immune system and then replacing it with either their own previously collected stem cells (autologous) or a donor's stem cells (allogeneic). Transplanted stem cells must then engraft and proliferate to reconstitute the immune system. The majority of morbidity and mortality in HSCT patients is caused by infectious complications (243), most often related to profound neutropenia, prolonged lymphopenia, immunosuppressive medications, graft-versus-host disease (GVHD), mucosal barrier disruption, and central venous catheters (243,244). HSCT may be indicated for patients with PI, bone marrow failure syndromes, and relapsed or refractory cancer; often this patient population has a history of OIs prior to HSCT.

The OIs that affect HSCT recipients change throughout the course of the transplantation process due to evolving immunosuppression of the recipient. The pre-engraftment period (lasting 4–6 weeks) includes conditioning (myeloablative chemotherapy) and the subsequent prolonged neutropenia that occurs prior to engraftment. The early postengraftment period (lasting 1–3 months) involves resolution of neutropenia, removal of the central catheter, and slow reconstitution of cell-mediated immunity. Cell-mediated immune recovery occurs more quickly in autologous transplant recipients than in allogeneic transplant recipients (244). The late postengraftment period begins 3 months after transplantation and is characterized by a lowered risk of infection but persistent cell-mediated and humoral immune defects. If no complications of HSCT interfere, immune recovery should be complete by 1 year posttransplant (Table 16.27).

GVHD occurs in allogeneic transplant recipients and is associated with several infectious risks. Specifically, GVHD causes dysregulation of cell-mediated immunity and inherent T-lymphocytes deficiency, it disrupts skin and/or mucosal barriers, and it requires the use of prolonged immunosuppressive therapy (243,244). Patients with GVHD are at particularly high and prolonged risk for OIs.

Solid Organ Transplant

The scope and survival of solid organ transplantation (SOT) has expanded and improved significantly since the onset of routine use of calcineurin inhibitors (cyclophosphamide, tacrolimus) (246). In the United States, solid organs transplanted include heart, lungs, combination heart and lungs, kidney, liver, small intestine, and pancreas. SOT, similar to HSCT, is a process that involves several different stages of infection risk. Infectious risk to the recipient begins with the donor organ, which may be from a cadaveric or live donor. Donor organs, and donors themselves, are routinely screened for syphilis, HIV, HTLV-1, CMV, hepatitis B virus, hepatitis C virus, and bacteremia. Donors are additionally screened for symptoms of pneumonia or encephalitis, as well as any regionally endemic infections, such as trypanosomiasis, *Strongyloides*, or WNV (247). Recipients are similarly screened for infections prior to undergoing transplant and immunosuppressive therapy (Table 16.28) (248).

In the immediate posttransplant period, recipients are at risk for surgical site infections, bacteremia associated with central venous catheters (CVC), and certain donor- and recipient-derived infections. One to 6 months following transplant, recipients are maximally iatrogenically immunosuppressed and at risk for reactivation of latent herpesvirus infections, *Pneumocystis carinii* and other fungal infections, respiratory viral infections, and opportunistic bacterial infections such as *Nocardia*. Six months and later following transplantation, recipients should be receiving less immunosuppression, although their immunosuppressive therapy will likely be lifelong. The late infectious complications of SOT include *P carinii* and mold, reactivatable herpesviruses, polyomaviruses, and EBV-associated posttransplant lymphoproliferative disorder (246).

The balance between risk of graft rejection and risk of infection is constantly being evaluated for SOT recipients. At certain times, even years following transplantation, recipients may experience an episode of graft rejection necessitating increased immunosuppressive therapy and therefore higher risk for infection.

HIV

HIV selectively infects and destroys CD4+ T-lymphocytes. Patients with HIV have varying levels

■ **Table 16.27** Time Periods of Infectious Risk in HSCT Recipients

Transplant phase	Time Period Following HSCT Initiation	Specific Immune Deficiencies	Infections	Common Prophylaxis
Pre-engraftment	4–6 weeks	Profound neutropenia, lymphopenia, CVC, mucosal barrier disruption	Bacteria (Gram-positive and Gram-negative), fungus (*Candida, Aspergillus*), HSV reactivation	Antibiotic (quinolones are common), acyclovir, antifungal (fluconazole, voriconazole, caspofungin)
Early postengraftment	1–3 months	Cell-mediated deficiency, GVHD	Bacteria, fungus (*Aspergillus*, PCP), CMV, EBV, BK virus, VZV	Trimethoprim-sulfa, antifungal (fluconazole, voriconazole), ganciclovir or foscarnet, acyclovir
Late postengraftment	3 months–1 year or end of immunosuppressive therapy (dependent on presence of GVHD)	Humoral immune deficiency, GVHD	Encapsulated bacteria, fungus (*Aspergillus, Pneumocystis carinii*), CMV, VZV, EBV, respiratory viruses	Acyclovir, trimethoprim-sulfa, vaccination

Abbreviations: CVC, central venous catheter; GVHD, graft-versus-host disease; HSCT, hematopoietic stem cell transplant.
Source: Adapted from Refs. 243–245.

of immunodeficiency based primarily on their CD4+ T-lymphocyte count; a CD4+ count less than 200 cells/mm^3 defines AIDS, and a CD4+ count less than 200 cells/mm^3 confers increased risk for OIs. Specific OI frequently encountered in HIV/AIDS include but are not limited to TB and atypical mycobacteria, cryptococcal meningitis and other disseminated fungal disease, parasitic disease, *Pneumocystis jiroveci*, herpesvirus infections, and *Polyomavirus* infections. Risk of infection decreases with immune reconstitution, most commonly achieved by starting combined antiretroviral therapy. Prophylactic antimicrobials should be administered in parallel with immune reconstitution. Immune reconstitution is imperative for patients who have infections for which there is no effective antibiosis available, such as PML (249) (see Slow Virus section). Initiation of antiretroviral therapy for patients with OIs may result in IRIS, a paradoxical inflammatory response resulting in worsened clinical symptoms of a previously recognized or unrecognized infection. The clinical symptoms of IRIS may be treated by NSAIDS or corticosteroids, but in severe cases IRIS is fatal (250).

Primary Immunodeficiency

Most PIs present in childhood with recurrent or severe infections, although some may not affect a given individual until later in life. PIs are rare, affecting approximately 1 in 10,000 people (251). The incidence is higher in children of consanguineous parents because most PIs are monogenic and inherited in an autosomal recessive pattern. PI may affect any compartment of the immune system and susceptibility to infection is determined by specific deficiencies.

X-Linked Agammaglobulinemia

X-linked agammaglobulinemia (XLA) was the first discovered inherited immunodeficiency. It is caused by a mutation in the Btk gene which results in deficient B-lymphocyte development and subsequent lack of immunoglobulin (252). Patients are at risk for infections with encapsulated bacteria and EVs (253). Given the nature of these organisms, patients with XLA are particularly at risk for encephalitis and meningitis.

■ **Table 16.28** Major Pathogens Transmitted by Donated Blood, Blood Products, and Tissue

Kidney, heart, liver, lung, bone marrow	CMV
Heart, kidney	Toxoplasmosis
Heart	*Trypanosoma cruzi*
Kidney, liver	HSV
Kidney	Human herpesvirus 8
Kidney, heart, liver	HIV, hepatitis B virus, hepatitis C virus, West Nile WNV
Kidney, liver, lung	Lymphocytic choriomeningitis virus, Old World *Arenavirus*
Kidney, liver, cornea	Rabies
Blood	CMV, Epstein-Barr virus, HIV, hepatitis B virus, hepatitis A virus, delta hepatitis virus, hepatitis C virus, human T-lymphotropic virus 1, WNV
Leukocytes	CMV, HIV

Source: Adapted from Mandell G, Bennett CL, Dolin R. Chapter 310: Risk factors and approaches to infections in transplant recipients. In: *Mandell, Douglas, and Bennett's Principles and Practice of Infectious Diseases.* Churchill Livingstone, an Imprint of Elsevier, Philadelphia, PA; 2009.

Chronic Granulomatous Disease

Chronic granulomatous disease (CGD) is caused by a mutation in one of the genes encoding a protein contained in the nicotinamide adenine dinucleotide phosphate (NADPH) oxidase complex necessary for functional killing by phagocytes. This results in a neutrophil function defect and predisposes patients to infection with one of several pathogens, including *S aureus, Burkholderia cepacia, Nocardia, Serratia marcescens,* mycobacteria, *Aspergillus,* and *Candida* (251, 254). Other pathogens may be responsible for disease in these patients, but are rare compared to those listed. CGD has a spectrum of immunodeficiency depending on the particular genetic defect (251).

Severe Combined Immunodeficiency

Severe combined immunodeficiency (SCID) encompasses a group of genetic mutations that result in severe deficiency of T-lymphocyte development and, to varying degrees, B-lymphocyte development. There are several phenotypes of SCID, the most critical of which results in complete lack of T- and B-lymphocytes (T-B-). T-B+ phenotype occurs when an adequate number of B-lymphocytes exist, but may not appropriately produce immunoglobulins due to lack of CD4+ T-lymphocyte costimulatory activity. Patients with SCID typically present with overwhelming mycobacterial and viral infections in infancy (251). SCID can be cured be HSCT early in life prior to acquisition of invasive infection and during active thymic development (255).

Other

Asplenia

Asplenia can be congenital, elective, or traumatic. Congenital asplenia occurs in patients with sickle cell anemia, congenital heart disease, and other genetic disorders. Splenectomy may be performed electively in hemolytic or immune-mediated hematologic diseases. The spleen normally functions to filter encapsulated bacteria (*H influenza, S pneumoniae, N meningitidis,* and others) out of the blood stream, and serves as a site for opsonization and IgM production. Without a functioning spleen, a child has a 3% to 5% increased risk for invasive bacterial infection (such as sepsis and meningitis) caused by encapsulated organisms (256); this risk is highest in the first 3 years following splenectomy, but remains elevated throughout a child's lifetime. Individuals with asplenia should receive penicillin prophylaxis for at least the first 3 years following splenectomy, and should be fully vaccinated (257).

Malnutrition

Protein is required for development and activation of all arms of the immune response, cell regeneration, and

■ **Table 16.29** Bacterial Pathogens Affecting Immunocompromised Individuals

Bacteria	Risk Group	Risk Factors	Treatment	Diagnosis	Clinical Notes
Gram-negative bacteria	Cancer, HSCT, PID, asplenia, malnutrition	Neutropenia, CVC, mucositis, GVHD	Empiric treatment with third or fourth generation cephalosporin, carbapenem, or quinolone. Definitive therapy is targeted to specific organism.	Blood and CSF cultures.	
Pneumococcus	HSCT, asplenia	Poor opsonization (late HSCT with GVHD)	Empiric vancomycin and third generation cephalosporin. Definitive therapy is targeted to susceptibility testing.	Blood and CSF cultures.	
Coagulase-negative *Staphylococcus* and *Staphylococcus aureus*	Brain tumors, PID	CVC, ventriculoperitoneal shunt	Vancomycin (intravenous and intrathecal).	CSF/VP shunt cultures.	
Viridans-group *streptococcus*	HSCT	Mucositis, poor dentition	Empiric vancomycin	Blood and CSF cultures.	High mortality in early HSCT
Tuberculosis	PID, HIV, SOT, HSCT, malnutrition	T-lymphocyte deficiency	Multidrug regimen based on organism susceptibility. Traditional 4 drug induction therapy includes INH, rifampin, pyrazinamide, ethambutol. Steroids for meningitis.	Brain imaging, PPD.	
Legionella	HSCT	Water exposure	Prolonged antibiotics (quinolone), until immune reconstitution.	Brain imaging, serum serologic testing, urine antigen.	Pulmonary nodules and pneumonitis, cerebellar lesions, meningoencephalitis.

(continued)

■ **Table 16.29** Bacterial Pathogens Affecting Immunocompromised Individuals (*continued*)

Bacteria	Risk Group	Risk Factors	Treatment	Diagnosis	Clinical Notes
Nocardiosis	HSCT, HIV, PID, SOT, malnutrition, immunosuppressive therapy	T lymphocyte deficiency. Plants and soil.	Prolonged antibiotics (TMP-sulfa, carbapenem) until immune reconstitution; abscess drainage.	Abscess drainage and culture.	Brain abscess, may also have skin and pulmonary lesions.

Abbreviations: : INH, isoniazid; PID, primary immunodeficiency; PPD, purified protein derivative; SOT, solid organ transplantation; VP, ventriculoperitoneal.
Source: Adapted from Refs. 96, 250, 263–265.

■ **Table 16.30** Viral Pathogens Affecting in Immunocompromised Hosts

Virus	Risk Group	Diagnosis	Treatment	Clinical Notes
CMV	HIV, HSCT, SOT, immunosuppressive therapy	Quantitative CMV PCR of CSF and blood.	Ganciclovir. Foscarnet is second line. Immune reconstitution.	CMV encephalitis is most common clinical manifestation, but CMV also causes meningitis, radiculopathy, and other CNS symptoms
VZV	HIV, HSCT, cancer, SOT, immunosuppressive therapy	VZV PCR of CSF and blood.	Acyclovir, decrease immunosuppression.	CNS manifestations: meningitis, encephalitis; other manifestations: rash, pneumonia.
EBV	HSCT, SOT	EBV PCR of blood and CSF.	Rituximab for patients with high viral load or PTLD.	Associated with posttransplant lymphoproliferative disorder.
Polyomaviruses (JC and BK)	HIV, SOT, cancer, HSCT, PID	BK virus PCR from urine, blood, and CSF or brain biopsy. JCV PCR from CSF low yield, brain biopsy PCR and histopathology higher yield. MRI with white matter changes.	Immune reconstitution	BK virus CNS manifestations: meningoencephalitis; other manifestations: hemorrhagic cystitis, renal graft rejection. JCV CNS manifestations: progressive multifocal leukoencephalopathy (demyelinating disease).
HHV6	HSCT, HIV, SOT	HHV6 PCR from CSF and blood.	No definitive benefit to antiviral therapy. Ganciclovir and foscarnet have been used.	Encephalitis, rash, hepatitis.
LCMV	SOT	Serologic testing of blood and CSF. PCR less widely available.	Supportive. Efficacy of ribavirin exists in vitro but not proven in vivo.	Encephalitis. Transmitted by rodents.
WNV	SOT	WNV PCR of CSF and blood.	Supportive. Efficacy of ribavirin exists in vitro but not proven in vivo.	Transmitted by mosquitoes.

Abbreviations: PTLD, post-transplant lymphoproliferative disorder; JCV, JC virus.
Source: Adapted from Refs. 169, 249, 266–273.

■ **Table 16.31**	Fungal Pathogens Affecting Immunocompromised Hosts			
Fungus	**Risk Group**	**Diagnosis**	**Treatment**	**Clinical Notes**
Cryptococcus	Immunosuppressive therapy, cancer, HIV, SOT, PID	Latex agglutination for cryptococcal antigen and fungal culture, CSF and blood.	Immune reconstitution. Induction: amphotericin[a] + flucytosine or fluconazole for at least 2 weeks. Maintenance: fluconazole (duration to be determined in consultation with infectious diseases specialist). Treatment should be monitored by serial CSF evaluations.	
Candida	Immunosuppressive therapy, cancer, HSCT, HIV, PID	Fungal culture of blood and CSF. Radiographic imaging of CNS and other organs.	Immune reconstitution. Consider donor granulocyte transfusion in neutropenic patients. Amphotericin[a] + fluconazole or flucytosine. Treatment should be monitored by serial CSF evaluations.	Meningoencephalitis, parenchymal brain lesions. May be widely disseminated to other visceral organs and retinas.
Aspergillus	Immunosuppressive therapy, HSCT, HIV	CSF fungal culture is low yield. Radiographic imaging of CNS. Galactomannan antigen from blood.	Immune reconstitution. Consider donor granulocyte transfusion in neutropenic patients. First line antifungal therapy is voriconazole. Amphotericin[a] is second line.	Very high mortality.
Zygomycetes	HSCT, cancer	CSF fungal culture is low yield. Biopsy of lesion. Radiographic imaging of sinuses and CNS.	Immune reconstitution. Consider donor granulocyte transfusion in neutropenic patients. Amphotericin[a] Surgical resection of lesion.	Higher risk of disease in hyperglycemic patients. Very high mortality.

[a] Amphotericin or liposomal formulation. Ambisome has superior CNS penetration.
Source: Adapted from Refs. 246, 274–279.

■ **Table 16.32**	Other Opportunistic Infections Affecting Immunocompromised Patients				
Pathogen	**Risk Group**	**Risk Factors**	**Diagnosis**	**Treatment**	**Clinical Notes**
Trypanosoma cruzi (Chagas disease)	Heart transplant, HIV	Multiple mammalian reservoirs, triatomine bug vector. Endemic in Mexico, Central and South America.	Direct identification of trypomastigotes in stained CSF or blood smears. Histopathology of biopsy specimens. Characteristic ring-enhancing lesions on brain radiography (undistinguishable from those of toxoplasmosis).	Benznidazole, nifurtimox. Allopurinol is second line.	CNS manifestations only occur in immunocompromised hosts.
Strongyloides stercoralis	HIV, malnutrition, immunosuppressive therapy, SOT, cancer	Corticosteroid therapy.	Protozoal evaluation of CSF demonstrating filariform larvae. Peripheral blood serology.	Thiabendazole, ivermectin. Immune reconstitution, specifically discontinuation of corticosteroid therapy.	Often comorbid with Gram-negative bacteremia and meningitis.
Toxoplasma gondii (toxoplasmosis)	HSCT, HIV, SOT	Cat feces exposure	Protozoal evaluation of CSF demonstrating tachyzoites. *Toxoplasma* antigen detection (ELISA) in blood and CSF. *Toxoplasma* PCR from CSF, blood, biopsy specimen. Histopathology of brain biopsy. Characteristic ring-enhancing lesions on brain radiography.	Pyrimethamine + sulfadiazine, or atovaquone. Immune reconstitution.	Encephalitis, focal cerebral lesions

Abbreviation: ELISA, enzyme-linked immunosorbent assay.
See Encephalitis and Myelitis section for list of amebic infections.
Source: Adapted from Refs. 246, 247, 280–284.

health of mucosal barriers. In addition, nutrients such as zinc and vitamin D are essential for immune function (258,259). Children with protein malnutrition are at risk for bacterial infection with Gram-negative organisms due to poor integrity of intestinal mucosa, and Gram-positive organisms due to weakened skin barriers. The rate of sepsis has been reported as 15% to 60% in children with acute, severe malnutrition (260). These children are routinely treated with empiric broad-spectrum antibiotics (261). Malaria, intestinal parasites, and nosocomial infections also pose significant infectious disease problems in this population (262).

An overview of specific bacterial, viral, fungal, and other pathogens affecting the immunocompromised host is presented in Tables 16.29 to 16.32.

■ CONCLUSIONS

In conclusion, infections of the pediatric CNS are a diverse set of disorders affecting the brain and spinal cord with heterogeneous clinical presentations, diagnostic criteria, therapies, and prognoses. Most children with CNS infections will require intensive care monitoring and treatment at some point during their course. This chapter aims to provide a framework for consideration of the appropriate initial evaluation and management of selected CNS infections.

■ ACKNOWLEDGMENTS

We thank Samir S. Shah, MD, MSCE (Cincinnati Children's Hospital Medical Center) and Daniel J. Licht (the Children's Hospital of Philadelphia, Division of Neurology) for reading and editing drafts of this chapter.

■ REFERENCES

1. Addy DP. When not to do a lumbar puncture. *Arch Dis Child*. 1987;62:873–875.
2. Tunkel AR et al. Practice guidelines for the management of bacterial meningitis. *Clin Infect Dis*. 2004;39:1267–1284.
3. Adler MD, Comi AE, Walker AR. Acute hemorrhagic complication of diagnostic lumbar puncture. *Pediatr Emerg Care*. 2001;17:184–188.
4. Edelson RN, Chernik NL, Posner JB. Spinal subdural hematomas complicating lumbar puncture. *Arch Neurol*. 1974;31:134–137.
5. Fleisher GR, Ludwig S, ed. Textbook of Pediatric Emergency Medicine. Philadelphia, PA: Lippincott, Williams, and Wilkins; 2000.
6. Straus SE, Thorpe KE, Holroyd-Leduc J. How do I perform a lumbar puncture and analyze the results to diagnose bacterial meningitis? *JAMA*. 2006;296:2012–2022.
7. Abo A et al. Positioning for lumbar puncture in children evaluated by bedside ultrasound. *Pediatrics*. 2010;125:e1149–e1153.
8. Nigrovic LE, Kuppermann N, Neuman MI. Risk factors for traumatic or unsuccessful lumbar punctures in children. *Ann Emerg Med*. 2007;49:762–771.
9. Boon JM et al. Lumbar puncture: Anatomical review of a clinical skill. *Clin Anat*. 2004;17:544–553.
10. Avery RA et al. Patient position during lumbar puncture has no meaningful effect on cerebrospinal fluid opening pressure in children. *J Child Neurol*. 2010;25:616–619.
11. Whiteley W et al. CSF opening pressure: reference interval and the effect of body mass index. *Neurology*. 2006;67:1690–1691.
12. Avery RA et al. Reference range for cerebrospinal fluid opening pressure in children. *N Engl J Med*. 2010;363:891–893.
13. Strupp M, Brandt T, Müller A. Incidence of post-lumbar puncture syndrome reduced by reinserting the stylet: a randomized prospective study of 600 patients. *J Neurol*. 1998;245:589–592.
14. Flaatten H, Kråkenes J, Vedeler C. Post-dural puncture related complications after diagnostic lumbar puncture, myelography and spinal anaesthesia. *Acta Neurol Scand*. 1998;98:445–451.
15. Scheld WM, Whitley RJ, Durack DT. *Infections of the Central Nervous System*. 2nd ed. Philadelphia, PA: Lippincott-Raven; 1997.
16. Vermeulen M, van Gijn J. The diagnosis of subarachnoid haemorrhage. *J Neurol Neurosurg Psychiatry*. 1990;53:365–372.
17. Ahmed A et al. Cerebrospinal fluid values in the term neonate. *Pediatr Infect Dis J*. 1996;15:298–303.
18. Kestenbaum LA et al. Defining cerebrospinal fluid white blood cell count reference values in neonates and young infants. *Pediatrics*. 2010;125:257–264.
19. Conly JM, Ronald AR. Cerebrospinal fluid as a diagnostic body fluid. *Am J Med*. 1983;75:102–108.
20. Hines EM et al. Adjustment of cerebrospinal fluid protein for red blood cells in neonates and young infants. *J Hosp Med*. 2012;7:325–328.
21. Johnson KS, Sexton DJ. Cerebrospinal fluid: physiology and utility of an examination in disease states. In: Thorner AR, ed. *UpToDate*; 2010.
22. Fishman RA. Studies of the transport of sugars between blood and cerebrospinal fluid in normal states and in meningeal carcinomatosis. *Trans Am Neurol Assoc*. 1963;88:114–118.
23. Nigrovic LE et al. Relationship between cerebrospinal fluid glucose and serum glucose. *N Engl J Med*. 2012;366:576–578.
24. Spanos A, Harrell FE, Durack DT. Differential diagnosis of acute meningitis. An analysis of the predictive value of initial observations. *JAMA*. 1989;262:2700–2707.
25. Byington CL, Kendrick J, Sheng X. Normative cerebrospinal fluid profiles in febrile infants. *J Pediatr*. 2011;158:130–134.
26. Shah SS et al. Age-specific reference values for cerebrospinal fluid protein concentration in neonates and young infants. *J Hosp Med*. 2011;6:22–27.
27. Chávez-Bueno S, McCracken GH. Bacterial meningitis in children. *Pediatr Clin North Am*. 2005;52:795–810, vii.
28. DeBiasi RL, Tyler KL. Viral Meningitis and Encephalitis. *CONTINUUM Lifelong Learning Neurol*. 2006;12:58–94.
29. Bamberger DM. Diagnosis, initial management, and prevention of Meningitis. *Am Fam Physician*. 2010;82:1491–1498.
30. Kim KS. Neurological diseases: pathogenesis of bacterial meningitis: from bacteraemia to neuronal injury. *Nat Rev Neurosci*. 2003;4:376–385.
31. Nigrovic LE, Kuppermann N, Malley R. Children with bacterial meningitis presenting to the emergency department during the pneumococcal conjugate vaccine era. *Acad Emerg Med*. 2008;15:522–528.
32. Dubos F et al. Clinical decision rules for evaluating meningitis in children. *Curr Opin Neurol*. 2009;22:288–293.
33. Brouwer MC et al. Corticosteroids for acute bacterial meningitis. *Cochrane Database Syst Rev*. 2010:CD004405.
34. Carlson RW, Gehab MA, ed. Principles and Practice of Medical Intensive Care. Philadelphia, PA: Saunders; 1993: 454–466.
35. Sande MA, Smith AL, Root RK, ed. Bacterial Meningitis (Contemporary Issues in Infectious Disease Vol 3). New York, NY: Churchill Livingstone; 1985:37.

36. Roos KL. Meningitis and encephalitis. Paper presented at: American Academy of Neurology Annual Meeting; April 2010; Toronto, Canada.

37. Valmari P et al. Childhood bacterial meningitis: initial symptoms and signs related to age, and reasons for consulting a physician. *Eur J Pediatr.* 1987;146:515–518.

38. Gururaj VJ et al. To tap or not to tap. What are the best indicators for performing a lumbar puncture in an outpatient child? *Clin Pediatr (Phila).* 1973;12:488–493.

39. Green SM et al. Can seizures be the sole manifestation of meningitis in febrile children? *Pediatrics.* 1993;92:527–534.

40. Kimia AA et al. Utility of lumbar puncture for first simple febrile seizure among children 6 to 18 months of age. *Pediatrics.* 2009;123:6–12.

41. Klein JO, Feigin RD, McCracken GH. Report of the Task Force on Diagnosis and Management of Meningitis. *Pediatrics.* 1986;78:959–982.

42. Bonadio WA et al. Distinguishing cerebrospinal fluid abnormalities in children with bacterial meningitis and traumatic lumbar puncture. *J Infect Dis.* 1990;162:251–254.

43. Feigin RD, McCracken GH, Klein JO. Diagnosis and management of meningitis. *Pediatr Infect Dis J.* 1992;11:785–814.

44. Nichols DG, ed. Textbook of Pediatric Intensive Care, 4th ed. Baltimore, MD: Lippincott, Williams, and Wilkins; 2008.

45. Neuman MI, Tolford S, Harper MB. Test Gram stain in children. *Pediatr Infect Dis J.* 2008;27:309–313.

46. Brizzi K et al. Diagnostic accuracy of cerebrospinal fluid gram stain in children with suspected bacterial meningitis. *Pediatr Infect Dis J.* 2012;31:195–197.

47. Nigrovic LE et al. Clinical prediction rule for identifying children with cerebrospinal fluid pleocytosis at very low risk of bacterial meningitis. *JAMA.* 2007;297:52–60.

48. Chandran A et al. Long-term sequelae of childhood bacterial meningitis. *Pediatr Infect Dis J.* 2011;30:3–6.

49. Baraff LJ, Lee SI, Schriger DL. Outcomes of bacterial meningitis in children: a meta-analysis. *Pediatr Infect Dis J.* 1993;12:389–394.

50. Pomeroy SL et al. Seizures and other neurologic sequelae of bacterial meningitis in children. *N Engl J Med.* 1990;323:1651–1657.

51. Koomen I et al. Hearing loss at school age in survivors of bacterial meningitis: assessment, incidence, and prediction. *Pediatrics.* 2003;112:1049–1053.

52. Kanegaye JT, Soliemanzadeh P, Bradley JS. Lumbar puncture in pediatric bacterial meningitis: defining the time interval for recovery of cerebrospinal fluid pathogens after parenteral antibiotic pretreatment. *Pediatrics.* 2001;108:1169–1174.

53. Nigrovic LE et al. Effect of antibiotic pretreatment on cerebrospinal fluid profiles of children with bacterial meningitis. *Pediatrics.* 2008;122:726–730.

54. Girgis NI et al. Dexamethasone treatment for bacterial meningitis in children and adults. *Pediatr Infect Dis J.* 1989;8:848–851.

55. Mongelluzzo J et al. Corticosteroids and mortality in children with bacterial meningitis. *JAMA.* 2008;299:2048–2055.

56. Peltola H et al. Adjuvant glycerol and/or dexamethasone to improve the outcomes of childhood bacterial meningitis: a prospective, randomized, double-blind, placebo-controlled trial. *Clin Infect Dis.* 2007;45:1277–1286.

57. Tan TQ. Chronic meningitis. *Semin Pediatr Infect Dis.* 2003;14:131–139.

58. Davis LE. Subacute and chronic meningitis. *CONTINUUM Lifelong Learning Neurol.* 2006;12:27–57.

59. Ginsberg L, Kidd D. Chronic and recurrent meningitis. *Pract Neurol.* 2008;8:348–361.

60. Ellner JJ, Bennett JE. Chronic meningitis. *Medicine.* 1976;55:341–369.

61. Hildebrand J, Aoun M. Chronic meningitis: still a diagnostic challenge. *J Neurol.* 2003;250:653–660.

62. Tuygun N, Tanir G, Aytekin C. Recurrent bacterial meningitis in children: our experience with 14 cases. *Turk J Pediatr.* 2010;52:348–353.

63. Cho TA, Venna N. Management of acute, recurrent, and chronic meningitides in adults. *Neurol Clin.* 2010;28:1061–1088.

64. Calfee DP, Wispelwey B. Brain abscess. *Semin Neurol.* 2000;20:353–360.

65. Canale DJ. William Macewen and the treatment of brain abscesses: revisited after one hundred years. *J Neurosurg.* 1996;84:133–142.

66. Frazier JL, Ahn ES, Jallo GI. Management of brain abscesses in children. *Neurosurg Focus.* 2008;24:E8.

67. Mathisen GE, Johnson JP. Brain abscess. *Clin Infect Dis.* 1997;25:763–779; quiz 780–761.

68. Brook I. Microbiology and antimicrobial treatment of orbital and intracranial complications of sinusitis in children and their management. *Int J Pediatr Otorhinolaryngol.* 2009;73:1183–1186.

69. Foy P, Sharr M. Cerebral abscesses in children after pencil-tip injuries. *Lancet.* 1980;2:662–663.

70. Tay JS, Garland JS. Serious head injuries from lawn darts. *Pediatrics.* 1987;79:261–263.

71. Mandell G, Bennett JE, Dolin R. Chapter 88: Brain abscess. In: *Mandell, Douglas, and Bennett's Principles and Practice of Infectious Diseases.* 7th ed. Philadelphia, PA: Churchill Livingstone, an Imprint of Elsevier; 2009.

72. Seydoux C, Francioli P. Bacterial brain abscesses: factors influencing mortality and sequelae. *Clin Infect Dis.* 1992;15:394–401.

73. Carpenter J, Stapleton S, Holliman R. Retrospective analysis of 49 cases of brain abscess and review of the literature. *Eur J Clin Microbiol Infect Dis.* 2007;26:1–11.

74. Quartey GR, Johnston JA, Rozdilsky B. Decadron in the treatment of cerebral abscess. An experimental study. *J Neurosurg.* 1976;45:301–310.

75. Venkatesh MS et al. Pediatric infratentorial subdural empyema: analysis of 14 cases. *J Neurosurg.* 2006;105:370–377.

76. Gupta S et al. Neurosurgical management of extraaxial central nervous system infections in children. *J Neurosurg Pediatr.* 2011;7:441–451.

77. Dill SR, Cobbs CG, McDonald CK. Subdural empyema: analysis of 32 cases and review. *Clin Infect Dis.* 1995;20:372–386.

78. Osborn MK, Steinberg JP. Subdural empyema and other suppurative complications of paranasal sinusitis. *Lancet Infect Dis.* 2007;7:62–67.

79. Leotta N, Chaseling R, Duncan G, Isaacs D. Intracranial suppuration. *J Paediatr Child Health.* 2005;41:508–512.

80. Bockova J, Rigamonti D. Intracranial empyema. *Pediatr Infect Dis J.* 2000;19:735–737.

81. Adame N, Hedlund G, Byington CL. Sinogenic intracranial empyema in children. *Pediatrics.* 2005;116:e461–e467.

82. Banerjee AD et al. Pediatric supratentorial subdural empyemas: a retrospective analysis of 65 cases. *Pediatr Neurosurg.* 2009;45:11–18.

83. Legrand M et al. Paediatric intracranial empyema: differences according to age. *Eur J Pediatr.* 2009;168:1235–1241.

84. Pradilla G et al. Epidural abscesses of the CNS. *Lancet Neurol.* 2009;8:292–300.

85. DeMuri GP, Wald ER. Complications of acute bacterial sinusitis in children. *Pediatr Infect Dis J.* 2011;30:701–702.

86. Ziai WC, Lewin JJ. Advances in the management of central nervous system infections in the ICU. *Crit Care Clin.* 2006;22:661–694; abstract viii–ix.

87. Tasher D et al. Cat scratch disease with cervical vertebral osteomyelitis and spinal epidural abscess. *Pediatr Infect Dis J.* 2009;28:848–850.

88. Lemierre A. On certain septicaemias due to anaerobic organisms. *Lancet.* 1936;1:701–703.

89. Chirinos JA et al. The evolution of Lemierre syndrome: report of 2 cases and review of the literature. *Medicine (Baltimore).* 2002;81:458–465.

90. Hagelskjaer LH et al. Incidence and clinical epidemiology of necrobacillosis, including Lemierre's syndrome, in Denmark 1990–1995. *Eur J Clin Microbiol Infect Dis.* 1998;17:561–565.

91. Vargiami EG, Zafeiriou DI. Eponym: the Lemierre syndrome. *Eur J Pediatr.* 2010;169:411–414.

92. Hagelskjaer Kristensen L, Prag J. Human necrobacillosis, with emphasis on Lemierre's syndrome. *Clin Infect Dis.* 2000;31:524–532.

93. Laupland KB. Vascular and parameningeal infections of the head and neck. *Infect Dis Clin North Am.* 2007;21:577–590, viii.

94. Sell B, Evans J, Horn D. Brain abscess and hereditary hemorrhagic telangiectasia. *South Med J.* 2008;101:618–625.

95. Kennedy KJ et al. A cluster of nocardial brain abscesses. *Surg Neurol.* 2007;68:43–49; discussion 49.

96. Lin Y-J et al. Nocardial brain abscess. *J Clin Neurosci.* 2010;17:250–253.

97. Panichpisal K, Nugent K, Sarria JC. Central nervous system pseudallescheriasis after near-drowning. *Clin Neurol Neurosurg.* 2006;108:348–352.

98. Doran TI. The role of *Citrobacter* in clinical disease of children: review. *Clin Infect Dis.* 1999;28:384–394.

99. Eckburg PB, Montoya JG, Vosti KL. Brain abscess due to *Listeria monocytogenes*: five cases and a review of the literature. *Medicine (Baltimore).* 2001;80:223–235.

100. Sánchez-Portocarrero J. The central nervous system and infection by *Candida* species. *Diagn Microbiol Infect Dis.* 2000;37:169–179.

101. Long SS, Pickering LK, Prober CG. Chapter 134: *Mycobacterium tuberculosis.* In: *Principles and Practice of Pediatric Infectious Disease.* 3rd ed. New York, NY: Churchill Livingstone, an Imprint of Elsevier; 2009.

102. Thwaites GE, Tran TH. Tuberculous meningitis: many questions, too few answers. *Lancet Neurol.* 2005;4: 160–170.

103. Organization WH. Health topics: tuberculosis. World Health Organization Web site. http://www.who.int/topics/tuberculosis/en/.

104. Berger JR. Tuberculous meningitis. *Curr Opin Neurol.* 1994;7:191–200.

105. Farinha NJ et al. Tuberculosis of the central nervous system in children: a 20-year survey. *J Infect.* 2000;41:61–68.

106. Council MR. Streptomycin treatment of tuberculous meningitis: report of the committee on Streptomycin in Tuberculosis Trials. *Lancet.* 1948;1:582–597.

107. Sinner SW. Approach to the diagnosis and management of tuberculous meningitis. *Curr Infect Dis Rep.* 2010;12:291–298.

108. Mahadevan B et al. Tuberculin reactivity in tuberculous meningitis. *Indian J Pediatr.* 2005;72:213–215.

109. Kilpatrick ME, Girgis NI, Tribble D, Farid Z. The value of the tuberculin skin test in patients with tuberculous meningitis. *J Egypt Public Health Assoc.* 1996;71:1–8.

110. Sleiman R, Al-Tannir M, Dakdouki G. Interpretation of the tuberculin skin test in bacilli Calmette-Guerin vaccinated and nonvaccinated school children. *Pediatr Infect Dis J.* 2007;26:134–138.

111. Menzies D. What does tuberculin reactivity after bacilli Calmette-Guerin vaccination tell us? *Clin Infect Dis.* 2000;31:S71–S74.

112. Garg RK. Tuberculous meningitis. *Acta Neurol Scand.* 2010;122:75–90.

113. Mandell G, Bennett JE, Dolin R. Chapter 250: *Mycobacterium tuberculosis.* In: *Mandell, Douglas, and Bennett's Principles and Practice of Infectious Diseases.* 7th ed. Philadelphia, PA: Churchill Livingstone, an Imprint of Elsevier; 2009.

114. van Well GTJ et al. Twenty years of pediatric tuberculous meningitis: a retrospective cohort study in the western cape of South Africa. *Pediatrics.* 2009;123:e1–8.

115. Verhagen LM et al, Hermans PWM. Human immunodeficiency virus and tuberculosis coinfection in children: challenges in diagnosis and treatment. *Pediatr Infect Dis J.* 2010;29:e63–70.

116. Schutte CM. Clinical, cerebrospinal fluid and pathological findings and outcomes in HIV-positive and HIV-negative patients with tuberculous meningitis. *Infection.* 2001;29:213–217.

117. Satishchandra P, Sinha S. Seizures in HIV-seropositive individuals: NIMHANS experience and review. *Epilepsia.* 2008;49 Suppl 6:33–41.

118. Zein TM, Fletcher PS, Mirghani ZM. Intracranial tuberculoma. *Saudi Med J.* 2000;21:196–199.

119. Gardam M, Lim S. Mycobacterial osteomyelitis and arthritis. *Infect Dis Clin North Am.* 2005;19:819–830.

120. Puthezhath K, Zacharia B, Mathew TP. Gluteal abscess: diagnostic challenges and management. *J Infect Dev Ctries.* 2010;4:345–348.

121. Vilar FC et al. [Spinal tuberculosis (Pott's disease) associated to psoas abscess: report of two cases and a literature review]. *Rev Soc Bras Med Trop.* 2006;39:278–282.

122. Mizumura K et al. Tuberculous retropharyngeal abscess associated with spinal tuberculosis well controlled by fine-needle aspiration and anti-tuberculous chemotherapy. *Intern Med.* 2010;49:1155–1158.

123. Benzagmout M et al. Pott's disease in children. *Surg Neurol Int.* 2011;2:1.

124. Organization WH. The use of rapid syphilis tests. World Health Organization Web site. http://www.who.int/std_diagnostics/publications/manuals. Accessed May 16.

125. Sung L, MacDonald NE. Syphilis: a pediatric perspective. *Pediatr Rev.* 1998;19:17–22.

126. Ghanem KG. Review: neurosyphilis: a historical perspective and review. *CNS Neurosci Ther.* 2010;16:e157–e168.

127. Mandell G, Bennett JE, Dolin R. Chapter 238: *Treponema pallidum*. In: *Mandell, Douglas, and Bennett's Principles and Practice of Infectious Diseases*. 7th ed. Philadelphia, PA: Churchill Livingstone, an Imprint of Elsevier; 2009.
128. Darville T. Syphilis. *Pediatr Rev*. 1999;20:160–164; quiz 165.
129. Hotson JR. Modern neurosyphilis: a partially treated chronic meningitis. *West J Med*. 1981;135:191–200.
130. Marra CM. Neurosyphilis. *Curr Neurol Neurosci Rep*. 2004;4:435–440.
131. Bonthius DJ, Karacay B. Meningitis and encephalitis in children. An update. *Neurol Clin*. 2002;20:1013–1038, vi–vii.
132. Lewis P, Glaser CA. Encephalitis. *Pediatr Rev*. 2005;26:353–363.
133. Tunkel Allan R et al. The management of encephalitis: clinical practice guidelines by the Infectious Diseases Society of America. *Clin Infect Dis*. 2008;47:303–327.
134. Galanakis E et al. A prospective multicenter study of childhood encephalitis in Greece. *Pediatr Infect Dis J*. 2009;28:740–742.
135. Koskiniemi M et al. Epidemiology of encephalitis in children. A prospective multicentre study. *Eur J Pediatr*. 1997;156:541–545.
136. Granerod J et al. Challenge of the unknown. A systematic review of acute encephalitis in non-outbreak situations. *Neurology*. 2010;75:924–932.
137. Glaser CA et al. Beyond viruses: clinical profiles and etiologies associated with encephalitis. *Clin Infect Dis*. 2006;43:1565–1577.
138. Mailles A, Stahl J-P, Group SCaI. Infectious encephalitis in France in 2007: a national prospective study. *Clin Infect Dis*. 2009;49:1838–1847.
139. Jeha LE et al. West Nile virus infection: a new acute paralytic illness. *Neurology*. 2003;61:55–59.
140. Tyler KL. Emerging viral infections of the central nervous system: part 1. *Arch Neurol*. 2009;66:939–948.
141. Glaser C, Christie L, Bloch KC. Rickettsial and ehrlichial infections. *Handb Clin Neurol*. 2010;96:143–158.
142. Bravo FG, Alvarez PJ, Gotuzzo E. Balamuthia mandrillaris infection of the skin and central nervous system: an emerging disease of concern to many specialties in medicine. *Curr Opin Infect Dis*. 2011;24:112–117.
143. Visvesvara GS. Amebic meningoencephalitides and keratitis: challenges in diagnosis and treatment. *Curr Opin Infect Dis*. 2010;23:590–594.
144. Kimberlin DW. Herpes simplex virus infections in neonates and early childhood. *Semin Pediatr Infect Dis*. 2005;16:271–281.
145. Brunette GW et al, eds. *The Yellow Book 2012*. New York, NY: Oxford University Press; 2012.
146. Bloch KC, Glaser C. Diagnostic approaches for patients with suspected encephalitis. *Curr Infect Dis Rep*. 2007;9:315–322.
147. Granerod J, Crowcroft NS. The epidemiology of acute encephalitis. *Neuropsychol Rehabil*. 2007;17:406–428.
148. Hollidge BS, González-Scarano F, Soldan SS. Arboviral encephalitides: transmission, emergence, and pathogenesis. *J Neuroimmune Pharmacol*. 2010;5:428–442.
149. Fowler A et al. Childhood encephalitis in Sweden: etiology, clinical presentation and outcome. *Eur J Paediatr Neurol*. 2008;12:484–490.
150. Kolski H et al. Etiology of acute childhood encephalitis at the Hospital for Sick Children, Toronto, 1994–1995. *Clin Infect Dis*. 1998;26:398–409.
151. Steiner I et al. Viral encephalitis: a review of diagnostic methods and guidelines for management. *Eur J Neurol*. 2005;12:331–343.
152. Kamei S. Evaluation of combination therapy using aciclovir and corticosteroid in adult patients with herpes simplex virus encephalitis. *J Neurol Neurosurg Psychiatry*. 2005;76:1544–1549.
153. Nakano A et al. Beneficial effect of steroid pulse therapy on acute viral encephalitis. *Eur Neurol*. 2003;50:225–229.
154. Färkkilä M, Tiainen T, Koskiniemi M. Epidemiology and prognosis of acute myelitis in Southern Finland. *J Neurol Sci*. 1997;152:140–146.
155. Kincaid O, Lipton HL. Viral myelitis: an update. *Curr Neurol Neurosci Rep*. 2006;6:469–474.
156. Solomon T, Willison H. Infectious causes of acute flaccid paralysis. *Curr Opin Infect Dis*. 2003;16:375–381.
157. Chen CY et al. Acute flaccid paralysis in infants and young children with enterovirus 71 infection: MR imaging findings and clinical correlates. *AJNR Am J Neuroradiol*. 2001;22:200–205.
158. Sigurdsson B. Observations on three slow infections of sheep. I. Maedi, slow progressive pneumonia of sheep: epizoological and pathological study. II. Paratuberculous (Johne's disease) of sheep in Iceland: immunological studies and observations on its mode of spread. III. Rida, chronic encephalitis of sheep, with general remarks on infections which develop slowly and some of their special characteristics. *Brit Vet J*. 1954;110:225–270, 307–322, 341–354.
159. Gilden DH. Slow virus diseases of the CNS. 1. Subacute sclerosing panencephalitis, progressive rubella panencephalitis, and progressive multifocal leukoencephalopathy. *Postgrad Med*. 1983;73:99–101, 104–108.
160. Gajdusek DC. Slow-virus infections of the nervous system. *N Engl J Med*. 1967;276:392–400.
161. Johnson RT. Slow infections of the central nervous system caused by conventional viruses. *Ann N Y Acad Sci*. 1994;724:6–13.
162. Boothpur R, Brennan DC. Human polyoma viruses and disease with emphasis on clinical BK and JC. *J Clin Virol*. 2010;47:306–312.
163. Weber T. Progressive multifocal leukoencephalopathy. *Neurol Clin*. 2008;26:833–854, x–xi.
164. Angelini L et al. Progressive multifocal leukoencephalopathy in a child with hyperimmunoglobulin E recurrent infection syndrome and review of the literature. *Neuropediatrics*. 2001;32:250–255.
165. Tan CS, Koralnik IJ. Progressive multifocal leukoencephalopathy and other disorders caused by JC virus: clinical features and pathogenesis. *Lancet Neurol*. 2010;9:425–437.
166. Gheuens S et al. Progressive multifocal leukoencephalopathy in individuals with minimal or occult immunosuppression. *J Neurol Neurosurg Psychiatr*. 2010;81:247–254.
167. Dawson JR. Cellular inclusions in cerebral lesions of epidemic encephalitis. *Arch Neurol Psychiatry*. 1934;31:685–700.
168. Payne FE, Baublis JV, Itabashi HH. Isolation of measles virus from cell cultures of brain from a patient with subacute sclerosing panencephalitis. *N Engl J Med*. 1969;281:585–589.
169. Reuter D, Schneider-Schaulies J. Measles virus infection of the CNS: human disease, animal models, and approaches to therapy. *Med Microbiol Immunol*. 2010;199:261–271.
170. Gutierrez J, Issacson RS, Koppel BS. Subacute sclerosing panencephalitis: an update. *Dev Med Child Neurol*. 2010;52:901–907.

171. Garg RK. Subacute sclerosing panencephalitis. *J Neurol.* 2008;255:1861–1871.

172. Gascon GG. Subacute sclerosing panencephalitis. *Semin Pediatr Neurol.* 1996;3:260–269.

173. Campbell H et al. Review of the effect of measles vaccination on the epidemiology of SSPE. *Int J Epidemiol.* 2007;36:1334–1348.

174. Jabbour JT et al. Subacute sclerosing panencephalitis. A multidisciplinary study of eight cases. *JAMA.* 1969;207:2248–2254.

175. Dyken PR, Swift A, DuRant RH. Long-term follow-up of patients with subacute sclerosing panencephalitis treated with inosiplex. *Ann Neurol.* 1982;11:359–364.

176. Wolinsky JS, Berg BO, Maitalnd CH. Progressive rubella panencephalitis. *Arch Neurol.* 1976;33:722–723.

177. Wolinsky JS et al. Progressive rubella panencephalitis: immunovirological studies and results of isoprinosine therapy. *Clin Exp Immunol.* 1979;35:397–404.

178. Townsend JJ et al. Progressive rubella panencephalitis. Late onset after congenital rubella. *N Engl J Med.* 1975;292:990–993.

179. UNAIDS. *Global Summary of the AIDS Epidemic 2009.* Geneva, Switzerland: World Health Organization; 2009.

180. Berger JR et al. Progressive multifocal leukoencephalopathy in patients with HIV infection. *J Neurovirol.* 1998;4:59–68.

181. Cohen BA. Neurologic complications of HIV infections. *Prim Care.* 1997;24:575–595.

182. Manns A, Hisada M, La Grenade L. Human T-lymphotropic virus type I infection. *Lancet.* 1999;353:1951–1958.

183. Olindo S et al. Natural history of human T-lymphotropic virus 1–associated myelopathy: a 14-year follow-up study. *Arch Neurol.* 2006;63:1560–1566.

184. Bittencourt AL, Primo J, Oliveira M. Manifestations of the human T-cell lymphotropic virus type I infection in childhood and adolescence. *J Pediatr (Rio J).* 2006;82:411–420.

185. Whitley RJ, MacDonald N, Asher DM. American Academy of Pediatrics. Technical report: transmissible spongiform encephalopathies: a review for pediatricians. Committee on Infectious Diseases. *Pediatrics.* 2000;106:1160–1165.

186. Ironside JW. Variant Creutzfeldt-Jakob disease: an update. *Folia Neuropathol.* 2012;50:50–56.

187. Norrby E. Prions and protein-folding diseases. *J Intern Med.* 2011;270:1–14.

188. Imran M, Mahmood S. An overview of human prion diseases. *Virol J.* 2011;8:559.

189. Snow RW et al. The global distribution of clinical episodes of *Plasmodium falciparum* malaria. *Nature.* 2005;434:214–217.

190. Idro R et al. Risk factors for persisting neurological and cognitive impairments following cerebral malaria. *Arch Dis Child.* 2006;91:142–148.

191. Newton CR, Taylor TE, Whitten RO. Pathophysiology of fatal falciparum malaria in African children. *Am J Trop Med Hyg.* 1998;58:673–683.

192. Thuma PE et al. Distinct clinical and immunologic profiles in severe malarial anemia and cerebral malaria in Zambia. *J Infect Dis.* 2011;203:211–219.

193. Mishra SK, Newton CRJC. Diagnosis and management of the neurological complications of falciparum malaria. *Nat Rev Neurol.* 2009;5:189–198.

194. Aikawa M et al. The pathology of human cerebral malaria. *Am J Trop Med Hyg.* 1990;43:30–37.

195. Idro R, Jenkins NE, Newton CRJC. Pathogenesis, clinical features, and neurological outcome of cerebral malaria. *Lancet Neurol.* 2005;4:827–840.

196. Newton CR et al. Coma scales for children with severe falciparum malaria. *Trans R Soc Trop Med Hyg.* 1997;91:161–165.

197. Molyneux ME et al. Clinical features and prognostic indicators in paediatric cerebral malaria: a study of 131 comatose Malawian children. *Q J Med.* 1989;71:441–459.

198. Molyneux ME. Cerebral malaria in children: clinical implications of cytoadherence. *Am J Trop Med Hyg.* 1990;43:38–41.

199. Birbeck GL et al. Identification of malaria retinopathy improves the specificity of the clinical diagnosis of cerebral malaria: findings from a prospective cohort study. *Am J Trop Med Hyg.* 2010;82:231–234.

200. Idro R et al. Burden, features, and outcome of neurological involvement in acute falciparum malaria in Kenyan children. *JAMA.* 2007;297:2232–2240.

201. Taylor TE et al. Differentiating the pathologies of cerebral malaria by postmortem parasite counts. *Nat Med.* 2004;10:143–145.

202. Jakka SR et al. Characteristic abnormalities in cerebrospinal fluid biochemistry in children with cerebral malaria compared to viral encephalitis. *Cerebrospinal Fluid Res.* 2006;3:8.

203. Boivin MJ et al. Developmental outcomes in Malawian children with retinopathy-positive cerebral malaria. *Trop Med Int Health.* 2011;16:263–271.

204. Kennedy PGE. The continuing problem of human African trypanosomiasis (sleeping sickness). *Ann Neurol.* 2008;64:116–126.

205. WHO. Human African Trypanosomiasis (Sleeping Sickness): Epidemiological Update. *Weekly Epidemiological Record* 2006;81(71–80).

206. Cattand P, Jannin J, Lucas P. Sleeping sickness surveillance: an essential step towards elimination. *Trop Med Int Health.* 2001;6:348–361.

207. Welburn SC, Odiit M. Recent developments in human African trypanosomiasis. *Curr Opin Infect Dis.* 2002;15:477–484.

208. Brun R et al. Human African trypanosomiasis. *Lancet.* 2010;375:148–159.

209. Barrett MP et al. The trypanosomiases. *Lancet.* 2003; 362:1469–1480.

210. Chimelli L, Scaravilli F. Trypanosomiasis. *Brain Pathol.* 1997;7:599–611.

211. Walker M, Kublin JG, Zunt JR. Parasitic central nervous system infections in immunocompromised hosts: malaria, microsporidiosis, leishmaniasis, and African trypanosomiasis. *Clin Infect Dis.* 2006;42:115–125.

212. Lejon V, Büscher P. Review Article: cerebrospinal fluid in human African trypanosomiasis: a key to diagnosis, therapeutic decision and post-treatment follow-up. *Trop Med Int Health.* 2005;10:395–403.

213. Carod-Artal FJ. Neurological complications of *Schistosoma* infection. *Trans R Soc Trop Med Hyg.* 2008;102:107–116.

214. Betting LE et al. Seizures and cerebral schistosomiasis. *Arch Neurol.* 2005;62:1008–1010.

215. Roberts M et al. Cerebral schistosomiasis. *Lancet Infect Dis.* 2006;6:820.

216. Garcia HH, Del Brutto OH, Peru CWGI. Neurocysticercosis: updated concepts about an old disease. *Lancet Neurol.* 2005;4:653–661.

217. García HH et al. Taenia solium cysticercosis. *Lancet*. 2003;362:547–556.

218. Moskowitz J, Mendelsohn G. Neurocysticercosis. *Arch Pathol Lab Med*. 2010;134:1560–1563.

219. Kalra V, Suri M, Jailkhani BL. A profile of childhood neurocysticercosis. *Indian J Pediatr*. 1994;61:33–42.

220. Willingham AL, Engels D. Control of Taenia solium cysticercosis/taeniasis. *Adv Parasitol*. 2006;61:509–566.

221. Wallin MT, Kurtzke JF. Neurocysticercosis in the United States: review of an important emerging infection. *Neurology*. 2004;63:1559–1564.

222. Bien CG et al. The natural history of Rasmussen's encephalitis. *Brain*. 2002;125:1751–1759.

223. Rasmussen T, Olszewski J, LloydSmith D. Focal seizures due to chronic localized encephalitis. *Neurology*. 1958;8:435–445.

224. Bauer J, Bien CG, Lassmann H. Rasmussen's encephalitis: a role for autoimmune cytotoxic T lymphocytes. *Curr Opin Neurol*. 2002;15:197–200.

225. Tekgul H et al. T-cell subsets and interleukin-6 response in Rasmussen's encephalitis. *Pediatr Neurol*. 2005;33:39–45.

226. Muto A et al. Nationwide survey (incidence, clinical course, prognosis) of Rasmussen's encephalitis. *Brain Dev*. 2010; 32:445–453.

227. Aarli JA. Rasmussen's encephalitis: a challenge to neuroimmunology. *Curr Opin Neurol*. 2000;13:297–299.

228. Granata T et al. Experience with immunomodulatory treatments in Rasmussen's encephalitis. *Neurology*. 2003;61:1807–1810.

229. Janeway CA et al. *Immunobiology: The Immune System in Health and Disease*. 8th ed. New York, NY: Garland Science; 2011.

230. Long SS, Pickering LK, Prober CG. *Principles and Practice of Pediatric Infectious Disease*. New York, NY: Churchill Livingstone, an Imprint of Elsevier; 2009.

231. Furst DE. The risk of infections with biologic therapies for rheumatoid arthritis. *Semin Arthritis Rheum*. 2010;39:327–346.

232. Anderson RJ et al. Infectious risk factors in the immunosuppressed host. *Am J Med*. 1973;54:453–460.

233. Marcén R. Immunosuppressive drugs in kidney transplantation: impact on patient survival, and incidence of cardiovascular disease, malignancy and infection. *Drugs*. 2009;69:2227–2243.

234. Hofflin JM et al. Infectious complications in heart transplant recipients receiving cyclosporine and corticosteroids. *Ann Intern Med*. 1987;106:209–216.

235. Pirsch JD. Cytomegalovirus infection and posttransplant lymphoproliferative disease in renal transplant recipients: results of the U.S. multicenter FK506 Kidney Transplant Study Group. *Transplantation*. 1999;68:1203–1205.

236. Kang I, Park SH. Infectious complications in SLE after immunosuppressive therapies. *Curr Opin Rheumatol*. 2003; 15:528–534.

237. Gabardi S et al. Induction immunosuppressive therapies in renal transplantation. *Am J Health Syst Pharm*. 2011;68:211–218.

238. Issa NC, Fishman JA. Infectious complications of antilymphocyte therapies in solid organ transplantation. *Clin Infect Dis*. 2009;48:772–786.

239. Wagner M et al. Prospective study on central venous line associated bloodstream infections. *Arch Dis Child*. 2011;96:827–831.

240. Guenier C, Ferreira J, Pector JC. Prolonged venous access in cancer patients. *Eur J Surg Oncol*. 1989;15:553–555.

241. Elting LS et al. The burdens of cancer therapy. Clinical and economic outcomes of chemotherapy-induced mucositis. *Cancer*. 2003;98:1531–1539.

242. van Vliet MJ et al. The role of intestinal microbiota in the development and severity of chemotherapy-induced mucositis. *PLoS Pathog*. 2010;6:e1000879.

243. Styczynski J, Gil L, Party EPDW. Prevention of infectious complications in pediatric HSCT. *Bone Marrow Transplant*. 2008;42(suppl 2):S77–S81.

244. Wingard JR, Hsu J, Hiemenz JW. Hematopoietic stem cell transplantation: an overview of infection risks and epidemiology. *Hematol Oncol Clin North Am*. 2011;25:101–116.

245. Mandell G, Bennett CL, Dolin R. Chapter 311: Infections in recipients of hematopoietic cell transplantation. In: *Mandell, Douglas, and Bennett's Principles and Practice of Infectious Diseases*. Philadelphia, PA: Churchill Livingstone, an Imprint of Elsevier; 2009.

246. Fishman JA. Infection in solid-organ transplant recipients. *N Engl J Med*. 2007;357:2601–2614.

247. Delmonico FL. Cadaver donor screening for infectious agents in solid organ transplantation. *Clin Infect Dis*. 2000;31:781–786.

248. Mandell G, Bennett CL, Dolin R. Chapter 310: Risk factors and approaches to infections in transplant recipients. In: *Mandell, Douglas, and Bennett's Principles and Practice of Infectious Diseases*. Philadelphia, PA: Churchill Livingstone, an Imprint of Elsevier; 2009.

249. Gasnault J et al. Improved survival of HIV-1-infected patients with progressive multifocal leukoencephalopathy receiving early 5-drug combination antiretroviral therapy. *PLoS ONE*. 2011;6:e20967.

250. Mofenson LM et al. Guidelines for the prevention and treatment of opportunistic infections among HIV-exposed and HIV-infected children: recommendations from CDC, the National Institutes of Health, the HIV Medicine Association of the Infectious Diseases Society of America, the Pediatric Infectious Diseases Society, and the American Academy of Pediatrics. *MMWR Recomm Rep*. 2009;58:1–166.

251. Notarangelo LD. Primary immunodeficiencies. *J Allergy Clin Immunol*. 2010;125:S182–S194.

252. Gambineri E. New frontiers in primary immunodeficiency disorders: immunology and beyond.... *Cell Mol Life Sci*. 2012;69:1–5.

253. Winkelstein JA et al. X-linked agammaglobulinemia: report on a United States registry of 201 patients. *Medicine (Baltimore)*. 2006;85:193–202.

254. Kang EM et al. Chronic granulomatous disease: overview and hematopoietic stem cell transplantation. *J Allergy Clin Immunol*. 2011;127:1319–1326; quiz 1327–1318.

255. Savides C, Shaker M. More than just infections: an update on primary immune deficiencies. *Curr Opin Pediatr*. 2010;22:647–654.

256. Price VE, Blanchette VS, Ford-Jones EL. The prevention and management of infections in children with asplenia or hyposplenia. *Infect Dis Clin North Am*. 2007;21:697–710, viii–ix.

257. Pediatrics AAO. Immunocompromised children. In: *Red Book: Report of the Committee on Infectious Diseases.* Elk Grove Village, IL: American Academy of Pedaitrics; 2009:72–86.

258. Hewison M. Vitamin d and the immune system: new perspectives on an old theme. *Rheum Dis Clin North Am.* 2012;38:125–139.

259. Lassi ZS, Haider BA, Bhutta ZA. Zinc supplementation for the prevention of pneumonia in children aged 2 months to 59 months. *Cochrane Database Syst Rev.* 2010:CD005978.

260. Christie CD, Heikens GT, McFarlane DE. Nosocomial and community-acquired infections in malnourished children. *J Trop Med Hyg.* 1988;91:173–180.

261. Manary MJ, Sandige HL. Management of acute moderate and severe childhood malnutrition. *BMJ.* 2008;337:a2180.

262. Berkowitz FE. Infections in children with severe protein-energy malnutrition. *Ann Trop Paediatr.* 1983;3:79–83.

263. Morelli N, Battaglia E, Lattuada P. Brainstem involvement in Legionnaires' disease. *Infection.* 2006;34:49–52.

264. Mamelak AN et al. Nocardial brain abscess: treatment strategies and factors influencing outcome. *Neurosurgery.* 1994;35:622–631.

265. Blyth CC, Adams DN, Chen SCA. Diagnostic and typing methods for investigating *Legionella* infection. *N S W Public Health Bull.* 2009;20:157–161.

266. Pahud BA et al. Varicella zoster disease of the central nervous system: epidemiological, clinical, and laboratory features 10 years after the introduction of the varicella vaccine. *J Infect Dis.* 2011;203:316–323.

267. Hirsch HH. BK virus: opportunity makes a pathogen. *Clin Infect Dis.* 2005;41:354–360.

268. Lopes da Silva R. Polyoma BK virus: an emerging opportunistic infectious agent of the human central nervous system. *Braz J Infect Dis.* 2011;15:276–284.

269. Verhelst X et al. Progressive multifocal leukoencephalopathy in liver transplant recipients: a case report and review of the literature. *Transpl Int.* 2011;24:e30–e34.

270. Caserta MT, Mock DJ, Dewhurst S. Human herpesvirus 6. *Clin Infect Dis.* 2001;33:829–833.

271. Lautenschlager I, Razonable RR. Human herpesvirus-6 infections in kidney, liver, lung, and heart transplantation: review. *Transpl Int.* 2012;25:493–502.

272. Fischer SA et al. Transmission of lymphocytic choriomeningitis virus by organ transplantation. *N Engl J Med.* 2006;354:2235–2249.

273. Razonable RR. Rare, unusual, and less common virus infections after organ transplantation. *Curr Opin Organ Transplant.* 2011;16:580–587.

274. Perfect JR et al. Clinical practice guidelines for the management of cryptococcal disease: 2010 update by the Infectious Diseases Society of America. *Clin Infect Dis.* 2010;50:291–322.

275. Pappas PG et al. Clinical practice guidelines for the management of candidiasis: 2009 update by the Infectious Diseases Society of America. *Clin Infect Dis.* 2009;48:503–535.

276. Liou J et al. Cryptococcal meningitis in pediatric systemic lupus erythematosus. *Mycoses.* 2003;46:153–156.

277. McCullers JA et al. Candidal meningitis in children with cancer. *Clin Infect Dis.* 2000;31:451–457.

278. Walsh TJ et al. Treatment of aspergillosis: clinical practice guidelines of the Infectious Diseases Society of America. *Clin Infect Dis.* 2008;46:327–360.

279. Roilides E, Zaoutis TE, Walsh TJ. Invasive zygomycosis in neonates and children. *Clin Microbiol Infect.* 2009;15(suppl 5):50–54.

280. Pentreath VW. Royal Society of Tropical Medicine and Hygiene Meeting at Manson House, London, 19 May 1994. Trypanosomiasis and the nervous system. Pathology and immunology. *Trans R Soc Trop Med Hyg.* 1995;89:9–15.

281. Yoo TW et al. Concurrent cerebral American trypanosomiasis and toxoplasmosis in a patient with AIDS. *Clin Infect Dis.* 2004;39:e30–e34.

282. Heyworth MF. Parasitic diseases in immunocompromised hosts. Cryptosporidiosis, isosporiasis, and strongyloidiasis. *Gastroenterol Clin North Am.* 1996;25:691–707.

283. Dutcher JP et al. Disseminated strongyloidiasis with central nervous system involvement diagnosed antemortem in a patient with acquired immunodeficiency syndrome and Burkitt's lymphoma. *Cancer.* 1990;66:2417–2420.

284. Barratt JLN et al. Importance of nonenteric protozoan infections in immunocompromised people. *Clin Microbiol Rev.* 2010;23:795–836.

17 *Neurotoxicology*

COLLEEN M. RIVERS, FRED HENRETIG, and LEWIS S. NELSON

This chapter reviews toxic influences on the central nervous system (CNS) with special reference to those classes of toxins that are significant, direct causes of critical illness likely to present to a pediatric intensive care unit (PICU). Many severe intoxications are capable of causing impaired or inadequate substrate delivery to the brain, for example, secondary to profound respiratory depression with consequent hypoxia (e.g., alcohols, barbiturates, opioids, other sedative-hypnotics); circulatory failure and shock (calcium channel antagonists, β-adrenergic blockers); hypoglycemia (ethanol, sulfonylureas); or status epilepticus (lead, tricyclic antidepressants [TCAs], camphor, isoniazid) with resulting neurotoxic syndrome. Additionally, innumerable specific neurotoxins have been described in the toxicology and neurology literature; the focus here is on postnatal exposure to those toxins that are most representative of agents with high risk for life-threatening effects.

■ GENERAL PRINCIPLES OF PEDIATRIC NEUROTOXICOLOGY

Poisoning is an important cause of significant acute injury in children, with toddlers and adolescents most frequently affected due to exploratory ingestions in the former and intentional overdoses in the latter. Estimates of poisoning episodes in children are in the millions annually in the United States. Fortunately, the vast majority of these result in little significant morbidity. This chapter focuses on those exceptional cases that result in critical pediatric illness.

The interaction between various exogenous toxic compounds and the CNS is predictably complex. This is particularly true when considering the prolonged developmental sequence for human brain architecture and function. The neurotoxic effects of exposure to a particular xenobiotic will vary greatly depending on total dose, acuity, and timing of exposure. These principles may be better conceptualized after a brief review of human neurovascular anatomy and brain ontogeny.

The CNS is relatively protected from some toxic influences by the blood-brain barrier. Highly polar compounds tend to be excluded, whereas lipid-soluble, nonpolar compounds cross the barrier more easily. The integrity of the barrier varies with age, and more substances cross in the immature brain. Thus inorganic lead poisoning can cause severe encephalopathy in young children but primarily a peripheral neuropathy in adults. The anatomic substrate of the blood-brain barrier is not fully understood, but 3 major concepts include (1) the function of glial cells wrapped around capillary endothelium; (2) unique properties of the capillary endothelium of the brain, particularly the finding of zonulae occludentes, or structures joining the endothelial cells together into tight junctions; and (3) the extracellular basement membrane between endothelial cells and glia and neurons. A blood-cerebrospinal fluid barrier also exists with analogous choroidal tight epithelial junctions.

Not all areas of the brain are equally affected by a given toxin, even if it does cross the blood-brain barrier. Variation can result from different vascular patterns and unique sensitivities of different cell types related to differing neurochemistry. Thus, a considerable degree of selectivity occurs in the neuropathologic effects of any given potential neurotoxin.

An additional consideration is the rapid prenatal and postnatal developmental changes in brain structure, which may be adversely impacted by toxins. The development of the brain begins as early as 3 weeks of gestation, when the neural plate is formed from the ectoderm. The neural plate then undergoes axial fusion, developing into the neural tube, with closure occurring by simultaneous cranial and caudal progression. After neurulation, subsequent sequential developments are neuronal proliferation, migration, differentiation, synaptogenesis, apoptosis, and myelination. These begin after gestational age of 28 days and continue into postnatal life, with active glial and synapse evolution until about 3 years of age. All of these processes may be impacted upon by toxic exposures (1,2). At birth, all large neuronal cell bodies are in place in the cerebral cortex and basal ganglia. However, synaptic connections are relatively sparse. Over the first 2 years of life, there is tremendous growth of these connections, such that by age 2 years, synaptic density is almost twice that of adulthood. Over the next few preschool-age years, these synapses are "pruned" selectively, presumably on the basis of sensory and motor stimulation. This process may be altered in the presence of even subtle toxic influences that affect neurotransmitter function, as well as more overt neuronal damage from global insults such as hypoxia or hypoglycemia. Alteration of dendritic architecture may result in difficulties with fine neurocognitive function such as memory, attention, and problem-solving skills. Such a paradigm has been invoked, with experimental evidence in animal models, for the effects of low-level lead toxicity on intellectual function (3).

Several mechanisms of neurotoxicity are recognized (4). An overarching concept is that of excitotoxicity, the process resulting in cell death from an energy imbalance when neuronal metabolic demands are not met. This is typically mediated by an oxidant stress and excessive stimulation of the N-methyl-D-aspartate (NMDA) receptors by glutamate, intracellular calcium influx, and resultant mitochondrial injury, and follows multiple classes of neurologic injury including those due to ischemic, infectious, and traumatic insults as well as intoxications. More specific classes of neurotoxicity include those mediated by the ability of various toxins to impact adversely on neurotransmitter function, direct receptor interactions, enzyme and transporter function,

axonal conduction, and neuronal intracellular metabolism. Neurotransmitter and direct receptor dysfunction, in particular, are common underlying mechanisms for many of the cases of critically ill children resulting from the ingestion of pharmaceutical and recreational drugs. Enhanced transmission occurs via one of several mechanisms, including inhibition of neurotransmitter presynaptic metabolism (e.g., monoamine oxidase inhibitors [MAOIs]), stimulation of release (e.g., amphetamines), reuptake inhibition (e.g., cocaine, many classes of antidepressants), and decreased synaptic degradation (e.g., organophosphates). Diminished synaptic transmission may result from inhibition of presynaptic release of neurotransmitter (e.g., botulinum and tetanus toxins), competitive receptor blockade (e.g., anticholinergic agents), and altered postsynaptic membrane potentials (e.g., tetrodotoxin). Common examples of toxin-mediated receptor dysfunction include those caused by agonism of opioids on opioid receptors, benzodiazepines and numerous sedative-hypnotic agents on γ-aminobutyric acid (GABA) receptors and lithium on serotonin receptors, or conversely by direct antagonism of receptors such as occurs in phencyclidine and ketamine toxicity with direct inhibition of NMDA receptors.

■ UNIQUE PEDIATRIC VULNERABILITIES TO TOXINS

Children may be relatively more vulnerable to many toxic agents than adults for multiple reasons beyond the prolonged neurologic developmental sequence, including greater relative exposure, immature metabolism, and longer life span to manifest chronic toxic effects including carcinogenesis. They have greater body-surface to mass ratios, higher metabolic rates, and higher minute ventilation for body size than adults do. Thus, for an inhalational exposure (e.g., carbon monoxide) they breathe more toxin per kilogram of body weight per minute than an adult counterpart exposed to the same degree of air contamination—for example, a higher dose. Children "live closer to the ground," with many toxins being heavier than air and thus more concentrated in a child's breathing zone than in that of an adult. For ingested toxins, the same body size and metabolic considerations mean that children will ingest relatively higher doses of toxin from contaminated food or water. Children also tend to have more hand-to-mouth activity than adults, so when their hands become contaminated, the risk of toxin ingestion also increases proportionally. Children may have immature metabolic pathways, especially in early infancy. This may mitigate, or exacerbate, certain toxic exposures. For example, some toxins are detoxified by intact metabolic pathways (e.g., organophosphate pesticides) and thus may be relatively more toxic to young children. Lastly, though of less concern for the acute intoxications discussed here, it is worth noting that many toxic effects require years or decades to manifest fully. This is particularly true for suspected carcinogens and agents linked to neurodegenerative diseases.

BASIC APPROACH TO THE CRITICALLY ILL POISONED CHILD

The initial evaluation of the poisoned child mirrors that of any critically ill child, and begins with a swift and thorough assessment of the "ABCs" (airway, breathing, and circulation.) After the patient's airway is deemed patent or is secured by an endotracheal tube, the clinician should evaluate the patient's respiratory effort. If either the respiratory rate or tidal volume is insufficient for the child's age, one should supplement the patient's breathing with a bag-valve-mask or mechanical ventilator. Next, the clinician assesses circulation by palpating central and peripheral pulses as well as time to capillary refill. The blood pressure and heart rate should be measured. If the patient is found to be hypotensive with a clear pulmonary exam, an intravenous (IV) line should be established and a fluid challenge of 20 mL/kg crystalloid should be administered.

In addition to the ABCs of basic life support, the poisoned child requires prompt evaluation of her blood glucose concentration, electrocardiogram (ECG), core temperature and consideration of gastrointestinal decontamination options (the latter are initiated infrequently in patients after PICU admission, and so are not discussed here, but toxicology consultation in this regard may be warranted for special cases). Thus, the "ABC"s are expanded to "ABCDEF"s, with *D* for dextrose and decontamination, *E* for ECG, and *F* for "fever" or hyperthermia. A rapid bedside capillary fingerstick should be obtained and the hypoglycemic child should be treated with hypertonic dextrose: 0.5 to 1.0 g/kg of $D_{10}W$ for an infant or $D_{25}W$ for a child. Due to immature energy pathways and smaller glycogen

stores, children are predisposed to hypoglycemia in the setting of agents that alter cellular metabolism. Common exposures that may result in hypoglycemia include sulfonylureas, meglitinides, β-adrenergic antagonists, pentamidine, propoxyphene, salicylates, ethanol, quinidine, and valproic acid (5). Lastly, a prompt core temperature reveals poisoned patients with hyperthermia, a potentially fatal feature of multiple toxicities. As detailed below, these patients require rapid cooling in order to maintain homeostasis and avoid multi-organ-system failure.

An ECG, often dubbed "the poor man's tox screen," offers valuable insight about the potential agents, clinical effects, and prognosis following an exposure. Particular attention should be focused on the ECG intervals and considered in the context of the cardiac action potential. (See Figure 17.1.) The QRS complex of a surface ECG correlates with phase 0 ventricular myocyte depolarization. This depolarization is mediated by sodium (Na⁺) influx through the voltage gated fast sodium channels (I_{Na^+}). Thus, agents that block this sodium channel cause a slowing of depolarization and result in a widened (> 100 milliseconds) QRS complex (6). Some such agents include cyclic antidepressants, propranolol, carbamazepine, cocaine, and diphenhydramine as well as quinidine and other type IA and IC antidysrhythmics. The PR interval or time between atrial and ventricular depolarization should also be measured. It is generally less than 200 milliseconds in a child and can be prolonged by agents such as β-adrenergic receptor antagonists, calcium channel blockers, or digoxin. These drugs inhibit electrical conduction between the atria and ventricles, sometimes resulting in complete heart block. The QT interval represents the time from ventricular depolarization through repolarization, and should be corrected for ventricular rate (QTc). The QTc is generally less than 450 milliseconds in young infants, 440 milliseconds in older infants and children, 440 milliseconds for adult men, and 460 milliseconds in adult women. Agents that block the outward potassium delayed rectifier channels during phase 2 and phase 3 of the action potential can prolong this interval and predispose the patient to ventricular dysrhythmias such as torsades de pointes. Common QTc prolonging agents include methadone, haloperidol, erythromycin, and ketoconazole. In addition to checking an ECG, all critically ill poisoned patients require continuous cardiac monitoring.

No set panel of laboratory tests should be ordered for every case of potential poisoning. Rather, one should tailor studies to assess for proof of exposure, to uncover

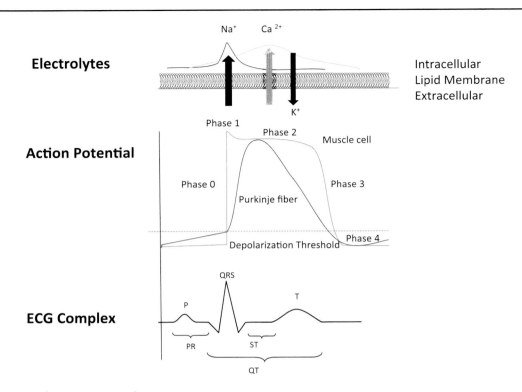

FIGURE 17.1 Cardiac action potential.

possible complications, or for prognostic reasons. However, in the case of the child ill from an unknown poison, evaluation of the basic metabolic panel often provides a useful first step toward narrowing the differential diagnosis. First, electrolyte abnormalities commonly associated with certain exposures might suggest a diagnosis in the proper clinical setting. For example, altered mental status with hyponatremia commonly results from binging with MDMA (3,4-methylenedioxymethamphetamine or "ecstasy"), which causes the syndrome of inappropriate antidiuretic hormone release (SIADH) (7,8).

Additionally, calculation of an anion gap (AG) helps distinguish common toxicologic causes of a metabolic acidosis. Patients with a metabolic acidosis in whom the AG ($Na-[Cl+HCO_3]$) is elevated (> 12 mmol/L) have an unmeasured anion present in their serum. A mnemonic to remember the potential causes of an elevated AG is KULTS: ketoacids, uremia, lactic acid, toxic alcohols, and salicylates. Ketones often result from an alcoholic or a starvation ketoacidosis. Uremia results from any toxin that causes renal insufficiency, and the diagnosis is confirmed by finding a markedly elevated blood urea nitrogen. Metabolic acidosis with an elevated lactate concentration accounts for most cases of toxin-induced elevated AG metabolic acidosis and etiologies range from cellular asphyxiants, such as cyanide, to antidiabetics, such as metformin. Toxic alcohols, such as ethylene glycol, undergo metabolism to an organic acid. In the case of ethylene glycol, the metabolites glycolic acid and oxalic acid result in an AG metabolic acidosis and renal failure may occur. Salicylate derivatives, such as aspirin or oil of wintergreen (methyl salicylate), cause both an AG metabolic acidosis and a primary respiratory alkalosis.

■ SYNDROMIC APPROACH TO POISONED PATIENTS

Given the vast array of potential poisons, the complex clinical findings they produce, and the limitation of the analytical laboratory in identifying specific toxins in real time, the ability to discern the nature of a toxic exposure on clinical grounds becomes critical. However, through recognition of toxicological syndromes, or "toxidromes," a clinician can identify the largest threats to a patient's life and institute empiric therapy while additional diagnostic strategies continue. The following paragraphs are intended to provide a framework with which to consider common poisonings and to highlight the related critical interventions and potential antidotes.

Altered Mental Status

While "altered mental status" frequently constitutes the entirety of a documented chief complaint, it fails to distinguish between the distinct clinical entities such as sedation, agitation, confusion, and hallucinations. Within these descriptors are a range of etiologies and severities with differing implications. For example, depressed mental status may range from sleepiness to coma, and this is often accompanied by progressive respiratory depression. An agitated patient, on the other hand, may present with a subtle delirium or an obvious psychosis. Some of these patients may be a danger to themselves or others and require physical and chemical restraint. Implicit in the described management strategies is that the fundamentals are addressed for each patient. These include acting on cardiorespiratory vital sign abnormalities, core body temperature, and rapid bedside testing such as glucometry and ECG.

Opioid Toxidrome

While most commonly noted for its associated "pinpoint pupils," decreased ventilation resulting from both decreased respiratory rate and decreased tidal volume remain the most consequential effects of this poisoning (Table 17.1). Implicated drugs are agonists at the opioid μ receptor in the CNS and include oxycodone and heroin. Due to the contemporary ubiquity of these analgesics, unintentional poisonings in children have reached epidemic levels (9). Other effects include mild hypotension and bradycardia but these findings are typically less concerning than the respiratory effects.

The primary intervention in an opioid poisoned child is to provide ventilatory support. Naloxone, an opioid antagonist, may be administered to reverse the clinical effects of an opioid agonist (Table 17.2). The usual pediatric starting dose of naloxone in an opioid naive child is 0.1 mg/kg IV, with a first dose maximum of 2 mg. This is paradoxically higher than the dose typically recommended for adults, but most children who are exposed to opioids are indeed opioid naive and thus not at risk of opioid withdrawal following naloxone

treatment. In addition, often the offending agent is a synthetic opioid or semisynthetic opiate derivative that may require higher dosing for reversal. In children or adolescents who are believed at risk for opioid dependence, the starting dose should be 0.001 mg/kg (maximum 0.04 mg). These starting doses can be administered and swiftly escalated as needed to as much as 2 to 4 mg in toddlers and 8 to 10 mg in adolescents if opioid toxicity is suspected or confirmed. Buprenorphine, a recently popularized partial-agonist at the opioid μ receptor, may be particularly resistant to reversal by naloxone (10–12). If the patient requires more than 1 dose of naloxone or the drug effect is expected to outlast the antidote effect, a naloxone infusion may be preferred, with a starting rate of two-thirds of the effective dose infused per hour, titrated to normal respiratory rate.

Sedative-Hypnotic Toxidrome

Patients poisoned by sedative hypnotics present with coma, generally associated with normal vital signs. Common causes of this relatively benign toxidrome include benzodiazepines, such as diazepam or clonazepam, newer sleep agents, such as zolpidem or eszopiclone, and ethanol. All of these enhance inhibitory tone in the CNS through GABA agonism. Most children exposed to one of these drugs in isolation tend to preserve their respiratory drive and hemodynamics. On the other hand, patients with mixed exposures (e.g., benzodiazepine with ethanol) often require airway protection and other supportive care. Additionally, γ-hydroxybutyric acid is a popular club drug that results in the sedative-hypnotic toxidrome.

Most patients demonstrating the sedative-hypnotic toxidrome are managed expectantly and do not require any specific treatment. Flumazenil, a competitive antagonist at the benzodiazepine receptor, should only be administered to patients with acute benzodiazepine exposure who have absolutely no history of chronic benzodiazepine use. When given to patients with chronic exposure to benzodiazepines, it can precipitate the benzodiazepine withdrawal syndrome including status epilepticus (13). As a result, flumazenil is not generally recommended for benzodiazepine intoxication in adults or teenagers due to the inability to exclude a history of chronic use with certainty. In young children, however, the drug may be used diagnostically to confirm and treat benzodiazepine overdose as a suspected cause of altered mental status. The recommended starting dose of flumazenil is 0.01 mg/kg (max 0.2 mg) IV at 0.1 per

■ Table 17.1 Toxidrome Vital Sign Findings

Toxidrome	Examples	Blood Pressure	Heart Rate	Respiratory Rate	Temperature	Pupils	Diaphoresis
Anticholinergic	Diphenhydramine Jimsonweed	+/−	↑	+/−	↑	↑	↓
Opioid	Heroin Oxycodone	↓	↓	↓	↓	↓	–
Sympathomimetic	Cocaine Methylphenidate	↑	↑	↑	↑	↑	↑
Sedative-hypnotic	Clonazepam Ethanol	↓	↓	↓	↓	–	–

minute. In this very specific treatment niche, flumazenil may save a child with a clear history of benzodiazepine naiveté from extensive testing such as a computerized tomography imaging of the head or a lumbar puncture, or unnecessary endotracheal intubation.

Agitated Delirium

Agitation poses unique challenges that are not encountered with other medical presentations. It requires that the provider take active measures to protect the patient with little opportunity to gather data or perform a thorough physical examination. Once these emergent interventions are implemented, close consideration of the patient's clinical findings enables identification of a likely cause and the initiation of therapy.

Sympathomimetic Toxidrome

Causes of sympathomimetic effects range from use of illicit drugs, such as cocaine and ecstasy, to overdoses of commonly prescribed attention deficit hyperactivity disorder medications, such as methylphenidate and dextroamphetamine. By different mechanisms, drugs in this class are agonists at adrenergic receptors in the sympathetic nervous system. Vital sign abnormalities include tachycardia, hypertension, and hyperthermia. On physical examination, patients exhibit mydriatic pupils that are reactive to light, diaphoresis, and normal bowel sounds.

Management of these patients centers on controlling their agitation with benzodiazepines and promptly diagnosing and treating any vital sign abnormalities, particularly hyperthermia. Importantly, physical restraints, which are often needed initially, should serve only as a

bridge to chemical restraint. Physical restraint without chemical sedation allows the patient to struggle and potentially develop hyperthermia, metabolic acidosis, and cardiac dysrhythmias (14,15). While various drugs have been used for sedation of the sympathomimetic patient, benzodiazepines offer the greatest safety profile and have the most logical pharmacologic mechanism (i.e., GABA agonism). As a result, the patient's heart rate and blood pressure improve and seizures are prevented. Diazepam starting at 0.1 mg/kg IV or midazolam starting at 0.025 mg/kg IV or intramuscular (IM) (max 5 mg) is recommended to gain behavioral control of the agitated sympathomimetic patient. Haloperidol, a butyrophenone

■ Table 17.2 Common Antidotes and Dosing

Antidote	Recommended Starting Dose
Dextrose	0.5 to 1.0 g/kg of $D_{10}W$ (0.1 g/mL) for an infant 0.5 to 1.0 g/kg of $D_{25}W$ (0.25g/mL) for a child
Naloxone	0.1 mg/kg IV (non-opioid-dependent) 0.001 mg/kg, max 0.04 mg (opioid-dependent) Escalate as indicated
Flumazenil	0.01 mg/kg (max 0.2 mg) IV Escalate as indicated
Diazepam	0.1 mg/kg IV Titrate as indicated
Midazolam	0.025 mg/kg (max 5 mg) IV or IM Titrate as indicated
Physostigmine	0.02 mg/kg (max 0.5 mg) IV
Pyridoxine	70 mg/kg (max of 5 g) IV empirically

Abbreviations: IM, intramuscular; IV, intravenous; Max, maximum.

antipsychotic that functions by blockade of dopamine receptors, is commonly utilized as a chemical restraint agent. However, haloperidol is not the drug of choice in this patient population due to its tendency to lower the seizure threshold, its ability to cause hyperthermic syndromes, and its association with torsades de pointes.

Hyperthermia is a primary contributor to death in these patients and necessitates rapid cooling (16,17). In cases of mild temperature elevation, IV benzodiazepines to control agitation coupled with external measures such as fans and ice packs typically result in prompt cooling. In cases of severe hyperthermia (> 105°F), these simple interventions are often inadequate and ice water immersion becomes the intervention of choice. If unable to obtain a tub or cholera bed in which to submerge the patient, cooling in bed may be effected by circumferentially covering the patient with a sheet and packing it with ice directly on the entire trunk. One should move quickly to paralysis and endotracheal intubation along with ice water immersion if unable to rapidly cool an awake patient (18).

It is important to consider the patient's particular complaints and the potential therapies within the context of their sympathomimetic toxidrome. For example, an otherwise healthy teenager who uses methamphetamine is at increased risk for subarachnoid hemorrhage, myocardial infarction, and also aortic, vertebral, and carotid dissection. While these disease processes classically spare the pediatric population, they must be considered in symptomatic patients with recent use of a sympathomimetic substance. Additionally, therapy must be guided to avoid unintended clinical effects; for example, β-blockers are contraindicated in patients with a sympathomimetic toxidrome. By blocking the β_2 receptor in the coronary vasculature, they may lead to unopposed α_1 receptor agonism causing worsened vasoconstriction and cardiac ischemia (19). Judicious treatment with IV benzodiazepines leads to well-controlled blood pressure and relief of chest pain in most cases.

Anticholinergic Toxidrome

More accurately called the antimuscarinic toxidrome, this syndrome results from any drug that is an antagonist to acetylcholine at muscarinic receptors. Common causative pharmaceuticals include diphenhydramine, tricyclic antidepressants (TCAs), and first generation antipsychotics such as haloperidol. Jimsonweed (*Datura stramonium*), a natural source of atropinelike chemicals can also cause this

toxidrome (20–22). The agitation of the anticholinergic patient is classically milder than that of the sympathomimetic patient. They typically mumble quietly to themselves with a characteristic dysarthria often termed "cotton ball mouth" and appear to be hallucinating as they pick with their fingers into the air and on their bed sheets. Their physical examination can also be distinguished from that of the sympathomimetic patient by their lack of diaphoresis. Due to muscarinic blockade at salivary and sweat glands, these patients have dry mucous membranes as well as difficulty dissipating heat by sweating, resulting in cutaneous vasodilation and a flushed appearance of their skin. Loss of vagal tone results in tachycardia. Decreased cholinergic input results in dilated pupils that are poorly reactive to light. The classic prose taught to students highlights the pertinent physical findings of this toxidrome: "Red as a beet (flushed), hot as a hare (hyperthermic), mad as a hatter (hallucinating), dry as a bone (anhydrotic), and full as a flask (urinary retention)."

Initial management of the anticholinergic patient mirrors that of the sympathomimetic patient. A core body temperature identifies hyperthermic patients in need of rapid cooling. Agitation is managed with IV benzodiazepines and patients are otherwise supported until toxicity resolves. Alternatively, known or suspected anticholinergic patients who have normal ECGs can be safely reversed with the antidote physostigmine. This drug inhibits acetylcholinesterase in the neurosynaptic junction allowing the accumulation of acetylcholine and the ability to overcome competitive antagonism at the muscarinic receptor. The starting dose is 0.02 mg/kg (max 0.5 mg) infused over at least 5 minutes. Atropine should be at the bedside and administered if symptoms of cholinergic toxicity occur (i.e., bradycardia, hypersalivation.) It is contraindicated in patients with a wide QRS complex or who have taken a TCA (23). Anticholinergic patients treated with physostigmine tend to normalize their vital signs and mental status within minutes. This intervention may provide a definitive diagnosis in the altered child with an anticholinergic toxidrome, thereby alleviating the anxiety of family members and sparing the child further invasive testing.

Toxin-Induced Seizures

Toxins that enhance excitatory input or decrease inhibitory tone can lead to seizure. Glutamate is the most pertinent excitatory neurotransmitter in the brain and acts via agonism at the NMDA receptor and others. Ibotenic acid, for example, a poison found in the mushroom *Amanita muscara* is an NMDA receptor agonist, and causes neuroexcitation and seizures (24). Alternatively, tetramethylenedisulfotetramine, an illegal rodenticide colloquially known as "tetramine," inhibits GABA in a noncompetitive fashion (chloride channel blocker), causing unopposed neuroexcitation and resulting in refractory seizures (25). Adenosine, a third critical neurotransmitter, is released by the presynaptic neuron during seizure activity and autoregulates further ictal discharge. Methylxanthines such as theophylline and caffeine, a once commonly prescribed asthma medication, inhibit endogenous adenosine and can lead to status epilepticus in overdose patients. While consideration of the crucial balance between neuroexcitation and neuroinhibition provides a framework with which to consider the poisoned seizure patient, one must keep in mind that any alteration of neuronal homeostasis can result in seizure. As such, toxins that lead to hypoglycemia, hypoxia, electrolyte abnormalities, or any other metabolic derangement may also cause seizure. Thus, the list of drugs that has been reported to cause seizure is too long to provide much clinical utility. Instead, the subsequent paragraphs highlight a select few toxins that characteristically cause consequential seizure activity in overdose or exposure.

Camphor, an essential oil once commonly found in mothballs, is a natural extract now used in nasal decongestant rubs and insect repellants. Children exposed to camphor often exude its unique aromatic odor. They may become symptomatic following ingestion or inhalation as well as through intranasal or transdermal absorption. Seizure is often the first manifestation of toxicity and occurs from minutes to hours after ingestion. It is typically short and self-limited although multiple seizures have been reported (26–29). The exact mechanism of camphor toxicity remains unclear but this lipophilic cyclic terpene may cause other neurologic manifestations such as CNS depression, agitation, headache, and hyperreflexia. The management strategy remains supportive, including administration of standard seizure medications starting with benzodiazepines.

Isoniazid, a commonly prescribed antituberculous medication, can cause refractory seizures in overdose and should be considered in any case of status epilepticus. It inhibits the enzyme pyridoxine phosphokinase, which is needed to activate pyridoxine to pyridoxal phosphate. Without this activated pyridoxine, GABA cannot be generated from glutamic acid, leading to a lack of physiologic inhibitory tone and status epilepticus. The treatment for this poisoning is IV pyridoxine (vitamin B_6), of which 1 gram should be administered for every 1 gram of isoniazid ingested. If the amount of ingested isoniazid is unknown or if the antidote is administered empirically for status epilepticus, a dose of 70 mg/kg IV (maximum of 5 g) should be administered at 0.5 g/min until the seizure stops and the remainder given IV over 4 to 6 hours. Benzodiazepines should also be administered as they work synergistically with pyridoxine to increase GABA agonism. Hydrazines, chemicals found in *Gyromitra* mushrooms ("false morel") or in rocket fuel, are structurally similar to isoniazid and can cause seizures by comparable mechanisms, also requiring treatment with pyridoxine (30).

While many commonly prescribed antidepressants have been reported to cause seizure in overdose, two drugs in this class deserve special attention. Citalopram, a selective serotonin reuptake inhibitor (SSRI), frequently causes seizure early after overdose. It may also cause QT prolongation on the ECG, which may be delayed up to 33 hours following ingestion (31,32). These effects appear to be dose-related and become more likely with larger overdoses. Bupropion, an atypical antidepressant often prescribed for smoking cessation, inhibits reuptake of norepinephrine and dopamine. It is associated with seizures at both therapeutic doses and in overdose, with an increased risk of delayed seizures and status epilepticus following ingestions of sustained release preparations. These patients are managed supportively with at least 24 hours of observation due to a consequential risk of delayed seizure following overdose.

Toxicologists are occasionally called to the pediatric intensive care unit to consult on previously healthy, school-aged children with abrupt onset of intractable seizures, typically occurring after a mild febrile prodrome, as described in a cohort of such children by Mikaeloff and colleagues (33). In addition to the induced pyridoxine deficiency-related intoxications noted above, a few additional relatively exotic toxic compounds are also associated with prolonged seizures that may be refractory to routine anticonvulsant therapy (34). These include the metals lead (e.g., lead encephalopathy, often associated with cerebral edema, and anemia with basophilic stippling) (35) and arsenic (especially in the context of acute arsenic poisoning, typically associated with severe gastroenteritis; cardiotoxicity with shock and /or

QTc prolongation and torsades de pointes; and acute lung, liver, and renal injury) (36), methylxanthine medications such as caffeine and theophylline, and the biologic toxins cicutoxin (from the water hemlock plant), and domoic acid (in amnestic shellfish poisoning) (4). Thus, such patients warrant a careful medication, environmental, dietary, and parental occupational history and complete physical examination, with emphasis on seeking evidence of multiorgan system dysfunction, and notation of unusual physical findings such as alopecia and abnormal fingernails (e.g., Mees lines, suggestive of heavy metal exposure). Comprehensive laboratory analysis (e.g., complete blood count, comprehensive metabolic panel with renal and hepatic function tests, urinalysis, and ECG, as well as specific toxicological testing) should be considered, perhaps best effected in conjunction with toxicology or poison center consultation. Unfortunately, in the authors' experience, such an evaluation, though reassuring in eliminating several potentially treatable conditions, has been unrevealing in most such patients.

Serotonin Syndrome

The serotonin syndrome, or serotonin toxicity is a constellation of signs and symptoms that result from excess stimulation of the serotonin type 1A receptors. This excess serotonergic agonism often results from the additive effects of drugs that enhance serotonin modulation. Some such drugs include those that inhibit serotonin metabolism (i.e., MAOIs), those that prevent reuptake of serotonin (i.e., SSRIs,) those that enhance serotonin release (i.e., MDMA), and those that directly act as agonists at serotonin receptors (i.e., lithium). Affected patients present with some combination of salient features including altered mental status, tremor, hyperreflexia of the lower extremities, muscle rigidity, diaphoresis, diarrhea, shivering, autonomic instability, and hyperthermia (37). The serotonin syndrome is a diagnosis made purely on clinical grounds, is one of exclusion, and often manifests on a spectrum with varying degrees of severity. The management of these patients mirrors that of the sympathomimetic patient, with special attention paid to actively cooling hyperthermic patients and providing benzodiazepines for agitation, tachycardia, and hypertension. The commonly cited antidote for this syndrome, cyproheptadine, acts as a serotonin antagonist but is not considered a first line therapy. It has not demonstrated clear benefits in patients with the serotonin syndrome and may cause anticholinergic effects including hyperthermia. It might be considered in patients who have failed to respond to good supportive care and benzodiazepines.

Neuroleptic Malignant Syndrome

The neuroleptic malignant syndrome, another drug-related hyperthermic syndrome, differs from serotonin syndrome both by the implicated drugs and by the insidious nature of its onset. While serotonin syndrome typically manifests within minutes to hours of treatment with a serotonergic agonist, neuroleptic malignant syndrome tends to evolve over the course of days following exposure to an implicated drug. Neuroleptic malignant syndrome results from dopamine antagonism in the CNS most commonly secondary to antipsychotic therapy. Higher potency agents such as haloperidol are more commonly causative especially in the setting of rapidly increasing doses and depot forms of administration (i.e., haloperidol decanoate). Clinical manifestations, similar to the serotonin syndrome, include altered mental status, hyperthermia, autonomic instability, tremor, and myoclonus. Increased muscle tone, also a finding common to both syndromes, can be distinguished in cases of neuroleptic malignant syndrome by its "lead pipe" quality. Treatment requires active cooling in the setting of hyperthermia and muscle relaxation with benzodiazepine therapy. If the patient fails to respond to these initial interventions, bromocriptine, a centrally acting dopamine agonist, should be considered.

Salicylism

Salicylism results from a wide variety of salicylate derivatives including acetylsalicylic acid (aspirin), methyl salicylate (oil of wintergreen), or occasionally bismuth subsalicylate (Pepto-Bismol.) While classically noted for its relatively unique acid-base derangement, a primary respiratory alkalosis coupled with a primary metabolic acidosis, close observation of the salicylate poisoned patient reveals a much more complex toxidrome than that found on a blood gas. Affected patients are both tachypneic and hyperpneic leading to the appearance of increased work of breathing in the setting of a clear pulmonary exam. Additionally they may complain of tinnitus or decreased hearing and exhibit nausea and vomiting along with diaphoresis and hyperthermia. The primary goal of therapy should be to prevent salicylic acid from crossing the blood brain barrier and entering the CNS where it can lead to cerebral edema and death. Alkalinization of the patient's serum with sodium bicarbonate accomplishes this, causing the salicylic acid to remain in an ionized form that cannot permeate the blood brain barrier. In turn, the patient's urine is alkalinized, similarly preventing reabsorption of this ionized acid in the distal tubule and enhancing elimination. The patient's spontaneous respiratory alkalosis should also be preserved if possible, with avoidance of sedation and intubation if practical. In cases where endotracheal intubation is clinically necessary, the ventilator should be set to maintain an appropriately large minute ventilation, maintaining the respiratory alkalosis.

The recommended treatment of symptomatic salicylate poisoned patients includes alkalinization of the blood and urine, starting with 1 to 2 mEq/kg IV push over 1 to 2 minutes and followed by an infusion of 3 ampules sodium bicarbonate in 1 L of D_5W run at twice maintenance. The infusion should be adjusted to reach a goal urine pH of 7.5 to 8 and a serum pH of 7.45 to 7.55. Serum potassium should be repleted and serial salicylic acid concentrations obtained until the concentration clearly trends down toward normal. Hemodialysis should be initiated if the patient cannot tolerate bicarbonate therapy (i.e., fluid overload), shows signs of end organ toxicity (i.e., altered mental status), has renal failure, or has an acute salicylate concentration of greater than 100 mg/dL or a chronic salicylate concentration of greater than 60 mg/dL (38). Of course, general signs of clinical deterioration in the setting of alkalinization also warrant drug removal by hemodialysis.

Tricyclic Antidepressant (TCA) Toxicity

TCA poisoned patients present with altered mental status and can rapidly deteriorate with the development of seizures, coma, cardiovascular collapse, and death. The ECG remains the cornerstone of diagnostic and prognostic significance of these patients. TCAs cause direct myocardial toxicity by binding to rapidly inactivating sodium channels on the myocardium, inhibiting sodium influx and slowing the phase 0 depolarization of the myocyte (Figure 17.1). In patients with a limb lead QRS interval of 100 milliseconds or longer, 33% have seizures. When the limb lead QRS interval is greater than 160 milliseconds, 50% develop ventricular dysrhythmias (6). Given this prognostic potential, all TCA poisoned patients should have an immediate ECG. If the QRS interval is 100 milliseconds or greater, the

patient should receive a sodium bicarbonate bolus of 1 to 2 mEq/kg IV push over 1 to 2 minutes. If the QRS narrows in response to this therapy, repeat boluses of sodium bicarbonate should be given or an infusion titrated to keep a narrow QRS interval while maintaining the serum pH between 7.45 and 7.55. Seizures should be treated with benzodiazepines at standard doses.

■ CONCLUSION

The poisoned patient shares much in common with other critically ill patients. Such patients require the same attention to airway support, breathing, circulation, and core body temperature. They require a sound clinical approach which is not overcome by an all-consuming preoccupation with reversing the toxin. As is commonly quipped by toxicologists, "Treat the patient, not the poison." The vast majority of poisoned patients do not require a specific antidote to ensure an optimal outcome, but rather they require both toxin specific therapy and general supportive care. Once the ABCDEFs have been addressed, contact with a regional poison center or institutional medical toxicologist is advised. Such consultation might be especially advisable in several recurring scenarios, based on the authors' experience: any child known to be poisoned who requires escalating supportive care, antidotal therapy or enhanced elimination interventions; an undiagnosed critical illness of acute onset, with significant alteration of mental status, especially if accompanied by multi-organ system dysfunction; protracted or recurrent neurologic dysfunction that is not diagnosed after the "usual suspects" have been evaluated for and excluded; and any particularly puzzling clinical picture, especially in toddlers and adolescents (or, if such occurs in young infants, or school-aged children, the possibility of a toxic etiology for Munchausen syndrome by proxy might be considered). The medical toxicology service in these situations may be able to narrow the differential diagnosis of the poisoned patient and can offer specific management strategies for particular poisonings.

■ REFERENCES

1. Mendola P et al. Environmental factors associated with a spectrum of neurodevelopmental deficits. *Ment Retard Dev Disabil Res Rev.* 2002;8(3):188–197.

2. Schmid C, Rotenberg JS. Neurodevelopmental toxicology. *Neurol Clin.* 2005;23(2):321–336.

3. Goldstein GW. Neurologic concepts of lead poisoning in children. *Pediatr Ann.* 1992;21(6):384–388.

4. Rao RB. Neurologic principles. In: *Goldfrank's Toxicological Emergencies.* 9th ed. New York, NY: The McGraw Hill Companies; 2011:275.

5. Bosse GM. Antidiabetics and hypoglycemics. In: Nelson LS et al, eds. *Goldfrank's Toxicological Emergencies.* 9th ed. New York, NY: McGraw Hill Companies; 2011:714.

6. Boehnert MT, Lovejoy FH Jr. Value of the QRS duration versus the serum drug level in predicting seizures and ventricular arrhythmias after an acute overdose of tricyclic antidepressants. *N Engl J Med.* 1985;313(8):474–479.

7. Ajaelo I, Koenig K, Snoey E. Severe hyponatremia and inappropriate antidiuretic hormone secretion following ecstasy use. *Acad Emerg Med.* 1998;5(8):839–840.

8. Hartung TK et al. Hyponatraemic states following 3,4-methylenedioxymethamphetamine (MDMA, 'ecstasy') ingestion. *QJM.* 2002;95(7):431–437.

9. Okie S. A flood of opioids, a rising tide of deaths. *N Engl J Med.* 2010;363(21):1981–1985.

10. Gal TJ. Naloxone reversal of buprenorphine-induced respiratory depression. *Clin Pharmacol Ther.* 1989;45(1):66–71.

11. van Dorp E et al. Naloxone reversal of buprenorphine-induced respiratory depression. *Anesthesiology.* 2006;105(1):51–57.

12. Sarton E, Teppema L, Dahan A. Naloxone reversal of opioid-induced respiratory depression with special emphasis on the partial agonist/antagonist buprenorphine. *Adv Exp Med Biol.* 2008;605:486–491.

13. Spivey WH. Flumazenil and seizures: analysis of 43 cases. *Clin Ther.* 1992;14(2):292–305.

14. Otahbachi M et al. Excited delirium, restraints, and unexpected death: a review of pathogenesis. *Am J Forensic Med Pathol.* 2010;31(2):107–112.

15. Schrag B, de Froidmont S, Lesta MD. Positional asphyxia, a cause of death insufficiently known. *Rev Med Suisse.* 2011;7(303):1511–1514.

16. Catravas JD, Waters IW. Acute cocaine intoxication in the conscious dog: studies on the mechanism of lethality. *J Pharmacol Exp Ther.* 1981;217(2):350–356.

17. Marzuk PM et al. Ambient temperature and mortality from unintentional cocaine overdose. *JAMA.* 1998;279(22):1795–1800.

18. Armstrong LE et al. Whole-body cooling of hyperthermic runners: comparison of two field therapies. *Am J Emerg Med.* 1996;14(4):355–358.

19. Lange RA et al. Potentiation of cocaine-induced coronary vasoconstriction by beta-adrenergic blockade. *Ann Intern Med.* 1990;112(12):897–903.

20. Bouziri A et al. *Datura stramonium* L. poisoning in a geophagous child: a case report. *Int J Emerg Med.* 2011;4(1):31.

21. Centers for Disease Control and Prevention (CDC). Jimsonweed poisoning associated with a homemade stew—Maryland, 2008. *MMWR Morb Mortal Wkly Rep.* 2010; 59(4):102–104.

22. Honey BL et al. Jimson weed abuse in an Oklahoma teen. *J Okla State Med Assoc.* 2009;102(12):351–353.

23. Pentel P, Peterson CD. Asystole complicating physostigmine treatment of tricyclic antidepressant overdose. *Ann Emerg Med.* 1980;9(11):588–590.

24. Benjamin DR. Mushroom poisoning in infants and children: the *Amanita pantherina/muscaria* group. *J Toxicol Clin Toxicol.* 1992;30(1):13–22.

25. Barrueto F Jr et al. Status epilepticus from an illegally imported Chinese rodenticide: "tetramine". *J Toxicol Clin Toxicol.* 2003;41(7):991–994.

26. Pillay VV. Camphor ingestion: an unusual cause of seizure. *J Assoc Physicians India.* 2009;57:216; author reply 216–217.

27. Peters AL, Dekker E, Michels WM. Camphor poisoning following ingestion of mothballs 'for headache'. *Ned Tijdschr Geneeskd.* 2011;155(39):A3676.

28. Khine H et al. A cluster of children with seizures caused by camphor poisoning. *Pediatrics.* 2009;123(5): 1269–1272.

29. Skoglund RR, Ware LL Jr, Schanberger JE. Prolonged seizures due to contact and inhalation exposure to camphor. A case report. *Clin Pediatr (Phila).* 1977;16(10):901–902.

30. Lheureux P, Penaloza A, Gris M. Pyridoxine in clinical toxicology: a review. *Eur J Emerg Med.* 2005;12(2):78–85.

31. Mohammed R et al. Prolonged QTc interval due to escitalopram overdose. *J Miss State Med Assoc.* 2010;51(12): 350–353.

32. Tarabar AF, Hoffman RS, Nelson L. Citalopram overdose: late presentation of torsades de pointes (TdP) with cardiac arrest. *J Med Toxicol.* 2008;4(2):101–105.

33 Mikaeloff Y et al. Devastating epileptic encephalopathy of school-aged children (DESC): a pseudo-encephalitis. *Epilepsy Res.* 2006;69:67–79.

34. Osterhoudt KC, Henretig FM. Refractory seizures. *Pediatr Emerg Care.* In press, 2012.

35. Henretig FM. Lead. In: Nelson LS et al, eds. *Goldfrank's Toxicologic Emergencies.* 9th ed. New York, NY: McGraw-Hill Companies; 2011:1266.

36. Munday SW, Ford MD. Arsenic. In: Nelson LS et al, eds. *Goldfrank's Toxicologic Emergencies.* 9th ed. New York, NY: McGraw-Hill Companies; 2011:1214.

37. Boyer EW, Shannon M. The serotonin syndrome. *N Engl J Med.* 2005;352(11):1112–1120.

38. Flomenbaum N. Salicylates. In: Nelson LS et al, eds. *Goldfrank's Toxicologic Emergencies.* 9th ed. New York, NY: McGraw-Hill Companies; 2011:508.

18 Hyperthermic Drug-Induced Disorders

SABA AHMAD and NICHOLAS S. ABEND

■ INTRODUCTION

Core body temperature is highly regulated. Afferent inputs from the body project to the central nervous system, in particular to the preoptic and anterior hypothalamic regions, to trigger heat-loss responses (vasodilation and sweating) or heat-gain responses (vasoconstriction and shivering). These mechanisms involve norepinephrine, dopamine, serotonin, acetylcholine, prostaglandins, and neuropeptides.

Elevated temperature may be classified as fever or hyperthermia (1). Fever, often defined as a temperature of 38.3°C or above, refers to an elevated hypothalamic temperature set point and generally occurs with infection, inflammation, or hypothalamic injury. Hyperthermia results from unbalanced heat generation and dissipation, but generally the hypothalamic set point is normal. Heat generation may occur with an increased metabolic rate, increased muscle activity (shivering, seizure, increased muscle tone, or rigidity), or increased sympathetic activity. Impaired heat dissipation may occur with elevated external temperatures (heat stroke) or reduced sweating.

Hyperthermia is a core feature of multiple drug reaction syndromes which have overlapping features (2). Distinguishing tests are not available, so diagnosis of these conditions is based on the clinical signs and symptoms, attention to medications being used, and details regarding when medications were initiated or had dosage adjustments relative to symptom onset. A toxidrome may lead to hospital admission or may start in the hospital in response to a new medication or change in dose

of a drug. Prompt recognition is important in order to institute specific therapy and provide the proper supportive measures. Close monitoring is required since these conditions are often associated with encephalopathy, disseminated intravascular coagulation, rhabdomyolysis, hepatic dysfunction, and dysautonomia.

This chapter reviews the neuroleptic malignant syndrome (NMS), malignant hyperthermia (MH), serotonin syndrome, and baclofen withdrawal syndrome. The anticholinergic and sympathomimetic toxidromes, which also involve hyperthermia and other overlapping features, are discussed in the Neurotoxicology chapter.

■ NEUROLEPTIC MALIGNANT SYNDROME

The NMS is a potentially fatal reaction to dopamine receptor antagonists. *Neuroleptic* originally referred to the effects on behavior and cognition of antipsychotic medications. While the estimated incidence of this disorder is 0.2% (3), the ubiquitous use of neuroleptic medications makes this an important problem to recognize and treat in its early stages. The neurotransmitter dopamine is involved in cognition, motor function, reward, and motivation. It is important in the function of the basal ganglia. The basal ganglia are nuclei deep in the cerebral hemisphere, include the substantia nigra and striatum, play an important role in movement, and comprise the extrapyramidal system. D2 receptor blockade can result in significant adverse effects in some patients, including parkinsonism, tardive dyskinesia, and NMS. NMS is thought to result from a reduction in dopamine in central nervous system nigrostriatal and hypothalamic pathways although the exact mechanism is not known. It can occur soon after the start of or increased dosage of medications that block dopaminergic transmission and, less often, after the prolonged use of a causative medication. These medications include the typical and atypical antipsychotic medications, antiemetics that are dopamine receptor antagonists, antidepressants, and others (Table 18.1). NMS may occur when changing from one neuroleptic or antiemetic to another. NMS or an NMS-like parkinsonism-hyperpyrexia syndrome (4) may also occur following withdrawal of L-dopa or dopamine agonists. It has also been reported after deep brain stimulation surgery (5).

The typical clinical NMS tetrad includes: (1) altered mental status, (2) extrapyramidal symptoms, (3) hyperthermia, and (4) autonomic dysfunction. The early manifestations of the disorder may be subtle, so a high level of suspicion for NMS is required in a patient receiving potentially causative medications

■ **Table 18.1** Drugs That Cause Neuroleptic Malignant Syndrome[a]

1. Typical neuroleptics (first generation antipsychotic drugs)
   A. Phenothiazines: chlorpromazine, thioridazine, fluphenazine, perphenazine, trifluoperazine
   B. Butyrophenone: haloperidol
   C. Thiothixene
2. Atypical neuroleptics (second generation antipsychotics drugs): Aripiprazole, clozapine, iloperidone, lurasidone, olanzapine, paliperidone, quetiapine, risperidone, ziprasidone
3. Antiemetics: domperidone, droperidol, metachlopramide, prochlorperazine, promethazine
4. Others: pimozide, loxitane, reserpine, tetrabenazine, phenelzine, amoxapine, desipramine. Lithium may be associated with NMS when used with neuroleptic medications. Tricyclics may be associated with NMS when used with metaclopramide. Cocaine might cause or predispose to an NMS-like variant.
5. Drug withdrawal associated with NMS-like condition: levodopa, amantadine, bromocriptine, ropinirole, pramipexole.

Abbreviation: NMS, neuroleptic malignant syndrome.
[a] Drugs not marketed in the United States are not included. There is controversy or incomplete data about some medications.

who presents with mildly altered mental status and/or mild hyperthermia. Onset is generally within 1 to 7 days of medication initiation or a dose increase, in contrast to the onset of MH and serotonin syndrome which usually have more rapid onset (Table 18.2). NMS is an evolving disorder, and in one review 82% of 340 patients presented with only 1 clinical sign (6). Typically, all of the signs occur within 24 hours and peak in 72 hours. Mental status may range from mild confusion to coma, and encephalopathy precedes other NMS symptoms in the majority of patients (6). The most common extrapyramidal signs are generalized lead-pipe rigidity (joint stiffness that is present throughout the range of passive motion) or dystonia (involuntary persistent abnormal postures of a limb or the torso sometimes with superimposed small repetitive movements), but tremor and myoclonus can also occur. Rarely, NMS may occur without hyperthermia (7). Dysautonomia is common and can include blood pressure lability, tachycardia, tachypnea, and diaphoresis. Patients may also have sialorrhea, incontinence, dysarthria, and dysphagia. As the disorder progresses, a severe hypermetabolic syndrome can ensue, resulting in multi-organ system derangement including cardiorespiratory collapse, renal failure, thromboembolic disease, hyperthermia, and hypoxemic end-organ injury.

Diagnostic criteria have been proposed (8). Major criteria include hyperthermia, rigidity, and elevated creatine kinase. Minor criteria include tachycardia, abnormal blood pressure, tachypnea, altered consciousness, diaphoresis, and leukocytosis. NMS is very likely if all three major or two major and four minor criteria are present. A recent literature review by a panel of multispecialty NMS experts used the Delphi process to reach consensus regarding which elements were most important in diagnosing NMS. The panel reached consensus regarding the importance of eight elements in diagnosing NMS: (1) recent dopamine antagonist exposure or dopamine agonist withdrawal, (2) hyperthermia, (3) rigidity, (4) mental status alteration, (5) creatine kinase (CK) elevation, (6) sympathetic nervous system lability, (7) tachycardia plus tachypnea, and (8) a negative workup for other causes. There was consensus regarding critical values for hyperthermia (> 38.0°C on at least two measurements), CK elevation (at least four times the upper limit of normal), hypertension (> 25% above baseline), blood pressure fluctuation (≥ 20 mmHg diastolic or ≥ 25 mmHg systolic change within 24 hours), tachycardia

	Neuroleptic Malignant Syndrome	Malignant Hyperthermia	Serotonin Syndrome
■ Table 18.2 Comparison of Neuroleptic Malignant Syndrome, Malignant Hyperthermia, and Serotonin Syndrome			
Drug	Dopamine antagonist Withdrawal of dopamine agonist	Succinylcholine Inhalational anesthetics	Serotonergic agents
Common time to onset after drug initiation or dose increase	1–7 days	Minutes to a few hours	A few hours to 1 day
Vital signs	Elevated HR, BP, RR Hyperthermia	Elevated HR, BP, RR Hyperthermia Elevated CO_2	Elevated HR, BP, RR Hyperthermia
Mental status	Any degree of encephalopathy; delirium is common	Any degree of encephalopathy	Any degree of encephalopathy; delirium is common
Movement abnormality	Rigidity, bradykinesia	Rigidity (often masseter, can be generalized)	Clonus, hyperreflexia, rigidity, tremor, restlessness, myoclonus
Other exam features	Sialorrhea, pallor, diaphoresis, decreased bowel sounds	Diaphoresis, decreased bowel sounds	Increased pupil size, diaphoresis, sialorrhea, increased bowel sounds, diarrhea
Management		Discontinue offending agent. ICU supportive care. Manage hyperthermia. Monitor for rhabdomyolysis.	
	Dopaminergic agents Benzodiazepines Dantrolene	Benzodiazepines Dantrolene	Benzodiazepines Cyproheptadine

Abbreviations: BP, blood pressure; ICU, intensive case unit, HR, heart rate; RR, respiratory rate.

($\geq 25\%$ above baseline), and tachypnea ($\geq 50\%$ above baseline). These criteria have not been validated (9).

The differential diagnosis for NMS will sometimes include encephalitis and meningitis, structural brain lesions, sepsis, serotonin syndrome, MH, heat stroke, diencephalic storm, intoxication (anticholinergic agents, MDMA (3,4-methylenedioxy-N-methylamphetamine, ecstasy), amphetamines, phenycyclidine), withdrawal (alcohol, sedatives, L-dopa, amantadine, baclofen), or endocrine abnormalities (thyrotoxicosis or pheochromocytoma). In many instances, testing to exclude other diagnoses will be needed. Malignant catatonia is a serious behavioral syndrome with altered movement including bradykinesia (slow, limited movement) or immobility, mutism, stuporlike state, and many of the features of NMS. In some cases, it cannot be distinguished from NMS except that malignant catatonia can occur in the absence of a provoking drug.

NMS is fatal in about 10% of patients (10). Given the progressive nature and severity of the disorder, all patients with suspected NMS should be admitted to a closely monitored critical care setting. Immediate withdrawal of the antidopaminergic agent and avoidance of further dopamine receptor blockade are required. While there is no controlled trial data regarding NMS management, early intervention and prevention of the more severe systemic problems that result from the hypermetabolic syndrome is important. In some cases, all that is needed is withdrawal of the provoking agent and general support. Treatment is typically individualized based on clinical severity. In mild cases, such as with a low-grade hyperthermia and mild hypokinesis or rigidity, parenteral benzodiazepines such as lorazepam can be administered. If the patient develops more worrisome hyperthermia or extrapyramidal signs (rigidity or dystonia), then a dopamine agonist such as bromocriptine should be administered orally or via a feeding tube. While bromocriptine is often the drug of choice, other dopaminergic agents include carbidopa/levodopa, ropinirole, and pramipexole. If there is moderate hyperthermia and rigidity, then dantrolene (a muscle relaxant that causes excitation-contraction decoupling) can be administered. Dantrolene helps reduce core body temperature by reducing skeletal muscle contraction and hypermetabolism (11). These agents can be coadministered. Treatment is often required for about a week, depending on the half-life of the causative medication. If NMS is caused by a depot injection, then continued treatment may be required for several weeks.

Along with the targeted treatment of the NMS described above, supportive treatment is the mainstay. The goal of supportive treatment is to reduce the damaging effects of the severe hypermetabolism. Adjunctive therapies to maintain normothermia include ice packs, cold intravenous fluids, or surface cooling systems (cooling blankets). Cardiopulmonary monitoring and support is needed, and fluid replacement is important, particularly if rhabdomyolysis occurs. Monitoring for disseminated intravascular coagulation, electrolyte abnormalities, CK elevation, and renal dysfunction is imperative.

If the symptoms of NMS are refractory to pharmacological treatment, particularly if there are prominent catatonic features, electroconvulsive therapy may be used. This may also be a treatment option if there are ongoing catatonic and parkinsonian features after NMS has resolved (11,12).

In patients who recover from NMS, there remains a significant risk of recurrence (up to 30%) if the patient is given a subsequent neuroleptic challenge (3). Starting a neuroleptic after recovery from NMS depends on the degree of need for such a medication and education of the patient about the risks and benefits. If feasible, the patient should not be treated with a neuroleptic for at least several weeks following recovery, drug selection should be based on both efficacy and low incidence of causing NMS, and the drug should be introduced at a low dose and escalated slowly.

■ MALIGNANT HYPERTHERMIA

MH is a life-threatening syndrome that occurs in susceptible patients after depolarizing neuromuscular blockade with succinylcholine or administration of halogenated inhalational anesthetics (halothane, sevoflurane, isoflurane, desflurane). Rarely, MH may occur after exposure to extreme heat or with vigorous exercise. MH typically presents immediately after exposure to the causative medication, but there can be a delay of several hours.

Clinical features of MH involve a hypermetabolic state. A high clinical suspicion is necessary in order to make the diagnosis. A 1994 consensus conference led to the formulation of a set of diagnostic criteria. The more criteria met (especially > 6), the more likely a reaction constitutes MH (13). The criteria included (1) respiratory acidosis (end-tidal CO_2 above 55 mmHg or arterial P_{CO_2} above 60 mmHg), (2) cardiac involvement (unexplained sinus tachycardia, ventricular tachycardia, or ventricular fibrillation), (3) metabolic acidosis (base deficit > 8, pH < 7.25), (4) generalized muscle rigidity, (5) rhabdomyolysis (CK > 20,000/L units, myoglobinuria, hyperkalemia), (6) hyperthermia (rapidly increasing temperature, > 38.8°C), (7) other (rapid reversal of MH signs with dantrolene, elevated resting serum CK levels), and (8) a family history of MH (autosomal dominant pattern).

The first manifestation is often a rise in end-tidal CO_2 due to muscle hypermetabolism. Other early symptoms include tachycardia and tachypnea in response to catecholamine release and muscle rigidity (often at masseter muscle). The initial presentation may be subtle making diagnosis difficult. Hyperthermia often develops later and rigidity develops in only about half of patients. Rhabdomyolysis, disseminated intravascular coagulation, and cardiac arrest may occur.

The hypermetabolic state and subsequent end-organ dysfunction are similar to what occurs in NMS. A major distinguishing factor between NMS and MH is the exposure itself, but there are some patients who perioperatively receive anesthetic agents as well as dopamine receptor blocking agents, making distinctions more difficult. In MH, the time from the drug exposure to severe hyperthermia and rigidity can be minutes to hours, while the time course for NMS is hours to days (Table 18.2). The differential diagnosis of MH is similar to that of NMS (see above).

MH is a disorder or calcium homeostasis in which calcium accumulation within the sarcolemma causes sustained muscle contraction. MH is an autosomal dominant inherited disorder. The majority of cases (50%–70%) are thought to be caused by a mutation in the ryanodine receptor gene (RYR1). The protein encoded by this gene is located on the sarcoplasmic reticulum and is responsible for excitation-contraction coupling. With abnormal RYR1 protein, calcium release is excessive and sustained skeletal muscle contraction ensues (14). Patients with MH may describe a family history of similar reactions. RYR genetic testing is available, but since there is heterogeneity a normal test does not prove absence of MH. An in vitro contracture test has been developed, in which the response of a muscle fiber to halothane or caffeine is investigated, but this requires a surgical procedure and is not widely available.

The mortality of untreated MH is high, but it is less than 5% with modern pharmacological intervention and supportive care (15). Guidelines for management are available from the malignant hyperthermia society (www.MHAUS.org). The provoking agent must be discontinued immediately. If the patient is still in the operating room then intravenous anesthesia should be initiated. Close observation in an intensive care unit (ICU) is required. One hundred percent oxygen should be administered. Ventilation rate may be increased to normalize $Paco_2$. Sedation using benzodiazepines is often required. Body cooling may be required involving ice packs, cold intravenous fluids, or surface cooling system (cooling blankets). Rhabdomyolysis management involves fluid hydration to maintain a high urine output. If pharmacologic paralysis is required for intractable rhabdomyolysis or hyperthermia, then nondepolarizing neuromuscular blocking medications should be used such as vecuronium. Monitoring for signs of disseminated intravascular coagulation is important. Potassium levels may rise. Parenteral dantrolene is the only specific treatment for MH, and it should be initiated immediately upon recognition of the disorder (16). Dantrolene 2.5 mg is given by intravenous bolus (17). Since the introduction of dantrolene, mortality related to MH has decreased. Dantrolene antagonizes RYR-mediated calcium release. Guidelines addressing the transfer of patients from ambulatory surgical centers to higher level facilities should MH occur recommend dantrolene administration prior to transfer (18). Recurrence may occur, usually within 1 day of the initial reaction, so prolonged monitoring well past the start of improvement is important.

Some patients with myopathy may have an increased risk for MH (19). These include central core disease, multiminicore disease, nemaline rod myopathy, a sodium channel form of myotonia, or hypokalemic periodic paralysis. Central core disease is the most linked

to MH and is a congenital myopathy with autosomal dominant transmission related to glycolytic enzyme deficiency that presents with generalized weakness in early infancy.

MH diagnosis has implications for both the patient and family members. Patients and their families must be informed of the diagnosis and implications, and the drug reaction should clearly be listed in the permanent medical record since it impacts future anesthetic use. Many patients with known MH risk wear a medical alert bracelet. If anesthesia is needed, then agents should include nondepolarizing neuromuscular blocking agents (such as vecuronium and rocuronium), nitrous oxide, and intravenous anesthetics (benzodiazepines, barbiturates, propofol, thiopental, ketamine, etomidate).

■ SEROTONIN SYNDROME

Serotonin syndrome has also been referred to as serotonin toxicity, serotonin behavioral syndrome, and serotonin hyperactivity syndrome. This toxidrome was initially described in 1960 in patients who were using monoamine oxidase inhibitors (MAOIs) and tryptophan concurrently (20). It is caused by medications that augment serotonin transmission. It can occur when a single serotonergic medication is used at an appropriate therapeutic dose, but it is more common when an overdose occurs (19) or when two or more serotonergic medications are used simultaneously. Combined use should be avoided, but if necessary, the two drugs should be kept at as low dose as feasible. The patient must be particularly well-educated about recognizing and reporting toxicity symptoms. Complete documentation of prescribed and over-the-counter medications and knowledge of medication effects with careful prescribing practices will minimize the risk of this sometimes fatal disorder. Table 18.3 is a list of medications that affect serotonin metabolism. There are various mechanisms by which serotonin activity can be increased in the central nervous system. These include direct serotonin agonists, inhibitors of serotonin reuptake from the synaptic terminal, serotonin release augmenting medications, and medications that prevent serotonin degradation. Dopamine agonists are also implicated in serotonin syndrome; it is thought that increased concentrations of dopamine in the central nervous system

■ **Table 18.3** Drugs That Augment Serotonin Transmission and Their Mechanisms of Action

SSRIs
- Citalopram
- Escitalopram
- Fluoxetine
- Fluvoxamine
- Paroxetine

- Sertraline
- Vilazodone
- Trazodone

Selective serotonin and norepinephrine reuptake inhibitors
- Venlafaxine
- Desvenlafaxine
- Duloxetine

Tricyclic antidepressants (inhibit serotonin reuptake)
- Amitriptyline
- Amoxapine
- Desipramine
- Doxepin
- Imipramine
- Maprotiline
- Nortriptyline
- Protriptyline
- Trimipramine

Other serotonin reuptake inhibitors
- Amphetamines
- Cocaine
- Dextromethorphan
- Tramadol

Drugs increasing serotonin release
- Cocaine
- Amphetamines
- Reserpine
- MDMA (3, 4-methylenedioxy-N-methylamphetamine, ecstasy)

Drugs that decrease serotonin metabolism (MAOIs)
- Phenelzine
- Isocarboxazid
- Selegiline
- Tranylcypromine

Direct agonists of serotonin
- Buspirone
- LSD
- Triptans

Dopamine agonists
- Amantadine
- Bromocriptine
- Bupropion
- Levodopa

Other drugs reported to cause serotonin syndrome
- Carbamazepine
- Linezolid
- Baclofen withdrawal

Factors that cause a nonspecific increase in serotonin
- Lithium
- Electroconvulsive therapy
- St Johns wort

Abbreviations: LSD, lysergic acid diethylamide; MAOI, monoamine oxidase inhibitor; SSRI, selective serotonin reuptake inhibitor.

contribute to serotonin release. Note that Table 18.3 includes illicit drugs. This adds to the need for obtaining a complete history.

Serotonin is widespread in the body. It plays a role in appetite, mood, cognition, autonomic function, motor function, gastrointestinal motility, blood pressure control, and coagulation. In the central nervous system, it is located primarily in the midline raphe nuclei, which play an important role in regulation of hunger, behavior, nociception, motor tone, and thermoregulation. Serotonin is synthesized from the amino acid tryptophan, one of the essential amino acids. It is degraded by monoamine oxidase (MAO).

The symptoms of serotonin syndrome involve mental status, autonomic function, and neuromuscular function. Any degree of encephalopathy may be present, from mild confusion to coma, with a combination of confusion, hypomania, and agitation being common. Autonomic features can include hyperthermia,

hypertension, tachycardia, nausea, skin flushing, diaphoresis, enteric dysmotility (with diarrhea), and pupillary dilation. The neuromuscular elements may include rigidity, tremor, hyperreflexia, clonus, and myoclonus. Hyperthermia is common, resulting from the increased heat generation of the hypermetabolic state and excess neuromuscular activity. It is only minimally related to changes in hypothalamic set point (fever) and thus is not well treated with antipyretics.

Criteria for diagnosis have been developed (21–23). The Hunter criteria found that the presence of clonus, agitation, diaphoresis, tremor, and hyperreflexia predicted serotonin toxicity (22). Serotonin symptoms have been described as (1) mild (may or may not concern the patient), (2) moderate (toxicity which causes distress but is not life-threatening), or (3) severe (medical emergency involving the rapid onset of severe hyperthermia, muscle rigidity, and multiple organ failure) (23,24).

It is important to distinguish NMS and serotonin syndrome. There is overlap of symptoms, but the provoking drugs and the time of onset of the symptoms in relation to starting the medication are different, and there are substantial differences in the movement abnormalities (Table 18.2). Other differential diagnosis is similar to that for NMS (see above).

Treatment of serotonin syndrome is largely supportive. The offending drug(s) must be discontinued. This often leads to substantial improvement over 24 hours. Close monitoring, cardiopulmonary support, and maintaining hydration and normothermia are important. Temperature control with ice packs, cold intravenous fluids, and surface cooling (cooling blankets) are considerations. Antipyretics are not effective since the hyperthermia is not related to a hypothalamic set point alteration. Testing for and treating rhabdomyolysis are important. Sedation with benzodiazepines such as lorazepam may be useful for agitation. Paralysis with vecuronium may be helpful for rhabdomyolysis, extreme rigidity, and intractable hyperthermia. Hypertension should be treated with short-acting medications. Hypotension should be treated with direct catecholamines such as phenylephrine, norepinephrine, or epinephrine. If an MAOI is potentially responsible for serotonin syndrome, then indirect catecholamines like dopamine may be ineffective since they require MAO activity for conversion.

In severe cases, nonspecific serotonin receptor blockade with cyproheptadine has been recommended, at a dose of 0.25 mg/kg/day (up to 12 mg daily) (25). Cyproheptadine is an antihistamine and serotonin antagonist. It may be crushed and given by nasogastric tube since no intravenous form is available. Olanzapine and chlorpromazine have been considered, but there is little supportive data. Dantrolene is often used in NMS and may reduce muscle contraction, but there is little data to guide use in serotonin syndrome. Anecdotal evidence suggests that electroconvulsive therapy may be helpful in refractory cases.

■ BACLOFEN WITHDRAWAL

Baclofen is a gamma-aminobutyric acid type B (GABA$_B$) receptor agonist used to treat spasticity associated with cerebral and spinal cord injuries. It is administered orally or via an intrathecal catheter and pump. When oral administration is ineffective, intrathecal administration allows for achievement of high cerebrospinal fluid levels which may improve spasticity with fewer adverse effects than with high oral dosing. Abrupt discontinuation of baclofen may cause baclofen withdrawal syndrome (26). While often only considered with intrathecal baclofen withdrawal, many cases associated with oral baclofen withdrawal have also been described (27). Symptoms often present within a day of intrathecal baclofen withdrawal and within several days of oral baclofen withdrawal (27). In a review of 23 adult cases of reported baclofen withdrawal, the most common psychiatric symptoms included hallucinations (auditory or visual or tactile), delusions, confusion, agitation, disorientation, fluctuations in consciousness, insomnia, and anxiety (27). In addition to the psychiatric manifestations, this potentially fatal syndrome may involve hyperthermia, autonomic dysfunction, altered mental status, spasticity, seizures, rhabdomyolysis, and disseminated intravascular coagulation. It often begins within a day or few days after intrathecal baclofen cessation, which may be caused by pump malfunction, failure to refill the pump, or catheter dysfunction (kinking or dislodgement). Onset of symptoms may take longer when oral baclofen has been discontinued. ICU monitoring and support are needed. Reinstituting baclofen often seems to lead to improvement. Patients who had been on intrathecal treatment may have a better response to restarting intrathecal therapy than administering oral baclofen. A temporary intrathecal catheter to administer baclofen may be useful (28). Treatment with benzodiazepines, cyproheptadine, and dantrolene has been attempted but there is no proven value. In most cases, symptoms resolve within 4 to 72 hours (27). If baclofen is to be discontinued, it should be tapered slowly to avoid baclofen withdrawal.

■ CONCLUSIONS

Diagnosis of these hyperthermic toxidromes requires awareness of the conditions and clinical acumen because of their overlapping features. This set of conditions places emphasis on always gathering complete drug lists, including prescription, over-the-counter, and illicit drugs. The list should be reviewed with the patient, family, and friends. While knowing what medications are being administered is often key to diagnosis of these syndromes, there are patients in whom the clinical features are so strongly suggestive that a working diagnosis might lead to further investigation of medications in use.

■ REFERENCES

1. Benarroch EE. Thermoregulation: recent concepts and remaining questions. *Neurology*. 2007;69:1293–1297.

2. McAllen KJ, Schwartz DR. Adverse drug reactions resulting in hyperthermia in the intensive care unit. *Crit Care Med*. 2010;38:S244–S252.

3. Caroff SN, Mann SC. Neuroleptic malignant syndrome. *Med Clin North Am*. 1993;77:185–202.

4. Newman EJ, Grosset DG, Kennedy PG. The parkinsonism-hyperpyrexia syndrome. *Neurocrit Care*. 2009;10:136–140.

5. Kim JH et al. Parkinsonism-hyperpyrexia syndrome after deep brain stimulation surgery: case report. *Neurosurgery*. 2010;66:E1029.

6. Velamoor VR et al. Progression of symptoms in neuroleptic malignant syndrome. *J Nerv Ment Dis*. 1994;182:168–173.

7. Lev R, Clark RF. Neuroleptic malignant syndrome presenting without fever: case report and review of the literature. *J Emerg Med*. 1994;12:49–55.

8. Levenson JL. Neuroleptic malignant syndrome. *Am J Psychiatry*. 1985;142:1137–1145.

9. Gurrera RJ et al. An international consensus study of neuroleptic malignant syndrome diagnostic criteria using the Delphi method. *J Clin Psychiatry*. 2011;72:1222–1228.

10. Ahuja N, Cole A. Hyperthermia syndromes in psychiatry. *Adv Psychiatr Treatment*. 2009;15:181–191.

11. Caroff SN, Mann SC, Keck PE Jr. Specific treatment of the neuroleptic malignant syndrome. *Biol Psychiatry*. 1998;44:378–381.

12. Caroff SN et al. Residual catatonic state following neuroleptic malignant syndrome. *J Clin Psychopharmacol*. 2000;20:257–259.

13. Larach MG et al. A clinical grading scale to predict malignant hyperthermia susceptibility. *Anesthesiology*. 1994;80:771–779.

14. Yang T et al. Functional defects in six ryanodine receptor isoform-1 (RyR1) mutations associated with malignant hyperthermia and their impact on skeletal excitation-contraction coupling. *J Biol Chem*. 2003;278:25722–25730.

15. Rosenberg H et al. Malignant hyperthermia. *Orphanet J Rare Dis*. 2007;2:21.

16. Krause T et al. Dantrolene—a review of its pharmacology, therapeutic use and new developments. *Anaesthesia*. 2004;59:364–373.

17. Lerman J. Perioperative management of the paediatric patient with coexisting neuromuscular disease. *Br J Anaesth*. 2011;107(suppl 1):i79–i89.

18. Larach MG et al. Special article: creation of a guide for the transfer of care of the malignant hyperthermia patient from ambulatory surgery centers to receiving hospital facilities. *Anesth Analg*. 2011;114:94–100.

19. Klingler W et al. Core myopathies and risk of malignant hyperthermia. *Anesth Analg*. 2009;109:1167–1173.

20. Oates JA, Sjoerdsma A. Neurologic effects of tryptophan in patients receiving a monoamine oxidase inhibitor. *Neurology*. 1960;10:1076–1078.

21. Sternbach H. The serotonin syndrome. *Am J Psychiatry*. 1991;148:705–713.

22. Dunkley EJ et al. The Hunter Serotonin Toxicity Criteria: simple and accurate diagnostic decision rules for serotonin toxicity. *QJM*. 2003;96:635–642.

23. Radomski JW et al. An exploratory approach to the serotonin syndrome: an update of clinical phenomenology and revised diagnostic criteria. *Med Hypotheses*. 2000;55:218–224.

24. Isbister GK, Buckley NA, Whyte IM. Serotonin toxicity: a practical approach to diagnosis and treatment. *Med J Aust*. 2007;187:361–365.

25. Graudins A, Stearman A, Chan B. Treatment of the serotonin syndrome with cyproheptadine. *J Emerg Med*. 1998;16:615–619.

26. Mohammed I, Hussain A. Intrathecal baclofen withdrawal syndrome—a life-threatening complication of baclofen pump: a case report. *BMC Clin Pharmacol*. 2004;4:6.

27. Leo RJ, Baer D. Delirium associated with baclofen withdrawal: a review of common presentations and management strategies. *Psychosomatics*. 2005;46:503–507.

28. Bellinger A et al. Prevention of intrathecal baclofen withdrawal syndrome: successful use of a temporary intrathecal catheter. *Reg Anesth Pain Med*. 2009;34:600–602.

19 | *Acute Metabolic Encephalopathy*

CAN FICICIOGLU

■ INTRODUCTION

Acute metabolic encephalopathy (AME) results from diffuse failure of brain metabolism whose causes (Table 19.1) include not only metabolic and endocrine diseases but also hepatic and uremic coma, hypoxia, seizure disorders, and central nervous system infections that sometimes clinically resemble acute metabolic brain disease. Inborn errors of metabolism (IEMs) constitute a small but significant subset of diseases causing AME. IEMs can result in accumulation of toxic metabolites and/or insufficient energy production that can trigger a sequence of metabolic events leading to pronounced central nervous system dysfunction and encephalopathy. Because IEMs are rare disorders, which tend to present with nonspecific clinical findings, they are easily and often overlooked (1). This is consequential for patients and their families. First, if diagnosed in a timely fashion, patients with some IEMs respond well to treatment and can avoid recurrent metabolic crises. Second, since all IEMs are genetic disorders, genetic counseling can play an important role in helping families make informed decisions about future pregnancies.

This chapter discusses IEMs which produce AME from the perspective of an intensivist and a pediatric neurologist caring for a patient with AME for whom routine biochemical test results are available (basic metabolic panel, ammonia, blood gases, urine analysis). It provides guidance about when to suspect and how to diagnose and treat IEMs. I summarize the general classification of IEMs and discuss the initial approach to them. I then explain when to suspect these disorders and provide a synopsis of some conditions with emphasis on clinical presentation, biochemical findings, and treatment. More extended descriptions of many of the individual disorders mentioned in this chapter can be found in other textbooks cited in the reference notes (1,2).

Which Classes of IEMs Sometimes Produce AME as Symptoms?

From a pathophysiologic perspective, IEMs can be classified into 3 groups (1):

Group 1—complex molecule: This group of disorders is caused by defects in the synthesis or catabolism of *complex molecules.* Symptoms of these disorders are progressive and permanent and are independent of any intercurrent illnesses or food intake. Lysosomal storage disorders (such as mucopolysaccharidosis, Gaucher, Fabry), peroxisomal biogenesis defects, and congenital disorders of glycosylation (CDG) belong to this group. The disorders in this group do not manifest with AME with a few exceptions. Fabry disease and CDG may present with strokelike episodes and seizures; Zellweger syndrome (peroxisomal defect) may present with a severe neurologic dysfunction in the newborn period. Group 1 disorders are not discussed in this chapter.

Group 2—intoxication: Inborn errors of intermediary metabolism lead to an acute and progressive *intoxication* due to accumulation of toxic metabolites proximal to biochemical defects. This group includes amino acid disorders (such as phenylketonuria (PKU), tyrosinemia, maple syrup urine disease [MSUD], homocystinuria), organic acidemias, urea cycle defects, galactosemia, and

■ **Table 19.1** Causes of Acute Encephalopathy

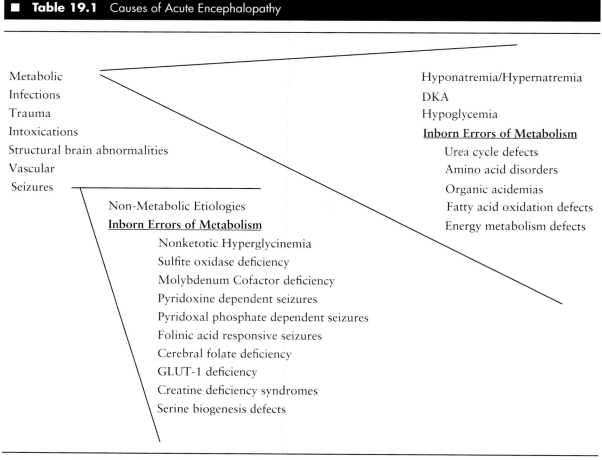

Metabolic
Infections
Trauma
Intoxications
Structural brain abnormalities
Vascular
Seizures

Hyponatremia/Hypernatremia
DKA
Hypoglycemia
<u>**Inborn Errors of Metabolism**</u>
    Urea cycle defects
    Amino acid disorders
    Organic acidemias
    Fatty acid oxidation defects
    Energy metabolism defects

Non-Metabolic Etiologies
<u>**Inborn Errors of Metabolism**</u>
    Nonketotic Hyperglycinemia
    Sulfite oxidase deficiency
    Molybdenum Cofactor deficiency
    Pyridoxine dependent seizures
    Pyridoxal phosphate dependent seizures
    Folinic acid responsive seizures
    Cerebral folate deficiency
    GLUT-1 deficiency
    Creatine deficiency syndromes
    Serine biogenesis defects

Abbreviations: DKA, Diabetic ketoacidosis; GLUT-1, glucose transporter type 1.

hereditary fructose intolerance. They present after a symptom-free interval either with acute symptoms such as vomiting, lethargy, acute encephalopathy, thromboembolic complications, liver failure, or chronic and progressive developmental delay. Some of these patients are at risk for recurrent metabolic crisis /encephalopathy.

Group 3—energy deficiency: These are the IEMs with symptoms due to a deficiency in *energy* production or utilization. In this group, there are glycogen storage disorders, gluconeogenesis defects, ketone utilization defects, fatty acid oxidation defects, primary lactic acidosis such as pyruvate dehydrogenase (PDH) or pyruvate carboxylase (PC) deficiency, as well as mitochondrial respiratory chain disorders. In energy deficiencies such as PDH, or PC deficiency there may be no symptom-free interval. The most frequent symptoms are generalized hypotonia, cardiomyopathy, and rapidly progressive neurologic deterioration.

This chapter focuses on group 2 and 3 disorders which can manifest with acute encephalopathy (Table 19.1).

■ INITIAL APPROACH TO DIAGNOSIS OF IEMs

Pediatric intensivists and neurologists are responsible for emergency care and stabilization of patients with IEMs and should be familiar with the fundamental aspects of such care and diagnostic approach.

Obtaining a careful past and current medical history including an assessment of diet, eating behaviors, and social, developmental, and family history is an essential first step (3). Historical features suggestive of IEMs include acute life-threatening symptoms in the newborn period, developmental delay, cardiomyopathy, episodic vomiting, liver dysfunction, hypoglycemia, acidosis, dehydration, and lethargy associated with minor illnesses. Diet history is crucial to determining food aversion. Patients with amino acid disorders or urea cycle defects may self-restrict their protein intake. A careful family history may reveal important clues that raise the possibility of IEM. Most IEMs are inherited as autosomal recessive traits, so there may be siblings with similar illnesses or deaths from sepsis with an unidentified pathogen or sudden infant death syndrome.

Routine biochemical tests such as basic metabolic panel and urine analysis can help to raise red flags for a possible IEM such as high anion gap acidosis or ketonuria. Once clinical suspicion is aroused based on the clinical presentation and basic laboratory investigation, more specific laboratory tests should be performed and supportive measures must be instituted immediately (4). The laboratory studies that should be obtained for a patient who has symptoms of a metabolic encephalopathy consistent with IEM are listed in Table 19.2.

How Does Newborn Metabolic Screening Help?

Since the early 1990s, tandem mass spectrometry has made screening possible for many IEM including amino acid, organic acid, and fatty acid oxidation disorders. The inclusion of these disorders in screening programs has enabled the timely diagnosis and treatment of these conditions and decreased complications such as mental retardation or death. Not all IEMs are screened in the newborn period. If the patient has symptoms and signs of a meta-

---

■ Table 19.2 Initial Investigation of Acute Encephalopathy

—Blood gases
—Electrolytes, glucose, CK
—Liver functions, PT, PTT
—Lactate, pyruvate
—Ammonia
—Plasma amino acids
—Plasma acylcarnitines
—Urine organic acids
—Urine analysis
—Blood and urine carnitine

Abbreviations: CK, Creatine kinase; PT, Prothrombin time; PTT, Partial thromboplastin time.

---

bolic disorder, further testing should be performed even if the result of the newborn screening test was normal.

Which Biochemical and Clinical Findings Should Trigger Suspicion of IEMs?

IEMs are difficult to distinguish from one another since the same symptoms and signs occur in many different diseases. Symptoms and signs of the clinical presentation (neurologic deterioration, seizures, presence or absence of symptom-free interval after birth) in combination with biochemical tests help differentiate IEMs. Figure 19.1 provides a flowchart guiding IEM differentiation.

While the symptoms and signs of each IEM vary considerably, I subdivide the most common disorders based mainly on their biochemical findings. Isolated persistent seizures causing encephalopathy do not have any biochemical findings in routine tests and they will be discussed under "seizures." The clinician, prepared with such knowledge, can narrow the range of diagnostic possibilities, select the appropriate laboratory tests and treatment, and request a metabolic consultation.

■ INTOXICATION (GROUP 2) DISORDERS ARRANGED BY BIOCHEMICAL FINDINGS (A-D)

A—Metabolic Acidosis with High Anion Gap + Ketosis

Metabolic acidosis with high anion gap (> 16) is an important laboratory abnormality of many IEMs during acute episodes of illness. It is easily demonstrated by arterial blood gases or basic metabolic panel. Ketonuria is an important indicator of a metabolic disorder. Neonates do not normally produce much acetoacetate; ketosis detected in neonates by dipstick is always abnormal and should prompt serious consideration of an organic acidemia. Among the inborn errors, the largest group associated with high anion gap metabolic acidosis and ketosis is the group of *organic acidemias* such as propionic acidemia (PA) and, methylmalonic acidemia (MMA) (5,6).

Organic acidemias: MMA and PA are the most frequent forms of branched-chain organic acidurias, and caused by enzymatic defects in the catabolism of branched-chain amino acids (BCAAs) valine and isoleucine (Figure 19.2) and of other propiogenic substrates, such as methionine, threonine, odd-chain fatty acids, and cholesterol.

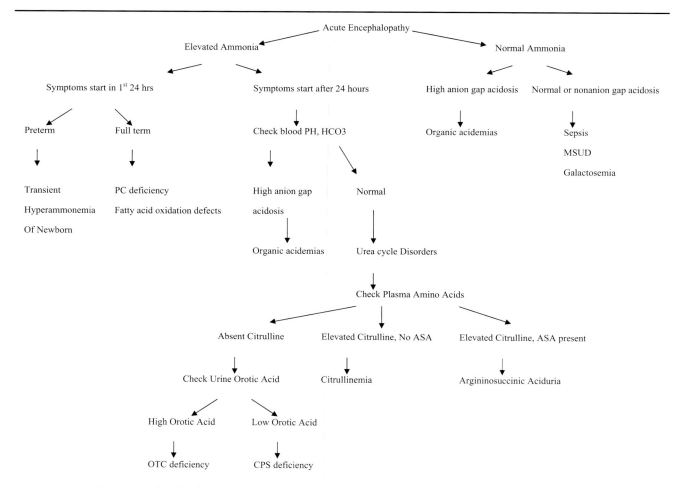

FIGURE 19.1 Diagnostic algorithm for acute metabolic encephalopathy.

PA is caused by a deficiency of propionyl CoA carboxylase (a biotin dependent enzyme). Isolated MMA results from either (1) deficient activity of the enzyme methylmalonyl-CoA mutase encoded by the *MUT* gene or (2) diminished synthesis of its cofactor adenosylcobalamine (cobalamin A or B disease). These autosomal recessive disorders can present with neurologic manifestations including acute progressive encephalopathy caused by the accumulation of toxic compounds proximal to the metabolic block. In most cases of PA and MMA, the onset of the disease is in the neonatal period but a later-onset presentation can occur.

Clinical and biochemical findings: The usual neonatal presentation is a sepsislike picture after an initial normal period of 24 to 48 hours: the neonate stops feeding well, begins vomiting, and becomes lethargic, which rapidly progresses to coma. Progressive neurologic findings include abnormal posturing and movements, hypotonia,

and seizures, often with a burst-suppression electroencephalographic (EEG) pattern. If left undiagnosed and untreated, most of these patients die in the newborn period. Some patients, especially those with some residual enzyme activity, may survive this crash and go on to have other acute metabolic crises or develop chronic developmental and neurologic sequelae.

In addition to metabolic acidosis, and ketosis, these patients may also have elevated lactate caused by secondary interference with coenzyme A metabolism. Neutropenia, thrombocytopenia, and anemia can occur during acute crisis and may lead to false diagnosis of sepsis (6). Hyperammonemia is commonly but not uniformly seen in these patients.

In about one-third of patients, the disease presents with late onset after a symptom-free interval longer than 1 year. The clinical picture of late onset forms is variable, ranging from acute encephalopathy to intermittent

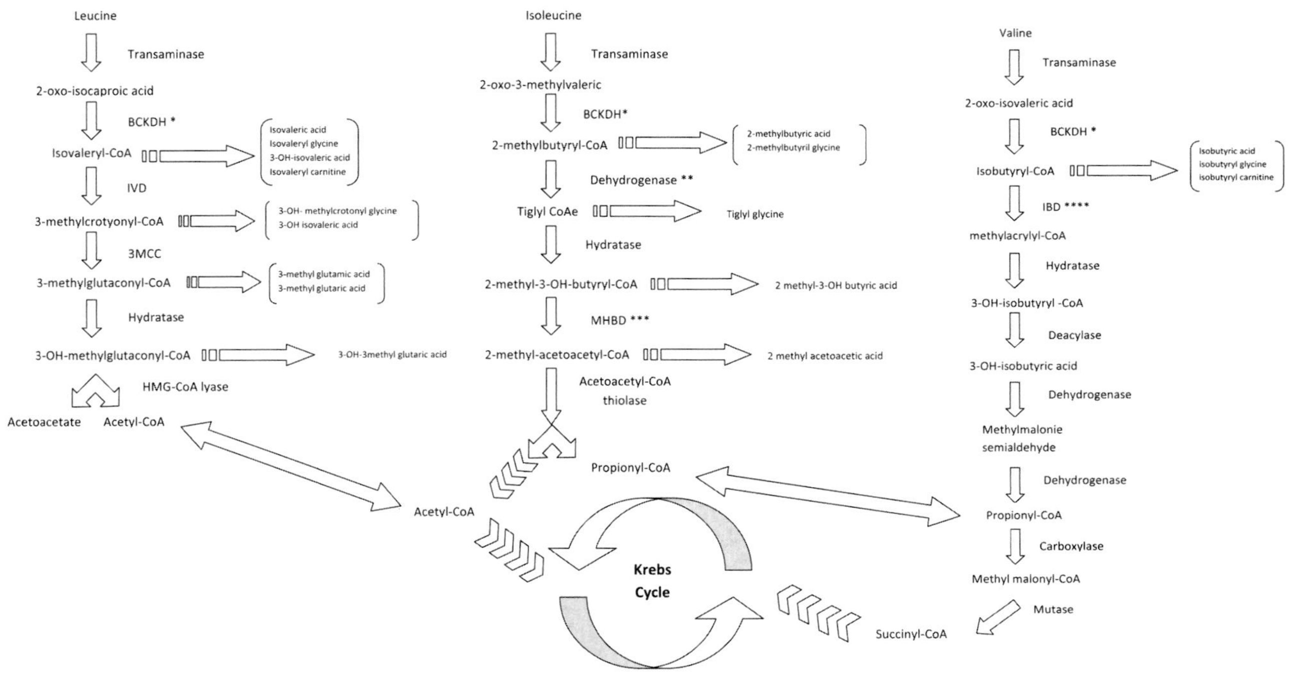

FIGURE 19.2 Pathways of branched-chain amino acids. *Branched-chain ketoacid dehydrogenase; **2-methylbutyryl Co-A dehydrogenase; ***2-methyl-3OH-butyryl Co-A dehydrogenase; ****Isobutyryl-Co-A dehydrogenase.

or chronic symptoms such as neurodevelopmental delay, recurrent vomiting, and ataxia. The recurrent attacks are usually triggered by catabolic stress such as infections or increased intake of protein rich foods. Patients may be entirely normal between attacks. These symptoms are associated with metabolic acidosis, ketosis, and hyperammonemia as seen in the neonatal onset form (5).

Early diagnosis and treatment is crucial for a better outcome. Patients who are not diagnosed and treated effectively develop mental retardation, seizures, and acute and progressive dystonic syndrome that result from insult to basal ganglia.

Magnetic resonance spectroscopy may show a decrease N-acetylaspartate (NAA) (a sign of neuronal injury) and increase lactate. Magnetic resonance imaging (MRI) findings of PA and MMA are brain atrophy and abnormal myelination.

Urine organic acid analysis and plasma acylcarnitine profile are the first line diagnostic tests that identify abnormal metabolites (7). Plasma amino acid analysis shows nonspecific abnormalities such as hyperglycinemia and hyperalaninemia. In PA, urine organic acid analysis shows elevated levels of propionic acid, propionylglycine, tyglylglycine, 3-hydroxyl-propionate, and methylcitrate.

Plasma acylcarnitine analysis shows elevated level of propionylcarnitine (7). Molecular genetic testing can be used to confirm the diagnosis. Propionyl CoA carboxylase enzyme activity can be measured in fibroblasts.

Patients with MMA show the same abnormal biochemical findings seen in PA patients in addition to elevated plasma and urine MMA level. Activity of methylmalonyl CoA mutase (Mut) can be assessed indirectly by measurement of incorporation of [1-14C] propionate into cellular macromolecules (C14 propionate tracer assay). Complementation analysis can determine the enzymatic block using heterokaryon rescue or enzymatic cross-correction (8).

B—Ketosis Without Acidosis or Hyperammonemia

Maple syrup urine disease: MSUD is caused by a deficiency of branched chain alpha ketoacid dehydrogenase (BCKD), which is the second enzyme in the degradation pathway of leucine, isoleucine, and valine (branched-chain amino acids [BCAAs]) (Figure 19.2). Accumulation of BCCAs, primarily leucine, is toxic and causes encephalopathy. Based on the clinical presentation, residual enzyme activity and thiamin responsiveness, 5 phenotypes have been described: (1) Classical MSUD is the most severe form and patients present with encephalopathy in the newborn period, (2) Intermediate MSUD with neurologic symptoms later in life but only rarely AME, (3) Intermittent MSUD with encephalopathy under catabolic stress intermittently, (4) Thiamine responsive MSUD, and (5) dihydrolipoamide dehydrogenase (E3) deficient MSUD with lactic acidosis and elevations of BCAAs and branched-chain keto-acid (BCKAs) (9). It is a combined deficiency of BCKD, PDH, and alpha ketoglutarate dehydrogenase complexes because E3 is a common component of these 3 enzymes (10).

Clinical and biochemical findings: Affected neonates with classical MSUD present with lethargy, poor suck, vomiting, and irritability after symptom-free interval of 2 to 3 days. If not diagnosed and treated, they develop opisthotonos, bicycling movements, and coma within 4 to 5 days. During acute encephalopathy, the EEG may demonstrate a V comb-like rhythm of 5 to 9 Hz spindle-like sharp waves over the central regions that are believed to be characteristic of MSUD.

Patients with MSUD do not have metabolic acidosis, hyperammonemia, or lactic acidosis (except E3 defects) but develop ketosis and ketonuria. Maple syrup odor is present in patients' urine and cerumen. The presence of 2-ketoacids can be detected in urine with the 2, 4-dinitrophenylhydrazine (DNPH) test. Plasma amino acid analysis shows an elevation of the BCAA; the presence of alloisoleucine is a definitive marker of MSUD (10).

Patients with intermediate MSUD have very high levels of BCAAs and present with developmental delay and/or seizures in the first years of life. Episodes of AME are rare in this form.

Patients with intermittent MSUD have normal early development and have normal BCAAs when they are well. They present with episodic ataxia, lethargy, and acute encephalopathy triggered by stress such as fever, infection, surgery in the first years of life. During metabolic crisis, plasma amino acids and urine organic acid profile show elevated levels of BCAAs and BCKAs.

C—Acidosis, Ketosis, or Hypoglycemia Accompanied by Neurologic Deterioration

Glutaric aciduria type I: Glutaric aciduria (GA) type I is caused by a deficiency of glutaryl CoA dehydrogenase enzyme, which is involved in the catabolism of L-lysine, L-hydroxylysine, and tryptophan. Early clinical diagnosis and treatment is important to prevent irreversible brain damage (11).

Clinical and biochemical findings: Patients are usually asymptomatic in the first year of life. Macrocepahly is a common finding. Soft neurologic signs such as jitteriness and irritability may be present. The most common presentation is acute encephalopathy precipitated by an intercurrent illness such as fever, diarrhea, or other stresses such as immunizations or surgery in a relatively healthy 1 to 2 year of child. Patients develop sudden onset of hypotonia, loss of head control, seizures, opisthotonos, fisting, rigidity, and dystonia. The sequela of the acute encephalopathic crisis is bilateral neuronal degeneration of the caudate and putamen, and subsequently, a movement disorder. Patients are at risk for recurrent metabolic crisis during fever or respiratory or gastrointestinal illnesses (11).

During acute metabolic crisis patients can have acidosis, ketosis, hypoglycemia, hyperammonemia, and mild liver disease (Reye-like syndrome). Plasma amino acid profile is normal. Plasma acylcarnitine analysis shows elevated glutarylcarnitine (C5-DC). Urine organic acid analysis shows elevated levels of glutaric acid and 3-hydroxyglutaric acid (12).

MRI shows frontotemporal atrophy, collections of fluid over frontal lobe and at the base of brain, and arachnoid or subdural cysts. The fluid collection between the brain and cranium stretches bridging vessels, making them vulnerable to a minor trauma, so subdural hematomas may occur (11).

It is very important to prevent catabolism during intercurrent illnesses because it is the only way to reduce the frequency of acute encephalopathic crisis and irreversible striatal injury. Emergency treatment follows the basic treatment principles of metabolic diseases of the "intoxication" type, which is discussed below.

D—Hyperammonemia

The breakdown of proteins and other nitrogen-containing molecules results in the production of free ammonia. The urea cycle (Figure 19.3) detoxifies ammonia by converting it to urea. Urea cycle disorders are the most common cause of hyperammonemia, but other IEMs, especially organic acidemias, can cause a comparable derangement (Table 19.3). The pathogenesis for hyperammonemia in some of these conditions is not fully understood.

Urea cycle disorders: The urea cycle includes 5 enzymes: (1) carbamyl phosphate synthetase (CPS),

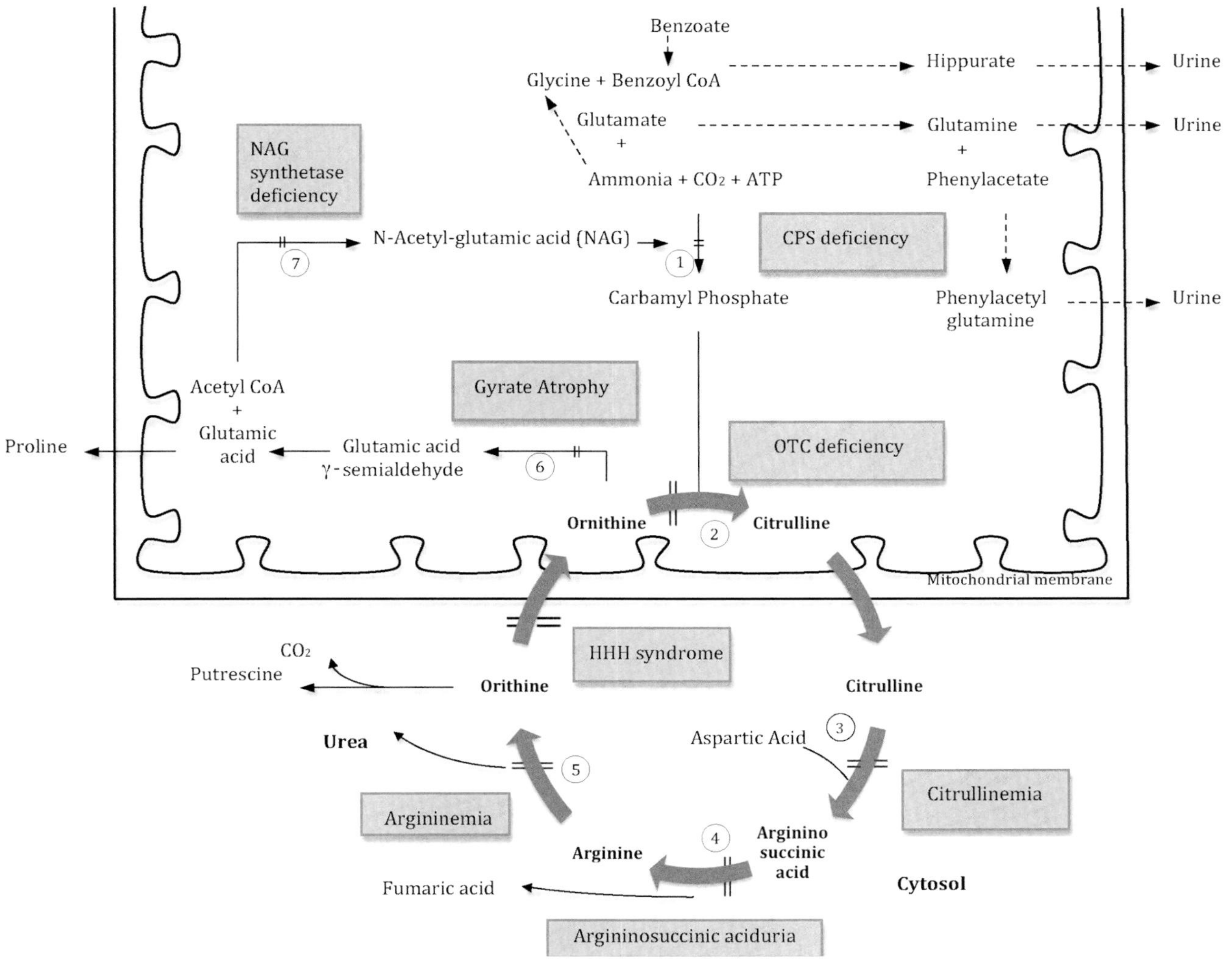

FIGURE 19.3 The urea cycle
Reactions shown with *interrupted arrows* are the alternate pathways for the disposal of ammonia. Enzymes: (1) carbamyl phosphate synthetase (CPS), (2) ornithine transcarbamylase (OTC), (3) argininosuccinic acid synthetase (AS), (4) argininosuccinic acid lyase (AL), (5) arginase, (6) ornithine 5-aminotransferase, (7) *N*-acetylglutamate (NAG) synthetase. Abbreviation: HHH syndrome, hyperammonemia-hyperornithinemia-homocitrullinemia syndrome.

(2) ornithine transcarbamylase (OTC), (3) argininosuccinate synthetase (AS), (4) argininosuccinate lyase (AL), and (5) arginase. In addition to these enzymes, *N*-acetylglutamate (NAG) synthetase is needed to produce NAG, a cofactor of the CPS enzyme (13).

Clinical and biochemical findings: The clinical symptoms may appear in the neonatal period, or they may appear any time thereafter with varying degrees of severity. In the neonatal onset form, the affected neonate is normal at birth but presents with a sepsis-like picture by 24 to 48 hours of life. The baby stops feeding, begins vomiting, and displays lethargy that quickly progresses to coma. Physical examination may reveal hepatomegaly in addition to the neurologic signs of coma. The encephalopathy is characterized by increased intracranial pressure with a bulging fontanel and dilated pupils, and seizures are common (14).

The late-onset form may present in infancy, childhood, and adulthood with vomiting and neurologic abnormalities such as ataxia, mental confusion, agitation, irritability, and combativeness. These manifestations usually occur during a high protein intake or catabolic stress such as infections.

■ **Table 19.3** Inborn Errors of Metabolism Causing Hyperammonemia

Urea Cycle Disorders
- N-acetylglutamate synthetase
- CPS
- OTC
- AS
- AL
- Arginase

Organic Acidemias
- Propionic acidemia
- Methylmalonic acidemia
- Multiple carboxylase deficiency
- 3-hydroxy-3-methylglutaric aciduria

Fatty Acid Oxidation Defects
- Medium chain acyl CoA dehydrogenase deficiency
- Multiple acyl CoA dehydrogenase deficiency

Other Inborn Errors of Metabolism
- Lysinuric protein intolerance
- HHH syndrome
- Pyruvate carboxylase deficiency
- Congenital hyperinsulinism with hyperammonemia
- Transient hyperammonemia of the newborn

Abbreviations: AL, argininosuccinate lyase; AS, argininosuccinate synthetase; CPS, carbamyl phosphate synthetase; HHH, hyperammonemia-hyperornithinemia-homocitrullinemia; OTC, ornithine transcarbamylase.

Routine laboratory tests often are normal. The blood urea is usually very low. Hyperammonemia may stimulate the brain stem respiratory center, leading to respiratory alkalosis. There may be mild increases in serum transaminases (alanine aminotransferase (ALT), aspartate aminotransferase (AST)), since ammonia can cause swelling of hepatic mitochondria (14).

It is imperative to measure plasma ammonia, amino acids, acylcarnitine levels, and urine organic acid levels in any ill infant whose clinical manifestations cannot be explained by sepsis. Brain ultrasound or computed tomographic imaging may show edema.

In infants with organic acidemias, hyperammonemia is commonly associated with high anion gap acidosis and ketonuria as discussed above.

The measurement of ammonia can be difficult with false elevations noted frequently. Ammonia should be measured in a free-flow blood sample and transferred to a laboratory on ice for immediate analysis to avoid artificial production from blood cells. In children and adults, the plasma ammonia concentration is usually less than 35 µmol/L. Blood concentrations in healthy newborns often can be as high as 100 µmol/L in a full-term baby and 150 µmol/L in a premature infant. The plasma ammonia concentration in the ill infant is usually more than 200 µmol/L.

A diagnostic algorithm for hyperammonemia is presented in Figure 19.1. The age of onset of symptoms, and presence or absence of acidosis help physicians to arrive at a diagnosis of hyperammonemia. Plasma amino acid analysis can help the diagnosis of different urea cycle disorders. Patients with deficiencies of CPS, OTC, or NAG synthetase have elevations in plasma glutamine and alanine with concurrent decrements in citrulline and arginine (14). A marked increase in urinary orotic acid in patients with OTC deficiency differentiates this defect from CPS deficiency. Differentiation in CPS vs. N-acetylglutamate (NAG) synthetase may require an assay of the respective enzymes, or mutation analysis. Clinical improvement occurring after oral administration of carbamylglutamate, however, may suggest NAG synthetase deficiency. Patients with deficiencies of AS, AL, or arginase have marked increases in the plasma levels of citrulline, argininosuccinic acid, or arginine, respectively (14).

General Aspects of Treatment of "Intoxication Type" Metabolic Disorders

The following principles of management are for all the disorders discussed above (group 2, subgroups A–D).

Management of acute metabolic decompensation: When IEMs are suspected, immediate treatment should be initiated even if the diagnosis is not yet established. AME, either at the onset or during a relapse of metabolic decompensation, is an emergency and patients should be managed in the intensive care unit. Delay in starting the emergency treatment results in rapid progression to encephalopathic crisis and irreversible brain damage. Serious neurologic damage is dependent on the duration of hyperammonemia and is very likely in infants with severe elevations in blood ammonia (> 300 µmol/L) for more than 12 hours.

There are 2 main goals of the acute treatment: (1) prevent catabolism by providing an adequate caloric intake and (2) remove toxic metabolites such as ammonia, organic acids, or leucine as quickly as possible.

After the first suspicion of an organic acidemia, urea cycle defect, or MSUD, protein intake should be discontinued and intravenous (IV) fluids containing glucose (glucose infusion rate at 10–15 mg/kg/min), electrolytes, and lipid (1–3 g/kg/day) should be started. It is essential to provide at least 1.5 times normal energy and fluid intake based on the patient's age. It is important to minimize exposure to hypotonic fluids and maintain sodium levels of 138 to 145 mEq/L. Insulin can be added to keep the blood glucose levels below 150 mg/dL. Whenever possible, protein-free formula with high calories can be started via nasogastric or gastrostomy tube. The total base deficit should be calculated and corrected aggressively using IV bicarbonate solutions. In MSUD, parenteral nutrition consisting of BCAA-free L-amino acid mixture can be used in combination with glucose, lipid, electrolyte, and vitamins. The plasma levels of isoleucine and valine drop much faster than that of leucine and it is important to supplement isoleucine and valine (20–120 mg/kg/day) after 1 day of MSUD treatment. Maintaining the normal levels of isoleucine and valine facilitates the normalization of plasma levels of leucine (9).

In critically ill patients with severe acidosis, hyperammonemia, or high leucine level who are unresponsive to treatment within the first few hours, hemodialysis should be initiated. All neonatal patients with severe neonatal hyperammonemic coma (plasma levels greater than 600 µmol/L) should be hemodialyzed. Continuous venovenous hemofiltration is more effective in ammonia, BCAAs/BCKAs, or organic acid removal than peritoneal dialysis.

Scavenger therapy offers an important way to decrease ammonia in a form other than urea. Compounds such as sodium benzoate and phenylacetate (250–500 mg/kg/day) lower blood ammonia by forming complexes with glycine and glutamine, respectively (13). Both are available in oral and IV forms.

Arginine is a nonessential amino acid in healthy individuals, who form it in the urea cycle, but it is essential in most patients with urea cycle disorders (except arginase deficiency). For this reason, patients with urea cycle defects are likely to need a supplementation of arginine (210–660 mg/kg/day) to maintain the levels within normal range (50–200 µmol/L). Patients with OTC deficiency benefit from supplementation with citrulline (170 mg/kg/day). Administration of arginine or citrulline is contraindicated in patients with arginase deficiency (13).

Sodium benzoate, sodium phenylacetate, and arginine can be administered together for maximal therapeutic effect. A priming dose of these compounds is followed by continuous infusion until recovery from the acute hyperammonemic crisis (Table 19.4). The recommended therapeutic doses of both compounds deliver a substantial amount of sodium to the patient that should be calculated as part of the daily sodium requirement. A commercial, parenteral preparation of sodium benzoate plus sodium phenylacetate is available (Ammonul). Sodium benzoate and sodium phenylbutyrate can also be used if hyperammonemia is persistent in organic acidemias. Recently, carbamylglutamate (50–100 mg/kg/day) has been shown to improve hyperammonemia in PA patients (15).

Vitamin therapy: Some forms of organic acidemias (usually late onset forms) are responsive to cofactor therapy. Biotin (cofactor of propionyl CoA carboxylase) 20 mg/day/oral and vitamin B_{12} (cofactor of MMA mutase) 1 mg/day/intramuscular should be started in all newly diagnosed patients in order to test their effect on stimulating the residual enzyme activity. Thiamin 100 to 300 mg/day/oral should be tried in all MSUD patients

■ Table 19.4 Treatment of Acute Hyperammonemia in an Infant

Medication	Loading dose/infusion over 1–2 hrs	Maintenance Dose/ Continuous infusion—24h
Sodium Benzoate*	250 mg/kg (5.5 g/m²)	250 mg/day (5.5 g/m²)
Sodium Phenylacetate*	250 mg/kg (5.5 g/m²)	250 mg/day (5.5 g/m²)
Arginine hydrochloride** (10%)	210–660 mg/kg/day (4.0–12.0 g/m²)	210–660 mg/kg (4.0–12.0 g/m²)

*These compounds are prepared as a 1% to 2% solution (10% glucose) for intravenous use. Sodium from these drugs should be included as part of the daily sodium requirement.
**The higher dose is recommended in the treatment of patients with citrullinemia and argininosuccinic aciduria. Arginine is not recommended in patients with arginase deficiency and in those whose hyperammonemia is caused by organic acidemia.

for 2 to 3 weeks to determine the responsiveness to thiamin (9). Although riboflavin responsiveness is an extreme rarity, it can be tried (50–300 mg/day/oral) in patients with GA type I (1). Carnitine supplementation (100 mg/kg/day IV or oral) helps to amplify physiologic detoxifying mechanism and prevent secondary carnitine deficiency.

In order to control brain edema, it is important to maintain normal sodium levels at the upper end of normal. Five percent saline can be used to replace urinary sodium losses and keep serum sodium between 140 and 145 mEq/L. Furosemide can prevent water retention, and urine specific gravity should remain below 1.010. Mannitol can be used to manage severe intracranial pressure elevation.

Long-term therapy: The principles of long-term treatment are to (1) decrease the accumulation of toxic metabolites by limiting certain amino acids which, if present in excess, are toxic or precursors of organic acids, (2) provide other essential/nonessential amino acids, and (3) provide adequate calories in diet. In general, all patients with urea cycle defects, regardless of the enzymatic defect, require some degree of protein restriction (1–2 g/kg/24 h). The concentrations of plasma amino acids should be monitored closely in order to prevent amino acid deficiencies. Long-term therapy should be directed by a metabolic physician working with a nutritionist.

In organic acidemias, during sick days complete protein intake should be decreased and special formula which does not contain the offending amino acids and protein-free food intake should be increased. In urea cycle defects, protein-free formula or food can be given during sick days for 24 to 48 hours. It is important to promote anabolism by providing adequate calories in diet. Catabolic states (infections, fasting) triggering metabolic decompensation should be avoided or treated vigorously.

Valproic acid should not be used because it may precipitate acute hyperammonemic attacks and it conjugates to carnitine, decreasing the availability of the later.

In patients with defects in the urea cycle, chronic administration of benzoate (250–500 mg/kg/24 h), phenylacetate or phenylbutyrate (250–500 mg/kg/24 h), and arginine (200–400 mg/kg/24 h) or citrulline (in patients with OTC deficiency, 200–400 mg/kg/24 h) is effective in maintaining blood ammonia levels within the normal range.

■ ENERGY DEFICIENCY (GROUP 3) DISORDERS ARRANGED BY BIOCHEMICAL FINDINGS (E–F)

E—Hypoglycemia With No or Minimal Ketonuria

Hypoketotic hypoglycemia is always abnormal and *fatty acid beta oxidation* (FAO) defects should be suspected. FAO fuels the synthesis of ketone bodies, which are utilized as an alternative source of energy by extrahepatic organs especially during periods of fasting or stress. There are 11 protein defects identified in FAO pathway in humans (16).

Clinical and biochemical findings: FAO disorders generally classified in 3 groups based on the organ system most involved: (1) hepatic, (2) cardiac, and (3) muscle phenotype (17). The hepatic group is mainly characterized by recurrent Reye-like illness including hypoketotic hypoglycemia leading to encephalopathy. Metabolic acidosis is unusual unless lactic acidosis occurs due to terminal illness. Hyperammonemia and liver dysfunction are usually observed. Liver biopsy may show micro or macrosteatosis. This presentation can be seen in patients with medium chain acyl-CoA dehydrogenase (MCAD), infantile carnitine palmitoyltransferase II (CPT-II), hypoglycemic form of very long chain acyl-CoA dehydrogenase (VLCAD), translocase, CPT-I deficiencies, or carnitine uptake defect. Patients with severe forms of CPT-II and VLCAD deficiencies can present with cardiomyopathy, myopathy, and liver disease in the newborn period. Muscular phenotype (CPT-II, VLCAD, trifunctional protein, long chain 3-hydroxyacyl-CoA dehydrogenase [LCHAD] deficiency) usually includes hypotonia, and recurrent rhabdomyolysis that occur during intercurrent illness or stress (17).

MCAD is the most common FAO disorder that can cause encephalopathy but other defects such as carnitine uptake defect, CPT-II deficiency, VLCAD deficiency, or LCHAD deficiency can cause hypoglycemia and present with acute encephalopathy. AME resembling Reye syndrome is a common presentation of MCAD deficiency. Affected children are usually well until they present with an episode of vomiting and lethargy precipitated by an intercurrent illness and poor feeding in the first 2 years of life. Lethargy progresses rapidly to stupor and coma. Hepatomegaly with evidence of hepatocellular dysfunction, hypotonia, hypoketotic hypoglycemia, and mild hyperammonemia are common findings during acute metabolic decompensation.

Acute encephalopathy can also develop with the absence of hypoglycemia or hepatocellular dysfunction suggesting that accumulation of fatty acid intermediates may be toxic and play a role in the pathogenesis. Plasma acylcarnitine analysis show elevated levels of hexanoyl carnitine (C6), octanoyl carnitine (C8), and decanoyl carnitine (C10). Urine organic acid analysis shows the presence of dicarboxylic acids (adipic, suberic, and sebacic acids) and hexanoylglycine (18). MCAD is an autosomal recessive disorder and A985G missense mutation is the most common disease causing mutation in Caucasians.

Conditions such as *glycogen storage disorders* or *gluconeogenesis defects* can present in infancy with altered mental status that may rapidly progress to coma and seizures. The presence of hypoglycemia generally directs the diagnostic workup.

Defects in ketone synthesis (*3-OH-3-methylglutaryl CoA synthase and 3-OH 3-methyl glutaryl CoA lyase deficiencies*) also present with episodes of hypoketotic hypoglycemia often with coma triggered by prolonged fasting or stress (18).

The mainstay of treatment of acute illnesses in patients with FAO defects is IV glucose at an infusion rate of 10 mg/kg/min or greater. Insulin can be added to maintain the glucose level less than 150 mg/dl. The goal is to provide sufficient glucose to stimulate insulin secretion that will suppress fatty acid oxidation and will block adipose tissue lipolysis. IV lipid is contraindicated.

F—Lactic Acidosis

Abnormal accumulation of lactate is one of the most common causes of metabolic acidosis in children. In the majority of cases, lactic acidosis is caused by tissue hypoxia, and it occurs in any situation in which the delivery of oxygen to tissues is impaired, such as shock, heart failure, congenital heart disease, or pulmonary hypertension (19). Lactic acidosis from hypoxemia may be severe, and it is associated with elevated lactate/pyruvate ratio in plasma. The cause of the lactic acidosis is obvious, and the acidosis is generally reversed within minutes to a few hours by correction of the hypoxic state. In contrast, lactic acidosis caused by IEM cannot be corrected easily. The lactic acidosis associated with cardiomyopathy presents a special diagnostic challenge because the cardiomyopathy itself may be due to an IEM.

A clinical classification of lactic acidosis and diagnostic algorithm are presented in Table 19.5 and Figure 19.4. Although diagnosing the underlying defect is usually a lengthy process and requires enzyme analysis in fibroblasts, tissue samples, or DNA analysis, the initial workup should include blood lactate, pyruvate, comprehensive metabolic panel, creatine kinase (CK), uric acid, 3-hydroxybutyrate, acetoacetate, plasma amino acids,

■ **Table 19.5** Causes of Lactic Acidosis

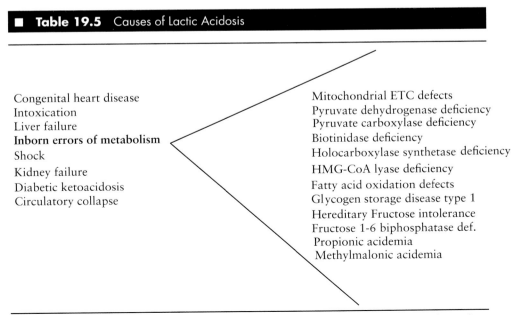

Congenital heart disease
Intoxication
Liver failure
Inborn errors of metabolism
Shock
Kidney failure
Diabetic ketoacidosis
Circulatory collapse

Mitochondrial ETC defects
Pyruvate dehydrogenase deficiency
Pyruvate carboxylase deficiency
Biotinidase deficiency
Holocarboxylase synthetase deficiency
HMG-CoA lyase deficiency
Fatty acid oxidation defects
Glycogen storage disease type 1
Hereditary Fructose intolerance
Fructose 1-6 biphosphatase def.
Propionic acidemia
Methylmalonic acidemia

Abbreviations: ETC, electron transport chain; HMG-CoA lyase, 3-hydroxy-3-methylglutaryl-CoA lyase.

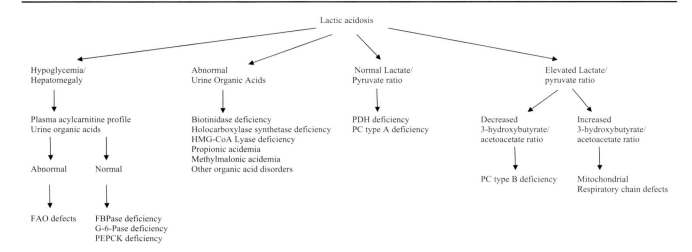

FIGURE 19.4 Algorithm for evaluation of a patient with lactic acidosis.

Abbreviations: FBPase, fructose-1, 6-bisphosphatase; G-6-Pase, glucose-6-phosphatase; HMG-CoA lyase, 3-hydroxy-3-methylglutaryl-coenzyme A lyase; PC, pyruvate carboxylase; PDH, pyruvate dehydrogenase; PEPCK, phosphoenolpyruvate carboxykinase.

plasma acylcarnitines, and urine organic acids. Brain MRI and magnetic resonance spectroscopy (MRS) are needed to pinpoint the diagnosis.

Lactate is always produced by reduction of pyruvate through lactate dehydrogenase and is removed by a reversal of this process. The oxidative metabolism of pyruvate is through PDH complex, the Krebs cycle, and the respiratory chain, whereas anabolic utilization proceeds primarily through PC. Pyruvate and lactate are the end products of glycolysis, the major source of energy when availability of oxygen is low. A defect in any of these pathways results in inadequate removal of pyruvate and lactate from circulation and leads to lactic acidosis (20).

Lactic acidosis can occur as a consequence of increased pyruvate production which is seen in patients with glycogen storage disease type 1 or hereditary fructose intolerance. It can also be caused by decreased oxidation of pyruvate. Pyruvate is oxidized to acetyl-CoA by the enzyme PDH or it is carboxylated to oxaloacetate which fuels the Krebs cycle.

Among IEMs, *PDH deficiency* is the one of the most common disorders causing lactic acidosis. The PDH complex is made up of 4 proteins: 2-ketoacid dehydrogenase (E1), dihyrolipoamide acyltransferase (E2), E3, and protein X (2). The most common defect is in the E1 component.

Clinical and biochemical findings of PDH deficiency: In its most severe form, patients present with a severe lactic acidosis and hypotonia at birth, and die within a few weeks or months. Some patient with PDH deficiency show subtle dysmorphic facial features that may resemble those of fetal alcohol syndrome (20). In PDH deficiency, plasma lactate levels are elevated and may worsen with carbohydrate ingestion. The lactate/pyruvate ratio is characteristically normal. The plasma alanine level is elevated due to increased pyruvate concentrations. Urine organic acids show elevated lactate level. The diagnosis is confirmed by measuring PDH enzyme in fresh lymphocytes, fibroblasts, or muscle. MRI findings correlate with the degenerative neuropathologic findings of subacute necrotizing encephalopathy. Some patients have congenital malformations of the brain, including agenesis of the corpus callosum.

There is no specific treatment for PDH deficiency. Some children improve on a ketogenic diet. When IV hydration is needed, it is important to keep the glucose concentration of IV fluids low (D5%) in order to prevent elevation of lactate. Some cases respond to thiamine (cofactor of E1 component) and it should be given in very large doses (300–2,000 mg/day) for all newly diagnosed cases, with concurrent monitoring of clinical symptoms and lactate levels (1).

Lactic acidosis is also a prominent feature of *PC* (a biotin dependent enzyme) deficiency, which presents in 2 ways.

Clinical and biochemical findings of PC deficiency: In the simple (type A) form of PC, patients present with mild to moderate lactic acidosis and developmental delay in the first months of life. Plasma amino acid analysis shows elevated levels of alanine and proline. The lactate to pyruvate ratio is normal. Urine organic acid analysis shows elevated lactate and 2-ketoglutarate. In the more complex (B) form of PC, patients present with a severe lactic acidosis and hypotonia at birth. Hyperammonemia, citrullinemia, and hyperlysinemia can also be observed. The lactate to pyruvate ratio is elevated. Patients usually die within the first months of life. Patients with both of these forms have hepatomegaly associated with lipid accumulation, and abnormal brain MRI findings including poor myelination and periventricular cysts. Despite the central role of PC enzyme in gluconeogenesis, hypoglycemia is rarely a prominent feature of this enzyme deficiency. The increase of blood lactate is usually more pronounced during fasting and improves after ingestion of carbohydrate (20).

The diagnosis is confirmed by measuring PC enzyme activity in fibroblast or by DNA analysis.

Patients with acute attacks of lactic acidosis can be treated with IV glucose (D10% or more). Persistent lactic acidosis may be corrected by bicarbonate. IV aspartate or citrate as an alternate source of 4-carbon intermediates may be beneficial.

Multiple carboxylase deficiency, either because of holocarboxylase synthetase or biotinidase deficiencies, presents with lactic acidosis due to the PC enzyme deficiency, 1 of the 4 biotin depended carboxylases. *Holocarboxylase synthetase deficiency* presents in the first weeks of life with poor feeding, hypotonia, seizures, metabolic acidosis, and hyperammonemia. *Biotinidase deficiency* manifests with seizures, developmental delay, dermatitis, alopecia in later infancy. Acute metabolic crisis with metabolic acidosis, respiratory distress, laryngeal stridor, developmental regression, ataxia, and lethargy can also be seen. The urine organic acids show elevated levels of lactate, methylcitrate, propionylglycine, 3-hydroxypropionate, 3-methylcrotonylglycine. Plasma acylcarnitine analysis shows elevated levels of propionylcarnitine (C3), 3-methylcrotonylcarnitine (C5-OH). The diagnosis is confirmed by the enzyme assay and DNA analysis. Both enzyme deficiencies can be treated with large dose of biotin (10 mg/day for biotinidase deficiency, 20–40 mg/day for holocarboxylase synthetase deficiency) (1).

Mitochondrial disorders are a clinically heterogeneous group of disorders that are caused by dysfunction of mitochondrial respiratory chain. Some mitochondrial disorders affect single organs but many involve multiple organ systems. Common clinical features include ptosis, developmental regression, seizures, external ophthalmoplegia, optic atrophy, pigmentary retinopathy, exercise intolerance, cardiomyopathy, deafness, fluctuating encephalopathy, strokelike episodes, ataxia (21). Some affected individuals have a cluster of clinical features that fall into one clinical syndrome, such as Kearns-Sayre syndrome, myoclonic epilepsy with ragged-red fibers, mitochondrial encephalomyopathy with lactic acidosis and strokelike episodes, or Leigh syndrome. However, there is considerable clinical variability in patients even with the same defects. The diagnosis of mitochondrial disorders are challenging and comprehensive workup including cerebrospinal fluid (CSF) amino acids, lactate, pyruvate, brain MRI and MRS, muscle biopsy for histopathology, and electron transport chain studies are needed. Patients with findings of a specific mitochondrial disorder can be diagnosed by molecular genetic testing. There is no specific treatment for mitochondrial diseases and the management is mainly supportive (21).

■ SEIZURES

G—Isolated Persistent Seizures

Seizures are not an isolated finding in many IEMs as discussed above, but there are some IEMs that present with "isolated" seizures and encephalopathy (22). For example: seizures are the main and only symptom in nonketotic hyperglycinemia (NKH), pyridoxine dependent seizures, sulfite oxidase (SO) deficiency, molybdenum cofactor deficiency, folinic acid responsive seizures, GLUT-1 deficiency, cerebral folate deficiency, 4-aminobutyrate aminotransferase deficiency, congenital neuronal ceroid lipofuscinosis, dihydropyrimidine dehydrogenase deficiency, creatine deficiency syndromes, and serine biogenesis defects.

Routine biochemical tests such as comprehensive metabolic panel, urine analysis, or ammonia level do not help physicians identify these disorders. Some may have findings of hypoxic ischemic encephalopathy on brain MRI, making accurate diagnosis difficult.

Table 19.6 provides a diagnostic evaluation. It includes step I and II tests to exclude defects in group 2 (intoxication type), and 3 (energy defects) categories and step III more specific test to rule out the disorders causing isolated seizures listed above. It is important to know that this diagnostic schema cannot rule out all metabolic disorders.

■ **Table 19.6** Initial Approach to Diagnosis of Inborn Errors of Metabolism in Neonatal Seizures

Step I
CMP
Ammonia
Check newborn screen
Step II
Plasma Amino acids
Plasma Acylcarnitines
Urine Organic Acids
Lactate, Pyruvate
Step III
Total Homocysteine
Pipecolic acid
CSF studies:
- Amino acids
- Lactate, Pyruvate
- Glucose
- Neurotransmitters

Urine
- Thiosulfate
- S-sulfocysteine
- Guanidinoacetate /Creatine
- Creatine/Creatinine
- α-AASA

Abbreviations: α-AASA, α-aminoadipic semialdehyde; CMP, comprehensive metabolic panel; CSF, cerebrospinal fluid.

Pyridoxine-dependent seizures: Pyridoxine-dependent seizures are due to the deficiency of α-aminoadipic semialdehyde (α-AASA) dehydrogenase, also known as antiquitin (23). This enzyme in the lysine degradation pathway converts α-AASA to L-2-aminoadipic acid. The deficiency of α-AASA dehydrogenase results in accumulation of α-AASA and pipecolic acid in body fluids, resulting in a severe secondary pyridoxal-5 phosphate (P5P) deficiency. P5P is a cofactor of various enzymes in the central nervous system and its deficiency causes seizures due to a perturbation of the metabolism of cerebral amino acids and neurotransmitters (24).

Clinical and biochemical findings: Patients generally present with seizures very shortly after birth or in the prenatal period, although atypical cases with late onset seizures have also been described. Almost all seizure types have been described, both generalized and partial. Some seizures may be completely or partially responsive

to standard antiepileptic drugs at first but become more difficult to control as the child ages.

Testing for serum, urine, and CSF α-AASA levels as well as specific genetic testing for ALDH7A1 is now commercially available, and thus a trial of pyridoxine withdrawal is no longer necessary to make the diagnosis of pyridoxine dependent seizures (25). If a therapeutic trial with pyridoxine will be done, plasma and urine samples for α-AASA should always be collected before the trial. If the patient is already receiving pyridoxine, genetic testing for ALDH7A1 can be performed.

All patients with unexplained treatment refractory neonatal seizures should be given a pyridoxine trial of 100 mg (about 30 mg/kg) IV while undergoing EEG monitoring if possible. There may not be an initial EEG response so it is important to continue the same dose at least 3 more days to assess the response. With the availability of specific genetic testing it is generally not necessary to perform a trial withdrawal of pyridoxine, and in fact this should be avoided if possible to prevent potential harm to the patient. If the diagnosis is confirmed, pyridoxine supplementation should be continued indefinitely. Gallagher and colleagues recommend consideration of treatment with both pyridoxine and folinic acid in patients with α-AASA dehydrogenase deficiency (26).

Folinic acid responsive seizures: Recent evidence suggests that most if not all cases of folinic acid responsive seizures are genetically and biochemically indistinguishable from pyridoxine dependent seizures, as both are associated with elevations of α-AASA and mutations in ALDH7A1 (26). It is recommended that patients with a clinical response to folinic acid undergo diagnostic testing as above for pyridoxine-dependent seizures and be treated simultaneously with folinic acid and pyridoxine (26).

Nonketotic hyperglycinemia: It is due to a defect in glycine cleavage complex. Glycine functions as a neurotransmitter which has an inhibitory effect in the brainstem and spinal cord but an excitatory effect in the cerebral cortex (27).

Clinical and biochemical findings: There are several forms of NKH and the majority of patients have the neonatal onset (classic) form. The neonatal onset form manifests with first hours to days of life with lethargy, hypotonia, apnea, and seizures. Patients usually die in the newborn period. If they survive, they develop severe mental retardation and continue to have intractable seizures. EEG shows a burst suppression pattern that may evolve to a hypsarrythmia pattern. MRI may be normal or show agenesis or thinning of the corpus callosum. Patients may develop cerebral atrophy and decreased myelination later. Simultaneous CSF and plasma samples are necessary to calculate CSF/plasma glycine ratio. An increased CSF/plasma glycine ratio (> 0.08; N < 0.02) suggests NKH (27,28). There is no effective treatment for NKH. Sodium benzoate 250 to 750 mg/kg/day can reduce plasma and CSF glycine levels (29). Phenobarbital, benzodiazepines, phenytoin may decrease seizures in some patients. Valproate increases glycine concentration and is contraindicated in NKH.

Sulfite oxidase and molybdenum cofactor deficiency: The catabolism of sulfur containing amino acids, namely, methionine and cysteine contributes to the bulk of sulfite load that requires SO enzyme and molybdenum cofactor for oxidation to sulfates. In SO deficiency, sulfites cannot be converted to sulfates and accumulation of toxic sulfites leads to neurologic disease. SO is one of the three enzymes that require molybdenum as a cofactor (30).

Clinical and biochemical findings: Patients with SO deficiency present with intractable seizures in the newborn period. In infants, who survive, lens dislocation may occur after 8 weeks of life. SO deficiency should be considered in all newborns with intrauterine/neonatal seizures and hypoxic ischemic findings in MRI, especially if there is no obvious hypoxic insult at the delivery (31).

Molybdenum cofactor deficiency manifests with similar presentation, including intractable seizures, hypotonia, feeding difficulties, developmental delay and lens subluxation, and low uric acid levels. EEG usually shows burst suppression. MRI findings are white matter (periventricular, central, and U fibers) and gray matter signal changes with rapid progression to cystic lesions in a symmetric pattern in the frontal, parietal, and temporal lobes. MRI findings may mimic those of hypoxic ischemic encephalopathy, but findings are usually more severe and show no subsequent recovery. Neonates with hypoxic ischemic encephalopathy usually clinically stabilize in a couple of weeks after birth. Patients with SO deficiency or molybdenum cofactor deficiencies get worse. MRS shows findings of energetic and metabolic imbalance with elevation of lactate, myoinositol, and reduction of NAA. In contrast to hypoxic ischemic encephalopathy, there is increased peak of choline probably due to undeveloped myelination and breakdown of membranes as part of atrophic process.

The biochemical findings of SO deficiency and molybdenum cofactor deficiency are the presence of urinary sulfites, elevation of urinary thiosulfate levels, increased plasma and urinary s-sulfocysteine, and reduced plasma total homocysteine and cysteine levels. The treatment is supportive.

Alpers-Huttenlocher syndrome, one of the most severe phenotypes of polymerase gamma (POLG)-related disorders, is characterized by childhood-onset progressive and ultimately severe encephalopathy with intractable epilepsy and hepatic failure (32). Onset is usually between ages 2 and 4 years, but ranges from 1 month to 36 years. Some patients have developmental delay prior to presentation with encephalopathy with intractable epilepsy. Valproic acid and sodium divalproate (divalproex) can cause the rapid onset of liver failure and must be avoided. The diagnosis can be confirmed with identification of disease-causing POLG mutations.

■ **REFERENCES**

1. Fernandes J et al, eds. *Inborn Metabolic Diseases*. 4th ed. New York, NY: Springer; 2006.
2. Scriver CR, Beaudet AL, Sly WS, eds. *The Metabolic and Molecular Bases of Inherited Disease*. 6th ed. New York, NY: McGraw-Hill; 1995.
3. Ficicioglu C, An Haack K. Failure to thrive: when to suspect inborn errors of metabolism. *Pediatrics*. 2009;124(3): 972–979.
4. Blau N et al. *Guide to the Laboratory Diagnosis of Metabolic Diseases*. 2nd ed. Berlin, Germany: Springer; 2003.
5. Fenton WA, Gravel RA, Rosenblatt DS. Disorders of propionate and methylmalonate metabolism. In: Scriver C et al, eds. *Metabolic and Molecular Bases of Inherited Disease*. 8th ed. New York, NY: McGraw Hill; 2001:2165–2193.
6. Ozand P, Gascon G. Organic acidurias: a review. Part 1 and part 2. *J Child Neurol*. 1991;6:196–215, 288–303.
7. Nyhan WL, Gibson MK. Disorders of Valine-Isoleucine metabolism. In: Blau et al, eds. *Physician's Guide to the Laboratory Diagnosis of Metabolic Diseases*. 2nd ed. Berlin, Germany: Springer; 2003:191–213.
8. Gravel RA et al. Genetic complementation in heterokaryons of human fibroblasts defective in cobalamin metabolism. *Proc Natl Acad Sci U S A*. 1975;72(8):3181–3185.
9. Strauss KA et al. Classical maple syrup urine disease and brain development: principles of management and formula design. *Mol Genet Metab*. 2010;99:333–345.
10. Gibson MK et al. Disorders of leucine metabolism. In: Blau et al, eds. *Physician's Guide to the Laboratory Diagnosis of Metabolic Diseases*. 2nd ed. Berlin, Germany: Springer; 2003:165–189.
11. Koelker S et al. Guideline for the diagnosis and management of glutaryl-CoA dehydrogenase deficiency (glutaric aciduria type I). *J Inherit Metab Dis*. 2007;30:5–22.

12. Pryzyrembel H. Disorders of ornitine, lysine, and tryptophan. In: Blau et al. eds. *Physician's Guide to the Laboratory Diagnosis of Metabolic Diseases.* 2nd ed. Berlin, Germany: Springer; 2003:277–290.
13. Brusilow SW, Horwich AL. Urea cycle enzymes. In: Scriver C et al, eds. *Metabolic and Molecular Bases of Inherited Disease.* 8th ed. New York, NY: McGraw Hill; 2001:1909–1963.
14. Bachmann C. Inherited hyperammonemia. In: Blau et al, eds. *Physician's Guide to the Laboratory Diagnosis of Metabolic Diseases.* 2nd ed. Berlin, Germany: Springer; 2003:261–276.
15. Ah Mew N et al. *N*-carbamylglutamate augments ureagenesis and reduces ammonia and glutamine in propionic acidemia. *Pediatrics.* 2010;126(1):208–214.
16. Rinaldo P, Matern D, Bennett MJ. Fatty acid oxidation disorders. *Annu Rev Physiol.* 2002;64:477–502.
17. Rinaldo P, Raymond K, Al-Odaib A, Bennett MJ. Clinical and biochemical features of fatty acid oxidation disorders. *Curr Opin Pediatr.* 1998;10:615–621.
18. Duran M. disorders of mitochondrial fatty acid oxidation. In: Blau et al, eds. *Physician's Guide to the Laboratory Diagnosis of Metabolic Diseases.* 2nd ed. Berlin, Germany: Springer; 2003:309–334.
19. Stern HJ. Lactic acidosis in pediatrics: clinical and laboratory evaluation. *Ann Clin Biochem.* 1994;31:410–419.
20. De Meirleir L. Defects of pyruvate metabolism and the Krebs cycle. *J Child Neurol.* 2002;17:3526–3534.
21. Di Donato S. Multisystem manifestations of mitochondrial disorders. *J Neurol.* 2009;256(5):693–710.
22. Ficicioglu C, Bearden D. Isolated neonatal seizures: when to suspect inborn errors of metabolism. *Pediatr Neurol.* 2011;45(5):283–291.
23. Plecko B et al. Biochemical and molecular characterization of 18 patients with pyridoxine-dependent epilepsy and mutations of the antiquitin (ALDH7A1) gene. *Hum Mutat.* 2007:28(1):19–26.
24. Baxter, P. Pyridoxine-dependent and pyridoxine responsive seizures. *Dev Med Child Neurol.* 2001;43:416–420.
25. A Bok et al. Pyridoxine-dependent seizures in Dutch patients: diagnosis by elevated urinary alpha-aminoadipic semialdehyde levels. *Arch Dis Child.* 2007;92:687–689.
26. Gallagher RC et al. Folinic acid–responsive seizures are identical to pyridoxine-dependent epilepsy. *Ann Neurol.* 2009;65:550–556.
27. Hoover-Fong JE et al. Natural history of nonketotic hyperglycinemia in 65 patients. *Neurology.* 2004;63(10):1847–1853.
28. Applegarth DA, Toone JR. Nonketotic hyperglycinemia (glycine encephalopathy): laboratory diagnosis. *Mol Genet Metab.* 2001;74:139–146.
29. Van Hove JL et al. Benzoate treatment and the glycine index in nonketotic hyperglycinemia. *J Inherit Metab Dis.* 2005;28(5):651–663.
30. Tan WH et al. Isolated sulfite oxidase deficiency: a case report with a novel mutation and review of the literature. *Pediatrics.* 2005;116(3):757–766.
31. Hoffmann C et al. Magnetic resonance imaging and magnetic resonance spectroscopy in isolated sulfite oxidase deficiency. *J Child Neurol.* 2007;10:1214–1221.
32. Hunter MF et al. Alpers syndrome with mutations in POLG: clinical and investigative features. *Pediatr Neurol.* 2011;45(5):311–318.

20 Movement Disorders

SABA AHMAD and NICHOLAS S. ABEND

■ INTRODUCTION

Movement disorders comprise a large group of conditions which cause one or more of the following: slowness or paucity of movement, difficulty in initiating movement, involuntary movements, and abnormal postures. They are not the result of weakness, spasticity, or sensory disturbance, but rather result from disorders of the higher level subcortical or cerebellar systems involved in movement planning, execution, inhibition, and coordination. Pediatric movement disorders range from simple motor tics to more serious conditions causing bradykinesia, tremor, myoclonus, chorea, athetosis, or dystonia. Some neurometabolic and neurodegenerative diseases may involve disordered movement in addition to other neurologic and nonneurologic problems. The majority of movement disorders present insidiously with slow progression and are managed in the outpatient setting. However, a smaller subset of movement disorders presents more urgently. This chapter addresses an important subset of movement disorders that are acute in onset and require urgent intervention.

Childhood acute movement disorders are uncommon and are often diagnosed clinically, although in some cases tests are helpful in confirming a diagnosis. A particular type of movement disorder can have multiple causes, and a particular etiology may have complex and variable presentations. In a recent prospective cohort of 52 children with acute movement disorders, the most common conditions were chorea, dystonia, tremor, myoclonus, and parkinsonism. Etiologic categories were (1) psychogenic (23%), most often tremor and myoclonus, (2) inflammatory-autoimmune (42%), and (3) noninflammatory (35%). Inflammatory disorders included N-methyl-D-aspartate (NMDA) receptor encephalitis, opsoclonus-myoclonus, Sydenham chorea, systemic lupus erythematosus, acute necrotizing encephalopathy, and other encephalitides. Noninflammatory etiologies include drug-induced movement disorders, post-pump (cardiac bypass) chorea, metabolic disorders, and vascular disorders including moyamoya disease. (1).

Prompt clinical evaluation is paramount in accurate diagnosis and guiding treatment. The medical history is very often helpful. For example, there may be history suggestive of infection or inflammatory disease, family history of neurologic disease, or use of medications, illicit drugs, or environmental exposures that suggest toxicity. Careful observation of the type of disturbance in voluntary movement and noting characteristics of involuntary movements usually allows designation of a movement disorder category and localization of the lesion, which then is helpful in considering the possible etiology. The general and neurologic examination, including assessment of mental status, will reveal whether there are other abnormalities accompanying the movement disorder which, if present, will usually aid in determining the etiology.

Brain Movement Control Centers

Movement control is distributed broadly in the central nervous system. The important centers include the cerebral cortex, basal ganglia, cerebellum, and thalamus.

The basal ganglia include the globus pallidus, putamen, caudate nucleus, and substantia nigra and are located deep in the cerebral hemispheres. Specific biochemical or strategically positioned structural lesions in the basal ganglia can result in parkinsonism, tremor, dystonia, chorea, athetosis, or ballismus. Disease of the cerebellum and cerebellar tracts results in wide-based unsteady gait and intention tremor of the limbs.

One of the important neurotransmitters of the basal ganglia is dopamine. Neuroleptic drugs used to treat psychiatric conditions block dopamine receptors in the basal ganglia, sometimes resulting in acute onset movement disorders, such as parkinsonism, abnormal movements, dystonia, and oculogyric crisis. Dopamine blockade can also result in neuroleptic malignant syndrome (see chapter on Hyperthermic Drug-Induced Disorders). Table 20.2 lists the most commonly implicated drugs. Any medication with properties of dopamine receptor blockade can produce these syndromes, but the atypical antipsychotics tend to be associated with a lower risk of these complications.

■ MOVEMENT DISORDER DESCRIPTION AND CLASSIFICATION

Movement disorders are often classified as (1) hyperkinetic, characterized by abnormal involuntary movement, or (2) hypokinetic (bradykinetic), characterized by paucity and slowness of movement. Some patients have mixed characteristics, such as slowness of voluntary movement with superimposed tremor. However, careful observation will usually lead to accurate diagnosis. In each of the following sections, a movement disorder will be described, the causes of acute onset calling for urgent evaluation will be listed, and for some disorders treatment will be reviewed. The more common causes of insidious nonurgent onset will either not be discussed or mentioned only to provide context. Key features of each movement disorder are provided in Table 20.1.

■ HYPOKINETIC MOVEMENT DISORDERS

Parkinsonism

Parkinsonism is the most common hypokinetic disorder. It is usually characterized by two or more of the usual parkinsonism signs: (1) rest tremor at 4 to 6 Hz that may also occur with sustained posture, (2) bradykinesia (slowness of movement) or more rarely akinesia, (3) rigidity in which muscle tone is increased in all directions of movement and which is not altered by movement velocity, and (4) postural instability in which dysregulation of postural reflexes may lead to retropulsion (multiple steps backward) when the patient is pulled backward (pull test). There are multiple causes of insidious onset parkinsonism. Parkinson's disease is common in adults and is a primary type of parkinsonism. Juvenile Parkinson's disease is rare, and it often presents with dystonia, rigidity, and bradykinesia without the classic rest tremor seen in adults (2,3). In children, parkinsonism is often secondary to other neurologic problems, and often presents along with other symptoms and signs (4).

A child presenting with parkinsonism that started in the preceding few days or weeks and is already

■ **Table 20.1**	Movement Disorder Features
Athetosis	Slow writhing/turning limb movements
Ballismus	Large amplitude, flinging movements (usually proximal joints)
Chorea	Rapid, brief, irregular, nonrhythmic, nonstereotyped movements
Dystonia	Involuntary sustained muscle contractions producing twisting and squeezing movements and often resulting in abnormal posture
Myoclonus	Sudden, brief, very fast (shocklike) movements
Parkinsonism	Bradykinesia, rigidity, tremor, and postural instability
Tic	Brief, paroxysmal, stereotyped movements (simple or complex) or vocalizations sometimes accompanied by premonitory urge
Tremor	Rhythmic, oscillatory movement of a body part

pronounced is unlikely to have a degenerative disease and urgent evaluation for acute or subacute illness causing secondary parkinsonism is indicated. There will often be clinical clues to the underlying diagnosis provided by the constellation of symptoms and signs. Subdural hematoma and hypothyroidism may mimic parkinsonism.

Drug-induced disease is most commonly caused by antiemetic medications including metoclopramide and neuroleptic medications (Table 20.2), but may also occur with amiodarone, calcium channel blockers, isoniazid, divalproex, and chemotherapeutic agents. In some cases, chemotherapy-induced parkinsonism is responsive to levodopa (5). Parkinsonism may occur as a delayed complication after bone marrow transplant in patients on chemotherapy (6).

Parkinsonism can be secondary to acute structural lesions such as stroke and tumor of the frontal lobes, substantia nigra, or thalamus (7–10). Parkinsonism may occur with hydrocephalus including due to ventriculoperitoneal shunt malfunction (8,11) and may also occur after shunt placement or third ventriculostomy procedures (12–14). Acute parkinsonism has been described following global hypoxemic injury (15–17). Demyelinating disorders including acute disseminated encephalomyelitis may cause parkinsonism (18). Subdural hematoma may present with parkinsonism (19).

Acute parkinsonism can also be a feature of toxic exposures. Carbon monoxide poisoning frequently causes necrosis of the globus pallidus. After recovery from the initial insult and coma, a phenomenon called delayed demyelination can result in profound, rapidly developing parkinsonism (20–22). Pallidal necrosis can also occur as a rare late complication of wasp stings (23). Acute parkinsonism was seen in a mini-epidemic of drug users who took the synthetic opiod desmethylprodine MPPP or 1-methyl-4-phenylproprionoxypiperidine, an analog of meperidine that was contaminated with MPTP (1-methyl-4-phenyl-1,2,3,6-tetrahydropyridine) (24).

Mycoplasma pneumoniae (25) and streptococcal pharyngitis (26) infections has been associated with parkinsonism. Similarly, many viral encephalitides can cause an acute parkinsonian syndrome: Epstein-Barr virus (EBV) (27), influenza (including H1N1) (28), coxsackie, measles, polio, St Louis encephalitis, and Western equine encephalitis. In HIV disease, acute parkinsonism can be seen with opportunistic infections including toxoplasmosis, Cryptococcus, progressive multifocal leukoencephalopathy, and tuberculosis. It can also be seen with the HIV associated encephalopathy spectrum (29,30). As

■ **Table 20.2** Medications With Properties of Dopamine Receptor Blockade

Typical antipsychotics

Low potency
- Chlorpromazine
- Thioridazine
- Mesoridazine
- Levomepromazine

Medium potency
- Loxapine
- Molindone
- Perphenazine
- Thiothixene
- Trifluoperazine

High potency
- Haloperidol
- Fluphenazine
- Droperidol
- Zuclopenthixol
- Flupentixol
- Prochlorperazine

Atypical antipsychotics
- Amisulpride
- Aripiprazole
- Asenapine
- Blonanserin
- Clotiapine
- Clozapine
- Iloperidone
- Lurasidone
- Mosapramine
- Olanzapine
- Paliperidone
- Perospirone
- Quetiapine
- Remoxipride
- Risperidone
- Sertindole
- Sulpiride
- Ziprasidone
- Zotepine

Antiemetics
- Metoclopramide
- Promethazine
- Domperidone
- Prochlorperazine
- Droperidol

Others
- Reserpine
- Pimozide
- Tetrabenazine

a historical note, in the early 20th century, von Economo described encephalitis lethargic, a disorder in which various acute forms including stupor or coma, hyperkinetic chorea and athetosis, or parkinsonism would often lead to death, and among survivors a postencephalitic parkinsonism would develop 5 to 10 years later (31–33). Recent cases have also been described (34).

Huntington's disease usually appears in adults and includes choreoathetosis and dementia. However, the Westphal variant occurs in childhood and includes bradykinesia, rigidity, seizures, and decline in mentation. This disorder is not acute in onset, but it can be more rapidly progressive than in adults and rarely presents in an urgent setting, eventually being diagnosed after secondary etiologies are ruled out.

Catatonia

Catatonia is characterized by extreme slowness of movement and altered responsiveness sometimes to the point of a stuporlike state. There may be catalepsy, in which the patient maintains unusual postures for prolonged periods of time, and "waxy flexibility," in which the patient maintains postures set by the examiner. Generally no structural disease is found and catatonia usually occurs in the setting of serious psychiatric disease, although it may also occur in the context of various neurodevelopmental and autoimmune disorders including childhood disintegrative disorder, Kleine-Levin syndrome, Prader-Willi syndrome, tic disorders, and autoimmune encephalitis (35,36). Malignant catatonia can mimic neuroleptic malignant syndrome and is discussed in other chapters (Hyperthermic Drug Induced Disorders and Neurotoxicology).

■ HYPERKINETIC MOVEMENT DISORDERS

Classifying a hyperkinetic movement disorder is challenging since there are many types. The initial assessment of these patients should distinguish between movements which are involuntary, abnormal, and excessive and other movements which may appear abnormal but are actually purposeful (such as guarding muscle contractions in the setting of pain). Once the movements are determined to be involuntary, they can be classified through careful observation, as discussed below.

Dystonia

Introduction

Dystonia is an involuntary abnormal posture of a limb or the torso. It is sometimes accompanied by twisting or repetitive movements or these movements may occur in isolation. Dystonia is caused by disease of the basal ganglia and is the result of abnormal persistent muscular contraction. An example is torticollis, where the head is persistently turned and tilted to one side or slow repetitive movements to the side or a combination of the two. Focal dystonia may occur at other locations along the torso, at a limb, the face, and the larynx. It can be widespread along the torso and all limbs. Some patients obtain temporary relief from sensory stimuli, as when the patient with torticollis has some neck relaxation in response to light touch to the face. Dystonia can resolve in sleep. Many of these conditions are hereditary, slow in onset, and progressive. This section focuses on acute dystonia requiring urgent assessment.

Acute Dystonic Reactions to Medications

Acute dystonic reactions to neuroleptics (Table 20.2) affect 2% to 3% of patients soon after initiation of dopamine receptor antagonist therapy (37), often within 1 to 5 days of starting therapy. Younger patients and males tend to be more susceptible, and the incidence of an acute dystonic reaction increases to almost 50% with high potency neuroleptic treatment (38,39). While dystonia can be one of the earliest side effects of dopamine receptor blockade, it can also be seen in the setting of chronic neuroleptic use, constituting tardive dystonia, where the incidence may be as high as 10% (40). It is often referred to as a toxic effect but can occur even with standard therapeutic doses. Other medications that occasionally cause dystonia include phenytoin, carbamazepine, levodopa, calcium channel blockers, and cetirizine. In addition to acute isolated dystonia, drug-induced neuroleptic malignant syndrome can include dystonia.

Acute dystonic reactions typically involve the muscles of the eyes, face, mouth, tongue, jaw, and neck. Less frequently the trunk and limbs are involved. For example, an acute prominent torticollis may appear. The sustained muscle contractions can be painful and severe. Cervical, oral, or laryngeal dystonia can be life-threatening if they affect respiration or result in dysphagia with aspiration. Oculogyric crisis is an acute dystonia that commonly includes forced eye deviation, jaw opening, tongue protrusion, and arching of the neck and/or trunk (41). Acute dystonic reactions have been associated with stridor, presumably due to dystonic involvement of the larynx or pharynx (42). In one patient acute dystonia led to self amputation of the tongue (43).

Treatment of acute dystonic reactions involves administration of oral, intramuscular, or intravenous anticholinergics or antihistamines such as benztropine or diphenhydramine (44). Intravenous diazepam has also been used as an effective alternative therapy (45). Even untreated, most acute dystonic reaction will resolve spontaneously within 12 to 48 hours after the last exposure to dopamine receptor antagonist. However, these reactions are often painful for the patient and potentially dangerous, so treatment is a consideration depending on the severity of the condition. Recurrence may occur, so often continued administration of an oral anticholinergic medication for 5 to 7 days or more is indicated.

Acute Dystonia—Other Etiologies

New structural disease in the basal ganglia and acute withdrawal of medications including intrathecal baclofen, tetrabenazine, and lithium may produce acute dystonia (46,47). Dystonia may occur in bacterial, viral, and fungal meningoencephalitis, including HIV, tuberculosis (TB), and celiac disease. Dystonia occurs in Wilson's disease, vitamin E deficiency, and autoimmune diseases. Organic acidemias may not present until a time of metabolic stress and then present with severe and rapid onset dystonia. Toxic disturbances caused by carbon monoxide, ethylene glycol, methanol, cyanide, stimulants such as amphetamines, and wasp stings may all involve dystonia. Dystonia can be psychogenic and occur as a component of a conversion disorder.

Initial management is with anticholinergics, benzodiazepines, dopamine receptor blockers. Rarely general anesthesia and paralysis are required as a temporizing measure. Management is mostly supportive and involves sedation, antipyretics, pain management, management of rhabdomyolysis, and appropriate cardiopulmonary support. In more refractory cases, particularly in patients with idiopathic torsion dystonia, management options include intrathecal baclofen or surgical interventions such as thalamotomy, pallidotomy, and deep brain stimulation (48).

There is a group of hereditary and acquired kinesigenic (provoked by movement especially exercise) and nonkinesigenic paroxysmal movement disorders that include dystonia or choreoathetosis and occur in children and adults. Episodes last from minutes to a few hours. Depending on the particular condition, there may be a response to antiepileptic drugs or benzodiazepines (49).

Status dystonicus (dystonic storm) is a rapidly developing and severe hyperkinetic movement disorder involving dystonia and chorea. It may occur in children with pre-existing dystonia, such as primary dystonia or dystonic cerebral palsy, who miss medications, undergo medication adjustments, or develop intercurrent infections. The condition is painful and may cause rhabdomyolysis or respiratory compromise. Treatment is difficult, and dystonic storm may persist for several months and recur with future infections. Trihexphenidyl and tetrabenazine may be tried, and anesthesia with paralysis is sometimes needed as a temporizing measure.

Pseudodystonia mimics dystonia. Atlantoaxial subluxation can cause pseudotorticollis (head tilt, contralateral neck rotation, and neck flexion), particularly in children with trisomy 21 or following head/neck trauma. The patient may not be able to rotate the head past midline. Neck muscles are found to be relaxed on palpation, as opposed to the usual hyperactive state noted in dystonia (50). Other structural disease in the posterior fossa or cervical spine and also diseases of the soft tissues of the neck (for example, pharyngitis, tonsillitis, mastoiditis) may simulate dystonia. Tetanus can mimic dystonia and delayed diagnosis can be potentially disastrous. In a patient who is unimmunized or underimmunized, it can present as focal spasm usually close to the site of injury. Trismus and other cephalic forms of tetanus may resemble oculogyric crisis. Focal tetanus of a limb may resemble a focal dystonia. The disorder is generally progressive, and a high degree of suspicion must exist. Treatment is with immunoglobulin and antibiotics (51). Other disorders that can produce pseudotorticollis are neoplastic or infectious processes of the head, neck, or spinal cord (52–54). Trochlear nerve palsy often results in head tilt. Sandifer syndrome is a childhood condition of dystonia associated with gastrointestinal reflux.

Chorea, Athetosis, and Ballismus

These are presented as a group because it is useful to compare the movements and etiologies, and because classification may be difficult with overlapping movements in a patient. Choreic movements are typically brief, rapid, small to moderate size movements that occur randomly at the limbs, torso, and face. The movements are involuntary, nonrhythmic, and direction-changing. The patient may try to mask a choreic movement by adding on a voluntary purposeful movement as the choreic movement ends, referred to as parakinesias. Athetosis is slower, more writhing, and continuous compared to chorea. Ballismus refers to large, brief, rapid, flinging irregularly timed movements at the shoulder or hip joint. It is often unilateral (hemiballismus). In some patients it is difficult to classify the movements in one of the three categories. Choreoathetoid movements have mixed characteristics. Chorea and athetosis and occasionally ballismus may be seen in the same patient, and they have a similar differential diagnosis.

Chorea and its related movements may occur with toxic, metabolic, vascular, infectious, postinfectious, and endocrine etiologies. Sydenham chorea is related to an autoimmune poststreptococcal process (see below). Focal lesions in the basal ganglia, including infarction, hemorrhage, tumor, and demyelination may produce acute onset or progressive chorea. Vascular etiologies include stroke, moyamoya disease, and vasculitis. Both hyperglycemia and hypoglycemia can present with chorea. Common systemic etiologies for chorea are the antiphospholipid antibody syndrome and systemic lupus erythematosus, both of which may present with neuropsychiatric symptoms including a variety of movement disorders often including chorea (55–59). Other systemic etiologies are hyperthyroidism, pheochromocytoma, Henoch-Schönlein purpura, and neuroacanthocytosis. Infections including Lyme disease, HIV, and mycoplasma may involve chorea. Medications that can cause these movements include anticholinergics, phenytoin, carbamazepine, stimulants including amphetamines and methylphenidate, tricyclic antidepressants, clonidine, L-dopa, lithium, and oral contraceptives. Toxins which may produce chorea include manganese, ethanol, toluene, and carbon monoxide. Neuroleptics sometimes cause chorea. Chorea may follow cardiac bypass (post-pump chorea) and may be transient or persistent. Chorea gravidarum usually occurs during the first or early second trimester and generally resolves later in the pregnancy or after delivery. Primary causes of nonacute chorea are unlikely to present for urgent care and include Huntington's disease and ataxia-telangiectasia.

Sydenham chorea should be considered in every child with chorea (60). It is the neurologic manifestation of rheumatic fever, as diagnosed by the Jones Criteria for Rheumatic Disease. It presents with a 1- to 8-month delay after group A beta hemolytic streptococcal infection. Onset is often over hours to days, and many families can identify the exact date of onset. Diagnosis of Sydenham chorea requires evidence of a prior clinical streptococcal infection or elevated antistreptolysin O or anti–DNase-B antibody titers as markers of prior infection. The typical age of presentation is 5 to 15 years, and there is a female preponderance. Brain magnetic resonance imaging (MRI) is typically normal but there are reports of reversible basal ganglia hyperintensities (61). There are often other psychiatric comorbidities seen, such as personality changes, attention deficit disorder, and obsessive compulsive features. It is critical to evaluate for the other rheumatic disease features including the systolic murmur characteristic of cardiac disease which generally prompts echocardiographic evaluation. Treatment goals are prevention of recurrence of rheumatic fever and management of the chorea. Antibiotics are used to prevent recurrence of rheumatic fever and may include several years of monthly injections of penicillin G, daily penicillin, or daily sulfadiazine. There are differences of opinion regarding treatment of the chorea. Benzodiazepines and valproic acid is sometimes helpful. Neuroleptics have also been used, but typically are used sparingly to avoid tardive abnormal movements (62,63). Depending on the severity of the chorea, immunomodulatory therapy with prednisone and more rarely intravenous immunoglobulin or plasmapheresis can be considered (64,65).

Hemiballismus may occur with stroke or other focal lesions in or near the subthalamic nucleus and with nonketotic hyperglycemia.

Myoclonus

Myoclonus is characterized by rapid, shocklike, involuntary, and irregularly timed movements of a limb, segment of the body, or large part of the body. The movements are much more rapid than in chorea. It may be physiologic as in sleep myoclonus, hereditary, part of a progressive degenerative condition, or secondary to other disease. It may be epileptic, cortical but not epileptic, or arise from disease of subcortical structures, the brainstem, or the spinal cord.

Myoclonus is a common component of neurodegenerative disorders including the progressive myoclonic epilepsies, in which case myoclonus occurs in the context of encephalopathy and other neurodevelopmental abnormalities, and does not present acutely. Additionally, myoclonic seizures are a common component of many epilepsy syndromes including juvenile myoclonic epilepsy, myoclonia with childhood absences, and Lennox-Gastaut syndrome. Rarely myoclonus can occur within the spectrum or jerking movements associated with epilepsia partialis continua.

Acute onset myoclonus or symptomatic myoclonus generally occurs in the context of encephalopathy and other neurologic problems (66). It may occur after severe brain injury, most commonly following hypoxic-ischemic brain injury. When myoclonic status epilepticus occurs after hypoxic ischemic encephalopathy, it suggests an unfavorable prognosis. However, nonepileptic myoclonus may occur after cardiac arrest and may be associated with favorable outcome (Lance-Adams syndrome) (67,68). Myoclonus may occur with stroke or tumor, infectious meningoencephalitis (including bacterial, arboviruses, herpes virus, EBV, Lyme disease, hepatitis, HIV, fungal) (69–71), autoimmune processes such as acute disseminated encephalomyelitis, hepatic and uremic encephalopathy, celiac disease, hypocalceima, hypomagnesemia, hypothyroidism, hyperglycemia, hypoglycemia, hyperthyroidism, vitamin E deficiency, and serotonin syndrome (discussed in the chapter on Hyperthermic Syndromes). It may be caused by medications including monoamine oxidase inhibitors, selective serotonin reuptake inhibitors, serotonin-norepinephrine reuptake inhibitors, tricyclic antidepressants, opiates, levodopa, triptans, some antibiotics (penicillin, cephalosporins, quinolones), and by illicit drugs including lysergic acid diethylamide, amphetamines, cocaine, and 3,4-methylenedioxymethamphetamine (ecstasy). Myoclonus may be caused by intoxication with lead, carbon monoxide, mercury, and bismuth. Wilson's disease should be considered. Psychogenic myoclonus occurs. A variety of epilepsy syndromes involve myoclonic seizures, and rarely some anticonvulsants (lamotrigine, carbamazepine, phenytoin, gabapentin, and vigabatrin) can worsen myoclonic seizures.

Myoclonus may occur as a component of opsoclonus-myoclonus syndrome. This syndrome may present with myoclonus that is diffuse, multifocal, and low amplitude. Opsoclonus, often considered the hallmark of the syndrome, may be intermittent, late occurring, or subtle, and this may not be readily apparent. Onset is often in children younger than 5 years of age. Consideration and evaluation is essential since it may be associated with neuroblastoma. Testing for urine catecholamines and a complete and often repeated evaluation for neuroblastoma is indicated. As described above, opsoclonus-myoclonus may also occur in the context of many infections and celiac disease.

Clonazepam, valproic acid, and levetiracetam are sometimes helpful for management, especially if the myoclonus is cortical, but their use is off label.

Tremor

Tremor is a rhythmic rapid oscillating movement at a fixed point caused by alternate contractions of antagonist muscles. It can be seen at rest (as in parkinsonism) or while maintaining a sustained posture (action tremor). Tremor can be divided into three broad categories. First, enhanced physiologic tremor refers to tremor which becomes enhanced or first visible in certain situations including emotional stress, fatigue, or stimulating medications/substances (such as caffeine, amphetamines, or thyroid hormones). Second, essential tremor which refers to a primary tremor that is often suppressed by alcohol. Third, symptomatic tremor in which tremor generally occurs in the context of other symptoms and signs.

Symptomatic tremor is generally caused by disorders affecting the corticostriatopallidothalamic or cerebellarthalamic circuits, and this involves generally subcortical and posterior fossa disorders. Lesions may include cerebellar malformations and cysts (72–74), neoplasms, stroke, and demyelinating disease. Rubral tremor may arise with lesions of the red nucleus. Systemic causes of symptomatic tremor include endocrine disorders [hyperthyroidism (75), hyperadrenalism], low magnesium, and hepatic encephalopathy. Drug-induced parkinsonism can include tremor. Other drugs that can cause tremor include tricyclic antidepressants, selective serotonin reuptake inhibitors (SSRI) medications, lithium, amiodarone, cyclosporine, divalproex, and some antiviral medications. Exposure to heavy metals such as lead or mercury as well as toxicity from recreational "sniffing" or inhalation of volatile vapors can cause tremor. Acute onset tremor can occur with Wilson's disease.

Tic Disorders

Tic disorders are seldom movement disorder emergencies, but they are important to recognize and distinguish from other movement disorders. They are involuntary, brief, rapid, and often stereotyped movements or vocalizations performed in response to an internal urge.

Tics differ from other movement disorders in that they can often be suppressed completely for a period of time. Simple tics that involve a sudden movement of a limb can often be confused with myoclonus, and the history of being suppressible is an important distinguishing factor. Tics can also involve a complex series of movements.

Ataxia

Ataxia is not typically classified as a movement disorder but is included here since it does involve abnormal movement and must be distinguished from other abnormal movements. Ataxia is usually due to disease of the cerebellum or tracts connecting the cerebellum to other structures. Ataxic movements are inaccurate volitional movements with incoordination of the multiple muscle contractions and multiple joint rotations that normally are carried out such that the terminal point of the limb is guided directly and smoothly to a target. Symptoms and signs are dysmetria, gait unsteadiness with a wide base, dysarthria, and titubation. Dysmetria, also called intention tremor, can be seen as inaccuracy, with repeated undershooting and/or overshooting of corrective movements, as the hand or foot approaches a target, often demonstrated with the "finger-nose" and "heal-shin" tests. Titubation is wavering movement of the trunk.

Primary ataxia is often genetic, including the spinocerebellar ataxias, ataxia-telangiectasia, and Friedreich ataxia. Secondary ataxias usually require urgent care. The most common etiologies of acute onset ataxia are ataxia due to intoxication or ataxia associated with a viral illnesses. Ataxia associated with intoxication may occur with exposure to alcohol, anticonvulsants, antihistamines, and benzodiazepines. Ataxia may occur after a variety of clinical and subclinical infections and generally presents with gait ataxia, and less commonly with truncal ataxia or nystagmus. Onset may be abrupt or slowly evolving. These are likely caused by autoimmune molecular mimicry between the cerebellum and viral proteins. MRI may demonstrate enhancement in the cerebellum consistent with a cerebellitis, and cerebrospinal fluid may show pleocytosis. Acute ataxia generally resolves, but this may take many months.

Other causes of acute ataxia include encephalitis, ataxic cerebral palsy, metabolic disorders (congenital disorders of glycosylation, mitochondrial disorders, urea cycle disorders, Refsum's disease, Hartnup's disease), vitamin E deficiency, and opsoclonus-myoclonus syndrome (which can also present with ataxia in the absence of opsoclonus or myoclonus), Wilson's disease, thiamine deficiency, Miller Fischer variant of Guillain-Barré disease, and hypothyroidism. Acute focal cerebellar lesions, for example due to stroke, tumor, and demyelination, may also present with acute ataxia, and neuroimaging is often indicated. These often present along with posterior fossa signs such as headache, emesis, and cranial nerve palsies, but may occur with just ataxia initially. Functional ataxia as a component of conversion disorder must also be considered.

Acute Torticollis

Acute torticollis may occur in children with processes involving the posterior fossa and cervical spine including tumors, hemorrhages, and infection. Acute infectious torticollis may occur after pharyngitis, tonsillitis, mastoiditis, or other infections involving the head or neck. Patients have a painful, fixed torticollis. Prompt recognition is required so specific therapy can be instituted. Management involves neuroimaging of the brain and cervical spine, infection evaluation of the head and neck structures as well as brain, and then specific therapy.

Bobble-Head Doll Syndrome

Persistent or episodic side-to-side or forward-and-back head movements like a bobble head doll can be seen in infants and children. These movements are often seen with third ventricular lesions and include third ventricular cysts, tumors, and aqueductal stenosis (76–78) and may occur with shunt malfunction (79). Neuroimaging is required.

Wilson's Disease

Wilson's Disease is often diagnosed when a movement disorder and neuropsychiatric symptoms appear. Usually liver disease is also present by that time. It requires a high degree of clinical suspicion and accurate tests are available. Treatment can alter the patient's outcome, particularly if initiated early. It is an autosomal recessive disorder characterized by copper accumulation. Clinically, there is elevated urinary copper excretion and low serum ceruloplasmin. Copper deposition is seen on liver biopsy. Ophthalmologic slit lamp exam reveals Kayser-Fleischer rings. The initial presentation is often subtle but progressive decline in cognitive and school performance, and behavioral changes are common. It is the movement disorder that often leads to medical attention. The abnormal movements are highly variable, involving tremor, bradykinesia, dystonia, dysarthria, dysphagia, incoordination, chorea, and athetosis (80). Tremor can be present at rest but often is much more prominent and proximal when the arms are held outstretched (wing beating tremor). There can be persistent grinning appearance (risus sardonicus), caused by dystonic facial muscles. Copper chelation therapy with penicillamine or trientine is standard, although both of these medications can make a patient's neurologic symptoms temporarily or persistently worse (81). Recently, penicillamine has fallen out of favor due to the side effect profile, and trientine is more widely used. Intestinal copper absorption may be reduced with zinc or tetrathiomolybdate (82,83).

Paraneoplastic Disorders With Prominent Movement Aspects

A brief review of the paraneoplastic disorders is presented here because these patients often present acutely. The presentation can be varied, so the clinician needs to have a high clinical suspicion for these disorders. In recent years anti-NMDA receptor antibody mediated encephalitis has been more widely recognized. In adults, this disorder was initially described in young women with ovarian teratomas (84), and recently it has been described in children with and without neoplasms (85). In children, the disorder should be suspected in patients who present with behavioral changes, abnormal movements, and seizures. These patients can have a nonspecifically abnormal electroencephalogram, a frequently mild CSF (cerebro-spinal fluid) lymphocytic pleocytosis, and typically a normal MRI, so diagnosis must be driven by clinical suspicion. Evaluation for tumors is essential, although none are identified in many children. Management may involve tumor removal, immunomodulation with corticosteroids and immunoglobulins, and, in more severe cases, cyclophosphamide and rituximab (62).

Opsoclonus myoclonus ataxia syndrome is another rare disorder that presents in children. This syndrome most commonly is associated with neuroblastoma, can be seen in up to 3% of patients with neuroblastoma, and may be the presenting sign (86). Rarely, it can precede the appearance of a tumor by up to 4 years. In some cases a tumor is never found and the disorder is hypothesized to be a parainfectious autoimmune process. Within the name of the diagnosis are the three cardinal features. Opsoclonus describes random, multidirectional, often "bouncing," conjugate eye movements. Myoclonus is often in the face and neck. Ataxia in these patients is often truncal and appendicular. Not all features need to be present, and some may be intermittent, lacking at presentation, or subtle. Treatment involves identifying and treating the neuroblastoma and immunomodulation for the symptoms of the disorder. Immunomodulation may include immunoglobulin and corticosteroids, as well as more aggressive therapies such as cyclophosphamide and rituximab (87).

Psychogenic Movement Disorders

Psychogenic movement disorders are common in children (1). These may have abrupt onset with severely abnormal looking movements, and thus may present to the acute setting. Identification is essential to avoid unnecessary testing and to rapidly initiate appropriate management. These are considered within the spectrum of conversion disorder, in which symptoms affecting motor or sensory function suggesting a neurologic cause are actually caused by psychological factors. Importantly, psychogenic movement disorders and organic disorders can coexist. Psychogenic movement disorders occur in about 2% to 5% of children with movement disorders (88–91). A review of 14 children with psychogenic movement disorders found that 29% presented with two or more movement disorders and 80% presented with unexplained symptoms in addition to the movement disorder. The most common movement disorders were tremor and dystonia (91). Although young children may present with psychogenic movement disorders, most children are aged 7 to 18 years (88–90). In general, outcome is favorable. Many resolve within several months, and most children achieve complete remission (92–94). Many children present with other psychiatric comorbidities including anxiety and mood disorders, and in about half of children a specific stressor can be identified. Involvement of psychologists, psychiatrists, and sometimes rehabilitation programs is essential.

■ CONCLUSIONS

Acute movement disorders are uncommon but they signal serious underlying disorders requiring rapid diagnosis and management. Careful observation and description of the movement abnormality (see Table 20.1) is important since identifying the specific movement abnormality will aid in differential diagnosis. A detailed history including focus on medication and toxic exposures is important, and brain MRI to search for an acute focal lesion is often indicated. For many of the conditions, outcome will be improved with early recognition and intervention.

■ REFERENCES

1. Dale RC et al. A prospective study of acute movement disorders in children. *Dev Med Child Neurol.* 2010;52:739–748.
2. Paviour DC, Surtees RA, Lees AJ. Diagnostic considerations in juvenile parkinsonism. *Mov Disord.* 2004;19:123–135.
3. Uc EY, Rodnitzky RL. Juvenile parkinsonism. *Semin Pediatr Neurol.* 2003;10:62–67.
4. Pranzatelli MR et al. Clinical spectrum of secondary parkinsonism in childhood: a reversible disorder. *Pediatr Neurol.* 1994;10:131–140.
5. Chuang C et al. Chemotherapy-induced parkinsonism responsive to levodopa: an underrecognized entity. *Mov Disord.* 2003;18:328–331.
6. Lockman LA, Sung JH, Krivit W. Acute parkinsonian syndrome with demyelinating leukoencephalopathy in bone marrow transplant recipients. *Pediatr Neurol.* 1991;7:457–463.
7. Dick JP et al. Simple and complex movements in a patient with infarction of the right supplementary motor area. *Mov Disord.* 1986;1:255–266.
8. Curran T, Lang AE. Parkinsonian syndromes associated with hydrocephalus: case reports, a review of the literature, and pathophysiological hypotheses. *Mov Disord.* 1994;9:508–520.
9. Kim JS. Delayed onset mixed involuntary movements after thalamic stroke: clinical, radiological and pathophysiological findings. *Brain.* 2001;124:299–309.
10. Kim JS. Involuntary movements after anterior cerebral artery territory infarction. *Stroke.* 2001;32:258–261.
11. Racette BA et al. Pathophysiology of parkinsonism due to hydrocephalus. *J Neurol Neurosurg Psychiatry.* 2004;75:1617–1619.
12. Akiyama T et al. Severe parkinsonism following endoscopic third ventriculostomy for non-communicating hydrocephalus—case report. *Neurol Med Chir (Tokyo).* 2011;51:60–63.
13. Prashantha DK et al. Reversible parkinsonism following ventriculoperitoneal shunt in a patient with obstructive hydrocephalus secondary to intraventricular neurocysticercosis. *Clin Neurol Neurosurg.* 2008;110:718–721.
14. Yomo S et al. Parkinsonism and midbrain dysfunction after shunt placement for obstructive hydrocephalus. *J Clin Neurosci.* 2006;13:373–378.
15. Hawker K, Lang AE. Hypoxic-ischemic damage of the basal ganglia. Case reports and a review of the literature. *Mov Disord.* 1990;5:219–224.
16. Straussberg R et al. Delayed parkinsonism associated with hypotension in a child undergoing open-heart surgery. *Dev Med Child Neurol.* 1993;35:1011–1014.
17. Li JY et al. Postanoxic parkinsonism: clinical, radiologic, and pathologic correlation. *Neurology.* 2000;55:591–593.
18. Dimova PS et al. Acute reversible parkinsonism in Epstein-Barr virus–related encephalitis lethargica–like illness. *Mov Disord.* 2006;21:564–566.
19. Gelabert-Gonzalez M, Serramito-Garcia R, Aran-Echabe E. Parkinsonism secondary to subdural haematoma. *Neurosurg Rev.* 2012;35(3):457–468.
20. Choi IS. Carbon monoxide poisoning: systemic manifestations and complications. *J Korean Med Sci.* 2001;16:253–261.
21. Choi IS. Parkinsonism after carbon monoxide poisoning. *Eur Neurol.* 2002;48:30–33.
22. Sohn YH et al. The brain lesion responsible for parkinsonism after carbon monoxide poisoning. *Arch Neurol.* 2000;57:1214–1218.
23. Leopold NA, Bara-Jimenez W, Hallett M. Parkinsonism after a wasp sting. *Mov Disord.* 1999;14:122–127.
24. Langston JW et al. Chronic parkinsonism in humans due to a product of meperidine-analog synthesis. *Science.* 1983;219:979–980.
25. Kim JS, Choi IS, Lee MC. Reversible parkinsonism and dystonia following probable mycoplasma pneumoniae infection. *Mov Disord.* 1995;10:510–512.
26. McKee DH, Sussman JD. Case report: severe acute parkinsonism associated with streptococcal infection and antibasal ganglia antibodies. *Mov Disord.* 2005;20:1661–1663.
27. Roselli F et al. Reversible parkinsonian syndrome associated with anti-neuronal antibodies in acute EBV encephalitis: a case report. *Parkinsonism Relat Disord.* 2006;12:257–260.
28. Gonzalez-Duarte A et al. Hypothalamic abnormalities and parkinsonism associated with H1N1 influenza infection. *J Neuroinflammation.* 2010;7:47.
29. Nath A, Jankovic J, Pettigrew LC. Movement disorders and AIDS. *Neurology.* 1987;37:37–41.
30. Mirsattari SM, Power C, Nath A. Parkinsonism with HIV infection. *Mov Disord.* 1998;13:684–689.
31. von Economo C. Encephalitis lethargica. *Weiner Klinische Wochenschrift.* 1917;30:581–585.
32. von Economo C. *Encephalitis Lethargica, Its Sequelae and Treatment.* Oxford University Press, London; 1931:I–XIV, 1–200.
33. Duvosin RC, Yahr MD. Encephalitis and parkinsonism. *Arch Neurol.* 1965;12:227–239.
34. Dale RC et al. Encephalitis lethargica syndrome: 20 new cases and evidence of basal ganglia autoimmunity. *Brain.* 2004;127:21–33.
35. Dhossche DM, Wachtel LE. Catatonia is hidden in plain sight among different pediatric disorders: a review article. *Pediatr Neurol.* 2010;43:307–315.
36. Florance-Ryan N, Dalmau J. Update on anti–N-methyl-D-aspartate receptor encephalitis in children and adolescents. *Curr Opin Pediatr.* 2010;22:739–744.
37. Ayd FJ Jr. A survey of drug-induced extrapyramidal reactions. *JAMA.* 1961;175:1054–1060.
38. Boyer WF, Bakalar NH, Lake CR. Anticholinergic prophylaxis of acute haloperidol-induced acute dystonic reactions. *J Clin Psychopharmacol.* 1987;7:164–166.
39. Yoshida I et al. Acute accidental overdosage of haloperidol in children. *Acta Paediatr.* 1993;82:877–880.

40. Sachdev PS, Singh S. Dyskinesia presenting as a respiratory emergency. *Med J Aust.* 1994;161:726–727.
41. Rupniak NM, Jenner P, Marsden CD. Acute dystonia induced by neuroleptic drugs. *Psychopharmacology.* 1986;88:403–419.
42. Koek RJ, Pi EH. Acute laryngeal dystonic reactions to neuroleptics. *Psychosomatics.* 1989;30:359–364.
43. Pantanowitz L, Berk M. Auto-amputation of the tongue associated with flupenthixol induced extrapyramidal symptoms. *Int Clin Psychopharmacol.* 1999;14:129–131.
44. Smith MJM, Miller MM. Severe extrapyramidal reaction to perphenazine treated with diphenhydramine. *N Engl J Med.* 1961;264:396–397.
45. Korczyn AD, Goldberg GJ. Intravenous diazepam in drug-induced dystonic reactions. *B J Psychiatry.* 1972;121:75–77.
46. Manji H et al. Status dystonicus: the syndrome and its management. *Brain.* 1998;121 (pt 2):243–252.
47. Marsden CD, Marion MH, Quinn N. The treatment of severe dystonia in children and adults. *J Neurol Neurosurg Psychiatry.* 1984;47:1166–1173.
48. Krack P, Vercueil L. Review of the functional surgical treatment of dystonia. *Eur J Neurol.* 2001;8:389–399.
49. Demirkiran M, Jankovic J. Paroxysmal dyskinesias: clinical features and classification. *Ann Neurol.* 1995;38:571–579.
50. Subach BR et al. Current management of pediatric atlanto-axial rotatory subluxation. *Spine.* 1998;23:2174–2179.
51. Jagoda A, Riggio S, Burguieres T. Cephalic tetanus: a case report and review of the literature. *Am J Emerg Med.* 1988;6:128–130.
52. Berry DS, Moriarty RA. Atlantoaxial subluxation related to pharyngitis: Grisel's syndrome. *Clin Pediatr.* 1999;38:673–675.
53. Bredenkamp JK, Maceri DR. Inflammatory torticollis in children. *Arch Otolaryngol Head Neck Surg.* 1990;116:310–313.
54. Visudhiphan P et al. Torticollis as the presenting sign in cervical spine infection and tumor. *Clin Pediatr.* 1982;21:71–76.
55. Reiner P et al. Long-term outcome of 32 patients with chorea and systemic lupus erythematosus or antiphospholipid antibodies. *Mov Disord.* 2011;26:2422–2427.
56. Kiechl-Kohlendorfer U, Ellemunter H, Kiechl S. Chorea as the presenting clinical feature of primary antiphospholipid syndrome in childhood. *Neuropediatrics.* 1999;30:96–98.
57. Sunden-Cullberg J, Tedroff J, Aquilonius SM. Reversible chorea in primary antiphospholipid syndrome. *Mov Disord.* 1998;13:147–149.
58. Olfat MO, Al-Mayouf SM, Muzaffer MA. Pattern of neuropsychiatric manifestations and outcome in juvenile systemic lupus erythematosus. *Clin Rheumatol.* 2004;23:395–399.
59. Sibbitt WL Jr et al. The incidence and prevalence of neuropsychiatric syndromes in pediatric onset systemic lupus erythematosus. *J Rheumatol.* 2002;29:1536–1542.
60. Oosterveer DM, Overweg-Plandsoen WC, Roos RA. Sydenham's chorea: a practical overview of the current literature. *Pediatr Neurol.* 2010;43:1–6.
61. Giedd JN et al. Sydenham's chorea: magnetic resonance imaging of the basal ganglia. *Neurology.* 1995;45:2199–2202.
62. Pena J et al. Comparison of the efficacy of carbamazepine, haloperidol and valproic acid in the treatment of children with Sydenham's chorea: clinical follow-up of 18 patients. *Arquivos de Neuro-Psiquiatria.* 2002;60:374–377.
63. Daoud AS et al. Effectiveness of sodium valproate in the treatment of Sydenham's chorea. *Neurology.* 1990;40:1140–1141.
64. Garvey MA et al. Treatment of Sydenham's chorea with intravenous immunoglobulin, plasma exchange, or prednisone. *J Child Neurol.* 2005;20:424–429.
65. Paz JA, Silva CA, Marques-Dias MJ. Randomized double-blind study with prednisone in Sydenham's chorea. *Pediatr Neurol.* 2006;34:264–269.
66. Borg M. Symptomatic myoclonus. *Neurophysiol Clin.* 2006;36:309–318.
67. Lee HL, Lee JK. Lance-Adams syndrome. *Ann Rehabil Med.* 2011;35:939–943.
68. English WA, Giffin NJ, Nolan JP. Myoclonus after cardiac arrest: pitfalls in diagnosis and prognosis. *Anaesthesia.* 2009;64:908–911.
69. Ertekin V, Tan H. Opsoclonus-myoclonus syndrome attributable to hepatitis C infection. *Pediatr Neurol.* 2010;42:441–442.
70. Smyth P, Sinclair DB. Multifocal myoclonus following group A streptococcal infection. *J Child Neurol.* 2003;18:434–436.
71. Verma A, Brozman B. Opsoclonus-myoclonus syndrome following Epstein-Barr virus infection. *Neurology.* 2002;58:1131–1132.
72. Heller AC et al. Posterior fossa arachnoid cyst associated with an exertional tremor. *Mov Disord.* 2000;15:746–749.
73. Morgan JT et al. Resting tremor secondary to a pineal cyst: case report and review of the literature. *Pediatr Neurosurg.* 2008;44:234–238.
74. Colnat-Coulbois S, Marchal JC. Thalamic ependymal cyst presenting with tremor. *Childs Nerv Syst.* 2005;21:933–935.
75. Sherman J et al. Surgical management of Graves disease in childhood and adolescence: an institutional experience. *Surgery.* 2006;140:1056–1061; discussion 61–62.
76. de Brito Henriques JG et al. Bobble-head doll syndrome associated with Dandy-Walker syndrome. Case report. *J Neurosurg.* 2007;107:248–250.
77. Zamponi N et al. Bobble head doll syndrome in a child with a third ventricular cyst and hydrocephalus. *Childs Nerv Syst.* 2005;21:350–354.
78. Bhattacharyya KB et al. Bobble-head doll syndrome: some atypical features with a new lesion and review of the literature. *Acta Neurol Scand.* 2003;108:216–220.
79. Ahn Y, Cho BK, Wang KC. Bobble-head doll syndrome associated with subduroperitoneal shunt malfunction. *Childs Nerv Syst.* 1997;13:234–237.
80. Brewer GJ, Yuzbasiyan-Gurkan V. Wilson's disease. *Medicine.* 1992;71:139–164.
81. Walshe JM. Treatment of Wilson's disease with trientine (triethylene tetramine) dihydrochloride. *Lancet.* 1982;1:643–647.
82. Brewer GJ et al. Treatment of Wilson's disease with zinc: XV long-term follow-up studies. *J Lab Clin Med.* 1998;132:264–278.
83. Brewer GJ et al. Treatment of Wilson's disease with ammonium tetrathiomolybdate: III. Initial therapy in a total of 55 neurologically affected patients and follow-up with zinc therapy. *Arch Neurol.* 2003;60:379–385.
84. Dalmau J et al. Paraneoplastic anti–N-methyl-D-aspartate receptor encephalitis associated with ovarian teratoma. *Ann Neurol.* 2007;61:25–36.
85. Florance NR et al. Anti–N-methyl-D-aspartate receptor (NMDAR) encephalitis in children and adolescents. *Ann Neurol.* 2009;66:11–18.

86. Rudnick E et al. Opsoclonus-myoclonus-ataxia syndrome in neuroblastoma: clinical outcome and antineuronal antibodies—a report from the Children's Cancer Group Study. *Med Pediatr Oncol.* 2001;36:612–622.

87. Gorman MP. Update on diagnosis, treatment, and prognosis in opsoclonus-myoclonus-ataxia syndrome. *Curr Opin Pediatr.* 2010;22:745–750.

88. Ferrara J, Jankovic J. Psychogenic movement disorders in children. *Mov Disord.* 2008;23:1875–1881.

89. Schwingenschuh P et al. Psychogenic movement disorders in children: a report of 15 cases and a review of the literature. *Mov Disord.* 2008;23:1882–1888.

90. Fernandez-Alvarez E. Movement disorders of functional origin (psychogenic) in children. *Rev Neurol.* 2005;40(suppl 1): S75–S77.

91. Canavese C et al. Phenomenology of psychogenic movement disorders in children. *Mov Disord.* 2012;27(9):1153–1157.

92. Fritz GK, Fritsch S, Hagino O. Somatoform disorders in children and adolescents: a review of the past 10 years. *J Am Acad Child Adolesc Psychiatry.* 1997;36:1329–1338.

93. Turgay A. Treatment outcome for children and adolescents with conversion disorder. *Can J Psychiatry.* 1990;35:585–589.

94. Grattan-Smith P, Fairley M, Procopis P. Clinical features of conversion disorder. *Arch Dis Child.* 1988;63:408–414.

21 *Neuromuscular Disorders*

BASIL T. DARRAS and H. ROYDEN JONES, JR.

■ INTRODUCTION

Acute neuromuscular disorders occasionally confront the pediatric intensivist and/or the pediatric neurologist. Many of these are primary disorders of the motor unit that present acutely and may require urgent admission to an intensive care unit (ICU). Because of the somewhat differing presentations of sometimes similar disorders, as well as some illnesses that are particularly unique to infants and toddlers, in comparison to older children, we will discuss these various processes apropos to these two respective age groups. Although this creates somewhat artificial categories, it provides a practical format for evaluating acute weakness in a child. The third category relates to those processes that develop in a child with an acute systemic illness that requires ICU management and, therefore, concomitantly predisposes the child to another set of acute motor unit disorders.

There is a rather unique differential diagnosis specific to both newborns and toddlers. These disorders present either at birth, or shortly thereafter with lesions at each level of the peripheral motor unit. Typical examples seen at or shortly after birth include Werdnig-Hoffman disease (spinal muscular atrophy [SMA], type I), neonatal congenital polyneuropathies, an intrauterine onset of Guillain-Barré syndrome (GBS), and congenital myotonic dystrophy (MD) or glycogen/lipid storage myopathies. In contrast, previously healthy infants may develop infantile botulism, other unique genetically determined congenital neuromuscular transmission disorders, and, now, very rarely, postvaccine poliomyelitis. Most of these disorders usually present during the first 3 to 6 months of life, although some may not occur until the infant is almost 1 year old.

The older child and adolescent are predisposed to a set of certain critical care peripheral motor unit disorders usually quite similar to the adult patient. These particularly include GBS and myasthenia gravis (MG), which have an increased incidence among older children. However, when GBS and MG affect children, both may vary significantly from their traditional presentation. The pseudoencephalopathic form of GBS is a good example. Additionally some very uncommon entities, such as tick paralysis, always deserve careful consideration in the differential diagnosis of an acutely paretic child. The neuromuscular complications of extended intubation and sepsis affecting either the peripheral nerve, or muscle cell, also occur in children. Careful review of the clinical records, by someone as junior as an astute intern, or the nondiagnostic results of an imaging study, often lead the clinicians to pursue further diagnostic testing. The differential diagnosis of these various motor unit disorders is also significantly aided by utilizing clinical neurophysiology techniques, particularly nerve conduction studies (NCSs) and electromyography (EMG) or electroencephalography (EEG), and cerebrospinal fluid (CSF) analysis. These studies provide the clinician an objective means to appropriately assign a specific pathoanatomic or neurophysiologic site for the child's illness.

Lastly, there is an interesting but relatively uncommon set of neuromuscular disorders that develop in a child predominantly in association with the following three conditions: (1) treatment with a nondepolarizing neuromuscular blocking agent, (2) high-dose systemic glucocorticoid treatment, or (3) sepsis or other severe illness. These processes may independently affect each primary portion of the peripheral motor unit from the anterior horn cell, to the peripheral nerve, neuromuscular junction, or muscle fiber per se. Thus, in comparison to the other disorders discussed in this chapter wherein a primary individual motor unit disorder presents in an acute fashion requiring intensive care management, this set of illnesses is usually serious but self-limited, and somehow secondary to a toxic process related to the underlying illness (1).

The acute care motor unit disorders discussed in this chapter illustrate a broad anatomic spectrum from the anterior horn cell to the muscle cell. This review is based on our 32-year experience (1979 to 2011) evaluating children, ages newborn through 18 years, at the Boston Children's Hospital (BCH) Neuromuscular Program, ICUs, and EMG laboratory. Because the clinical spectrum of motor unit diseases appears to involve a somewhat different clinical set for infants and toddlers (2,3) in comparison to older children, this report separately discusses each age group.

■ ACUTE NEUROMUSCULAR CRISES IN THE INFANT

Babies may present during the neonatal period with the floppy infant syndrome, or acutely with a flaccid paralysis after being healthy during the first few months of their life (4). Some newborns, presenting primarily with an acute respiratory compromise during the immediate neonatal period, are concomitantly observed to be hypotonic, sometimes to the degree of being identified as a floppy baby. A variety of congenital or developmental lesions at any level of the peripheral motor unit may lead to this picture (Table 21.1).

Another subset during the first year of life includes those previously healthy infants who unexpectedly develop a precipitous neuromuscular crisis. Specific clinical mechanisms, that require consideration in this instance, include a previously unrecognized SMA, GBS, infantile botulism, congenital myasthenic syndromes, or, very rarely, postvaccine poliomyelitis.

Anterior Horn Cell

The Werdnig-Hoffmann form of SMA or SMA type I is one of the most common causes of the floppy infant syndrome as well as the most common anterior horn cell

■ Table 21.1 Conditions Leading to Acute Neuromuscular Crises in the Infant

Anterior Horn Cell
— Spinal muscular atrophy, type 0, type I
— Vaccine-associated poliomyelitis

Peripheral Nerve
— Congenital hypomyelinating or axonal polyneuropathies
— Guillain-Barré syndrome[a]

Neuromuscular Junction
— Transient neonatal myasthenia gravis
— Congenital myasthenic syndromes
— Infantile botulism
— Magnesium treatment in the mother

Muscle
— Congenital myotonic dystrophy
— Congenital myopathies
— Metabolic/mitochondrial myopathies

[a] Guillain-Barré syndrome rarely occurs during infancy.

disorder of infancy (2,3). Usually, these infants either present as a floppy baby, or with failure to develop or loss of early motor milestones between 1 and 3 months of age. Rarely, SMA (classified as type 0) may present at birth with profound hypotonia, severe weakness, and respiratory failure (5,6). Eventually some SMA type I infants will later require neonatal ICU. Their diagnosis is usually made by a combination of EMG and DNA analysis or just DNA analysis (2). Occasionally, their SMA is not initially recognized and it is not until they are unable to cope with a respiratory illness that they present to the ICU requiring pulmonary support or cannot be weaned from a ventilator.

Case 1: Werdnig-Hoffman Disease Presenting With Respiratory Distress

This previously "healthy" 4-month-old first child was admitted with an acute bronchiolitis and required intubation. Subsequently, when his pulmonary status had significantly improved his pediatricians had unexpected difficulty weaning him from the respirator. Neurologic consultation demonstrated generalized hypotonia and absent muscle stretch reflexes.

An EMG was performed because of its ability to provide a rapid means to localize the anatomic site for the baby's motor unit abnormality. This demonstrated low amplitude compound muscle action potentials (CMAPs), normal motor conduction velocities (MCVs), and distal latencies (DLs), as well as sensory nerve action potentials (SNAPs). Needle EMG demonstrated a marked decrease in the number of motor unit potentials (MUPs) with widespread active denervation characterized by many fibrillation potentials and positive waves. Subsequent to the EMG, DNA analysis for the SMA defect at 5q11-13 was positive (homozygous deletion of exon 7 of the survival of motor neuron 1 [SMN1] gene, which is the most common mutation in SMA patients).

Comment

Infants with SMA are usually easily recognized because of their typical clinical presentation as a floppy baby with an alert facies, absent muscle stretch reflexes, and fasciculations of their tongue. In this instance, DNA analysis of the *SMN1* gene is the appropriate means to make the diagnosis today. Occasionally, however, parents and pediatricians have not recognized a relatively subtle clinical presentation until an acute illness leads to hospitalization. In the intensive care setting, as above, one may need to make a more rapid diagnosis, utilizing EMG, to provide appropriate clinical management as well as counseling of the parents. Rarely, infants with non-5q SMAs may have similar clinical and EMG findings (7).

Another form of acute anterior horn cell disease, vaccine-associated poliomyelitis, deserves mention in the differential diagnosis of any infant or child with an acute weakness (8).

Case 2: Acute Postimmunization Poliomyelitis

A previously healthy 11-week-old boy presented with a 2-day history of fever, irritability, lethargy, and head lag. Computerized tomographic (CT) examination of the head and brain was normal. CSF analysis demonstrated 580 white blood cells (WBCs), 41% polymorphonuclear leukocytes, 59% lymphocytes; glucose 59 mg/dL, and protein 143 mg/dL. Although intravenous antibiotics were initiated, the baby soon developed apneic spells requiring intubation. This infant soon developed a weak cry and asymmetric skeletal muscle weakness particularly sparing left plantar flexor and extraocular muscles.

On the seventh day of his illness an EMG was performed demonstrating an anterior horn cell disease pattern. Subsequently, repetitive motor nerve stimulation (RMNS) failed to identify a neuromuscular transmission defect (NMTD).

Review of this baby's immunization records documented that he had received type 3 Sabin live poliomyelitis vaccine 3 weeks prior to onset of his illness. His recovery was poor; he was ventilator dependent more than 2 years later.

Comment

Three cases of acute flaccid paralysis occurring in infants, secondary to immunization-related poliomyelitis, became known to one of the authors (HRJ) within just a few years during the mid-1990s (8,9; J. Goldstein, personal oral and written communication, 1995). All three babies were 3 to 4 months old, each having received type 3 polio immunization less than 1 month earlier. An acute febrile illness preceded a progressive asymmetric extremity weakness, head lag, irritability, and lethargy. A CSF pleocytosis with 100 to 580 WBCs was associated with protein values between 82 and 143 mg/dL in all and glucose of 49 mg/dL in 1 (8). EMG demonstrated classic electrophysiologic evidence of an acute asymmetric anterior horn cell disorder.

Most instances of paralytic poliomyelitis from the attenuated live Sabin oral vaccine occurred among infants less than age 1 year usually subsequent to their first polio vaccine, and within 2 weeks of immunization (10). Revised Center for Disease Control guidelines require that the initial immunization protocol utilize Salk's killed vaccine as the primary immunization method for all children (11). This new infantile immunization protocol has made postvaccination related poliomyelitis of historical interest in North America. However, the live vaccine is still being utilized in underdeveloped countries.

Peripheral Nerve

Some congenital hypomyelinating or axonal polyneuropathies present in the newborn period with a clinical phenotypic appearance similar to SMA I, Werdnig-Hoffman disease. These infants may be so ill that they require intensivist support (2).

Case 3: Severe Newborn Infantile Demyelinating Polyneuropathy

A 2-week-old old infant was delivered after what the mother perceived as a normal pregnancy with normal fetal movements in utero. Since birth, he had a "paucity of spontaneous movements," and a weak cry.

His mom stated that he was still able to breast-feed although he did not hold the pacifier tightly. His gag was weak. Fasciculations of the tongue were present. This alert baby was markedly hypotonic with frog leg posture, no spontaneous movements of the legs, wrist drops, weak palmar grasp, and arthrogryposis multiplex. He assumed the inverted U posture when held prone. He was areflexic and the plantar responses were mute. He responded to noxious stimuli applied to all extremities.

The CSF protein was elevated at 190 mg/dL. Sensory NCS failed to demonstrate any median SNAP. Median and peroneal CMAPs were widely dispersed, of very low amplitude 0.05 and 0.02 mV, had prolonged latencies 3.6 and 8.2 ms and very slow MCV of 6 and 8 m/sec. EMG demonstrated mild diminution in the number of MUPs which were of slightly longer duration, polyphasic, normal amplitude, and firing at increased frequency. The only areas with occasional fibrillations and positive waves were present in the most distal muscles. These findings were compatible with an acquired, diffuse, predominantly demyelinating, peripheral neuropathy.

Sural nerve biopsy demonstrated hypomyelination with abortive onion bulb formation. These findings did not provide a base to distinguish between an inborn error of myelination or an unusual acquired autoimmune demyelinating peripheral neuropathy, such as intrauterine GBS. A trial of prednisone was unsuccessful. Subsequently, progressive respiratory failure ensued. The baby died at age 2 months; an autopsy was declined.

Comment

Any floppy infant presenting with a frog leg posture and tongue fasciculations most likely has SMA type 0 or type I. In contradistinction, this baby's EMG findings of very slow MCVs, with dispersed low amplitude CMAPs, and absent SNAPs were diagnostic of an acquired demyelinating polyneuropathy and not an abnormality primarily at the motor neuron level. The incidence of peripheral neuropathies was 6% in our BCH review of over 100 floppy babies seen in our EMG lab (2,3). These were more common among the infants who also had arthrogryposis (3,12). The absence of sensory responses is the most important pediatric EMG clue to the appropriate diagnostic conclusion that the baby has one of these rare neonatal neuropathies. The nerve pathologies included primary axonal, demyelinating, and widespread neuronal degeneration.

GBS rarely affects newborn infants. It needs consideration in the differential diagnosis of neonatal flaccid paralysis (13–15). In one instance, GBS onset was soon after birth (13). The baby's mother had an autoimmune disease, chronic ulcerative colitis. During the 30th week of her pregnancy she had observed significantly decreased fetal movements (13). Her baby was quadriparetic when delivered at 37 weeks with an Apgar score of 6 at 10 minutes. At age 3 days, neurologic exam demonstrated severe leg and moderate proximal arm weakness, with generalized absence of muscle stretch reflexes. The CSF protein was normal, 38 mg/dL. In contrast, motor NCS demonstrated profound motor nerve conduction velocity (NCV) slowing between 3 and 15 m/sec, with conduction block and temporal dispersion in many nerves. Needle EMG revealed active denervation in many muscles. He had gradual and complete recovery by age 1 year without any specific treatment (13).

Another pregnant mother, aged 33, developed severe GBS during the 29th week of her pregnancy (14). She became tetraplegic and was still respirator dependent when her baby was born at the 38th week. He developed hypotonia, marked respiratory distress, and feeding problems 12 days postpartum although he was well at birth. His CSF protein was 243 mg/dL. An EMG was typical for GBS. Both the mother and child had immunoglobulin G (IgG) antibodies positive for recent cytomegalovirus infection. Intravenous immunoglobulin therapy was associated with a complete symptomatic resolution in 2 weeks (14). One presumes his GBS developed in utero (14).

GBS affected another pregnant woman. Her baby had poor spontaneous ventilation at delivery requiring brief intubation. During the next 5 days of observation, there were no other signs of GBS (15). Despite such, both this infant and his mother had high antibody titers to human peripheral nerve myelin glycolipids (15).

Even without any known intrauterine events, GBS may occur shortly after birth, as early as age 3 weeks. These previously healthy babies present with an acute, rapidly progressive, and often severe hypotonia, with possible respiratory distress, and feeding difficulties (16,17). Chronic inflammatory demyelinating polyneuropathy subsequently developed in a 7-week-old infant with acute GBS (18). An EMG is particularly helpful for the differentiation of GBS from other acute floppy infant syndromes (16). Absent SNAPs, profound motor conduction slowing, and dispersed CMAPs are the quintessential EMG clues for the diagnosis of neonatal

GBS. In our BCH EMG review of more than 100 floppy babies, there was a 6% incidence of peripheral neuropathies (3). Only one of these six infants had EMG findings commensurate with GBS (3).

Although tick paralysis mimics acute GBS in children, we are unaware of an infantile case. Nonetheless, any baby with an acute onset of generalized muscle weakness needs to be searched for a tick, particularly in the scalp (19).

Neuromuscular Junction

Various neuromuscular junction (NMJ) disorders are occasionally encountered during infancy. Autoimmune maternal associated MG is the most easily recognized and probably most common NMJ pathologic entity occurring in this age group. This relatively short-lived disorder typically occurs at birth in 15% to 20% of infants whose mothers have MG (20–22). Rarely, infants born to mothers who had eclampsia and received magnesium treatment, also have the potential to develop an acute infantile presynaptic NMJ disorder (23,24). These two neuromuscular transmission disorders only occasionally come to the attention of the pediatric neurologist as pediatricians are well versed in the management of these infants.

There are also a number of relatively rare congenital myasthenic syndromes with a primary pathophysiologic site of difficulty varying between the presynaptic NMJ, the synapse, or the postsynaptic NMJ. An endplate deficiency of choline acetyltransferase is a congenital myasthenic syndrome that predisposes the baby to an acute onset NMJ disorder (25). Typically, these babies have recurrent episodic apnea. In contrast, it is unusual for other congenital myasthenic syndrome forms to have such an acute presentation.

Infantile botulism is the one other presynaptic neuromuscular transmission disorder that will acutely affect previously healthy babies and toddlers. Clinical suspicion, with subsequent EMG, is crucial to making this diagnosis. Because of its somewhat varied presentation we are concerned that possibly infantile botulism is more common than recognized.

Case 4: Infantile Botulism

A previously healthy, 4-month-old baby was admitted to another hospital with a 1-week history of constipation, and subsequently poor feeding, lethargy, a weak cry, and dehydration. She had lost her ability to roll over, lift her head, or sit up. A full septic evaluation was unremarkable including CSF examination. After she developed cyanosis with an acute apneic spell, and subsequent increasing lethargy, she was transported to BCH.

Attempt to wean her from the ventilator was unsuccessful. Neurologic examination here demonstrated no extraocular muscle movements, absent corneal responses, and no gag reflex. At this time she still had movement in all extremities, and intact muscle stretch reflexes. The initial clinical impression was an "indeterminate encephalopathy." This conclusion was based on nonspecific EEG findings in the right occipital lobe, as her brain magnetic resonance imaging (MRI), CSF, bacterial and viral cultures, and metabolic evaluations were all normal. During this evaluation, she became increasingly hypotonic and areflexic. Seven days after onset of symptoms and subsequent to further clinical review, at change of service a diligent intern requested an EMG for possible infantile botulism.

The EMG evaluation, in the ICU, demonstrated low amplitude median and peroneal CMAPs (0.56 mV and 0.2 mV respectively; normal > 3.5 mV and 1.6 mV) with normal motor NCV, and DLs. RMNS of the median nerve at 2 Hz demonstrated an 11% decrement, and with 20 Hz stimulation a 160% facilitation. MUPs were very "myopathic." These EMG findings were consistent with a diagnosis of infantile botulism. Subsequently, a stool sample, as well as an assay of a honey specimen from home, were both positive for type A botulinum toxin. She gradually improved, with supportive treatment, during the next few months.

Comment

Infantile botulism usually has a stereotyped clinical presentation. Typically, a previously healthy infant, between ages 10 days and 12 months, has the acute onset of hypotonia, generalized descending weakness, poor feeding, oculomotor and pupillary abnormalities, dysphagia, and constipation (26–33). However, one also needs to consider this diagnosis in the setting of unexplained respiratory distress in any baby under 12 months of age. Infantile botulism has been linked to honey ingestion. In its most severe state the presentation may be acute and require ventilatory support. Treatment with human botulinum antitoxin can expedite the infant's recovery (34,35).

Bacteriologic confirmation usually requires a few weeks, but a mouse bioassay and real-time polymerase chain reaction (PCR) assays can provide a rapid confirmation of the diagnosis (36). EMG is the most useful early diagnostic tool. Most babies with infantile botulism have clear-cut evidence of a neuromuscular transmission disorder. Low-rate RMNS, at 2 to 5 Hz, often but not always demonstrates a decremental response (37). More rapid RMNS rates of 20 to 50 Hz provide the primary electrophysiologic technique for diagnosing infantile botulism (37). A posttetanic facilitation varying between 23% and 313%, with a mean of 73%, was documented in 23 of 25 babies (37). A longer period of posttetanic facilitation is also observed. One may not always be able to confirm a diagnosis of infantile botulism with EMG as not all cases have a documented facilitation with RMNS (37,38). However, in most instances of infantile botulism, babies will have a typical EMG diagnostic triad (39). This includes: (1) low amplitude CMAPs (beware normal maturation standards for age), (2) posttetanic facilitation, and (3) absence of posttetanic exhaustion (38).

Muscle

Congenital myopathies typically present as a floppy infant syndrome but most babies are not ill enough to require neonatal ICU monitoring. In addition, myopathies do not typically cause acute infantile flaccid paralysis and/or respiratory distress. However, occasionally we are asked to see a neonatal ICU baby who is found to have a primary myopathy.

Case 5: Neonatal MD

Respiratory distress developed soon after birth in this baby girl, with clubfeet. She required intubation for her first month of life. An EMG was requested for evaluation of her generalized hypotonia when she was 2 months old. Motor NCS demonstrated low amplitude CMAPs but other parameters were normal including SNAPs. Profound and prolonged decrescendo myotonic discharges occurred during her EMG. These were associated with rare fibrillation potentials. Her MUPs were normal. The mother had no myotonia detectable by physical examination or on EMG but she recalled that her father had difficulty releasing his grip when driving a car.

Comment

MD is one of the few dystrophies that presents as a severely floppy infant. Babies with congenital MD may have severe generalized hypotonia requiring intubation

at birth for their associated respiratory compromise. Sometimes, the diagnosis is suspected clinically by their classic facies with "tenting" of the mouth that appears like an upside down letter V. Most all MD infants have a family history of MD, however it is often unrecognized in the parent. Typically, the mother has a milder form requiring premature cataract removal or has evidence of mild subclinical myotonia and/or distal weakness on clinical exam (40).

Today when confronted with the typical clinical phenotype, DNA testing is 98% to 99% accurate in both infants with MD as well as their symptomatic or asymptomatic mothers. Myotonia detectable by EMG may be present in the hypotonic newborn infant, as early as age 5 days, although it sometimes is not always evident this early on (41,42). Occasionally, one finds that a maternal EMG will detect previously unsuspected myotonia (2). Nowadays, a DNA test will quickly establish the diagnosis.

Case 6: Metabolic Myopathy: Phosphofructokinase Deficiency

A 39-week gestation newborn infant had a history of diminished fetal movement and developed immediate respiratory distress at birth. He had severe generalized and bifacial weakness, a high arched palate, absent muscle stretch reflexes, and marked distal arthrogryposis. At 2 days of age, NCS demonstrated low amplitude to absent CMAPs with otherwise normal motor and sensory conduction parameters. EMG demonstrated very low amplitude, short duration MUPs primarily in proximal muscles typical of a myopathy. Muscle biopsy demonstrated an absence of the glycolytic enzyme phosphofructokinase. Swoboda and colleagues (43) suggested that a ketogenic diet might be beneficial. This commenced at age 4 months. He gained some clinical motor improvement through age 2 years; however, he died of other complications later that year.

Comment

Metabolic myopathies rarely present with severe hypotonia and respiratory weakness in the newborn period. A fatal case of phosphorylase deficiency presented at 4 weeks of age with feeding difficulties, tiring easily, and severe respiratory distress. This infant had a rapidly progressive course, becoming very hypotonic with generalized weakness (44). A muscle biopsy shows an excess of glycogen accumulation in infants with phosphofructo-kinase deficiency; the diagnosis is confirmed with enzyme assay and/or genetic analysis.

■ ACUTE NEUROMUSCULAR CRISES IN THE TODDLER AND THE OLDER CHILD

Anterior Horn Cell

We are pleased to comment that since the inception of our EMG lab in 1979 at BCH we are not aware of the occurrence of any acute poliomyelitis, beyond infancy. However, one needs to keep this possibility always in mind, as there are some parents who reportedly still decline to have their children appropriately immunized. In addition, with the increased use of air travel and children being adopted, immigrating, or visiting from all parts of the world, one always needs to be alert to the possibility of poliomyelitis in countries with less than ideal immunization standards. However, we do see a few instances of subacute polio in children coming from those nations where standard immunization is not routinely available (45). Physicians must keep poliomyelitis within the differential diagnosis of any child with an acute, particularly asymmetric, flaccid paralysis.

Peripheral Nerve

Today, GBS is the most common cause for an acute generalized paralysis in the older child. A few rare other primary pediatric polyneuropathies occasionally develop. In addition, some of these clinical settings are caused by some unusual neuromuscular transmission defects as noted later in this chapter. In the ICU setting, an EMG is particularly important for rapid localization of the acute motor unit lesion. It may also prove helpful for making prognostic judgments. The following case examples illustrate some of the interesting GBS variants.

Case 7: Guillain-Barré Syndrome: Pseudoencephalopathy, Painful Weakness, and Meningismus

Two weeks prior to evaluation at BCH, this previously healthy 5-year-old boy participated in an Audubon field trip to collect insects along the Rhode Island coast. He soon developed a fine papular rash on his face and neck that was followed 24 hours later by headache, nausea, and vomiting during a family sailing cruise. Bilateral pain developed in his knees, posterior thighs, and popliteal fossa 4 days prior to our evaluation. A viral syndrome was diagnosed and the pediatrician treated him symptomatically. Subsequently he lay in his bunk complaining of headaches and occasional vomiting but no fever. He was brought to BCH 1 week later.

Here he was extremely uncomfortable, groaning and writhing. His conjunctivae were injected, and his neck stiff. Muscle strength was "grossly" normal, and capable of supporting his weight to stand. Sensation seemed intact, however, his muscle stretch reflexes were not elicitable. Brain CT was normal. Subsequent CSF analysis demonstrated a protein of 145 mg/dL, glucose 65 mg/dL, and 1 WBC/dL. On neurologic examination the next morning he was listless with bilateral Babinski signs. Muscle strength was still difficult to assess.

Motor NCSs were of variably low amplitude with dispersed CMAPs, and multifocal asymmetric prolongation of DLs. Motor NCV varied from 22 m/sec for median to 38 m/sec for ulnar and 50 m/sec for peroneal fibers. Peroneal F waves were absent. No median or ulnar SNAPs were elicited. Needle EMG was normal. This EMG was compatible with an acute demyelinating polyneuropathy typical for GBS.

Comment

With the history of headache and rash, in an agitated child with Babinski signs, an encephalopathic process was the initial diagnostic consideration. After the brain CT was normal, a spinal fluid examination was performed. The high CSF protein led to the consideration of an atypical form of GBS. Other neurologic considerations included a transverse myelitis, an entity that also occasionally mimics GBS, however, there was no evidence of a cord level in this instance. Spinal MRI was therefore not performed. Some individuals with GBS appear to occasionally have an associated, but indeterminate central nervous system process such as locked-in syndrome, indicated by the presence of acute tetraplegia, areflexia, and cranial nerve involvement despite otherwise typical clinical and EMG findings for GBS. These patients, however, are fully conscious (46).

Severe pain was the primary presenting symptom of GBS in 21% (5 of 24) of children seen at BCH (47). A significant degree of pain was present in 67% of our GBS cases (47). At times, as in this instance, this discomfort was so bothersome and led to such irritability, that a number of these children were initially thought to have a meningoencephalopathy (48). Because of the severity of the pain, three of the children, each younger than this boy, were unable to participate in formal muscle testing. Thus the actual muscle weakness related to their GBS was difficult to clinically appreciate. A total of nine youngsters seen here at BCH were thought to be encephalopathic during their initial emergency room evaluations but later proven to have GBS (48). Initially each one received either brain CT or MRI, and when normal, this was followed by CSF exam anticipating an infection. When the albuminocytologic dissociation was found, neurologic consultation followed. The elevated CSF protein with areflexia and severe pain provided the clinical clues suggesting GBS. EMG was requested for further definition.

A reduced CMAP, in 83%, with absent or prolonged long latency waves, in 81%, were the two most common EMG findings in children with the demyelinating form of GBS (also known as acute inflammatory demyelinating polyneuropathy [AIDP]) seen at BCH (47). Specific findings consistent with demyelination, including conduction block, temporal dispersion, or MCV slowing, occurred in 70% to 74% of these children. MRI of the spinal cord may show enhancement of the nerve roots. In addition to GBS, the differential diagnosis of an acute demyelinating peripheral neuropathy in children includes some toxins, in particular glue sniffing, and rarely buckthorn wild cherry ingestion, insecticides, and thallium (16, 49). Porphyria, arsenic, lead, or mercury poisoning also enter the differential diagnosis when there is concomitant gastrointestinal distress (16). The differential diagnosis of children living in agricultural communities also includes organophosphate pesticide poisoning (50). Interestingly, in Paraguay a 30% incidence of organophosphate pesticide exposure was noted with otherwise typical childhood GBS (51). A few inborn metabolic errors, porphyria or Leigh disease (52), enhanced by medications, particularly barbiturates, may also precipitate symptoms resembling childhood GBS.

The clinical course and eventual prognosis of either the demyelinating or axonal forms is determined by the extent of primary or secondary axonal damage. There is a primary axonal variant of GBS that has been predominantly reported from China (53,54) but also occurs in America (particularly in Latin America), Europe, and Japan. In this instance, there is an initial immunologic reaction against epitopes specific to the axonal membrane. Axonal GBS has been classified into two subtypes: acute

motor axonal neuropathy (AMAN) and acute motor and sensory axonal neuropathy (AMSAN) (55). EMG and NCSs are the main method for distinguishing AMAN, AMSAN, and AIDP; however, in certain cases, the distinction between AMSAN and AIDP may be difficult. Both AMAN and AMSAN may follow *Campylobacter jejuni* enteritis. Anti-GM1, anti-GM1b, and anti-GD1a IgG antibodies can be detected in patients with AMAN and AMSAN and can be used to differentiate these axonal forms of GBS from AIDP (56,57).

Case 8: Axonal GBS With "Brain Death" Presentation

A 6-year-old boy presented with a 2-week history of headaches and 2 days with difficulty walking. He had surgery and chemotherapy for a medulloblastoma 8 months previously, and subsequently was feeling fine. His last vincristine, cisplatin, and cyclophosphamide were completed 2 months earlier. Suddenly, he developed acute gasping and shortly thereafter had a respiratory arrest. On admission to the hospital he had no spontaneous movements and he was unresponsive to all noxious stimuli. He had total external ophthalmoplegia and his pupils were fixed and dilated. No muscle stretch reflexes or corneal, oculocephalic, and gag responses were elicitable. Plantar stimulation was mute. Initially he was thought to be "brain dead." His CSF had a protein 167 mg/dL with just 6 WBCs. When an EEG was unexpectedly normal, a toxic screen and testing for heavy metals and porphyrins were also unremarkable.

An EMG was first performed on the fifth day of his illness. No motor or sensory responses, or MUPs were identified. However, fibrillations and positive waves were present in all muscles. Subsequent trial of intravenous immunoglobulin therapy did not result in any improvement for a few weeks. Eventually his cranial nerve function slowly recovered followed by respiratory and limb movements. One year later he was able to ambulate with a walker. His arm strength was then normal.

Comment

It is very rare to see fixed dilated pupils with GBS as occurred here. Both diphtheria and botulism are diagnostic considerations with this clinical set particularly when there is predominant bulbar involvement (58). MG or poliomyelitis also enters into this differential diagnosis but in these instances the pupillary responses are preserved.

Rarely, infectious diseases also need consideration in the differential diagnosis of GBS. In adults, GBS may be the presenting manifestation of AIDS. A 6-year-old boy with congenital AIDS has also developed GBS (59). However, to date based on a complete National Library of Medicine computer search, GBS has not been the presenting illness leading to a diagnosis of childhood AIDS. Lyme disease may be associated with a painful neuropathy, but this review also did not uncover an instance of a GBS-like illness in children. Diphtheria still occurs in those geopolitical settings without access to modern immunizations. Bulbar symptoms usually predominate early on. Usually these children have had a recent severe sore throat, and fever before the onset of the bulbar palsy. The acute peripheral neuropathy symptoms always occur subsequent to the onset of the bulbar symptoms. Once again as with the rare instance of infantile polio, the investigation of an immunization history is of significant importance in this clinical setting. Rarely one may see this constellation of findings in an older child. Diphtheria occurred in a teenager, presenting with bulbar symptoms, who was seen by one of us (HRJ). He had inadvertently received only one diphtheria, pertussis, and tetanus (DPT) immunization early in life (Table 21.2).

An acute vincristine exacerbation of an underlying polyneuropathy may occur if this chemotherapeutic agent is prescribed to children with a mild, subtle, or even unrecognized Charcot-Marie-Tooth type 1 (CMT1) hereditary neuropathy. This toxic neuropathy may be relatively severe when superimposed on this underlying genetic neuropathic process. As sometimes CMT1 is unsuspected early in life, it is important to query the parents before any vincristine therapy is initiated, as to the presence of any personal or family history of CMT1 by asking about the presence of high arches and weak feet. Testing for the specific genetic defect (a 17p11.2-12 duplication of the PMP22 gene) needs consideration in any child where there is any clinical suspicion of CMT1 prior to treatment with vincristine. One clinical example of such a severe neuropathy occurred in an immunocompromised child with an unrecognized family history of CMT1 (60).

Additionally, as mentioned earlier, children very occasionally present with one of two very rare, acute axonal forms of GBS. One of these, acute *motor* axonal neuropathy (AMAN), occurs predominantly in China (53), although it does have a much less common worldwide distribution. We have seen a few instances of this at BCH. Additionally, as discussed earlier, there is also an even

■ **Table 21.2** Conditions Leading to Acute Neuromuscular Crises in the Toddler and Older Child

Anterior Horn Cell
— Spinal muscular atrophies (5q and non-5q)
— Poliomyelitis in the nonimmunized child

Peripheral Nerve
— Guillain-Barré syndrome
  – Acute demyelinating
  – Axonal forms
— Glue sniffing
— Buckthorn wild cherry ingestion
— Insecticides
— Heavy metal poisoning
— Vincristine treatment in patient with Charcot-Marie-Tooth type 1
— Diphtheria
— Acute mononeuritis multiplex

Neuromuscular Junction
— Autoimmune myasthenia gravis
— Congenital myasthenic syndromes
— Tick paralysis

Muscle
— Channelopathies/periodic paralyses
— End-stage muscle disease
— Inflammatory myopathies
— Metabolic myopathies

Other
— Transverse myelitis
— Spinal cord injury

less common acute *motor sensory* axonal neuropathy (AMSAN), which we have not diagnosed at BCH thus far. Another very rare pediatric form of GBS, originally defined by Miller-Fisher, also occurs in children (61). These children typically present primarily with gait ataxia, extraocular muscle palsies, and areflexia. Such a presentation occurred in about 5% of our BCH experience (47). Overlap cases, in which the clinical features of GBS and Miller-Fisher syndrome are intermixed, do occur. Miller-Fisher syndrome is also a postinfectious syndrome, frequently triggered by *C jejuni* enteritis. Sera from more than 90% of pure Miller-Fisher syndrome and GBS overlap patients, collected during the acute phase of the illness, contain high titers of antibodies to GQ1b ganglioside (62–65). These antibodies tend to disappear during clinical recovery. Strains of *C jejuni* isolated from Miller-Fisher syndrome patients bear GQ1b epitopes, suggesting that the underlying mechanism is one of molecular mimicry (66).

Prognosis in these pediatric GBS variants is determined by a combination of clinical and/or EMG signs of very significant axonal damage. Often children with GBS have a relatively benign prognosis (47). In some clinical instances, however, a more prolonged recovery, or even rarely a fatality (67), may occur. Examples include the child who requires a respirator, those in whom one cannot evoke a CMAP with NCS during an EMG, and those children who have very widespread active denervation on needle EMG. This last group may often require more than a year for reinnervation and subsequent recovery (58).

The prognosis for recovery in children with GBS is far better than for adults; however, there is no universal agreement on this opinion (68). Approximately 15% of hospitalized children with GBS require mechanical ventilatory support during the course of their admission (69). It is important to emphasize the need for the intensive-care setting, where it is possible to monitor cardiovascular and autonomic function (70). Of nine patients who died of GBS, two were children, one of whom died of cardiac arrest; the other had periods of bradycardia and hypotension and became neurologically unresponsive (67). Fluctuating blood pressure and autonomic instability have been recognized as predictors of a potentially fatal cardiac arrhythmia (67). Careful monitoring of respiratory function, good management of fluid balance, and avoidance of bed sores and pressure neuropathies are other important areas for care of the child with GBS. A significant cause of death in adults is pulmonary embolism; however, the literature is not clear as to the value of subcutaneous heparin for the prophylaxis of venous thrombosis in a child (16).

Guidelines as to when to transfer a child with GBS to the ICU and when to proceed with intubation have not been developed. Respiratory failure should be expected in any GBS patient with progressive appendicular or bulbar weakness. In children with GBS cared for on a regular pediatric ward, pulmonary insufficiency may develop insidiously and remain clinically silent without obvious signs of respiratory failure. Hypoxemia may not be detected until the vital capacity has fallen significantly, and hypercarbia is a late finding; therefore, blood gases are not useful in monitoring the diaphragmatic weakness in GBS patients. In older children who can cooperate for pulmonary function testing, bedside measurements of vital capacity (VC) and maximal inspiratory (PImax) and expiratory (PEmax) pressures should be carried out every 6 to 8 hours. In the younger

uncooperative child, oxygen saturation, especially in sleep, should be monitored by pulse oximetry. It should be noted, however, that a fall in oxygen saturation is a late finding in children receiving oxygen.

Again, practice parameters allowing the prediction of need for mechanical ventilation have not been established in children. However, even in the adult literature the respective guidelines are not unanimous. A recent study summarizing 20 years of ICU experience from the Mayo Clinic, Rochester, Minnesota, provided some important guidelines which could be extrapolated to the pediatric age group (Table 21.3). Important clinical indicators of impending respiratory failure included bulbar dysfunction and autonomic instability, bilateral facial palsy, and rapid disease progression. The presence of these clinical parameters was associated with increased likelihood of mechanical ventilation. In our experience, however, bilateral facial palsy in children has not been a strong predictor of impending respiratory failure. Analysis of serial respiratory function measurements showed that a 30% reduction in VC, PImax, or PEmax were associated with subsequent progression to respiratory failure and intubation. Also, the following "threshold" respiratory values—VC less than 20 mL/kg, PImax less than 30 cm of H_2O, and PEmax less than

---

■ **Table 21.3** Indications for Transfer of Child With Guillain-Barré Syndrome (GBS) to the Intensive Care Unit

1. Bulbar dysfunction
2. Autonomic instability
3. Rapid disease progression
4. More than 30% reduction in vital capacity (VC) from baseline
5. VC less than 20 ml/kg
6. Maximal inspiratory pressure less than 30 cm H_2O
7. Maximal expiratory pressure less than 40 cm H_2O
8. Aspiration episode
9. Recurrent oxygen desaturation events with values below 90%[a]

4, 5, 6, and 7 should be considered indications for elective intubation.
8 is an indication for intubation.
[a] In a young child not receiving oxygen, however, a fall in oxygen saturation may be a late sign in patients with GBS. In older cooperative children, serial pulmonary function studies are far more reliable predictors of impending respiratory failure than pulse oximetry. (Adapted in part from Lawn ND et al. Anticipating mechanical ventilation in Guillain-Barré syndrome. *Arch Neurol.* 2001;58: 893–898.)

40 cm of H_2O—were shown to be highly associated with subsequent progression to respiratory failure. The use of the so-called 20/30/40 rule allows patients-at-risk to be identified and to be preemptively admitted to the ICU for close monitoring and elective intubation under optimal conditions. In the past, clinical signs of respiratory fatigue and severe bulbar weakness with aspiration, or fall of the VC to less than 15 mL/kg or arterial PO_2 values to less than 70 mmHg, had been defined as criteria for intubation (71). Although these criteria might be accurate in determining the need for intubation, they cannot be considered as practice guidelines for preemptive respiratory management of children with GBS. When serial bedside respiratory function testing shows constant decline of VC, PImax, PEmax, fulfilling criteria for the 20/30/40 rule, or more than 30% reduction in VC from baseline, the patient should be transferred to the ICU and elective intubation should be considered. It is also prudent to have young children with oxygen desaturation events with values falling below 90% and/or signs of dysautonomia, bulbar dysfunction, or aspiration transferred to the ICU for monitoring and possible intubation. One also needs to be aware of the fact that dysautonomia in GBS patients may also be triggered or accentuated by tracheal manipulation (i.e., intubation, suctioning). Because of the propensity of GBS patients for upper airway collapse, noninvasive methods of respiratory support such as continuous or bilevel positive airway pressure methods have probably a limited role in the respiratory management of severe GBS patients with borderline respiratory values. Nocturnal decompensation is also a common occurrence in patients with severe GBS due to a combination of reduction in VC related to the supine position and also impairment of central respiratory drive; thus the need for close respiratory monitoring during sleep. Immune therapies, plasma exchange, and high-dose intravenous immunoglobulin have been shown to be of equal efficacy and are known to expedite recovery from GBS (72).

Another major immediate diagnostic consideration in the differential diagnosis of GBS relates to excluding an acute spinal cord tumor or transverse myelitis. Children with either lesion may also be admitted to the medical ICU (73–76). Both of these disease entities may acutely produce a rapidly progressive paralysis, hyporeflexia, and back pain. More commonly spinal cord lesions, and rarely GBS, are associated with early sphincter dysfunction. However, in contrast to spinal lesions, these symptoms are usually transient with GBS

(47). Four children had severe pain, asymmetric lower extremity weakness, and a clear-cut sensory level on careful neurologic examination (73). MRI was abnormal in four of the eight children evaluated (73). Each child had a malignant spinal cord tumor (73). Even imaging studies may cause confusion. One 6-year-old child developed progressive weakness and areflexia (74). Both the clinical and EMG findings were commensurate with a GBS diagnosis. If there is enlargement of the spinal cord, swelling with increased signal intensity of the cord, and no contrast enhancement, a diagnosis of GBS is not excluded because, rarely, transverse myelitis and GBS may occur concurrently (74,75). Transverse myelitis is the primary spinal cord lesion that may occasionally produce significant confusion in the differential diagnosis of GBS (76).

Case 9: Transverse Myelitis With Acute Gait Difficulty and Back Pain

A 12-year-old boy had sudden problems walking, tending to waddle with his knees flexed, the night before coming to BCH. Initially, his parents thought he was actually clowning. Later that night he developed knife-like back pain. In the morning he was found paraplegic and unable to urinate. Neurologic evaluation here demonstrated a flaccid paraplegia, absence of muscle stretch reflexes, and "ambiguous" responses to plantar stimulation. Arm and hand strength as well as their respective muscle stretch reflexes were normal. Sensory examination was somewhat limited in accuracy; there was a questionable sensory level at T10-12. CSF evaluation demonstrated 30 WBCs with 90% monocytes, and protein of 175 mg/dL. Spinal imaging demonstrated a tethered cord. No peroneal or tibial F waves were defined; routine peroneal, tibial, and median motor nerve conduction velocities (MNCVs) and sural SNAPs were normal. Needle EMG was unremarkable. MRI of the spinal cord showed T2 hyperintensities extending longitudinally in the lower thoracic region.

Comment

The acute onset of leg weakness, areflexia, and back pain with the absent F waves on EMG initially suggested a diagnosis of GBS with predominant involvement at the nerve root level. However, the lack of subsequent arm involvement, the persistent sphincter involvement, and the more precise definition of a saddle sensory level led to the appropriate clinical diagnosis of transverse myelitis. It is important to emphasize that although the absence of F waves is one of the most common early signs of GBS, similar findings are also found with transverse myelitis if the segmental lesion affects the precise spinal level for the legs or arms (47). EMG is generally normal in this setting, however, if segmental anterior-horn cells are affected, both the CMAPs and F waves may be affected. This leads to neurophysiologic mimicking of the typical early GBS findings. MRI usually confirms the diagnosis.

Mononeuritis Multiplex

During our 32-year experience at BCH, we have evaluated just one child with an acute fulminating mononeuritis multiplex (MNM) affecting a very ill teenager in renal failure. We have seen only two instances of MNM in more than 32 years at BCH. A colleague at Johns Hopkins recalls just one case (T. Crawford, personal oral communication, March 2002). This limited experience has been reported; two of the three cases were related to systemic vasculitis and one possibly represented a case of non-systemic vasculitis (77–79).

Case 10: Acute MNM

This 16-year-old girl with systemic lupus erythematosus had dialysis dependent, membranous, proliferative glomerulonephritis associated with hypertension, pericardial effusion, and seizures. She was not a renal transplant candidate because of medication noncompliance. A sudden onset of left-hand numbness occurred just 1 month before we initially evaluated her. She developed an acute left foot drop shortly thereafter followed by an acute numbness in her right hand and an acute right foot drop the very next day. She became incapacitated. Neurologic examination demonstrated a left median and ulnar and bilateral asymmetric peroneal neuropathies.

EMG demonstrated an MNM. Sural nerve biopsy confirmed the clinical diagnosis of a vasculitis. Treatment with intravenous solumedrol (30 mg/kg, maximum 1 g) per day for 5 days followed by oral prednisone (80 mg/d) was initiated. Within just a few days, she developed an acute gastrointestinal distress with upper gastrointestinal bleeding. Gastroscopy demonstrated an active bleeding site. A gastric mucosa biopsy also demonstrated a vasculitis.

Comment

MNM is very uncommon in children and adolescents. Interestingly, although MNM is commonly seen in diabetics, we are not aware of such complication in the pediatric age group. However, this single case emphasizes that if a child has an underlying connective tissue disorder and presents with an acute mononeuropathy, especially with no evidence of a mechanical reason, the possibility of a systemic vasculitis needs to be considered early on in the differential diagnosis. Today, children with renal compromise much less commonly develop a polyneuropathy (80).

Neuromuscular Junction Disorders in the Older Child

The differential diagnosis of acute childhood bulbar and generalized weakness requires consideration of a neuromuscular transmission defect. MG and the Miller-Fisher variant of GBS are the primary considerations. When MG occurs in children, it is typically quite similar to its presentation in adults. However, occasionally one may see some clinical variants that lead to an intensive care admission before the diagnosis of MG is even entertained.

Another very rare, often unidentified, and unsuspected disorder is tick paralysis. This biologic toxin is a rare and dramatic neuromuscular transmission defect that always needs consideration in the differential diagnosis of GBS or MG, particularly among children from the preschool ages forward (19,81–85). Each child with acute weakness requires careful inspection of the scalp to exclude this unusual diagnosis. The pathophysiology here is also most likely a defect in neuromuscular transmission although this hypothesis is difficult to prove with standard EMG techniques.

Case 11: Tick Paralysis Presenting as Acute Quadriparesis, Dysarthria, and Neck Muscle Weakness

This 3-year-old girl had a recent upper respiratory infection. The night prior to admission to BCH she stubbed her toe and later asked her dad to carry her to the bathroom. The next morning she was unable to move well and had to be carried downstairs. When her parents realized that she could not lift her head to watch television they took her to the local pediatrician. She found the child to have a weak voice, quadriparesis, areflexia, and normal sensation.

Careful inspection of the scalp demonstrated a tick. The pediatrician removed the tick and referred the child to BCH. The next morning this little girl had a very significant improvement. She was able to sit up with support and walk to the bathroom. Although intellectually of interest, we did not feel an EMG was needed with her rapid improvement.

Comment

One of the most helpful clinical clues, allowing the clinician to differentiate tick paralysis from GBS or MG, is the finding of early pupillary involvement, as seen in four of six Australian cases (19). Total ophthalmoplegia occurred in two patients and all but one of six children had extraocular muscle paresis. Those findings may sometimes suggest the Miller-Fisher GBS variant. Nonreactive pupils also occur with diphtheria and rarely GBS (58).

Typical EMG findings in tick paralysis include very diminished CMAP amplitudes with preserved MCVs, motor DLs, and SNAPs (19,84,85). These findings are similar to AMAN or even some early demyelinating forms of GBS. Sequential NCS studies immediately prior to removal of a tick, a few days hence, and in 6 months demonstrated that the reduced CMAP improved dramatically after the tick was removed (84,85). No neuromuscular transmission defect has been demonstrated with standard EMG RMNS (84,85). However, experimental data do point to tick paralysis being related to the presynaptic NMJ with decreased acetylcholine release (86). In some children the early appearance of fibrillation potentials, as soon as 24 to 48 hours, may lead to diagnostic confusion if one does not pay close attention to the total constellation of neurophysiologic findings (84,85).

Tick paralysis evolves more slowly than other biologic toxins, however, it may actually be more deadly (19). Prolonged respiratory paralysis occurred in two of the six Australian children (19). There the responsible tick *Ixodes holocyclus* is a different species than *Dermacentor andersoni* or *Dermacentor variabilis* common to North America (19). The latter is associated with a rapid improvement once the tick is removed in contrast to a continued deterioration for up to 48 hours in the Australian variety. In that setting the physicians must be careful not to discharge the child too soon. Four of their six children deteriorated after initial hospital discharge (19).

Case 12: Myasthenia Gravis With Acute Dysphagia, Drooling, and Ptosis

This infant girl was very healthy through age 15 months when she developed drooling, irritability, and inability to finish her bottles. Her pediatrician, noting a red throat, performed a throat swab that proved to be rapid streptococcal negative. During this procedure, she developed acute respiratory distress. After emergent admission to a local hospital she had an otolaryngology evaluation during which she was intubated. She was diagnosed with middle lobe pneumonia and treated with ceftriaxone. Her fever resolved but she had continued difficulty swallowing liquids. While taking oral medication she suddenly became limp and lethargic, sustaining a respiratory arrest. She responded to positive pressure ventilation and corticosteroids. An emergent transfer was made to BCH. Although successfully extubated she had continued difficulties swallowing. When this child was extubated 4 days later, she was then noted to have bilateral ptosis, bifacial weakness, frequent cough after eating, and was unable to walk.

Tensilon (edrophonium chloride) testing with a dose of 1.6 mgm produced a dramatic improvement in her ptosis and facial appearance. A subsequent EMG, with 3 Hz RMNS, demonstrated 38% to 45% decrements in the CMAPs. There was no repetitive component to her CMAPs. Her initial, commercially performed acetylcholine receptor antibody was negative; however, it was then definitely positive at the Mayo laboratories. She was treated with Mestinon (pyridostigmine bromide), in gradually increased dosages to 10-mg tid, with gradual but variable improvement of her neuromuscular findings. Interestingly, the ptosis and bifacial weakness were the last to resolve. A thymectomy was considered but with her excellent course it was decided to await a recurrence of her symptoms. The medication was withdrawn during the second 6 months of her illness. She has been asymptomatic now for a number of years.

Comment

Autoimmune MG (AMG) is a rare but important consideration in the differential diagnosis of either acute respiratory distress or failure to wean from a respirator. This applies to children of any age, even in toddlers, as noted in this instance. The youngest child with non-neonatal AMG that we are aware of was a 9-month-old (87). Although most AMG children present with ptosis and/or diplopia (88), we occasionally see other clinical settings, some of which require urgent intensive care management (89). This is particularly so when there is any hint of airway compromise. For instance, we evaluated one teenager being followed by an otolaryngologist for progressive but variable speech difficulties when suddenly she developed severe dysphagia and increasing respiratory distress. The reader is referred to Andrews' (90) treatment outline.

■ MUSCLE

Channelopathies

Some of the various channelopathies, particularly hyperkalemic and hypokalemic periodic paralysis, always warrant consideration in the differential diagnosis of acute GBS. As these are autosomal dominant sodium or calcium channelopathies, there is usually a well-documented family history. Clinically the episodes of paralysis are relatively short-lived on most occasions. Routine NCS findings are normal; however, prolonged periods of exercise with EMG monitoring can evoke a diminution in CMAP amplitudes (91). Needle EMG often demonstrates significant myotonic-like discharges with the hyperkalemic variant.

We do call attention to a case of an 18-month-old, with a previously unrecognized sodium channel myotonia, who presented with respiratory stridor and increasing difficulty breathing, secondary to an acute bronchiolitis. She had trouble opening her eyes that was worsened with crying, as was her stridor. This child had somewhat elevated serum potassium presumably secondary to her increased respiratory effort. These findings were all compatible with a form of paramyotonia. This clinical combination exacerbated her underlying sodium channelopathy with vocal cord myotonia and led to ever increasing respiratory stridor.

Dermatomyositis

Very occasionally one may witness the acute onset of dermatomyositis in the pediatric age group. More commonly this illness has a slowly ingravescent temporal profile and does not require evaluation in the ICU.

■ CRITICAL ILLNESS NEUROMUSCULAR DISORDERS

The acute weakness or paralysis which may occasionally occur in children with critical illness is sometimes related to conditions involving the peripheral nerve, endplate, or muscle. Children with overwhelming sepsis or status asthmaticus may develop a critical illness neuromuscular syndrome that may mimic a hospital-acquired GBS presenting with a failure to wean from the respirator (92-94). Some of these syndromes had initially been felt to be secondary to a defect in neuromuscular transmission. Bolton was one of the first to emphasize the need for us to consider these various syndromes when we are called to the ICU (93). Subsequent to his initial report, defining the role of the peripheral nerve in some of these critical care failures to wean patients, further careful studies have led to the demonstration that most of these children may have a primary myopathy (95). These various critical illness neuromuscular disorders may affect each level of the motor unit (Table 21.4).

Segmental Anterior Horn Cell Disease (Hopkins Syndrome)

Hopkins syndrome or postasthmatic amyotrophy is a poliomyelitis-like illness that occurs following status asthmaticus and primarily in childhood, but it may also occur after puberty (96). It is characterized by rapidly progressive and permanent monoplegia or diplegia (Table 21.5) (97–106). The etiology of the syndrome remains unknown and, despite its resemblance to poliomyelitis, all 27 reported patients were appropriately immunized against polio (Table 21.6). Other viruses considered as possible etiologies include enteroviruses and herpes simplex virus type 1. CSF examination in one 7-year-old patient with Hopkins syndrome showed primary herpes simplex virus type 1 infection, supporting the hypothesis of a viral mechanism (107,108). An outbreak of poliomyelitis-like paralysis indistinguishable from Hopkins syndrome has been described in an

---

■ **Table 21.4** Critical Illness Neuromuscular Disorders

1. Segmental anterior horn cell disease (Hopkins syndrome)
2. Critical illness polyneuropathy
3. Persistent neuromuscular blockade
4. Acute quadriplegic myopathy
5. Acute necrotizing myopathy of intensive care

■ Table 21.5 Differentiating Features of Critical Illness Neuromuscular Disorders

Features	Critical Illness Polyneuropathy	Acute Quadriplegic/ Necrotizing Myopathy	Hopkins Syndrome
Age group	Elderly (reports in children)	Children, adolescents	Young children
Risk factors	Multiorgan failure/sepsis	Neuromuscular blocking agents and/or steroids	Status asthmaticus
Timing	> 2 weeks	Variable	< 2 weeks
Clinical findings	Sensory and motor	Purely motor	Purely motor
Limbs affected	Quadriparesis	Quadriparesis	Monoparesis
Pain	Unusual	Muscular tenderness	Mild
Reflexes	Absent or ↓	↓	Normal in unaffected limbs
Recovery	Good (slow, complete); may be incomplete	Good (slow, complete); may be rapid	Poor
Creatine kinase	< Twice upper normal value	Normal to ↑↑↑[a]	Normal
Nerve conduction studies	↓ SNAP and CMAP amplitudes	Normal SNAPs; ↓↓ CMAPs	Normal SNAPs
Electromyography	Neuropathic	Myopathic	Localized neuropathic
Muscle excitability	Normal	Absent or ↓↓	Normal
Spinal fluid	Normal	Not reported	Pleocytosis
Muscle biopsy	Grouped atrophy; axonal loss	Type II atrophy; myosin loss	Not reported

[a] Normal to mildly increased in acute quadriplegic myopathy; significantly increased in acute necrotizing myopathy.
Abbreviations: CMAPs, compound muscle action potentials; SNAPs, sensory nerve action potentials.

■ Table 21.6 Features of 27 Children With Hopkins Syndrome (Postasthmatic Amyotrophy)[a]

Age of onset	13 mo–11 y
Sex, male/female	19/8
Immunization (polio)	27/27
Days to pareses after asthma	1–11
Spinal fluid protein (mild elevation)	6/13 reported
Spinal fluid pleocytosis	13/13 reported
Denervation on electromyography	17/17 reported
Slowed conduction velocities	4/15
Virus isolation	
Enteroviruses	5/22
Herpes simplex virus type 1 (spinal fluid)	1/22
Permanent paralysis	27/27
Monoplegia	21
Diplegia	4
Hemiplegia	2

[a] Data derived from cases reported in the literature (98–105).
Source: Adapted from Sheth RD, Bolton CF. Neuromuscular complications of sepsis in children. *J Child Neurol.* 1995;10:346–352.

epidemic of enterovirus 71 (107); these patients, however, did not have acute asthma. Electrophysiological findings suggest segmental anterior horn cell disease. MRI of the cervical spine in Hopkins syndrome has revealed swelling and edema in the region of the clinically involved segments (103,108). Surgical exploration of the brachial plexus did not show any evidence of pathology (101). Since all patients who have developed Hopkins syndrome received steroids, the possibility of an immunologically mediated mechanism, perhaps an underlying immunodeficiency and/or steroid-mediated susceptibility of patients to invasion of the anterior horn cells by a virus, has also been postulated (105).

Critical Illness Polyneuropathy

Initially described by Bolton and colleagues in 1984 (93), critical illness polyneuropathy (CIP) is a sensorimotor axonal polyneuropathy that develops in association with sepsis and multiorgan failure. Although signs of CIP can usually be seen early in the ICU course (109), the onset of the neuropathy is difficult to recognize because of the frequently associated encephalopathy, the severity of the underlying illness, and the use of neuromuscular blocking agents in conjunction with ventilatory support (Table 21.5). It is usually noted when the patient cannot be weaned from the mechanical ventilator. The main clinical findings include distally predominant extremity weakness and loss of muscle stretch reflexes. Sensory loss is hard to demonstrate but is sometimes detectable in patients who can cooperate for a neurologic examination. Cranial nerves are involved only rarely, and therefore, predominant cranial nerve involvement suggests another condition. If the child exhibits facial grimacing in response to rigorous painful stimulation of the distal extremities, implying intact sensory pathways, a myopathic mechanism for the quadriparesis needs to be suspected; nonetheless, the differentiation cannot usually be made clinically.

CIP is a primarily distal axonopathy and its pathogenesis remains uncertain. It is possible that humoral and cellular processes result in disturbed or lack of vascular autoregulation with increased microvascular permeability, endoneural edema, and capillary occlusion (93,110). Serum creatine kinase (CK) levels are usually normal or mildly elevated. Electrophysiologic studies show evidence of an axonal neuropathy (110,111). NCSs show reduced amplitude of motor and sensory responses. Significant slowing of nerve conduction or nerve conduction blocks are not expected findings and, if present, suggest other diagnostic possibilities, particularly GBS. In CIP, needle EMG often demonstrates neurogenic MUPs as well as fibrillation potentials and positive sharp waves, in both the extremity musculature and the diaphragm (110). Phrenic NCSs show either absent or reduced responses (51). Nerve biopsy as well as autopsy studies are consistent with axonal degeneration of both motor and sensory fibers without evidence of significant inflammation or demyelination (110). The differential diagnosis here includes acute GBS, porphyria, botulism, myasthenic crisis, prolonged neuromuscular blockade, and CIP (111). Recovery may be slow and incomplete.

Persistent Neuromuscular Blockade

Neuromuscular blockade following the discontinuation of neuromuscular blocking agents may persist, resulting in prolonged weakness and inability to wean from the ventilator. This may occur more frequently in children with impaired renal or hepatic function and has been reported with all neuromuscular blocking agents,

including pancuronium, vancuronium, and atracurium (112–114). Serum CK levels are usually normal. RMNS demonstrates a decremental response of the CMAP, identifying the NMJ as the anatomic site of this physiologic abnormality. Rarely, however, no motor response is obtained in the child with severe prolonged blockade or in those with acute quadriplegic myopathy (AQM). In children with persistent neuromuscular blockade, the weakness typically lasts for only a few days and should not last for more than a week after the discontinuation of the neuromuscular blocking agents . If the weakness persists beyond 7 days, other conditions such as AQM need consideration. Thus the EMG studies must be repeated if the weakness persists, particularly in instances where no motor responses are present on initial evaluation. Normal motor conduction studies with a concomitant decrement on RMNS supports the diagnosis of prolonged blockade. In contrast, the presence of persistently reduced or absent motor responses is compatible with the possible diagnosis of AQM (114,115).

Acute Quadriplegic Myopathy

AQM was initially reported in 1977 in a woman with status asthmaticus treated with a combination of corticosteroids and neuromuscular blocking agents (116). A number of other names have been used in the literature to describe this syndrome, such as acute myopathy, critical illness myopathy, critical care myopathy, and acute myopathy with selective loss of myosin filaments (111). The most common predisposing condition is asthma in conjunction with the use of intravenous corticosteroids, nondepolarizing neuromuscular blocking agents, and aminoglycosides (115). However, AQM is also described in patients with sepsis who were not treated with neuromuscular blocking agents or corticosteroids (117–119). Other predisposing conditions for AQM include muscle unloading, pneumonia, organ transplantation (e.g., heart, liver, lung) (120), hepatic failure, and acidosis (111). In a study from the Hospital for Sick Children, Toronto, Canada, 8 of the 14 critically ill children with muscle weakness (57%) were solid organ or bone marrow transplant recipients (121). This study aimed to establish the incidence of muscle weakness in children admitted to pediatric ICU for > 24 hours. Fourteen of 830 (1.7%) children had generalized muscle weakness and most had received neuromuscular blocking agents, corticosteroids, or aminoglycoside antibiotics. In four of the five children who had an EMG performed, the study showed myopathic findings, and in the fifth it was normal. Seven patients underwent NCS. Overall, electrodiagnostic studies were myopathic in four children, normal in two, showed compressive neuropathies in one child, and a mild demyelinative polyneuropathy in one patient (121).

Most patients with AQM are severely affected, having significant weakness or even paralysis, as well as inability to be weaned from the ventilator. In contrast, a few patients may have only mild weakness. Extraocular movements are usually preserved, sensation is intact, and muscle stretch reflexes are decreased proportionate to the decrease in strength. Although rapid recovery is sometimes observed, the usual course of recovery is slow (weeks or months) and may be complete (95,122). In a series of eight adults with AQM associated with biopsy-proven loss of thick myofilaments, six patients died, one patient recovered fully in 1 month, and one patient remained quadriparetic at 1 year, probably due to concomitant CNS disease (123). In another study of five children with critical illness neuromuscular disease, both children with critical illness myopathy recovered completely within 3 weeks and 6 months (124).

In most patients with AQM, the CK is normal or mildly elevated (117,125,126). Nevertheless, in a small number of patients CK levels may be significantly elevated. Muscle biopsy shows loss of myosin ATPase staining which can be localized or be maximal in the center (core-like) of the myofibers; electron microscopy shows loss of myosin-thick filaments (121,123, 125–127). There is relative sparing of actin filaments and Z disks. Light microscopy commonly shows small angulated atrophic predominantly type 2 fibers, with basophilic staining of the cytoplasm with hematoxylin and eosin staining. The majority of core-like lesions are seen in type I fibers (123). Necrosis of myofibers is usually mild but in some cases can be quite severe.

NCSs in AQM are usually normal except for diminished CMAP amplitudes (115,117). Needle EMG often records early recruited low amplitude, short duration myopathic motor units, as well as fibrillation potentials (128). However, many patients may be unable to activate their muscles due to an associated encephalopathy or inability to generate any voluntary activity. The resulting lack of clear EMG findings, combined with the fact that either CIP or AQM may occur in septic patients who have not received corticosteroids or neuromuscular blocking agents, combined with the coexistence of these two syndromes in certain patients, sometimes make the differentiation of these two syndromes extremely difficult. The presence of normal SNAPs and small CMAPs suggests the presence of AQM, but small or absent SNAPs indicative of CIP do not necessarily exclude AQM (129). Also, the finding of low-amplitude CMAPs is not diagnostic of a polyneuropathy and may indicate AQM (123). Significant conduction slowing or conduction blocks are not consistent with either CIP or AQM. Myopathic MUPs with an early recruitment pattern are indicative of a myopathic process. However, myopathic potentials may also occur with prolonged neuromuscular blockade from the use of nondepolarizing neuromuscular blocking agents, and thus routine 2 Hz RMNS is required as part of the electrophysiological evaluation of these patients (111). Direct muscle stimulation may allow the diagnosis of AQM in patients with confusing electrophysiological findings. In very weak patients or patients whose EMG findings are hard to interpret, direct muscle stimulation has been employed to study muscle membrane excitability; the latter is normal in patients with CIP and reduced or absent in patients with AQM. Muscle is reported to be electrically inexcitable in AQM (117,130). Therefore in patients with AQM, direct muscle stimulation does not lead to action potentials. The membrane excitability does return with clinical recovery of patients.

Although muscle biopsy showing the classic pathological findings described above is diagnostic of AQM, this procedure does not always provide a definitive differentiation between AQM and CIP. This is because the characteristic loss of myosin is seen in only a fraction of patients with AQM. It should be noted that neither author of this chapter has personal experience in the performance of direct muscle stimulation and thus cannot comment on the utility of this test in a clinical setting.

Increased activation of specific proteases such as calpain, a calcium-activated protease, has been found in muscle of patients with AQM. This may be crucial in the pathogenesis of this disorder (118). The expression of ubiquitin and other proteases, as well as DNA fragmentation, was studied in muscle biopsies from three patients with AQM. All of these patients demonstrated significant overexpression of caspases, calpain, cathepsin B, and ubiquitin, and the presence of numerous apoptotic nuclei in over 70% of the muscle fibers (131). This study provides further evidence that proteolytic proteases are important in the pathogenesis of AQM; proteases seem to stimulate apoptosis, but why the thick filaments are preferentially involved remains to be elucidated (131). Published data generated by the same group provide additional evidence suggesting that stimulation of proapoptotic pathways may underlie, at least in part, the pathogenesis of AQM (132). A more recent study of myofibrillar protein and gene expression support the important role of transcriptional regulation of myofibrillar protein synthesis in the loss and resynthesis of contractile proteins, myosin in particular, in AQM (133).

AQM is probably a disorder of protein turnover in muscle. Corticosteroids and other conditions such as sepsis stimulate muscle catabolism, which is further amplified by muscle inactivity secondary initially to neuromuscular blockade and later on to lack of membrane excitability. Conditions such as sepsis and renal or respiratory failure, often associated with significant acidosis, may also result in high levels of cytokines that have a catabolic effect on muscle. The catabolic state usually persists despite treatment of sepsis and/or withdrawal of therapy with corticosteroids and neuromuscular blocking agents; it is possible that the paralysis that results from the lack of membrane excitability prevents muscle from switching to an anabolic state, and thus the recovery from AQM is usually a slow process (134).

Acute Necrotizing Myopathy of Intensive Care

Case 13: Severe Generalized Weakness After Intubation for Status Asthmaticus

This 12-year-old girl had an acute exacerbation of her asthma and required intubation. She required high-dose corticosteroid therapy and neuromuscular blocking agents. One of her arterial lines became infected, and she developed sepsis. When she was extubated she had severe generalized weakness. Her serum CK was markedly elevated with associated myoglobinemia and myoglobinuria. Motor NCVs were essentially normal initially. The median CMAP was mildly diminished in amplitude at 3 mV, however, the peroneal CMAP was normal. MUPs on needle EMG were myopathic with increased percentages of low amplitude, short duration, and at times polyphasic MUPs. Scattered fibrillation potentials were present on needle insertion. A week after the EMG, muscle biopsy demonstrated thick filament fiber loss typical of critical care AQM with extensive areas of panfascicular fiber necrosis. Her recovery was extremely slow.

Comment

These critical care myopathies most typically are associated with severe pulmonary disorders. Other clinical settings to consider in this scenario include patients with severe sepsis or those who have had an organ transplant. Most of these patients have received high-dose intravenous corticosteroids in conjunction with low to moderate doses of neuromuscular blocking agents. As was noted in case 13, in patients with acute necrotizing myopathy of intensive care, muscle biopsy shows panfascicular muscle fiber necrosis, suggesting that acute necrotizing myopathy may be a severe form of AQM. This pathology contrasts with the multiple pyogenic abscesses typical for pyomyositis, a condition also seen in septic patients but more endemic to the tropics. This is usually associated with significant CK elevation, myoglobinuria, and myopathic EMG findings (135). Serum CK levels are sometimes, but not uniformly, markedly elevated with AQM. Rarely this laboratory finding is associated with myoglobinemia that may be severe enough to result in acute renal failure (128,135). The CK level per se is not a very helpful tool for making the differentiation between a myopathic or neuropathic lesion. In a study of 14 patients with critical illness myopathy of the AQM variety, only 3 of 14 patients had an elevated CK (95). With these three instances there was only a mild change with a maximal value reported to be 331 IU/lt. In another study of eight adult patients with biopsy-proven AQM, only four patients had elevated serum CK levels (417–4770 U/L; normal, up to 295 U/L), but serial CK determinations were not performed in all patients; thus, transient hyperCKemia may not have been detected (123). The degree of enzyme elevation and disease severity did not correlate. The EMG may exclude a polyneuropathy and, as with case 13, often demonstrates typical myopathic findings; as discussed above, however, in certain cases the EMG findings are hard to interpret. The muscle biopsy defined the typical abnormalities of a primary loss of thick skeletal muscle filaments.

■ CONCLUSIONS

When infants and children develop an acute flaccid paralysis, there is a clinical differential diagnosis somewhat dissimilar to that considered in the older child. In newborns and during the first 6 months of life, certain unusual syndromes require careful consideration (136). Infantile botulism is a good example. We question whether this illness may be more common than currently recognized. This is particularly relevant among infants with acute indeterminate respiratory distress. GBS is another example of a possibly underrecognized or not considered illness in the evaluation of the floppy infant syndrome, particularly so with those infants who may have had an intrauterine onset. At times the clinical presentation of some acute pediatric motor unit disorders, such as GBS, mimics central nervous system lesions including various encephalopathies, even brain death, or acute myelopathies such as transverse myelitis or spinal cord tumors.

MRI provides an important diagnostic tool for making this differentiation. EMG is also very helpful for defining the presence of a number of primary motor unit lesions. Pediatric neurologic and intensive care colleagues need to be encouraged to increase their utilization of EMG in some of these ICU settings. This is especially true when the initial clinical suspicions are not supported by the various investigations. The important finding that infantile botulism, or a severe form of axonal GBS can clinically mimic brain death always needs top consideration in the emergency room and the ICU. An EMG may provide the important tool and information leading to consideration of these severe peripheral neuropathies or neuromuscular transmission defects.

■ REFERENCES

1. Darras BT, Jones HR Jr. Neuromuscular problems of the critically ill neonate and child. *Semin Pediatr Neurol.* 2004;11(2):147–168.
2. Jones HR Jr. Evaluation of the floppy infant. In: Jones HR Jr, Bolton CF, Harper CM, eds. *Pediatric Clinical Electromyography*. Philadelphia, PA: Lippincott-Raven; 1996:37–104.
3. David WS, Jones HRJ. Electromyography and biopsy correlation with suggested protocol for evaluation of the floppy infant. *Muscle Nerve.* 1994;17:424–430.
4. Jones HRJ et al. An approach to pediatric electromyography. In: Jones HRJ, Bolton CF, Harper CM, eds. *Pediatric Clinical Electromyography*. Philadelphia, PA-New York, NY: Lippincott-Raven; 1996:1–36.
5. MacLeod MJ et al. Prenatal onset spinal muscular atrophy. *Eur J Paediatr Neurol.* 1999;3(2):65–72.
6. Dubowitz V. Very severe spinal muscular atrophy (SMA type 0): an expanding clinical phenotype. *Eur J Paediatr Neurol.* 1999;3(2):49–51.
7. Darras BT. Non-5q spinal muscular atrophies: the alphanumeric soup thickens. *Neurology.* 2011;77(4):312–314.
8. David WS, Doyle JJ. Acute infantile weakness: a case of vaccine-associated poliomyelitis. *Muscle Nerve.* 1997;20(6), 747–749.
9. Beausoleil JL, Nordgren RE, Modlin JF. Vaccine-associated paralytic poliomyelitis. *J Child Neurol.* 1994;9(3):334–335.
10. Robbins FC. Eradication of polio in the Americas. *JAMA.* 1993;270(15):1857–1859.
11. Recommendations of the Advisory Committee on Immunization Practices: revised recommendations for routine poliomyelitis vaccination. *MMWR Morb Mortal Wkly Rep.* 1999;48(27):590.
12. Kang PB et al. Diagnostic value of electromyography and muscle biopsy in arthrogryposis multiplex congenita. *Ann Neurol.* 2003;54(6):790–795.
13. Jackson AH, Baquis GD, Shah BL. Congenital Guillain-Barré syndrome. *J Child Neurol.* 1996;11(5):407–410.
14. Luijckx GJ et al. Guillain-Barré syndrome in mother and newborn child. *Lancet.* 1997;349(9044):27.
15. Rolfs A, Bolik A. Guillain-Barré syndrome in pregnancy: reflections on immunopathogenesis. *Acta Neurol Scand.* 1994;89(5):400–402.
16. Jones HR. Childhood Guillain-Barré syndrome: clinical presentation, diagnosis, and therapy. *J Child Neurol.* 1996;11(1):4–12.
17. Gilmartin RC, Ch'ien LT. Guillain-Barré syndrome with hydrocephalus in early infancy. *Arch Neurol.* 1977;34(9):567–569.
18. Pasternak JF et al. An infant with chronic, relapsing polyneuropathy responsive to steroids. *Dev Med Child Neurol.* 1982;24(4):504–524.
19. Grattan-Smith PJ et al. Clinical and neurophysiological features of tick paralysis. *Brain.* 1997;120(pt 11):1975–1987.
20. Papazian O. Transient neonatal myasthenia gravis. *J Child Neurol.* 1992;7(2):135–141.
21. Lefvert AK, Osterman PO. Newborn infants to myasthenic mothers. A clinical study and an investigation of acetylcholine receptor antibodies in 17 children. *Neurology.* 1983;33:133–138.
22. O'Carroll P et al. Transient neonatal myasthenia gravis in a baby born to a mother with new-onset anti-MuSK-mediated myasthenia gravis. *J Clin Neuromuscul Dis.* 2009;11(2):69–71.
23. Lipsitz PJ. The clinical and biochemical effects of excess magnesium in the newborn. *Pediatrics.* 1971;47(3):501–509.
24. Sokal MM et al. Neonatal hypermagnesemia and the meconium-plug syndrome. *N Engl J Med.* 1972;286(15):823–825.
25. Mallory LA et al. Congenital myasthenic syndrome with episodic apnea. *Pediatr Neurol.* 2009;41(1):42–45.
26. Pickett J et al. Syndrome of botulism in infancy: clinical and electrophysiologic study. *N Engl J Med.* 1976;295(14):770–772.
27. Clay SA et al. Acute infantile motor unit disorder. Infantile botulism? *Arch Neurol.* 1977;34(4):236–243.
28. Hoffman RE, Pincomb BJ, Skeels MR. Type F infant botulism. *Am J Dis Child.* 1982;136(3):270–271.
29. Schwartz RH, Eng G. Infant botulism: exacerbation by aminoglycosides. *Am J Dis Child.* 1982;136(10):952.
30. Thompson JA et al. Infant botulism: clinical spectrum and epidemiology. *Pediatrics.* 1980;66(6):936–942.
31. Shukla AY et al. Neonatal botulism (abstr). *Neurology.* 1991;41(suppl 1):202.

32. Donley DK et al. A patient with infant botulism, improving with edrophonium (abstr). *Muscle Nerve*. 1991;41:201.

33. King LA et al. [Infant botulism in France, 1991–2009]. *Arch Pediatr*. 2010;17(9):1288–1292.

34. May ML, Corkeron MA, Stretton M. Infant botulism in Australia: availability of human botulinum antitoxin for treatment. *Med J Aust*. 2010;193(10):614–615.

35. Chalk C, Benstead TJ, Keezer M. Medical treatment for botulism. *Cochrane Database Syst Rev*. 2011;(3):CD008123.

36. Grant KA et al. Report of two unlinked cases of infant botulism in the UK in October 2007. *J Med Microbiol*. 2009;58(pt 12):1601–1606.

37. Cornblath DR, Sladky JT, Sumner AJ. Clinical electrophysiology of infantile botulism. *Muscle Nerve*. 1983;6:448–452.

38. Sheth RD et al. Infantile botulism: pitfalls in electrodiagnosis. *J Child Neurol*. 1999;14(3):156–158.

39. Gutierrez AR, Bodensteiner J, Gutmann L. Electrodiagnosis of infantile botulism. *J Child Neurol*. 1994;9(4):362–365.

40. Darras BT, Chad DA. Myotonic dystrophy. In: Basow DS, Shefner JM, Nordli DR Jr, eds. *UpToDate*. Waltham, MA: UpToDate, Inc., 2011. http://www.uptodate.com. Last updated: May 9, 2012. Last accessed: September 10, 2012.

41. Swift TR, Ignacio OJ, Dyken PR. Neonatal dystrophia myotonica. Electrophysiologic studies. *Am J Dis Child*. 1975;129(6):734–737.

42. Kuntz NL, Daube JR. *Electrophysiology of Congenital Myotonic Dystrophy*. Rochester, MN: AAEE Course E, American Association of Electromyography and Electrodiagnosis; 1984.

43. Swoboda KJ et al. Infantile phosphofructokinase deficiency with arthrogryposis: Clinical benefit of a ketogenic diet. *J Pediatr*. 1997;131:932–934.

44. DiMauro S, Hartlage P. Fatal infantile form of muscle phosphorylase deficiency. *Neurology*. 1978;28:1124–1129.

45. McMillan HJ et al. Pediatric monomelic amyotrophy: evidence for poliomyelitis in vulnerable populations. *Muscle Nerve*. 2009;40(5):860–863.

46. Medici C et al. Locked-in syndrome in three children with Guillain-Barré syndrome. *Pediatr Neurol*. 2011;45(2):125–128.

47. Bradshaw DY, Jones HRJ. Guillain-Barré syndrome in children: clinical course, electrodiagnosis, and prognosis. *Muscle Nerve*. 1992;15(4):500–506.

48. Bradshaw DY, Jones HRJ. Pseudomeningoencephalitic presentation of pediatric Guillain-Barré syndrome. *J Child Neurol*. 2001;16(7):505–508.

49. Jones HR Jr. Guillain-Barré syndrome: perspectives with infants and children. *Semin Pediatr Neurol*. 2000;7(2):91–102.

50. Dirik E, Uysal KM. Organophosphate-induced delayed polyneruopathy (abstr). *Pediatr Neurol*. 1994;11:111.

51. Hart DE et al. Childhood Guillain-Barré syndrome in Paraguay, 1990 to 1991. *Ann Neurol*. 1994;36(6):859–863.

52. Coker SB. Leigh disease presenting as Guillain-Barré syndrome. *Pediatr Neurol*. 1993;9(1):61–63.

53. McKhann GM et al. Clinical and electrophysiological aspects of acute paralytic disease of children and young adults in northern China. *Lancet*. 1991;338(8767):593–597.

54. Ho TW et al. Guillain-Barré syndrome in northern China. Relationship to *Campylobacter jejuni* infection and antiglycolipid antibodies. *Brain*. 1995;118(pt 3):597–605.

55. Griffin JW et al. Pathology of the motor-sensory axonal Guillain-Barré syndrome. *Ann Neurol*. 1996;39(1):17–28.

56. Kuwabara S et al. IgG anti-GM1 antibody is associated with reversible conduction failure and axonal degeneration in Guillain-Barré syndrome. *Ann Neurol*. 1998;44(2):202–208.

57. Yuki N et al. Acute motor axonal neuropathy and acute motor-sensory axonal neuropathy share a common immunological profile. *J Neurol Sci*. 1999;168(2):121–126.

58. Bakshi N et al. Fulminant demyelinating neuropathy mimicking cerebral death. *Muscle Nerve*. 1997;20(12):1595–1597.

59. Raphael SA et al. Inflammatory demyelinating polyneuropathy in a child with symptomatic human immunodeficiency virus infection. *J Pediatr*. 1991;118(2):242–245.

60. Graf WD et al. Severe vincristine neuropathy in Charcot-Marie-Tooth disease type 1A. *Cancer*. 1996;77(7):1356–1362.

61. Costiniuk CT et al. Miller Fisher syndrome in a toddler with influenza A (pH1N1) infection. *J Child Neurol*. 2011;26(3):385–388.

62. Chiba A et al. Serum IgG antibody to ganglioside GQ1b is a possible marker of Miller Fisher syndrome. *Ann Neurol*. 1992;31(6):677–679.

63. Chiba A et al. Serum anti-GQ1b IgG antibody is associated with ophthalmoplegia in Miller Fisher syndrome and Guillain-Barré syndrome: clinical and immunohistochemical studies. *Neurology*. 1993;43(10):1911–1917.

64. Willison HJ et al. Miller Fisher syndrome is associated with serum antibodies to GQ1b ganglioside. *J Neurol Neurosurg Psychiatry*. 1993;56(2):204–206.

65. Yuki N et al. Frequent presence of anti-GQ1b antibody in Fisher's syndrome. *Neurology*. 1993;43(2):414–417.

66. Jacobs BC et al. Serum anti-GQ1b IgG antibodies recognize surface epitopes on *Campylobacter jejuni* from patients with Miller Fisher syndrome. *Ann Neurol*. 1995;37(2):260–264.

67. Honavar M et al. A clinicopathological study of the Guillain-Barré syndrome. Nine cases and literature review. *Brain*. 1991;114(pt 3):1245–1269.

68. Kleyweg RP et al. The natural history of the Guillain-Barré syndrome in 18 children and 50 adults. *J Neurol Neurosurg Psychiatry*. 1989;52(7):853–856.

69. Sladky JT. Guillain-Barré syndrome. In: Jones JJ, De Vivo DC, Darras BT, eds. *Neuromuscular Disorders of Infancy, Childhood, and Adolescence: A Clinician's Approach*. Philadelphia, PA: Butterworth-Heinemann; 2003:407–424.

70. Ropper AH. The Guillain-Barré syndrome. *N Engl J Med*. 1992;326(17):1130–1136.

71. Ropper AH, Kehne SM. Guillain-Barré syndrome: management of respiratory failure. *Neurology*. 1985;35(11):1662–1665.

72. Lawn ND et al. Anticipating mechanical ventilation in Guillain-Barré syndrome. *Arch Neurol*. 2001;58(6):893–898.

73. Hesketh E et al. Spinal cord compression—do we miss it? *Acta Paediatr*. 1998;87(4):452–454.

74. Delhaas T, Kamphuis DJ, Witkamp TD. Transitory spinal cord swelling in a 6-year-old boy with Guillain-Barré syndrome. *Pediatr Radiol*. 1998;28(7):544–546.

75. Bajaj NP et al. Acute transverse myelitis and Guillain-Barré overlap syndrome with serological evidence for mumps viraemia. *Acta Neurol Scand*. 2001;104(4):239–242.

76. Knebusch M, Strassburg HM, Reiners K. Acute transverse myelitis in childhood: nine cases and review of the literature. *Dev Med Child Neurol*. 1998;40(9):631–639.

77. Ryan MM et al. Paediatric mononeuritis multiplex: a report of three cases and review of the literature. *Neuromuscul Disord.* 2003;13(9):751–756.

78. Srinivasan J et al. Pediatric sciatic neuropathies: a 30-year prospective study. *Neurology.* 2011;76(11):976–980.

79. Srinivasan J et al. Pediatric sciatic neuropathies due to unusual vascular causes. *J Child Neurol.* 2008;23(7):738–741.

80. Bolton CF, Young GB. *The Neurologic Complications of Renal Disease.* Boston, MA: Butterworths, 1990.

81. Haller JS, Fabara JA. Tick paralysis. Case report with emphasis on neurological toxicity. *Am J Dis Child.* 1972; 124(6):915–917.

82. Donat JR, Donat JF. Tick paralysis with persistent weakness and electromyographic abnormalities. *Arch Neurol.* 1981;38(1):59–61.

83. Kincaid JC. Tick bite paralysis. *Semin Neurol.* 1990;10(1): 32–34.

84. Swift TR, Ignacio OJ. Tick paralysis: electrophysiologic studies. *Neurology.* 1975;25(12):1130–1133.

85. Cherington M, Synder RD. Tick paralysis. Neurophysiologic studies. *N Engl J Med.* 1968;278(2):95–97.

86. Cooper BJ, Spence I. Temperature-dependent inhibition of evoked acetylcholine release in tick paralysis. *Nature.* 1976;263(5579):693–695.

87. Geh GH, Bradbury JA. Ocular myasthenia presenting in an 11-month-old boy. *Eye.* 1996;12(pt 2):319–320.

88. Mullaney P et al. The natural history and ophthalmic involvement in childhood myasthenia gravis at the hospital for sick children. *Ophthalmology.* 2000;107(3):504–510.

89. Chiang LM, Darras BT, Kang PB. Juvenile myasthenia gravis. *Muscle Nerve.* 2009;39(4):423–431.

90. Andrews PI. A treatment algorithm for autoimmune myasthenia gravis in childhood. *Ann N Y Acad Sci.* 1998;841: 789–802.

91. Bolton CF. Spinal muscular atrophies of childhood and adolescence. In: Jones HRJ, Bolton CF, Harper CM, eds. *Pediatric Clinical Electromyography.* Philadelphia, PA-New York, NY: Lippincott-Raven; 1996:105–122.

92. Sheth RD et al. Critical illness neuromuscular disease in children manifested as ventilatory dependence. *J Pediatr.* 1995;126(2):259–261.

93. Bolton CF et al. Polyneuropathy in critically ill patients. *J Neurol Neurosurg Psychiatry.* 1984;47(11):1223–1231.

94. Goulden KJ et al. Critical illness polyneuropathy: a reversible cause of paralysis in asthmatic children (abstr). *Ann Neurol.* 1989;26:451.

95. Lacomis D, Zochodne DW, Bird SJ. Critical illness myopathy. *Muscle Nerve.* 2000;23(12):1785–1788.

96. Horiuchi I et al. Acute myelitis after asthma attacks with onset after puberty. *J Neurol Neurosurg Psychiatry.* 2000; 68(5):665–668.

97. Hopkins IJ, Shield LK. Letter: Poliomyelitis-like illness associated with asthma in childhood. *Lancet.* 1974;1(7860):760.

98. Shapiro GG et al. Poliomyelitis-like illness after acute asthma. *J Pediatr.* 1979;94(5):767–768.

99. Blomqvist HK, Bjorksten B. Poliomyelitis-like illness associated with asthma. *Arch Dis Child.* 1980;55(1):61–63.

100. Manson JI, Thong YH. Immunological abnormalities in the syndrome of poliomyelitis-like illness associated with acute bronchial asthma (Hopkin's syndrome). *Arch Dis Child.* 1980;55(1):26–32.

101. Nihei K, Naitoh H, Ikeda K. Poliomyelitis-like syndrome following asthmatic attack (Hopkins syndrome). *Pediatr Neurol.* 1987;3(3):166–168.

102. Shahar EM et al. Poliomyelitis-like paralysis during recovery from acute bronchial asthma: possible etiology and risk factors. *Pediatrics.* 1991;88(2):276–279.

103. Wakamoto H et al. MRI in poliomyelitis-like syndrome. *Pediatr Radiol.* 1992;22(7):533–534.

104. Batley R, Johnson EW. Asthmatic amyotrophy. Three cases. *Am J Phys Med Rehabil.* 1991;70(6):332–334.

105. Sheth RD, Bolton CF. Neuromuscular complications of sepsis in children. *J Child Neurol.* 1995;10(5):346–352.

106. Liedholm LJ et al. Acute postasthmatic amyotrophy (Hopkins' syndrome). *Muscle Nerve.* 1994;17(7):769–772.

107. Hayward JC et al. Outbreak of poliomyelitis-like paralysis associated with enterovirus 71. *Pediatr Infect Dis J.* 1989; 8(9):611–616.

108. Kyllerman MG et al. PCR diagnosis of primary herpesvirus type I in poliomyelitis-like paralysis and respiratory tract disease. *Pediatr Neurol.* 1993;9(3):227–229.

109. Ahlbeck K et al. Signs of critical illness polyneuropathy and myopathy can be seen early in the ICU course. *Acta Anaesthesiol Scand.* 2009;53(6):717–723.

110. Bolton CF et al. Critically ill polyneuropathy: electrophysiological studies and differentiation from Guillain-Barré syndrome. *J Neurol Neurosurg Psychiatry.* 1986;49(5):563–573.

111. Gutmann L. Critical illness neuropathy and myopathy. *Arch Neurol.* 1999;56(5):527–528.

112. O'Connor M, Russell WJ. Muscle strength following anaesthesia with atracurium and pancuronium. *Anaesth Intensive Care.* 1988;16(3):255–259.

113. Partridge BL et al. Prolonged neuromuscular blockade after long-term infusion of vecuronium bromide in the intensive care unit. *Crit Care Med.* 1990;18(10):1177–1179.

114. Segredo V et al. Persistent paralysis in critically ill patients after long-term administration of vecuronium. *N Engl J Med.* 1992;327(8):524–528.

115. Bird SJ, Rich MM. Neuromuscular complications of critical illness. *Neurologist.* 2000;6:2–11.

116. MacFarlane IA, Rosenthal FD. Severe myopathy after status asthmaticus. *Lancet.* 1977;2(8038):615.

117. Rich MM et al. Direct muscle stimulation in acute quadriplegic myopathy. *Muscle Nerve.* 1997;20(6):665–673.

118. Showalter CJ, Engel AG. Acute quadriplegic myopathy: analysis of myosin isoforms and evidence for calpain-mediated proteolysis. *Muscle Nerve.* 1997;20(3):316–322.

119. Latronico N et al. Critical illness myopathy and neuropathy. *Lancet.* 1996;347(9015):1579–1582.

120. Perea M et al. Acute quadriplegic myopathy with loss of thick (myosin) filaments following heart transplantation. *J Heart Lung Transplant.* 2001;20(10):1136–1141.

121. Banwell BL et al. Muscle weakness in critically ill children. *Neurology.* 2003;61(12):1779–1782.

122. Salviati L et al. Acute quadriplegic myopathy in a 17-month-old boy. *J Child Neurol.* 2000;15(1):63–66.

123. Sander HW, Golden M, Danon MJ. Quadriplegic areflexic ICU illness: selective thick filament loss and normal nerve histology. *Muscle Nerve.* 2002;26(4):499–505.

124. Tabarki B et al. Critical illness neuromuscular disease: clinical, electrophysiological, and prognostic aspects. *Arch Dis Child.* 2002;86(2):103–107.

125. Lacomis D, Petrella JT, Giuliani MJ. Causes of neuromuscular weakness in the intensive care unit: a study of ninety-two patients. *Muscle Nerve.* 1998;21(5):610–617.

126. Lacomis D et al. Acute myopathy of intensive care: clinical, electromyographic, and pathological aspects. *Ann Neurol.* 1996;40(4):645–654.

127. Larsson L. Acute quadriplegic myopathy: an acquired "myosinopathy". *Adv Exp Med Biol.* 2008;642,:92–98.

128. Zochodne DW et al. Acute necrotizing myopathy of intensive care: electrophysiological studies. *Muscle Nerve.* 1994; 17(3):285–292.

129. Primavera A, Abbruzzese M. Case 11-1997: critical-illness myopathy. *N Engl J Med.* 1997;337(12):862–863.

130. Rich MM et al. Muscle is electrically inexcitable in acute quadriplegic myopathy. *Neurology.* 1996;46(3):731–736.

131. Di Giovanni S et al. Apoptotic features accompany acute quadriplegic myopathy. *Neurology.* 2000;55(6):854–858.

132. Di Giovanni S et al. Constitutive activation of MAPK cascade in acute quadriplegic myopathy. *Ann Neurol.* 2004;55(2):195–206.

133. Norman H et al. Myofibrillar protein and gene expression in acute quadriplegic myopathy. *J Neurol Sci.* 2009; 285(1-2):28–38.

134. Ruff RL. Why do ICU patients become paralyzed? *Ann Neurol.* 1998;43(2):154–155.

135. Lannigan R, Austin TW, Vestrup J. Myositis and rhabdomyolysis due to Staphylococcus aureus septicemia. *J Infect Dis.* 1984;150(5):784.

136. Jones HR, Darras BT. Acute care pediatric electromyography. *Muscle Nerve.* 2000;23(suppl):S53–62.

22 Neurosurgical Postoperative Monitoring and Complications

MICHAEL J. KRAMARZ, STACEY J. JACOVINI, and PHILLIP B. STORM

■ INTRODUCTION

The greatest risk of a postoperative neurosurgical complication is within the first 24 to 36 hours after surgery. This time frame holds for both intracranial and spinal surgery, although the complication etiologies differ. Neurosurgeons and intensivists must work closely to ensure early and correct identification of complications. Many neurosurgical patients leave the operating room (OR) with a known and expected neurologic deficit that needs to be clearly documented and communicated. Similarly, some patients are intact, but are at a high risk for developing a deficit based on the intraoperative findings. These patients cannot be sufficiently monitored for early and subtle new deficits without clear and concise dialogue between the neurosurgical and critical care teams.

■ INTRACRANIAL SURGERY COMPLICATIONS

Hydrocephalus

The most common pediatric neurosurgical procedure is diverting cerebral spinal fluid (CSF) in a patient who has hydrocephalus. There are two types of hydrocephalus: communicating (nonobstructive) and noncommunicating (obstructive). Communicating hydrocephalus is the most frequent type and often results from premature infants suffering a hypoxic/ischemic event leading to periventricular/intraventricular hemorrhages. These patients should be monitored with serial head ultrasounds, daily head circumference measurements, and palpation of the anterior fontanelle and the sutures. Apneas and bradycardias (As and Bs) should be recorded and reported to the neurosurgical team. Because of the open fontanelles and unfused sutures, the neonatal head is able to easily increase its volume, thereby keeping the pressure low without causing further damage. We prefer to wait for shunt placement until the patient weighs a minimum of 2 kg due to the high rate of infections in this patient population.

Shunts

The typical shunt procedure involves placing a burr hole in the skull (either frontal or parietal) and then passing a catheter through the brain and into the ventricular space. The proximal end of the shunt is connected to a valve and the distal tubing. There are many possible locations for the distal tubing. The three most common locations are peritoneum, pleura, and right atrium via the jugular or subclavian vein. Other potential locations are the gall bladder, urinary bladder, femoral vein, sagittal sinus, and direct right atrial placement after sternotomy.

Intraoperative complications from the original placement of a shunt are quite rare. In the brain, the possible complications are hemorrhage along the tract of the proximal catheter or in the subdural space from an avulsion of a bridging vein. Other possible complications can arise from a misplaced catheter. Frontal catheters can cause weakness from passing through or near the genu of the internal capsule, cranial nerve

(CN) injuries to CN2, CN3, and CN6, and short-term memory difficulty from forniceal injury. The most common complication of a misplaced catheter is failure to relieve—or early recurrence of—the signs and symptoms of hydrocephalus. Dialogue with the neurosurgeon is important. A proximal catheter that is passed one time with excellent egress of clear CSF is unlikely to have a complication.

The quality of CSF draining from the catheter is predictive of whether or not a complication occurred. Clear CSF is unlikely to be associated with an intraoperative or early postoperative complication with the valve. If there is blood, high protein, or particulate matter in the CSF, then there is the possibility of valve clogging. This scenario is a concern in a premature infant with an intraventricular hemorrhage, but otherwise is extremely uncommon when placing the first shunt in a patient.

Intraoperative complications of placing the distal end of the shunt in the peritoneum with a new shunt is also rare. However, tunneling of the shunt under the clavicle or ribs and into the chest has the potential to cause a pneumothorax or hemothorax, either of which may or may not be recognized in the OR. If tachypnea, hypoxia, hypotension, or respiratory distress develops in the pediatric intensive care unit (PICU), then these complications should be considered. In small premature infants, bleeding from tunneling can lower the baby's hemoglobin significantly, necessitating transfusion or even cardiac arrest from hypovolemic shock. A more likely, but still rare, complication is injury to the intestine. Making a hole in the small or large intestine is usually recognized intraoperatively and repaired, but a minor bowel perforation could go undiagnosed in the OR. A small amount of air on an immediate postoperative abdominal x-ray is the typical finding; however, if the patient develops a fever, elevated white blood count, or peritoneal air several days after placement of a peritoneal catheter, a perforated intestine needs to be considered.

The complication rate for a shunt revision procedure is much higher. Proximal shunt malfunctions are the most worrisome for complications. Patients with a proximal obstruction cannot have their pressure relieved by simply tapping the shunt because the ventricular catheter is clogged. Therefore the options are to (1) emergently place a new ventricular catheter in the emergency department or PICU, (2) insert a 20 gauge spinal needle through the skin, through the previous burr hole, and into the ventricle to remove excess CSF,

or (3) take the patient to the OR for a proximal revision. Fortunately, very few patients are so shunt dependent that they cannot be adequately managed with Decadron, Diamox, and Zantac and then taken to the OR for proximal shunt revision on an urgent or elective basis. Signs and symptoms of shunt malfunction are headache, nausea, and vomiting. More severe and worrisome signs are diplopia, decreased level of consciousness, sluggish pupillary light reflex, and bradycardia. Patients exhibiting signs of herniation secondary to shunt malfunction should be managed with emergent intubation, mannitol, or hypertonic saline, and emergent procedures should be performed to remove CSF, as described above. A common mistake is overestimating the bradycardia in a patient waiting to go to the OR for a proximal shunt revision who is wide awake and completely appropriate without any neurologic deficit.

When shunt malfunction is suspected, we perform a head computed tomography (CT). Additionally, we obtain a shunt series in most patients looking for a break or migration of the catheter to a nonfunctioning position. The diagnosis of a proximal shunt obstruction is easily made when the patient has signs and symptoms consistent with shunt malfunction, large ventricles, and a valve that pumps but does not refill. However, if the patient has small to slit ventricles, it is much more difficult to diagnose on head CT. Furthermore, if there is little to no CSF around the tip of the proximal catheter, then the shunt will pump and refill very slowly, even if it is optimally functioning. Pumping working shunts in patients with small ventricles also carries a putative risk of clogging the catheter. Thus, we discourage pumping shunts in the absence of head CT imaging documenting ventricle size.

Once a proximal shunt malfunction is identified, a proximal revision is performed in the OR. The complications that can result from a proximal revision are infection, hemorrhage, inability to remove the proximal catheter, inability to enter the ventricle with the new catheter, injury to surrounding structures such as the fornix, internal capsule, and all of the other risks associated with placing a new shunt. We prefer to place a metal stylette down the lumen of the clogged catheter and touch the stylette with the electrocautery to coagulate the tissue clogging the catheter. Theoretically, this decreases the risk of hemorrhage when the catheter is removed. Once the malfunctioning catheter is removed, the new catheter is then placed down the same tract into the ventricle. When the catheter is too stuck to be removed safely, it is often left in place and a new catheter is placed. Because the choroid plexus, which is very vascular, is usually the offending tissue clogging the catheter, the risk of hemorrhage is much higher with a revision than with the original placement. Most complications are identified in the OR, but the PICU team needs to be acutely aware that an uneventful procedure does not mean that the shunt is functioning well. The catheter is blindly placed in the OR and may not be in the ventricle. For example, if the catheter is interhemispheric, then the surgeon will see CSF flowing but it will not adequately drain CSF. Other possibilities are catheters that are slightly too short or too long. Regardless of the cause, patients without rapid resolution of signs and symptoms of hydrocephalus after a proximal revision need to be evaluated for suboptimal shunt functioning. Some institutions obtain a head CT after every shunt operation, but we prefer to use our clinical judgment to reduce the amount of radiation exposure (1).

Distal obstructions typically present similarly to proximal obstructions (headaches and vomiting), but the onset of symptoms is usually more insidious and the duration may be longer. The diagnosis is usually made when the shunt pumps and refills briskly and the shunt tap results in easy aspiration of CSF and rapid resolution of symptoms. As a result, distal obstructions are not as urgent as proximal obstructions. Distal catheters can also migrate to a myriad of locations. Peritoneal catheters can migrate through the diaphragm into the chest,

out of the peritoneum into the subcutaneous tissue (2); through the wall of the intestine and out the anus, or through the uterus and out the vagina. Moreover, distal catheters can break or be disconnected, which is why it is important to obtain not only a head CT but also a shunt series. If there is a lot of scarring then a distal revision is more difficult than the original insertion, but in general, the postoperative risk is the same as the initial insertion.

Externalized Ventriculostomy

Externalized ventriculostomies are very similar to proximal shunts except that they are tunneled out of the skin and drain into a bag rather than into a body cavity or vessel. The most common complication of an externalized ventriculostomy is a poorly placed catheter (Figure 22.1). No patient should leave the OR or arrive in the PICU with a ventriculostomy that is not working. If CSF is not draining, a head CT is required directly after leaving the OR. If the catheter is in good position and there is no CSF in the ventricles, then the patient can go to the PICU.

Unfortunately, some patients do leave the OR without a working ventriculostomy, do not get a CT scan, and arrive in the PICU with a malfunctioning ventriculostomy. The burden then falls to the PICU team. There are many reasons why a ventriculostomy would not drain CSF, but an externalized ventriculostomy that is

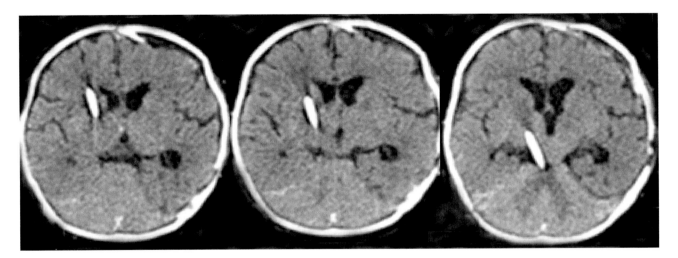

FIGURE 22.1 Nonenhanced head computed tomography (CT) obtained because of poor drainage from the ventriculostomy. The proximal catheter is suboptimally placed. Patient was taken back to the operating room for repositioning and returned with adequate cerebrospinal fluid drainage.

not draining CSF should be attributed to a malpositioned catheter until proven otherwise. The differential diagnosis of a nonfunctioning ventriculostomy includes (1) a malpositioned catheter, (2) stopcocks accidentally turned to the off position, (3) catheter clogged with blood, brain, or air, (4) no CSF in the brain, (5) very low pressure in the brain, or (6) a disconnected or kinked catheter. All of these potential etiologies can be easily assessed. First, confirm that all of the stopcocks are in the open position and there are no kinks. Second, inspect the tubing for debris blocking CSF flow. Third, drop the ventriculostomy bag to the floor to see if lowering the pressure results in drainage. These maneuvers can all be done in minutes. If there is still no CSF drainage, obtain a head CT. If the catheter is in good position and there is CSF in the ventricular system, the treatment is gentle flushing of the system. If the catheter is still not draining after flushing, then it may need to be replaced. Even when the orders from the neurosurgical team are to keep the catheter clamped, periodically checking the ventriculostomy is required to ensure that there is a good waveform and that dropping the bag several centimeters results in CSF flow. If these maneuvers do not result in either a good waveform or egress of CSF, then the neurosurgical team should be notified.

Lumbar Drains

Lumbar drains are most commonly placed in pediatric patients to stop CSF leaks after anterior skull base surgery or trauma, and in certain spine procedures.

Lumbar drains are not benign and can cause a myriad of complications. Complications begin at the time of insertion and can continue for several days after they are removed.

Lumbar drains are placed by inserting a Touhy needle (14 gauge) into the lumbar cistern and threading the catheter into the lumbar cistern. Patients can complain of radicular pain from injury during insertion or of severe back and leg pain every time the drain is opened. Lumbar drains are difficult to secure and can easily be accidentally dislodged. Low pressure headaches and infections are also not uncommon.

The most severe complication is tension pneumocephalus (Figure 22.2). The typical presentation is a patient who underwent an anterior skull base procedure and has lumbar drain placed to divert the CSF and allow the skull base repair to heal to a watertight seal. Air entering the nose is now in communication with the intracranial cavity and, because of the CSF flow out through the lumbar drain, a downward herniation of the brain can occur causing headache, obtundation, CN deficits, and even death. The signs and symptoms need to be recognized early and treated immediately. The treatment is clamping of the lumbar drain followed by removal of the drain with emergent placement of a blood patch (3). It is critical to recognize that this condition can develop and worsen even if the drain is clamped, or within 24 to 48 hours after the drain is removed. The treatment in this case is emergent blood patch.

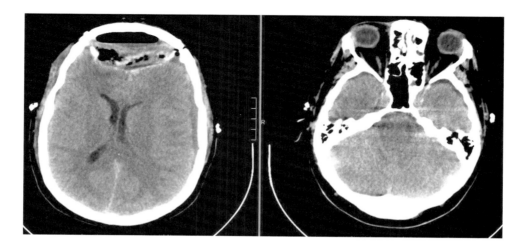

FIGURE 22.2 Nonenhanced head CT obtained because the patient became increasingly confused 24 hours after an anterior skull base procedure. The patient's lumbar drain was clamped; however, he continued to deteriorate. The image shows classic signs of low pressure changes. Patient improved hours after getting an emergent blood patch.

Posterior Fossa Brain Tumors

Approximately 50% of pediatric brain tumors are in the posterior fossa. The three most common tumors are medulloblastoma, juvenile pilocytic astrocytoma, and ependymoma. The most common presentation is secondary to the obstructive hydrocephalus which develops when these tumors block CSF flow through the fourth ventricle. Children present with headaches, nausea, and vomiting. Head CT or magnetic resonance imaging (MRI) will demonstrate a posterior fossa mass (Figure 22.3A and B). These tumors often need urgent (24–72 hours) treatment to relieve the pressure. In the absence of a hemorrhage into the tumor causing an acute increase of the hydrocephalus, these patients rarely need an emergent ventriculostomy.

Typically, these tumors are treated by placing an externalized ventriculostomy with or without an endoscopic third ventriculostomy. This is generally safe but, as discussed above, there are important postoperative considerations with externalized ventriculostomies. Next the patient undergoes a midline incision, the bone is removed (we advocate a craniotomy, but some surgeons do a craniectomy), and the dura opened. The vermis is divided to provide better visualization, but it is important to limit manipulation of the vermis because

of the postoperative complications of cerebellar mutism (also known as posterior fossa syndrome) (4,5). The tumor is then carefully removed with continuous inspection of the floor of the fourth ventricle. It is not uncommon for these tumors to become adherent to the floor of the fourth ventricle, especially in the case of juvenile pilocytic astrocytomas. These tumors can sometimes originate from the floor of the fourth where they are exophytic brainstem tumors filling the fourth ventricle (Figure 22.4). It is important for the PICU team and the neurosurgeon to discuss the extent of vermian and fourth ventricular floor involvement.

Splitting the vermis, especially the superior vermis in patients between the ages of 7 and 11 years of age who have a medulloblastoma, increases the risk of postoperative mutism. When severe, patients may not be able to be extubated, will be unable to speak or be hypophonic (speaking softly as if whispering), will have tremors and titubations, and will have severe strabismus and abnormal ocular movements. It is important to distinguish abnormal ocular movement abnormalities related to vermian involvement from those reflecting CN involvement, especially CN 6, but also CN 3 and CN 4. If the floor of the fourth ventricle is involved, then the patient is also at risk for CN 7 injury because of the dorsal location of the facial colliculus. Patients with injury to the

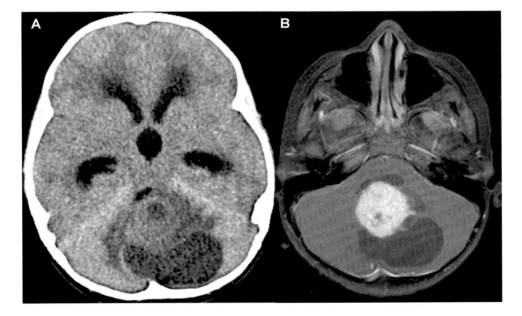

FIGURE 22.3 (A) Nonenhanced head CT showing obstructive hydrocephalus and a posterior fossa mass. (B) Axial magnetic resonance imaging (MRI) after gadolinium administration in the same patient. Tumor is originating in the cerebellum, strongly enhancing with multiple cysts. Patient underwent resection and the diagnosis was juvenile pilocytic astrocytoma.

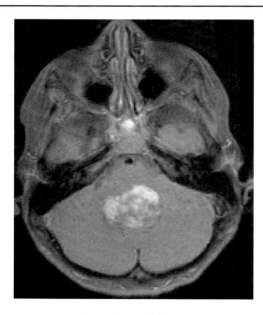

FIGURE 22.4 Axial MRI after gadolinium administration. The tumor is originating from the floor of the fourth ventricle. The tumor was unable to be completely resected, and the patient had transient intraoperative and postoperative hemodynamic instability.

facial colliculus will have a peripheral CN 7 palsy and may also have a CN 6 palsy. The presence of both CN 6 and CN 7 paresis or palsies localizes the injury to the brainstem, in contrast to the presence of both CN 7 and CN 8 injuries which localizes the lesion to the cerebellopontine angle.

Another concern with tumors invading the brainstem is possible postoperative hemodynamic instability if the nuclei of CN 9 and 10 are involved (6). Usually there are episodes of severe bradycardia and hypertension intraoperatively when this occurs, so the PICU team should carefully inspect the anesthesia record and ask the neurosurgeon about the extent of brainstem involvement and possible hemodynamic changes in the OR. It is unlikely that the nuclei of CN 12 would be injured but this may occur with inferior medullary exophytic tumors. In the unlikely event of bilateral CN 12 injuries the tongue will fall back into the pharynx and lead to severe airway obstruction. If this deficit is permanent, then tracheostomy is required.

The most common postoperative complications of a midline posterior fossa tumor are hemorrhage and hydrocephalus. Understanding the tumor location and the postoperative examination is important in evaluating any changes in the postoperative period. For example, if

the patient had a medulloblastoma that was not adherent to the floor of the fourth ventricle and several hours after surgery the patient became lethargic with hemodynamic instability, pinpoint pupils (pontine lesion), diplopia or sluggish pupils, then this is a hemorrhage until proven otherwise and emergent head CT is needed. A less likely explanation of these postoperative findings is a stroke, but that is extremely uncommon and the deficit would likely present immediately and be detected in the OR or in the PICU's initial examination. Our policy is that if the patient is unable to be extubated or has any unexpected change in exam immediately after extubation in the OR, then he or she goes directly for a head CT. A postoperative CT is key in identifying hemorrhage, poor ventriculostomy placement, hydrocephalus, pneumocephalus, and stroke. While head CT is likely to miss small strokes, it would be unlikely to miss any complication severe enough to produce an examination change. The other complication to consider is related to the reaccumulation of hydrocephalus. The signs and symptoms are the same as discussed above.

Some posterior fossa tumors extend out the foramen of Luschka and grow into the cerebellopontine angle. This is almost exclusively a feature of ependymomas, but can also occur in atypical teratoid rhabdoid tumors or medulloblastoma.

Patients with neurofibromatosis type 2 have bilateral seventh nerve schwannomas. Patients like these with tumors in the cerebellopontine angle are at risk for postoperative injuries to CNs 7, 8, 9, 10, 11, and 12 (Figure 22.5). Resection is performed with concurrent neuromonitoring of these nerves, but patients are at risk for postoperative aspiration even when the nerves stimulate normally at the end of the case. It is better to leave the endotracheal tube in for an extra day or two than to extubate prematurely and risk an aspiration or respiratory arrest. These patients require speech and swallowing evaluation prior to initiating oral nutrition.

Suprasellar Tumors

The two most common pediatric tumors in the sellar and suprasellar region are hypothalamic gliomas (with or without a neurofibromatosis type 1 diagnosis) and craniopharyngiomas. Hypothalamic tumors should be suspected in children under the age of 4 with tumors that do not have calcium on a head CT and are not cystic. Younger children often carry the diagnosis of failure to thrive (Russell syndrome) and may have nystagmus. Patients

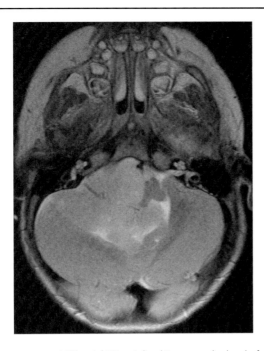

FIGURE 22.5 MRI axial T2-weighted image at the level of cranial nerves 7 and 8 showing a very large fourth ventricular ependymoma growing out into the right cerebellopontine angle, putting the patient at risk for postoperative lower cranial nerve dysfunction.

with neurofibromatosis type 1 and a hypothalamic glioma have a better prognosis than patients without neurofibromatosis type 1. Many patients with hypothalamic gliomas do not need surgery and are managed by the neurooncologists alone. However, if the tumors are very large and causing mass effect on the brainstem, obstructive hydrocephalus, or have radiographic features that are atypical or concerning for a more aggressive tumor, then they will be debulked. Because these tumors grow out of the optic nerves and chiasm, they cannot be completely removed surgically.

The postoperative complications here are ischemia related to vasospasm of the anterior and middle cerebral arteries and/or seizures related to hyponatremia. Children younger than 2 years of age are at greatest risk (7,8). If vasospasm is encountered in the OR, then papaverine is placed on the affected artery and the patient is managed by elevating the postoperative mean arterial pressure (MAP) and aggressive fluid goals. We usually aim for a MAP of 10% higher than the patient's baseline MAP during the start of the procedure. We also consider the calcium channel blocker nimodipine, but have to carefully weigh the risks and benefits in a young child

because nimodipine administration may lower MAPs. Intraoperative vasospasm is usually related to direct manipulation of the arteries. Postoperative vasospasm is often a result of arteries that were under severe stretch from a large tumor which develop vasospasm as they relax (Figure 22.6). These patients require frequent monitoring for signs and symptoms of vasospasm. The typical presentation is a waxing and waning neurologic exam that is exquisitely sensitive to blood pressure. In this situation, it is imperative to keep the patient in positive fluid balance and keep the blood pressure elevated with pressors. The duration of vasospasm for this patient population is not as well known. We typically monitor closely for 48 hours, and if there are no signs of vasospasm on exam or postresection MRI/A, then we relax the MAP goals and slowly wean fluids, while closely monitoring for subtle neurologic changes. If the patient is symptomatic, then we continue close monitoring, aggressive fluid goals, and an elevated MAP for 48 hours beyond the last symptoms, and then we slowly relax these strategies. However, there is no good literature on this patient population.

In general, we do not administer prophylactic anticonvulsants to any of our tumor patients since the risk of perioperative seizures is low, especially when controlling for hyponatremia (7,8). Children younger than 2 years of age are at higher risk for seizures, and although we do not currently provide prophylactic anticonvulsants, a trial of prophylactic anticonvulsants may be warranted.

Patients with lesions in the suprasellar region need to be closely monitored for sodium levels as hyponatremic seizures may occur. Additionally, diabetes insipidus occurs in almost every craniopharyngioma resection, producing hypernatremia and hypovolemia. Frequently the signs of diabetes insipidus begin in the OR or within a few hours of arriving in the PICU. Other endocrine abnormalities may also complicate suprasellar tumor resections.

With the development of endonasal surgery for craniopharyngiomas, there are a new set of postoperative complications. The main postoperative complication is a CSF leak (9–11). Because of the approach, the dura cannot be primarily closed. To prevent a CSF leak, vascularized nasal septal flaps are elevated and fat and tensor fascia lata is removed from the patient's thigh. The fat, fascia lata, and nasal septal flaps are all placed to prevent a CSF leak. Inevitably, the patient will have drainage from their nose, but it is not necessarily CSF. It is important to keep a test tube at the bedside to check the fluid for beta transferrin. Because of the

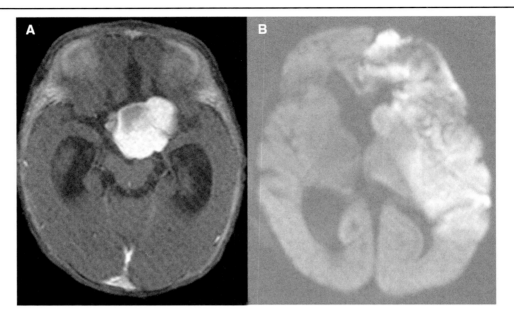

FIGURE 22.6 Preoperative (A) and postoperative (B) MRI of a chiasmatic hypothalamic glioma. (A) Axial MRI after gadolinium administration showing a large enhancing suprasellar tumor. (B) Diffusion weighted MRI showing a large left-sided stroke that occurred on postoperative day 4 from vasospasm.

trauma and edema immediately after surgery it is rare to see a CSF leak before postoperative day 4. It is only after the acute swelling starts resolving that CSF leaks occur. We currently do not place lumbar drains after endonasal procedures, but many surgeons do. Lumbar drains pose their own set of serious complications, as described above. Patients with CSF leak are initially managed with flat bed rest, Lasix, and Diamox. If that fails after 2 to 3 days, then the patient returns to the OR for revision of the nasal septal flaps and a ventriculostomy is placed (not a lumbar drain). If the patient fails a trial of ventriculostomy clamping, then we will again return to the OR for placement of a ventricular peritoneal shunt. Despite operating through the nose, the infection rate is low (10,12). Patients are placed on vancomycin and cefotaxime for several days and then transitioned to Augmentin until the second set of packing material is removed.

Supratentorial Tumors

Postoperative complications of supratentorial tumors usually result from hemorrhage or venous infarct. The vast majority of supratentorial complications occur in the OR and are present on arrival to the PICU. A large stroke would be detected with intraoperative monitoring or immediately after extubation in the OR. Postoperative hemorrhage usually occurs within the first 24 to 36 hours, but a venous infarct can occur in a much more delayed fashion. It is important to communicate with the neurosurgical team to understand the lesion location and which structures were at risk for injury. A detailed baseline exam is critical, and should be clearly documented to determine whether interval changes occur. While a general screening neurologic exam is important, it should be supplemented with detailed examination components related to the structures at risk for injury. For example, in the temporal lobe, language dysfunction and a field cut are possible. A formal test with naming, repeating, calculations, following multistep commands, and visual field testing are imperative. In the lateral ventricle, the exam needs to focus on short-term memory (fornix), weakness and aphasia (venous infarcts in the basal ganglia), and signs and symptoms of hydrocephalus.

Postoperative infections are very unlikely in elective craniotomies. They are more common in children with traumatic brain injury, subdural grids, or with externalized ventriculostomy. Our infection rate is approximately 8%. Infections are rarely evident during the initial surgery but may present approximately 7 days to 3 months after surgery.

Vascular Lesions

Arteriovenous malformations (AVMs) are the most common vascular lesions treated surgically (13). Depending on the location, severity of the hemorrhage, and the patient's exam, AVMs are not operated on acutely because unlike aneurysms, AVMs do not have a high rerupture rate. Typically, the patient undergoes a four-vessel angiogram to diagnose the AVM, but surgery is not performed immediately. The patient is then brought back for another angiogram with embolization the day before surgery. After embolization, the patient is at risk for a postembolization hemorrhage, especially if the embolization glue enters venous structures leading to AVM rupture. These patients often have headaches after embolization, which may be related to the changes in perfusion after the major feeding arteries are closed. After surgery, the complications are similar to those with tumors. Patients may also have a depressed level of consciousness from the dramatic changes in brain perfusion after the AVM is removed.

Aneurysms are much less common than AVMs (14) but are much more difficult to manage postoperatively because of the potential for vasospasm and hydrocephalus. Vasospasm may occur with ruptured aneurysms, but not with unruptured aneurysms, undergoing elective surgery. We found that our patients over the age of 2 years did not develop clinical and radiographic signs of vasospasm-induced ischemia. Regardless, we aggressively treat all of our patients with calcium channel blockers, daily transcranial Dopplers, hypervolemia, and close observation of a waxing and waning neurologic exam that responds to fluids and increased MAPs.

Epilepsy Surgery—Subdural Grids

Subdural grids may be needed to identify the exact seizure onset focus in patients with intractable epilepsy. Subdural grids are placed in the OR and then patients undergo several days of monitoring in the PICU or epilepsy monitoring unit. Patients with subdural grid are the most likely to develop a postoperative complication. Almost every grid patient complains of pain which is likely related to the grids irritating the dura. However, because the grids irritate the dura and bridging veins, they also put the patient at a significant risk for delayed postoperative hematomas (Figure 22.7). This makes evaluating postoperative patients with grids difficult. It is not prudent to get a head CT every time the patient complains of a headache, but it is important not to mistakenly attribute a growing subdural to typical postoperative pain. Every patient develops some subdural bleeding, but less than 5% of them require urgent evacuation. Additionally, the metal in the grids causes significant artifact and can make interpreting the CT scan difficult. Patients with severe or progressive headaches will undergo head CT, and it is important to focus on the bone windows more than the brain windows

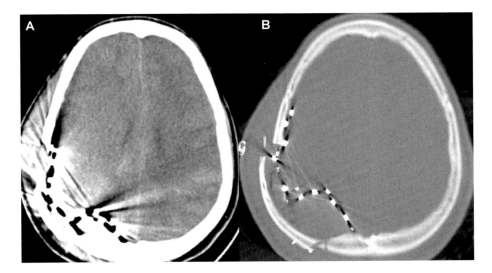

FIGURE 22.7 Nonenhanced head CT. (A) Brain window. (B) Bone window. Patient had subdural grids placed to localize the seizure focus and developed a severe headache and decreased level of consciousness on postoperative day 3. There is less artifact on the bone window (B) than on the brain window (A), making it easier to appreciate the extent of the mass effect of the subdural hematoma.

because there is less artifact in the former. A scan that does not look impressive on a brain window can look very impressive on the bone window when evaluating for the size of clot between the bone and grid. Some patients do require emergent clot evacuation in the OR. Warning signs are increasing headache, decreasing level of consciousness, and development of even a subtle focal deficit. The electroencephalogram (EEG) recordings may show attenuation in the region of subdural hemorrhage. If all of these findings are present, but the scan does not show an impressive hematoma and the patient has not had adequate seizure localization, then the grids are left in place. If the EEG recording is severely compromised, such that seizure localization would be affected, then the patient is taken back to the OR for evacuation, even if the scan and clinical exam are not impressive.

When a grid patient is taken to the OR for grid removal, the postoperative headache should reduce substantially. Any patient who complains of persisting or worsened severe headache after grid removal requires an urgent head CT.

Although unlikely, it is important to observe for signs of infection, which becomes more common if the grids are left in place for more than 1 week. Infections may not present until 3 to 7 days after grid removal. Published infection rates after grid implantation are around 3% to 10% (15–18).

■ SPINE PROCEDURE COMPLICATIONS

Spine procedures can be divided into different categories. For the purpose of this chapter, we will divide them into instrumented and noninstrumented spine procedures. Instrumented fusions in pediatric patients are done to correct acute deformities after trauma, subacute deformities after tumor or infection, and chronic deformities (scoliosis). They are also done to prevent deformities after tumor or trauma, or to stabilize deformities so that they do not progress. Uninstrumented spine surgeries typically only involve a few levels and are performed on well-balanced spines in both the sagittal and coronal planes.

The most likely complication in a patient with an instrumented fusion is a misplaced screw (19). It is important to know the indication for the procedure and the levels instrumented. Cervical spine traumas have a high likelihood of a vertebral artery dissection. Fortunately,

most of the dissections are asymptomatic and are either not treated or only treated with aspirin. If the patient developed brainstem symptoms or embolic events, then heparin may be indicated. Knowing preoperatively that one vertebral artery is injured may affect how the surgeon treats the injury to make sure the other vertebral artery is preserved.

A thorough neurologic exam with particular attention to the levels that were instrumented is paramount. An anterior approach may injure the esophagus, vagus nerve, spinal cord, vertebral artery, or nerve root. In the cervical spine, a misplaced screw can injure a nerve root, the vertebral artery, or the spinal cord. The best way to evaluate a potentially misplaced screw is to get a CT scan through the levels of the fusion and one level above and below. In the thoracic spine, a misplaced screw can injure the spinal cord, esophagus (upper-mid thoracic), or aorta. In the lumbar spine, the most likely injury is putting a screw into the neural foramen and injuring the exiting nerve root. These patients will complain of new radicular pain or new or worsening weakness. With improvement in intraoperative technology such as the O-Arm™ (Medtronic), misplaced screws are becoming less frequent, but remain a major complication.

Hematoma is the second most common complication in an instrumented fusion and the most common complication in an uninstrumented fusion. These patients typically have severe pain out of proportion to the procedure and will usually complain of weakness in particular muscle groups (if radicular or paraparesis [thoracic]). It is important to distinguish true weakness from weakness secondary to poor effort because of pain, which is why it is important to document a good exam on PICU arrival. Most patients will undergo intraoperative neuromonitoring. If the signals did not change during the procedure and the patient has good power in all muscle groups but then develops subtle but progressive weakness, then it is important to notify the surgeons and obtain an emergent MRI. An MRI is very good for an uninstrumented fusion, but the metal artifact in an instrumented fusion may distort the image too much to be helpful, especially in the thoracic spine. Depending on the symptoms, the patient may go directly to the OR for an exploration to rule out a clot without delaying the procedure to perform a MRI.

Occasionally a patient who does not undergo an instrumented fusion will have pain out of proportion to the procedure and not have a neurologic deficit, but may have a new acute or subacute instability. These

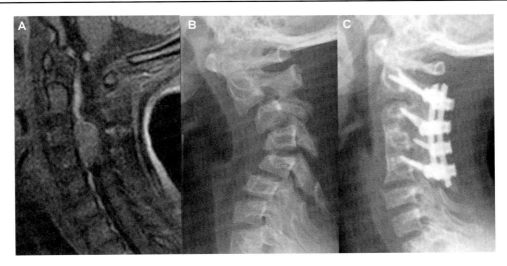

FIGURE 22.8 (A) Preoperative sagittal T1-weighted image in a patient with neurofibromatosis type 2. (B) Lateral plain x-ray 3 weeks after a 2 level cervical laminectomy for tumor resection. (C) Lateral plain x-ray after instrumented fusion. Surgery was unremarkable but the patient immediately complained of new onset severe neck pain. Pain completely resolved with instrumented fusion.

patients will have relatively few or no symptoms in the recumbent position but will experience worsening pain when upright that quickly resolves when lying flat (Figure 22.8). These patients should have anteroposterior and lateral plain x-rays and possibly dynamic flexion and extension films. If there is a new deformity or abnormal motion, then the patient would benefit from an instrumented procedure.

■ SUMMARY

Early and accurate identification of signs and symptoms of postoperative neurosurgical complications can significantly reduce the risk of permanent neurologic deficits. This requires a comprehensive understanding of the procedure and detailed discussion with the neurosurgical team regarding the preoperative exam, intraoperative findings, postoperative exam, expected postoperative changes, and potential postoperative complications.

■ REFERENCES

1. Brenner DJ, Hall EJ. Computed tomography—an increasing source of radiation exposure. *N Engl J Med.* 2007;357(22):2277–2284. doi:10.1056/NEJMra072149.

2. Samdani AF et al. Ventriculoperitoneal shunt malfunction presenting with pleuritic chest pain. *Pediatr Emerg Care.* 2005;21(4):261–263.

3. Samadani U et al. Intracranial hypotension after intraoperative lumbar cerebrospinal fluid drainage. *Neurosurgery.* 2003;52(1):148–151; discussion 151–142.

4. Doxey D et al. Posterior fossa syndrome: identifiable risk factors and irreversible complications. *Pediatr Neurosurg.* 1999;31(3):131–136.

5. Gudrunardottir T et al. Cerebellar mutism: review of the literature. *Childs Nerv Syst.* 2011;27(3):355–363. doi:10.1007/s00381-010-1328-2.

6. Heuer GG et al. Pulmonary edema and cardiac dysfunction after resection of a fourth ventricle tumor in a toddler: case report. *Childs Nerv Syst.* 2011;27(11):2005–2009. doi:10.1007/s00381-011-1573-z.

7. Hardesty DA, Kilbaugh TJ, Storm PB. Cerebral salt wasting syndrome in post-operative pediatric brain tumor patients. *Neurocrit Care.* 2011. doi:10.1007/s12028-011-9618-4.

8. Hardesty DA et al. Perioperative seizure incidence and risk factors in 223 pediatric brain tumor patients without prior seizures. *J Neurosurg Pediatr.* 2011;7(6):609–615. doi:10.3171/2011.3.PEDS1120.

9. Hadad G et al. A novel reconstructive technique after endoscopic expanded endonasal approaches: vascular pedicle nasoseptal flap. *Laryngoscope.* 2006;116(10):1882–1886. doi:10.1097/01.mlg.0000234933.37779.e4.

10. Kassam AB et al. Endoscopic endonasal skull base surgery: analysis of complications in the authors' initial 800 patients. *J Neurosurg.* 2011;114(6):1544–1568. doi:10.3171/2010.10.JNS09406.

11. Leng LZ et al. "Gasket-seal" watertight closure in minimal-access endoscopic cranial base surgery. *Neurosurgery.* 2008; 62(5 suppl 2):ONSE342-343; discussion ONSE343. doi:10.1227/01.neu.0000326017.84315.1f.

12. Fraser JF et al. Endoscopic endonasal minimal access approach to the clivus: case series and technical nuances. *Neurosurgery*. 2010;67(3 suppl operative):ons150–158; discussion ons158. doi:10.1227/01.NEU.0000383130.80179.41.

13. Lang SS et al. Follow-up imaging to detect recurrence of surgically treated pediatric arteriovenous malformations. *Journal of Neurosurgery. Pediatrics* 2012;9(5):497–504.

14. Stiefel MF et al. Endovascular and surgical treatment of ruptured cerebral aneurysms in pediatric patients. *Neurosurgery*. 2008;63(5):859–865; discussion 865–856. doi:10.1227/01.NEU.0000327573.42267.CC.

15. Johnston JM Jr et al. Complications of invasive subdural electrode monitoring at St. Louis Children's Hospital, 1994–2005. *J Neurosurg*. 2006;105 (5 suppl):343–347. doi:10.3171/ped.2006.105.5.343.

16. Lee WS et al. Complications and results of subdural grid electrode implantation in epilepsy surgery. *Surg Neurol*. 2000;54(5):346–351.

17. Onal C et al. Complications of invasive subdural grid monitoring in children with epilepsy. *J Neurosurg*. 2003;98(5):1017–1026. doi:10.3171/jns.2003.98.5.1017.

18. Wiggins GC, Elisevich K, Smith BJ. Morbidity and infection in combined subdural grid and strip electrode investigation for intractable epilepsy. *Epilepsy Res*. 1999;37(1):73–80.

19. Sarlak AY et al. Evaluation of thoracic pedicle screw placement in adolescent idiopathic scoliosis. *Eur Spine J*. 2009;18(12):1892–1897. doi:10.1007/s00586-009-1065-y.

23 Neurologic Complications in Pediatric Cardiac Disease

KIMBERLY Y. LIN, LAUREN A. BESLOW, and DANIEL J. LICHT

■ INTRODUCTION

Congenital heart defects are among the most common birth defects. Population-based registries in 16 European countries estimate the incidence of congenital heart disease (CHD) to be 5.36 to 15.32 per 1,000 births using data from 2000 to 2005 (1). Previously healthy children can suffer from acquired cardiac disorders including endocarditis and myocarditis. Others, including those with underlying neuromuscular disorders such as Becker muscular dystrophy and Pompe disease, may have an intrinsic abnormality of myocardial function referred to as a cardiomyopathy.

Children with cardiac disease often have neurologic complications that present while in the intensive care unit (ICU) or that lead to ICU admission. They are at risk for a variety of acute neurologic emergencies including seizures, hypoxic-ischemic injury, arterial ischemic stroke, cerebral venous sinus thrombosis, and intracerebral hemorrhage. Evaluation and management of these neurologic conditions may be complicated due to specific cardiac considerations and physiologic requirements.

■ ANATOMIC CONSIDERATIONS

From a neurologic perspective, CHDs may be categorized as either single ventricle lesions, biventricular lesions with intracardiac shunts, or biventricular lesions without intracardiac shunts. Single ventricle lesions, before the completion of staged palliation, allow direct access to the brain from the venous and systemic circulations. Biventricular lesions, on the other hand, allow blood flow to the brain only from the systemic circulation, or via shunts between the pulmonary and systemic circulations. The exact anatomy of CHDs is extremely variable, but examples of common lesions are provided in Table 23.1.

Understanding the series of operations that a child with single ventricle physiology may undergo can be daunting. Amidst the complex terminologies that accompany these procedures, the neurologist and intensivist should pay attention to how cerebral venous drainage is achieved, whether and where mixing of oxygenated and deoxygenated blood takes place, and what risk factors for thrombotic or hemorrhagic complications are present.

A summary of the classic three-staged surgical palliation for hypoplastic left heart syndrome (HLHS), a prototypical single ventricle CHD lesion, is provided in Table 23.2. With the first stage, a child's venous drainage is accepted into the actively pumping and relaxing ventricle, as with a normal child. With the second and third stages, venous drainage becomes a passive flow phenomenon wherein vena caval blood must empty directly into the pulmonary arteries. The resulting central venous pressure may be quite high, leading to frequent headaches and an increased risk of cerebral venous sinus thrombosis. Stasis of flow may also lead to thrombus formation in the cavopulmonary pathway itself. The acute increase in central venous pressure that results from the obligate passive venous return from the systemic vena cavae to the pulmonary vasculature may lead

■ **Table 23.1** Examples of Congenital Heart Defects by Physiology

Single Ventricle	Two Ventricle	Shunt Lesions
HLHS	Coarctation of the aorta	ASD
UAVC	CAVC	VSD
DORV	TGA	PDA
Tricuspid atresia	Tetralogy of Fallot	
Double inlet left ventricle	Total or partial anomalous pulmonary venous return	
PA/IVS	Valve disease with adequate chamber development	

Abbreviations: ASD, atrial septal defect; CAVC, common atrioventricular canal; DORV, double outlet right ventricle; HLHS, hypoplastic left heart syndrome; PA/IVS, pulmonary atresia with intact ventricular septum; PDA, patent ductus arteriosus; TGA, transposition of the great arteries; UAVC, unbalanced atrioventricular canal; VSD, ventricular septal defect.

to pleural effusions. Procoagulant and anticoagulant factors may be lost through a draining pleural effusion or via protein losing enteropathy. This, along with the loss of overall body fluid, may place the child after stage 2 or stage 3 palliative surgery at higher risk of thrombotic and thromboembolic complications. Careful monitoring of hydration status and serum levels of factors such as antithrombin III are warranted, and management with hydration and fresh frozen plasma administration may be indicated.

The first two stages of single ventricle palliation require mixing of the venous and systemic circulations in the heart, which means that venous blood may flow to the brain without the pulmonary bed as an intermediary filter. In the third stage, most venous blood flows through the pulmonary bed, but a communication called a *fenestration* may be created between the pulmonary and systemic circulations, allowing right-to-left shunting of venous blood to the arterial circulation. Such fenestrations are commonly created to aid in postoperative recovery by preserving cardiac output in the face of acutely

■ **Table 23.2** Staged Palliation Approach to Hypoplastic Left Heart Syndrome

	Stage 1	Stage 2	Stage 3
Alternate names	1. Norwood procedure 2. Sano procedure	1. Hemi-Fontan 2. Bidirectional Glenn 3. Partial caval-pulmonary anastomosis	1. Fontan (multiple variations) 2. Total caval-pulmonary connection
Typical age	Neonatal	4–6 months	2–5 years
Major components	1. Atrial septectomy (ensures complete mixing) 2. Aortic arch augmentation (allows systemic perfusion) 3. Anastomose pulmonary artery and aorta (provides ventricular outflow and coronary perfusion) 4. Blalock-Taussig shunt or right ventricle to pulmonary artery conduit (provides controlled blood flow to lungs)	1. Connect upper body venous return directly to pulmonary arteries	1. Connect remainder of venous return directly to pulmonary arteries
Source of pulmonary blood flow	Blalock-Taussig shunt (Norwood) or right ventricle to pulmonary artery conduit (Sano)	Superior vena cava	Superior and inferior vena cava
Notes	Hybrid approach possible (stent in ductus arteriosus, bands on bilateral pulmonary arteries to control pulmonary blood flow).	Acutely increased central venous pressure may lead to headaches and increased risk of thrombosis.	Fenestration commonly created to allow systemic venous blood to "pop off" to systemic circulation if central venous pressures are too high.

elevated central venous pressure. Many Fontan fenestrations endothelialize and close spontaneously, although those that do not can usually be closed later by percutaneous device in the cardiac catheterization laboratory.

Children with biventricular heart disease may warrant special neurologic attention as well. Those with ventricular dysfunction will be discussed further in the section on heart failure. Shunt lesions including septal defects and patent ductus arteriosus (see Table 23.1) can provide a conduit from the venous to the systemic circulation. Prosthetic material on either side of the circulation can serve as a nidus for infection (e.g., endocarditis) or thrombus formation. Current American Heart Association guidelines recommend antibiotic prophylaxis for bacterial endocarditis at times of increased risk for patients with prosthetic heart valves, with a history of infectious endocarditis, with unrepaired cyanotic CHD, in the first 6 months after completing a CHD repair using prosthetic material or device, with repaired CHD and a residual defect near prosthetic material, and in cardiac transplant recipients with valvulopathy (2). Anticoagulation is recommended for those with a mechanical prosthetic valve replacement, with a goal international normalized ratio (INR) of 2.5 (range 2.0–3.0) for those placed in the semilunar valve position (as with bioprosthetic valves in any position), and a goal INR of 3.0 (range 2.5–3.5) for those placed in the tricuspid or mitral valve positions (3).

■ PERIOPERATIVE CONSIDERATIONS

Surgical correction or palliation is often required to support infants and children with CHD. Given the variety of heart defects, surgical procedures are varied. The timing of intervention is linked closely to the severity of the heart lesion. A detailed discussion on the risks associated with each surgical intervention is beyond the scope of this chapter. Typical surgical risks involving anesthetics, mechanical ventilation, bleeding, or infections are present. Some perisurgical neurologic morbidity is specific to the type of heart defect or postoperative management, and not simply the conduct of the surgery itself. The following discussion will focus on specific risks related to the care of infants and children with CHD. The management of other complications such as arterial ischemic stroke, intracranial hemorrhage, and cerebral venous sinus thrombosis are discussed elsewhere in this text.

■ WHITE MATTER INJURY

Infant heart surgery refers to surgical procedures performed on children less than 30 days old with heart defects so severe that survival depends on surgical correction or palliation. For such patients, the mortality from these early surgeries has dropped dramatically since the late 1980s. In the more experienced centers with the highest surgical volumes, survival approaches 90% for the most complex and technically challenging surgeries (4). With this increase in survival, the focus of care has shifted to neurologic morbidity.

It has long been observed that the head circumferences in infants with severe CHD are smaller than infants of similar gestation ages without CHD (5,6). Infants with CHD are also prone to hypoxic-ischemic white matter injury that is not distinguishable from periventricular leukomalacia (PVL), an injury seen primarily in premature infants (Figure 23.1) (7,8). In infants with multiple forms of CHD, this injury is seen in 17% to 40% before surgery (9–11) and in over 50% after surgery (12,13). Research has now demonstrated that the primary risk for this injury is a brain-specific intrauterine growth retardation that arises as a consequence of the alterations in fetal hemodynamics created by the CHD (5,6,12). Fetal circulation in children with CHD has recently been reviewed (14).

Brain magnetic resonance imaging (MRI) is required to diagnose PVL because the lesions are typically of a volume that is below the resolution threshold for head computed tomography (HCT) or head ultrasound imaging. The typical PVL lesion occurs in the white matter watershed zone, is hyperintense on T1 imaging (Figure 23.1A), may demonstrate restriction of water motion if acute (Figure 23.1B), and may have susceptibility signal on T2* (Figure 23.1C) that reflects either hemorrhage or mineralization. The lesions may demonstrate restriction of water motion if acute (Figure 23.1B). The limitation of diffusion-weighted imaging is that pseudonormalization may occur as early as 7 days after injury. MRI slice thickness is also important since interslice gaps may cause obscuration of lesions. There is controversy in nomenclature of these white matter lesions. Some centers refer to white matter lesions with restriction of water motion on diffusion-weighted imaging as arterial ischemic stroke (see later discussion) while other centers consider these lesions part of the spectrum of PVL.

The risk for preoperative and postoperative injury is different for individual cardiac diagnoses. Higher preoperative risk is seen in transposition of the great arteries (TGA), and a higher rate of postoperative injury

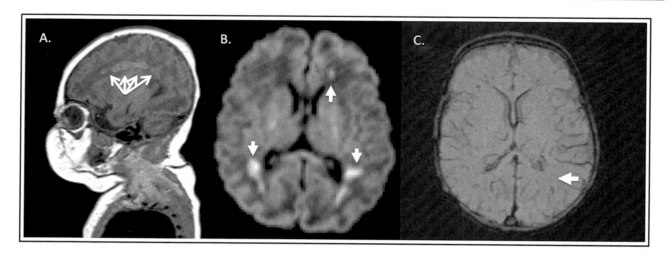

FIGURE 23.1 Magnetic resonance imaging of white matter injury (periventricular leukomalacia). (A), Sagittal plane, T1 hyperintensity in the white matter watershed (radial arrows). (B), Axial plane, diffusion weighted imaging—areas of periventricular restriction of water diffusion (arrows). (C), Axial plane, susceptibility weighted imaging (SWI) demonstrating the absence of hemorrhage within lesions (single arrow).

is seen in HLHS. Recent investigations (unpublished data from D.L. Licht) suggest that low arterial oxygen content coupled with increasing cerebral oxygen metabolic demand after either birth or cardiopulmonary bypass create the conditions that lead to the white matter injury in the form of PVL. For patients with TGA, the lowest oxygen saturations occur prior to surgery and should normalize after corrective surgery. Therefore proceeding to surgical correction at the earliest time possible as suggested by Petit and colleagues (11) should be protective against PVL. Conversely, for patients with HLHS or other single ventricle heart lesions, systemic oxygen saturations are typically in the mid 70% to 80% range before surgery and are not significantly higher after initial surgical palliation. Cerebral oxygen metabolism for these infants however, is greatest in the first 24 hours during the recovery from the moderate (~25°C) or deep (~18°C) hypothermia that is required for safe conduct of these intricate surgeries with cardiopulmonary bypass. Thus, the risk for PVL in HLHS and other infants with single ventricle physiology is increased after surgery (up to 75% risk) (12,13). Strategies to either reduce metabolic demand or increase oxygen delivery may thus be particularly useful in these populations.

In patients with HLHS and similar single ventricle lesions, the cerebral-systemic circulation is in series with the pulmonary circulation since all cardiac output is through the common pulmonary artery. Maintaining a balance of pulmonary to systemic blood flow ensures optimal systemic oxygen delivery. However, maintaining this balanced circulation is often difficult because the perinatal pulmonary vascular resistance drops after birth. Rising peripheral oxygen saturations in an HLHS patient may be a sign of pulmonary overcirculation and should thus prompt careful assessment of systemic perfusion. As a higher fraction of cardiac output flows to the lungs, organ ischemia may ensue with lactic academia and circulatory collapse. Early surgery may be warranted for those HLHS patients with peripheral oxygen saturations in the 90% range to prevent ischemic damage to other organs. Likewise, in the postoperative single ventricle patient after stage 1 palliation, permissive hypercarbia with slight respiratory acidosis is preferable to a respiratory alkalosis with overventilation to prevent pulmonary overcirculation through the systemic-to-pulmonary artery shunt.

■ ARTERIAL ISCHEMIC STROKE

The risk for arterial ischemic stroke in the perisurgical care of the infant with severe CHD is much debated, and controversy exists on how brain injury is defined in this setting. Classically, arterial ischemic stroke is defined by focal neurologic deficits that are referable to an arterial territory of the brain. In children, this definition has been expanded to include confirmatory neuroimaging. In infants, arterial ischemic stroke may be asymptomatic; thus the definition can be purely based on neuroimaging. McQuillen and colleagues (15) reported a very high incidence (30%) of preoperative arterial ischemic stroke in infants with TGA. Their group showed a higher risk of arterial ischemic stroke in those who underwent balloon atrial septostomy, a catheter-based procedure performed to rapidly improve arterial blood saturations by enhancing intracardiac mixing of oxygenated and deoxygenated blood. Two later publications by Petit and colleagues (11) and Beca and colleagues (9) both reported very low arterial ischemic stroke rates (0% and 4.5%, respectively) in patients with TGA. Petit and colleagues further argued that the performance of balloon atrial septostomy was necessary to protect infants with TGA from PVL and was not a risk for arterial ischemic stroke. It is possible that differences in lesion nomenclature (PVL versus arterial ischemic stroke) at different centers have led to the discrepancies in stroke incidence.

There is sparse literature on stroke in infants with severe CHD requiring infant heart surgery. In a retrospective study, Chen and colleagues (16) identified stroke in 12 of 122 infants (10%). Of these 12, 6 had arterial ischemic stroke and 6 had watershed stroke. This low prevalence rate is congruent with the rate of stroke seen by Beca and colleagues (9) and with our own experience of 2% to 4% preoperative and 8.6% postoperative, in mixed populations of infants with severe CHD (Goff et al. manuscript in preparation). With such small numbers, investigation of risk factors is not likely to be fruitful. Centrally placed catheters, such as umbilical catheters, right atrial catheters, and femoral catheters are potential thrombus sources.

Older children with single ventricle heart lesions are highly predisposed to arterial ischemic stroke due to their unique anatomy. Lower extremity access should be avoided if possible in patients with bidirectional Glenn physiology (stage 2) because the inferior vena cava remains in direct communication with the systemic circulation. Fenestrations placed surgically at the time of Fontan completion act as a pressure pop-off valve, but are obligate right-to-left shunts that may also allow for paradoxical emboli. Chylous effusions and protein losing enteropathy from high central venous pressures can result in a prothrombotic state due to protein losses. Adequate hydration and factor replacement with fresh frozen plasma may be required.

■ INTRACRANIAL HEMORRHAGE

Detection of intracranial hemorrhage prior to surgery is of obvious importance because the conduct of heart surgery with cardiopulmonary bypass requires aggressive anticoagulation. The term intracranial hemorrhage includes epidural, subdural, subarachnoid, intraventricular, and intraparenchymal hemorrhages. In contrast, the term intracerebral hemorrhage encompasses only intraparenchymal hemorrhage and intraventricular hemorrhage. At the time of birth, some amount of intracranial hemorrhage has been found to be very common (17). These include subdural hemorrhages along the tentorial membrane and choroid plexus hemorrhages, which may have intraventricular extension (Figure 23.2A). It is important to note that these hemorrhages do not usually extend during the conduct of infant heart surgery with cardiopulmonary bypass despite the requirement for systemic anticoagulation during cardiopulmonary bypass.

Intraparenchymal hemorrhages found on preoperative head ultrasound, or incidentally as part of a research protocol, must be managed on a case-by-case basis since there is a paucity of information on the risk of hemorrhagic extension on cardiopulmonary bypass. If an incidental intracranial hemorrhage is found that is not a subdural hemorrhage along the tentorial membrane or choroid plexus hemorrhage, our practice is to postpone surgery when possible by 1 week. The patient is reevaluated with a follow-up, preoperative brain MRI before proceeding.

Subdural hemorrhages are the most common clinically significant hemorrhages in the postsurgical patient, and these can occur acutely or subacutely after surgery. Anticoagulation, elevation in central venous pressures, and brain atrophy (from other injury) are all putative contributors to increased risk. Subdural hemorrhages requiring surgical intervention are uncommon in the cardiac ICU population.

Punctate microhemorrhages seen on brain MRI (Figure 23.2B, C, and D) after heart surgery with

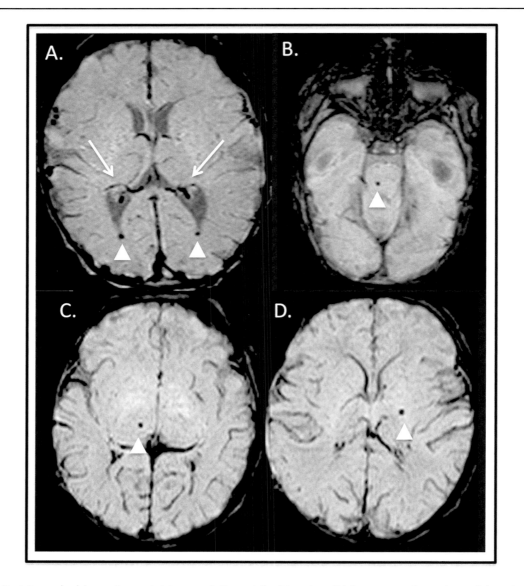

FIGURE 23.2 Intracerebral hemorrhage. Axial susceptibility weighted imaging. (A) Preoperative hemorrhage: bilateral choroid plexus hemorrhage (long arrows) with intraventricular extension (arrowheads). Postoperative punctate hemorrhages in the pons (B, arrowhead), right thalamus (C, arrowhead), and left globus pallidum (D, arrowhead).

cardiopulmonary bypass or after catheter-based interventional procedures are of unclear clinical significance. These microhemorrhages may be the result of microthromboembolic material from bypass cannulation. The lesions are common, occurring in 30% to 50% of postsurgical patients. There is a single report that these lesions may contribute to the neurodevelopmental impairment that is seen in survivors of infant heart surgery (18).

■ CEREBRAL VENOUS SINUS THROMBOSIS

Cerebral venous sinus thrombosis has been described in the CHD population, particularly in children or infants with dehydration and/or protein loss through pleural effusions or protein losing enteropathy. Management is described in Chapter 11, but in general includes hydration, elevation of the head of bed when possible to promote venous drainage, and systemic anticoagulation.

■ HEART FAILURE

Heart failure is the syndrome that results from the inability of the heart to meet the body's metabolic demands. Heart failure may be primary (due to intrinsic cardiomyopathy) or secondary to an underlying condition like valvulopathy (Table 23.3). A child in heart failure is at increased risk of neurologic complications due to several factors. First, a low cardiac output places a child at risk for decreased cerebral perfusion, a situation that can lead to watershed infarctions, hypoxic-ischemic brain injury, and secondary seizures or encephalopathy. Second, if the child's symptoms are due to decreased ventricular systolic function, the resulting stasis of blood may increase the child's risk of thromboembolic events. Third, arrhythmias may occur and may increase the risk of thromboembolism and thus arterial ischemic stroke. Some of those arrhythmias are secondary to the condition which has also caused heart failure, such as mitral valve stenosis and secondary atrial flutter. Some arrhythmias can result in complete circulatory collapse. This sudden complete cessation of circulation can result in hypoxic-ischemic injury to the deep gray nuclei, motor cortex, visual cortex, or other areas of the brain.

The degree of thrombotic risk associated with severe ventricular dysfunction is poorly defined. Anticoagulation and/or antiplatelet therapy is not universally recommended for children with heart failure due to the risk of bleeding and a lack of evidence to support its efficacy. Current American College of Cardiology/American Heart Association adult heart failure guidelines suggest giving anticoagulation to adults with heart failure and a history of atrial fibrillation or prior thromboembolic events (class IIb recommendation with level of evidence B) (19). A similarly lukewarm recommendation specifically aimed at the pediatric heart failure population suggests anticoagulation only for children with cardiomyopathy awaiting heart transplantation (20). Neither guideline specifies a threshold level of ventricular dysfunction below which antiplatelet or anticoagulant agents are strongly recommended. Further investigation is needed to help define the risk:benefit ratio of these therapies in various heart failure scenarios.

Several features of the cardiomyopathies may be of particular interest to the neurologist. Most of the cardiomyopathies carry an increased risk of atrial and ventricular arrhythmias for which a child should be regularly screened. When found, consideration for anticoagulation should be given. In some cases these arrhythmias are secondary to progressive myocardial dysfunction, but in others they are unrelated to the development of heart failure symptoms. For example, the form of hypertrophic cardiomyopathy which is inherited in an autosomal dominant fashion carries an increased risk of ventricular arrhythmias that may have more to do with disorganized myocardial architecture and fibrosis than simply the degree of left ventricular outflow tract obstruction. A child with hypertrophic cardiomyopathy should be regularly screened for risk factors that increase the risk of sudden cardiac arrest; if such risk factors are identified, an implantable cardioverter-defibrillator may be indicated as a primary prevention measure (21).

Left ventricular noncompaction is a form of cardiomyopathy that is characterized by deep trabeculations (also referred to as crypts) in the myocardium (Figure 23.3). Anecdotal reports of embolic strokes in patients with left ventricular noncompaction indicate that these crypts may serve as a nidus for thrombus formation (22). When left ventricular noncompaction is identified, consideration for primary prevention with an agent such as aspirin or even with anticoagulation should be given, especially in light of the risk of systemic embolism from the left ventricle.

Several neuromuscular conditions are commonly associated with a primary cardiomyopathy. Children with Duchenne and Becker muscular dystrophy may have a dilated cardiomyopathy, and their degree of ventricular

■ Table 23.3 Causes of Heart Failure	
Primary	**Secondary**
Dilated cardiomyopathy	Volume overload (e.g., ASD)
Hypertrophic cardiomyopathy	Pressure overload (e.g., aortic stenosis)
Restrictive cardiomyopathy	Surgical complications (e.g., impaired coronary perfusion after arterial switch)
Left ventricular noncompaction	Arrhythmias (e.g., complete heart block)
Arrhythmogenic right ventricular cardiomyopathy	Inflammatory (e.g., myocarditis)

Abbreviation: ASD, atrial septal defect.

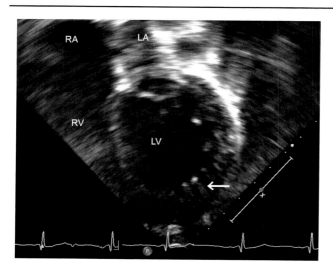

FIGURE 23.3 Apical 4 chamber view by echocardiogram of a heart with left ventricular noncompaction. Note the deep trabeculations near the apex (arrow) which may serve as a nidus for thrombus formation. Abbreviations: LA, left atrium; LV, left ventricle; RA, right atrium; RV, right ventricle.

dysfunction may progress independent of skeletal myopathy (23). Friedrich ataxia is associated with a hypertrophic cardiomyopathy. Careful assessment of the patient's current cardiac status, especially with respect to hydration, is warranted whenever such patients are admitted to the ICU.

For those children in heart failure secondary to CHD, the reader is directed to Table 23.1 as a guide for determining whether the brain is directly exposed to the venous circulation without the pulmonary bed as an intermediary filter. In mixing lesions, any thrombotic risk should also be considered an embolic stroke risk as well.

The treatment of decompensated heart failure, and therefore the treatment of neurologic comorbidities due to heart failure, includes a tailored regimen of diuretics, cardiac reverse remodeling agents, and inotropic support. Surgical intervention is often warranted for heart failure secondary to CHD. However, some of the surgical options for the treatment of decompensated heart failure, while often life-saving, may entail increased neurologic risk, as outlined in the following section on mechanical support devices.

■ MECHANICAL CIRCULATORY SUPPORT DEVICES

Children with severe heart failure may require support devices to maintain cardiopulmonary circulation. These support devices often require maintenance

on anticoagulation, antiplatelet agents, or both. Complications from the underlying cardiac failure, the device itself, or the medications used to maintain the device may arise, most commonly stroke (Table 23.4).

Extracorporeal Membrane Oxygenation

Extracorporeal membrane oxygenation (ECMO) has been the most commonly used form of mechanical cardiopulmonary support to date and is a form of heart-lung bypass. There are 2 types of ECMO, venoarterial and venovenous. In venoarterial ECMO, a catheter must be placed into an artery and into a vein, allowing support of the systemic circulation in addition to oxygenation of venous blood. In children, the right carotid artery is often used and subsequently sacrificed unless the surgeon chooses to repair the vessel at the time of decannulation. In venovenous ECMO, a single catheter with 2 lumens is placed into a vein. Venovenous ECMO is used for children without significant heart or blood pressure problems, and the carotid artery is not sacrificed. Neurologic complications can arise from ischemia due to carotid cannulation in venoarterial ECMO, hypoxic-ischemic injury, embolic arterial ischemic stroke, or intracranial hemorrhage. Sequelae including seizures and encephalopathy can arise in any of these settings.

Ventricular Assist Device

Ventricular assist devices (VADs) are a form of mechanical circulatory support without a membrane oxygenator that can be used to assist the left ventricle only, right ventricle only, or both ventricles. Most cases involve direct cannulation of the ventricle for VAD inflow, and aortic cannulation for VAD outflow. VADs are more compact than ECMO, thus providing a longer-term option for mechanical circulatory support on which the patient can be an active participant in rehabilitation (Figure 23.4). In pediatric centers, VADs are currently used almost exclusively as a bridge to cardiac transplantation. The VADs currently available for use in infants and small children are all pulsatile devices. In contrast, the adult heart failure and transplant community has seen a dramatic shift in recent years to the use of continuous flow devices. Such devices have shown improved overall survival and fewer adverse neurologic outcomes compared with pulsatile devices in adults (24, 25). Therefore, some centers now use continuous flow VADs in adult-sized children as well.

Children supported by VADs are at significant risk of neurologic complications including arterial ischemic

■ **Table 23.4** Neurologic Complications Reported in Children on Mechanical Circulatory Support Devices

Device	Series, Number of Patients	Neurologic Complications (N, %)

ECMO	Duncan (28), 70	22 (31%) total
		  4 arterial ischemic stroke
		  8 intracranial hemorrhage
		  5 seizures
		  2 anoxic encephalopathy
		  1 developmental delay
		  1 Horner's syndrome
		  1 abnormal EEG

VAD	Malaisrie (32), 8	5 (63%) total 4 arterial ischemic stroke or hemorrhage
	Hetzer (33), 62	4 of 36 survivors to transplant (11%), stroke
	Fan (34), 92[a]	22 (24%), stroke 4 of 34 deaths (12%) due to stroke
	Blume (26), 99	19 (19%), stroke 11 of 17 deaths (65%) due to stroke

	Reinhartz (27), 58	15 (26%) total
		  5 intracerebral hemorrhage
		  10 arterial ischemic stroke
		  3 transient ischemic attack
		5 of 17 deaths (29%) due to intracerebral hemorrhage
		1 of 17 deaths (6%) due to arterial ischemic stroke

Abbreviations: ECMO, extracorporeal membrane oxygenation; EEG, electroencephalogram; VAD, ventricular assist device.
[a] Some patients overlapped with Hetzer series.

stroke and intracerebral hemorrhage. The prevalence of neurologic complications varies by series. In one study, children with short-term VAD devices were significantly more likely to suffer a stroke than those with long-term VAD devices (35% versus 13%, $P = .02$) (26). In another series, children with left atrial cannulation were more likely to develop embolic arterial ischemic stroke than were those with left systemic apical cannulation (27). The Food and Drug Administration recently approved the Berlin Heart EXCOR Pediatric VAD under the Humanitarian Device Exemption Program.

As for neurologic complications in children supported with ECMO versus VAD, one nonrandomized study reported a higher rate of neurologic complications with ECMO than with VADs (28). However, in a different study that compared an institutional experience between ECMO and the Berlin EXCOR device, the incidence of stroke was not significantly different between the 2 devices (29). The choice between cannulation onto ECMO or VAD is therefore based on other factors, including technological capabilities at the center, potential for myocardial recovery, and anticipated duration of

need for mechanical circulatory support. VAD is generally favored over ECMO when long-term support is anticipated as a bridge to transplantation.

Treatment of Neurologic Complications of ECMO and VAD

For arterial ischemic stroke that occurs while on ECMO or a VAD, the presumption is that the source is cardioembolic. Therefore, optimizing anticoagulation levels is paramount, as is supporting cerebral perfusion with isotonic intravenous fluids, prevention of fevers, and prevention of hyperglycemia. For children who suffer intracranial or intracerebral hemorrhage, treatment is limited since cessation of anticoagulation is considered extremely high risk for thrombus formation while on mechanical circulatory support. Neurosurgical evacuation or placement of an intraventricular catheter to decompress hydrocephalus may be considered but is again limited by anticoagulation. If any type of intracranial hemorrhage does occur, if possible, the head of bed should be elevated to about 30°

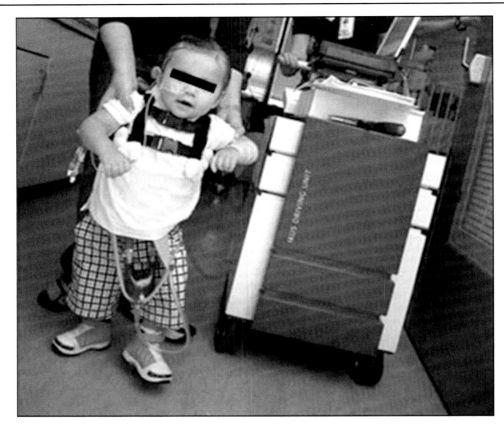

FIGURE 23.4   Ventricular assist device (Berlin EXCOR) being used by a child receiving physical rehabilitation. The device can be seen below his shirt. A computerized driver is wheeled behind his left shoulder.

to facilitate venous drainage, thereby lowering intracranial pressure. This cannot usually be accomplished if the child is on ECMO. Sequelae of stroke or hypoxic-ischemic damage like seizures should be treated with appropriate antiseizure medications. Continuous electroencephalography to monitor for subclinical seizures should be considered for any patient on ECMO or VAD with new brain injury, acute clinical seizures, altered mental status, or when clinical neurologic assessment is limited by sedation and/or neuromuscular blockade.

■ NEUROLOGIC MANAGEMENT SPECIFIC TO CARDIAC CARE

When managing neurologic complications of cardiac disease, the intensivist must choose medications and management with the child's underlying cardiac status

in mind. For example, a child with acute arterial ischemic stroke or cerebral venous sinus thrombosis is often placed on isotonic fluids at 1 to 1.5 times maintenance rate for age and weight. In the child with heart failure, the fluid rate may require modification in order to avoid iatrogenic worsening of heart failure. In the management of seizures with or without status epilepticus, anticonvulsant choices should take into account the child's cardiac status. While phenobarbital is often the medication of choice in infants and phenytoin or fosphenytoin is often used in older children, these medications can cause hypotension. Furthermore, phenytoin is a class 1B sodium channel blocker with both arrhythmogenic and antiarrhythmic properties. Therefore, in a child in whom hypotension is a concern or who has had or is at high risk for arrhythmias, intravenous levetiracetam may be preferred for both loading and maintenance purposes. Alternatively, the loading dose of phenobarbital or phenytoin may be administered in divided doses or more slowly than would otherwise be done.

While indwelling vascular catheters are the likely source for most clots in the cardiac ICU, a complete thrombophilia workup is still recommended for patients with arterial ischemic stroke (see Chapter 10). An echocardiogram is helpful to evaluate for residual clot or fibrin stranding in the heart, as can be seen after removal of a right atrial catheter. Rarely is a transesophageal approach required for this assessment because a transthoracic approach can usually provide adequate images in the pediatric population. For patients with significant residual right-to-left shunting, Doppler flow ultrasounds of the lower extremity veins are also indicated.

For patients with single ventricle physiology, at any stage in the surgical palliation, consideration should be given to lifelong anticoagulation with either low molecular weight heparin or warfarin. Further studies on the use of anticoagulation and antiplatelet agents are needed in the single ventricle population. Thus far there has been no demonstrated advantage to warfarin over aspirin for stroke prevention in Fontan patients, but there is no randomized trial data on either agent versus placebo (30). The risk for clot formation increases with time, and early clots (around stage 1) may herald an increased risk for clot formation during stages 2 and 3, regardless of a negative thrombophilia workup. For patients with single ventricle physiology, the risk for right atrial clots (systemic) increases dramatically 15 years after Fontan (complete cavopulmonary connections) completion (31). Factors such as protein losing enteropathy and increased central venous pressures may increase the risk of clot formation in these patients.

■ CONCLUSIONS

Children with congenital or acquired heart disease are at risk for many neurologic complications. Awareness of these complications ensures that any neurologic changes can be quickly assessed and managed.

■ REFERENCES

1. Dolk H, Loane M, Garne E. Congenital heart defects in Europe: prevalence and perinatal mortality, 2000 to 2005. *Circulation.* 2011;123:841–849.
2. Wilson W et al. Prevention of infective endocarditis: guidelines from the American Heart Association: a guideline from the American Heart Association Rheumatic Fever, Endocarditis, and Kawasaki Disease Committee, Council on Cardiovascular Disease in the Young, and the Council on Clinical Cardiology, Council on Cardiovascular Surgery and Anesthesia, and the Quality of Care and Outcomes Research Interdisciplinary Working Group. *Circulation.* 2007;116:1736–1754.
3. Salem DN et al. Valvular and structural heart disease: American College of Chest Physicians Evidence-Based Clinical Practice Guidelines (8th Edition). *Chest.* 2008;133:593S–629S.
4. Hirsch JC et al. Hospital mortality for Norwood and arterial switch operations as a function of institutional volume. *Pediatr Cardiol.* 2008;29:713–717.
5. Licht DJ et al. Brain maturation is delayed in infants with complex congenital heart defects. *J Thorac Cardiovasc Surg.* 2009;137:529-536; discussion 36–37.
6. Limperopoulos C et al. Brain volume and metabolism in fetuses with congenital heart disease: evaluation with quantitative magnetic resonance imaging and spectroscopy. *Circulation.* 2010;121:26–33.
7. Glauser TA et al. Acquired neuropathologic lesions associated with the hypoplastic left heart syndrome. *Pediatrics.* 1990;85:991–1000.
8. Kinney HC et al. Hypoxic-ischemic brain injury in infants with congenital heart disease dying after cardiac surgery. *Acta Neuropathol.* 2005;110:563–578.
9. Beca J et al. Pre-operative brain injury in newborn infants with transposition of the great arteries occurs at rates similar to other complex congenital heart disease and is not related to balloon atrial septostomy. *J Am Coll Cardiol.* 2009;53:1807–1811.
10. McQuillen PS et al. Temporal and anatomic risk profile of brain injury with neonatal repair of congenital heart defects. *Stroke.* 2007;38:736–741.
11. Petit CJ et al. Preoperative brain injury in transposition of the great arteries is associated with oxygenation and time to surgery, not balloon atrial septostomy. *Circulation.* 2009;119:709–716.
12. Andropoulos DB et al. Brain immaturity is associated with brain injury before and after neonatal cardiac surgery with high-flow bypass and cerebral oxygenation monitoring. *J Thorac Cardiovasc Surg.* 2010;139:543–556.
13. Galli KK et al. Periventricular leukomalacia is common after neonatal cardiac surgery. *J Thorac Cardiovasc Surg.* 2004;127:692–704.
14. McQuillen PS, Goff DA, Licht DJ. Effects of congenital heart disease on brain development. *Prog Pediatr Cardiol.* 2010;29:79–85.
15. McQuillen PS et al. Balloon atrial septostomy is associated with preoperative stroke in neonates with transposition of the great arteries. *Circulation.* 2006;113:280–285.
16. Chen J et al. Perioperative stroke in infants undergoing open heart operations for congenital heart disease. *Ann Thorac Surg.* 2009;88:823–829.
17. Tavani F et al. Incidental intracranial hemorrhage after uncomplicated birth: MRI before and after neonatal heart surgery. *Neuroradiology.* 2003;45:253–258.
18. Soul JS et al. Subtle hemorrhagic brain injury is associated with neurodevelopmental impairment in infants with repaired congenital heart disease. *J Thorac Cardiovasc Surg.* 2009;138:374–381.
19. Hunt SA et al. 2009 Focused update incorporated into the ACC/AHA 2005 Guidelines for the Diagnosis and

Management of Heart Failure in Adults A Report of the American College of Cardiology Foundation/American Heart Association Task Force on Practice Guidelines Developed in Collaboration with the International Society for Heart and Lung Transplantation. *J Am Coll Cardiol.* 2009;53:e1–e90.

20. Monagle P et al. Antithrombotic therapy in neonates and children: American College of Chest Physicians Evidence-Based Clinical Practice Guidelines (8th Edition). *Chest.* 2008;133:887S–968S.

21. Gersh BJ et al. 2011 ACCF/AHA Guideline for the Diagnosis and Treatment of Hypertrophic Cardiomyopathy: Executive Summary A Report of the American College of Cardiology Foundation/American Heart Association Task Force on Practice Guidelines Developed in Collaboration with the American Association for Thoracic Surgery, American Society of Echocardiography, American Society of Nuclear Cardiology, Heart Failure Society of America, Heart Rhythm Society, Society for Cardiovascular Angiography and Interventions, and Society of Thoracic Surgeons. *J Am Coll Cardiol.* 2011;58:2703–2738.

22. Pitta S, Thatai D, Afonso L. Thromboembolic complications of left ventricular noncompaction: case report and brief review of the literature. *J Clin Ultrasound.* 2007;35:465–468.

23. Romfh A, McNally EM. Cardiac assessment in Duchenne and Becker muscular dystrophies. *Curr Heart Fail Rep.* 2010;7:212–218.

24. Kirklin JK et al. Third INTERMACS Annual Report: the evolution of destination therapy in the United States. *J Heart Lung Transplant.* 2011;30:115–123.

25. Park SJ et al. Reducing adverse neurological events in LVAD patients: pulsatile vs. continuous flow? *J Heart Lung Transplant.* 2010;29:S51.

26. Blume ED et al. Outcomes of children bridged to heart transplantation with ventricular assist devices: a multi-institutional study. *Circulation.* 2006;113:2313–2319.

27. Reinhartz O et al. Multicenter experience with the thoratec ventricular assist device in children and adolescents. *J Heart Lung Transplant.* 2001;20:439–448.

28. Duncan BW et al. Mechanical circulatory support in children with cardiac disease. *J Thorac Cardiovasc Surg.* 1999;117:529–542.

29. Imamura M et al. Bridge to cardiac transplant in children: Berlin Heart versus extracorporeal membrane oxygenation. *Ann Thorac Surg.* 2009;87:1894–1901; discussion 901.

30. Monagle P et al. A multicenter, randomized trial comparing heparin/warfarin and acetylsalicylic acid as primary thromboprophylaxis for 2 years after the Fontan procedure in children. *J Am Coll Cardiol.* 2011;58:645–651.

31. Khairy P et al. Long-term survival, modes of death, and predictors of mortality in patients with Fontan surgery. *Circulation.* 2008;117:85–92.

32. Malaisrie SC et al. Pneumatic paracorporeal ventricular assist device in infants and children: initial Stanford experience. *J Heart Lung Transplant.* 2008;27:173–177.

33. Hetzer R et al. Improvement in survival after mechanical circulatory support with pneumatic pulsatile ventricular assist devices in pediatric patients. *Ann Thorac Surg.* 2006;82:917–925.

34. Fan Y et al. Predictors of in-hospital mortality in children after long-term ventricular assist device insertion. *J Am Coll Cardiol.* 2011;58:1183–1190.

24 Rehabilitation: Indications, Management, and Timing

TOM DRAKE

■ OVERVIEW

The concept of a patient's level of *function* and its implications are the lens through which the rehabilitation specialist evaluates and treats his patient. The actual act of rehabilitation is the process of "helping a person to reach the fullest physical, psychological, social, vocational, avocational, and educational potential consistent with his or her physiologic or anatomic impairment, environmental limitations, and desires and life plans" (1). With such a broad definition, the goals of rehabilitation are very diverse and differ vastly from patient to patient. Meanwhile, the goals for each patient can be very specific and can often only be met in the rehabilitation setting.

In the neurocritical care unit, the priority of these goals often shift due to many factors such as the acuity of the current illness, or the constraints that the current acute care places on rehabilitative therapy, the ability of the patient to tolerate rehabilitation therapy, or even the prognosis. In this chapter we will discuss the goals of rehabilitation, the timing of rehabilitation, some of the constraints of rehabilitation, and some of the specific rehabilitation issues relevant to children in a neurocritical care unit.

■ GOALS AND THE REHABILITATION TEAM

Ideally, the goal of all rehabilitation is to restore a patient to a premorbid level of function. This is often possible, but there are many neurocritical care patients who will have residual neurologic deficits even after an exhaustive rehabilitation course. These goals are set when the child is first evaluated in a critical care unit, and then revised throughout their stay on an acute rehabilitation unit.

It is helpful to discuss some general guidelines regarding appropriate goal setting for these patients. Take, for example, a boy with a new left middle cerebral artery infarction. This patient likely has any combination of the following: right hemiplegia, visual deficits, aphasia, sensory deficits, dysphagia, incontinence, attention problems, and a visuospatial neglect. He is very dependent on others for care. Initial family goals may be walking, talking, and using his right arm. In the child, recovery of function often appears more robust and quick as compared with the adult. Appropriate level of optimism and high expectations should be incorporated into the rehabilitative plan of care.

The rehabilitation specialist breaks down these goals into more steps. Doing so creates a more realistic series of manageable steps and this helps to document progress. These goals are primarily carried out by the therapists working intensively and intimately with the patients. Physical therapy (PT), occupational therapy (OT), and speech therapy are the primary services involved, but there are other critical members of a rehabilitation team that may also be involved (Table 24.1). Regarding the example of a boy with stroke, the rehabilitation team may begin work while the patient is in the neurocritical care unit and then continue work after the patient has transitioned to a rehabilitation unit or outpatient setting.

■ **Table 24.1**   Roles of Therapists

Physical therapy
  Functional restoration
  Restore/preserve range of motion
  Balance, transfers, mobility
  Gait training or wheelchair use
  Improve strength, endurance, coordination
  Edema management
  Application of different modalities (heat, cold, hydrotherapy, electrical stimulation, traction, massage)
  Wheelchair skills
  Proper ergonomics

Occupational therapy
  Functional activities
  Self-care
  Maximize independence
  Use of orthoses and adaptive equipment
  Home management
  Vocational activities
  Avocational activities
  Suggest home modifications
  Equipment and modified strategies
  Assistive technology

Speech/language therapy
  Language processing
  Impairments in speech, comprehension, reading, and writing
  Diagnoses include aphasia, dysarthria, apraxia, cognitive impairments, and language impairments
  Assessment and training in augmentative communication devices
  Evaluation of swallowing function
  Implementation of feeding strategies and programs
  Motor-speech impairment assessment and treatment

Recreation therapist and child life specialist
  Assess the patient's interests, cognitive and physical limitations, and emotional functioning
  Educate patients in recreation and leisure activities that are available, even in light of the patient's limitations
  Assist in the patient's and family's adjustment to illness and disability
  Community reintegration
  Reinforce the efforts and goals of the other therapies
  Increase independence
  Use play to help to normalize the hospital setting and foster continued development
  Help to explain medical information and procedures in a developmentally appropriate manner

Mental health professional
  Identify and treat behavioral issues

Pain specialist
  Assess, titrate, and treat pain to optimize analgesia and goals of rehabilitation

Case management
  Optimize the case to the third-party payers to optimize financial support of appropriate therapies

A speech and language therapist focuses on communication, swallowing, and speech production, and has a number of goals. One of the most basic goals is to find or create a way of identifying wants and needs.

For example, utilizing a series of pictures may be beneficial to a patient with a dense aphasia. Another communication goal would be the ability to call staff using a call bell. Further communication goals might be speech production and better strategies to articulate for a dysarthric patient. For the patient's dysphagia, there may be swallowing trials with different textures of food, so that the goal of swallowing safely can be pursued systematically. Adaptive equipment and strategies need to be developmentally appropriate. For instance, communication boards may utilize pictures to point to rather than letters.

PT usually focuses on gross motor activity and mobility goals, but this is not limited to safe ambulation or wheelchair use. For our stroke patient, PT goals would include bed mobility, transfers, posture, and mobility for self-care. Only after those initial goals are partially achieved can actual gait training begin. The PT would also eventually help order any needed bracing devices, assistive devices (e.g., cane, crutch, or walker) or mobility devices (e.g., wheelchair).

OT usually focuses on fine motor skills, but also works on specific vocational or recreational goals and academic strategies that would be helpful in almost any classroom. OT would work with our stroke patient to strengthen his hemiplegic arm as motor activity returns, but a more preliminary goal might be to develop strategies for managing activities of daily living in the setting of hemiplegia.

Many goals noted in the acute rehabilitation setting involve multiple members of the team. Memory-based tasks for example are reinforced in PT, OT, and speech therapy but are also stressed by nursing and with child life specialists or music or art therapists. Self-care goals and many activities of daily living are usually pursued in all of these settings as well. Cognitive retraining for children with new cognitive deficits is primarily addressed in OT, speech and language therapy, and with whatever classroom setting is available. However, all of the therapists ideally would reinforce the cognitive-based goals. This is the nature of this multidisciplinary rehabilitation team.

■ BASELINE STATUS

Understanding a patient's "baseline functional status" is of particular importance to rehabilitation. The goals of a rehabilitation plan of care hinge on baseline status. An example will help to illustrate its importance:

> Two 13-year-old girls who sustained moderate to severe traumatic brain injuries are stabilized in the intensive care unit (ICU). Both are left with cognitive deficits, confused, inappropriate at times, and are in need of assistance for activities of daily living. In terms of baseline functional status, one of the girls carries a diagnosis of tuberous sclerosis and was presumed to have moderate to severe intellectual disability, while the other reportedly had "some difficulty in school" prior to her accident but had no medical illness or syndrome. After a more careful evaluation of the situation it was found that the girl with tuberous sclerosis actually had an IQ of 80 at baseline and the other young woman labeled with "learning difficulties" had an IQ of 60, an individual education plan, and was in a life-skills classroom setting. Neurocognitive testing postacutely revealed that the girl with tuberous sclerosis was well below her baseline, yet many on the treating team mistakenly presumed she was at her baseline in 24 hours after her trauma. The same evaluation on the other girl revealed that she was actually at her baseline the day after her injury. She actually was never age appropriate for her activities of daily living even prior to her traumatic brain injury.

> The girl with tuberous sclerosis had almost been discharged without any potentially beneficial inpatient rehabilitation. The other girl actually was transferred to inpatient rehabilitation and it was not until a week later that her individualized educational plan was obtained, showing that she had been at her baseline the entire time.

For many children with a neurologic injury, however, there is a decline that may ultimately limit their neurocognitive potential. A careful and thoughtful evaluation of their projected *new* baseline status is required. When it can be predicted that a child will have new limitations on his neurocognitive potential following brain injury, then this must be taken into account when establishing goals for rehabilitation. This is perhaps most important for the family of that child, so that they can have a realistic view of the potential outcome and new needs of their child.

Alternately, a change in cognition can be easily overlooked by both the ICU team and the family. A common scenario where such changes go unrecognized occurs in patients with a spinal cord injury and coexisting traumatic brain injury. If subtle, the traumatic brain injury may go unrecognized because of the readily apparent (and distressing) paresis that may exist. These brain injuries may be missed, despite the fact that up to 60% of spinal cord injury patients also have evidence of a traumatic brain injury (2). Over 30% of these co-occurring traumatic brain injuries are mild, and this more subtle presentation may lead to lack of brain injury identification upon presentation.

■ EARLY REFERENCE POINTS

Clinical outcomes remain difficult to predict early in the course of a neurologic injury, when the patient is still in the critical care unit. The literature on spinal cord injury has provided some good evidence for predicting the functional status that may be attained by a patient (Table 24.2). This table may serve as an aid to early discussions about prognosis which may occur in the critical care unit. Translating medical terms regarding function into layman's terms is far more meaningful to a patient and his or her family.

Outcomes following brain injury often prove more difficult to predict. The complexity both in terms of pathophysiology and premorbid function, superimposed on developmental age make prognosticating a problem for both the clinician and the family. In the short term however, the Rancho Los Amigos Scale (Table 24.3) may be helpful in describing cognitive function. In the

■ Table 24.2 Functional Potential Outcomes for Cervical (SCI) spinal cord injury (Complete) Patients

	C3-C4	C5	C6	C7	C8-T1
Feeding	May be able with adapted equipment	Independent with equipment after setup	Independent with equipment	Independent	Independent
Grooming	Dependent	Independent with equipment after setup	Independent with equipment	Independent with equipment	Independent
UE dressing	Dependent	Requires assistance	Independent	Independent	Independent
LE dressing	Dependent	Dependent	Requires assistance	May be independent with equipment	Independent
Bathing	Dependent	Dependent	Independent with equipment	Independent	Independent
Bed mobility	Dependent	Requires assistance	Independent with equipment	Independent	Independent
Weight shifts	Independent with power Dependent in manual	Requires assistance	Independent	Independent	Independent
Transfers	Dependent	Requires assistance	Possible independent with transfer board	Independent with or without board except floor transfer	Independent
W/C propulsion	Independent with power Dependent in manual	Independent with power Short distances in manual with lugs or plastic rims on level surfaces	Independent manual with plastic rims on level surfaces	Independent except curbs	Independent
Driving	Unable	Unable	Specially adapted van	Car with hand controls or adapted van	Car with hand controls or adapted van
Bowel and bladder	Dependent	Dependent	Independent— bowel assists— bladder	Independent	Independent

Abbreviation: LE, lower extremity; SCI, spinal cord injury; UE, upper extremity; W/C, wheelchair.

Table 24.3 Rancho Los Amigos Revised Levels of Cognitive Functioning	
Level I:	No response
Level II:	Generalized response
Level III:	Localized response
Level IV:	Confused—agitated
Level V:	Confused—inappropriate
Level VI:	Confused—appropriate
Level VII:	Automatic—appropriate
Level VIII:	Purposeful—appropriate

presence of a noncommunicative patient, parental distress is often decreased in a small but significant way by thinking of "stages" of brain injury recovery. Progression in the levels represents improvement, even though the scale is nonlinear. Both clinicians and families often need to be reminded that there is not a clear duration for each of these levels, and that some levels can be bypassed by a patient, and some patients may plateau at certain levels. Lastly, these levels can be tracked by the care team to objectify some of the findings.

■ TIMING/WHEN TO CONSULT

While the immediate issues of medical management of a neurocritical care patient are the first priority, rehabilitation concerns can and must be addressed early. Several studies have shown worse outcomes with delays in rehabilitation. One study demonstrated that delays in admitting children with critical brain injuries from an ICU to an appropriate rehabilitation facility correlated with a less efficient rehabilitation course with significantly less measurable improvement in their functional measures (3). Early rehabilitation for adult brain injury patients has been shown to improve outcomes and decrease postacute rehabilitation duration (4) as well as reduce overall hospitalization costs (5). Similarly, earlier initiation of rehabilitation following adult stroke results in better functional outcome scores (6). Multiple adult studies have noted better outcome metrics with earlier or more intense rehabilitation.

Rehabilitation is not a separate phase of care that begins after medical management has been optimized and completed. Very little effective rehabilitation is likely to get done during the golden hour of trauma

resuscitation or during status epilepticus, but there are multiple reasons to involve the rehabilitation team early in the course of any critical care stay, especially in the neurocritical care setting. Furthermore, a large percentage of patients presenting to a neurocritical care unit have ongoing rehabilitation needs, but are admitted for other acute medical illnesses. One recent study of hospitalized children in neonatal and pediatric ICUs in France reported that the prevalence of preexisting chronic conditions and disability was 67% (7), and a similar study in the United States found that number to be slightly greater than 50% (8). This would imply that this subset of the patients in a neurocritical care unit have regular, ongoing need for rehabilitative services. These patients likely were getting some of these services prior to admission, and now there has been some neurologic decline which may warrant additional therapy.

■ WHOM TO CONSULT—THE COMPOSITION OF THE REHABILITATION TEAM

The rehabilitation team is composed of (but certainly not limited to) the rehabilitation physician (also known as a physiatrist or specialist in physical medicine and rehabilitation), speech therapist, occupational therapist (OT), physical therapist (PT), and a recreation specialist (sometimes referred to as a "child life specialist"). Others that are considered part of the team include nursing, family, social work, teacher/academic specialist, rehabilitation engineering specialist, orthotist, prosthetist, and mental health professional such as psychologist and psychiatrist.

Early consultation is recommended, but patient stability, access to the patient, and medical or diagnostic procedures each potentially delay how early this can occur. In many circumstances consultation by speech therapy, OT, and PT can be requested simultaneously with the physiatrist consultation. More often, however, in the early course of such an admission, the needs and goals are difficult to identify and consultation with the physiatrist can help to crystallize the initial rehabilitation plan and recommend which members of the team need to be involved most urgently. Furthermore, it has been reported that review by a rehabilitation physician significantly improves the chance of referral to formal rehabilitation (9).

■ REHABILITATION'S IMPACT DURING THE ICU COURSE

Involvement of the rehabilitation team in the ICU has important impact on the team and the course of an illness that is less direct and more difficult to quantify. Several of these benefits deserve mention:

1. Giving the patient and family a more active role in their recovery. Often there is little or no ability for the family to participate in their own care, but in PT, OT, or speech therapy, the patient and/or family are asked to participate.
2. Facilitating self-care. This leads to less helplessness and more independence.
3. Facilitating early communication. Helping to interpret when the ability to communicate is limited is an everyday occurrence for a skilled speech therapist and can be key in determining care as well as assuring caregivers.
4. Laying the groundwork for the rehabilitation over the subsequent months by informing the family about the timing and details of recommended therapies, and giving an example of the daily routine of a rehabilitation unit or an outpatient rehabilitation program.

■ FACTORS THAT LIMIT REHABILITATION

In the neurocritical care setting, there are many common medical and physical limitations that can be barriers for the rehabilitation team. For example, caution over blood pressure control and cerebral perfusion often limit the amount of physical activity, either active or passive, that a patient can tolerate. Positioning can also be an issue for many therapeutic interventions, such as when the patient is required to lay supine without any elevation of the head of the bed. Sometimes the patient is limited in terms of positioning for intracranial pressure monitoring or cerebrospinal fluid drainage.

Endotracheal intubation is another common limitation to early rehabilitation. While this is physically limiting and potentially uncomfortable for the patient, it does not always make them ineligible for PT, OT, or even speech therapy. While phonation is not a reasonable goal in this circumstance, communication may be achieved. A speech therapist can help to facilitate communication in an intubated patient using augmentative or alternative strategies. Often this evaluation benefits the entire care team because nonverbal communication might be the only means of assessing mental status. The consistency and the skill of a speech therapist often produces some of the most reliable insights into the patient's cognitive status, their wishes, and their psychological state in such a circumstance.

Another common limitation is patient tolerance of therapies. Pain, fatigue, nausea, weakness, mood disturbance, and many other issues make it difficult for a patient to tolerate therapy that will ultimately benefit them. Those problems must be addressed to both improve overall care and allow the earliest possible initiation of rehabilitation therapy. Regional anesthetic techniques such as nerve blocks can occasionally be utilized to minimize pain, maximize mobility, and minimize sedation.

Paroxysmal autonomic instability with dystonia syndrome, also referred to as "storming," is due to hypothalamic-midbrain dysregulation, diencephalic seizures, and sympathetic storming. This phenomenon is a common occurrence in a neurocritical care unit, and is most often seen following traumatic or anoxic brain injury. This is thought to be due to mesencephalic injury leading to dysregulation of normal autonomic function (10). It is sometimes responsive to medications, but it is often difficult to control, and not very well understood. Regardless of the name used, therapies are often discontinued when these episodes occur due to changes in blood pressure, heart rate, temperature, and the distressed appearance of the patient. Furthermore, episodes of this type can be initiated by noxious stimuli or relatively benign stimuli. Storming episodes can be initiated by something as seemingly innocuous as range of motion exercises from a PT or OT. Early on, this usually leads to stopping a therapeutic session until the symptoms subside, but for some, the dysautonomia persists and it must be decided how much stress the patient can tolerate. Labile blood pressure is undesirable during acute management, but if the primary manifestations are diaphoresis and changes in muscle tone, then often therapy can and should continue.

■ REHABILITATION-SPECIFIC MEDICAL ISSUES

Following is a brief overview of a few of the many medical issues that are commonly seen in acute rehabilitation, but that generally have their roots in the neurocritical care unit.

Seizure management is discussed in detail in Chapter 8. Most recommendations from the rehabilitation literature for management of seizures related to a traumatic brain injury do not recommend long-term prophylactic therapy. When seizures do need to be treated, anticonvulsants that do not significantly impair cognition or cause sedation are ideal for cognitive rehabilitation goals.

Heterotopic ossification (HO) is a form of abnormal calcification within soft tissues that can occur following spinal cord injury, traumatic brain injury, or burns, and can inhibit function. HO can be seen in up to 22% of severe pediatric traumatic brain injury cases. It can begin in the weeks after a traumatic brain injury, but usually does not have much clinical significance until after a patient is out of the neurocritical care unit. In approximately 20% of these patients the presence of HO may physically impede the rehabilitation process (11).

Deep-venous thrombosis is also a rare, but important problem following traumatic brain injury or spinal cord injury in the pediatric age groups. Medical prophylaxis with anticoagulants is effective, and recommended in some populations based on risk factors (12).

Fatigue and disturbance of normal sleep/wake cycle are common problems in any ICU that can persist as problems in an acute rehabilitation setting. In the traumatic brain injury population, these problems are particularly prevalent, even weeks after injury and it appears to be multifactorial (13). The initial treatment should be improved sleep hygiene, but medication may be needed. Melatonin can assist in optimizing sleep hygiene, and trazodone is widely used in the traumatic brain injury population.

Problems of arousal and attention are also common following many of the disorders seen in a neurocritical care unit that often continue to be problematic in the acute rehabilitation setting. This is a very complex issue and sedating medications are often a factor. The judicious uses of psychostimulants such as methylphenidate or dextroamphetamine often produce positive results. Current research in adults suggest that twice per day methylphenidate has clinically significant positive effects on processing speed in individuals with attentional complaints after traumatic brain injury (14). Early medical treatment of arousal issues and sleep disturbances is often problematic because of the environmental disturbances that cannot be avoided such as monitors, painful procedures, and the occurrence of around-the-clock care. Many of these disturbances are reduced or eliminated in a rehabilitation unit. In addition, the evaluation and treatment of these particular problems is much easier when there is a more routine schedule for these patients on a rehabilitation unit.

Immobilization's negative effects are many fold and can be profound. These effects can be seen in most organ systems (Table 24.4). Many of the effects of immobilization can be delayed or completely prevented with hard work from the entire team, and most specifically the therapists and nurses. Operating within the confines of procedures and constraints of neurocritical care, this generally consists of proper positioning, range of motion exercises, splinting, and pressure relief. Active exercise by the patient, good pulmonary toilet, and weight bearing are all elements of optimal care. Immobilization hypercalcemia can exacerbate other organ system dysfunction and can be minimized by weight bearing.

■ **Table 24.4** Adverse Effects of Immobilization by Organ System

Organ Systems	Conditions
Muscles	Reduced strength, endurance, flexibility, and bulk
Joints	Reduced flexibility; joint contractures
Bones	Osteopenia and osteoporosis, immobilization hypercalcemia
Heart	Reduced stroke volume, cardiac output, and exercise capacity tachycardia
Peripheral circulation	Reduced orthostatic tolerance and venous return; deep vein thrombosis
Lungs	Atelectasis and pneumonia; pulmonary embolism
Gastrointestinal tract	Reduced appetite and bowel motility; constipation
Urinary tract	Urolithiasis, infection
Skin	Pressure ulcers
Endocrine	Reduced endorphin production and insulin sensitivity; reduced lean body mass; obesity
Psychological	Reduced self-image and stress tolerance; anxiety and depression

■ SPASTICITY MANAGEMENT

In many centers, management of spasticity or upper motor neuron syndrome is the domain of the rehabilitation doctor. Spasticity is a common problem for patients admitted to the neurocritical care unit, both as a preexisting problem and one of new onset. This multifaceted topic deserves special mention here; however, seldom is it possible to optimize management of spasticity in the time frame of an admission to the unit. More often "tone" management is a project that will commence in the critical care period, but will need further adjustment for a period of weeks to months to gain the best outcome.

The first step in management is identifying where and when spasticity occurs. This increased tone may be specific to a hemiplegic side, just one limb, just a few muscles, or may affect all limbs or trunk. Is it focal or generalized? The tone may be purely in response to stimulus, only with purposeful movements, or present for much of the day. Does it present a problem for the entire day, just at night, or only a few brief episodes each day?

The next step is to identify spasticity management goals. A common goal is to relieve a positional issue that is either painful or leading to secondary complications such as joint dislocation. Alternately, spasticity can be painless and merely have functional implications. One very helpful way to categorize the issues for patients where pain is not the primary concern is by differentiating "active functions" from "passive functions." Active functions are the movements that the patient does (or attempts to do) for his or herself such as reaching, standing, or grasping. Passive functions are those that a caregiver performs on a patient such as dressing, hygiene, and positioning. When deciding which treatment and how aggressively to treat tone disorders in the neurocritical care unit it is essential to define which of these goals the therapies targets are, and how achieving these goals will help the patient to function. For example, treatment for a patient with a new stroke could include Botox injections to the finger flexors to help with overactive grasp. Alternately, treatment for a mentally retarded youngster with generalized hypertonia that prevents comfortable positioning in his wheelchair or even in bed might include enteral baclofen to allow for better passive positioning at the hips and trunk.

Management of spasticity can be divided into three categories: mechanical management, focal treatment, and more generalized treatments:

1. *Mechanical management* can be in the form of splinting, bracing, casting, and range-of-motion exercises. These are done with collaboration from physician, therapists, and orthotists. Often the main goals of these interventions when done in the critical care period are to prevent secondary complications such as contractures, dislocations, deformity, and skin breakdown.

2. *Focal treatment* for spasticity is the administration of Botox or alcohol (usually phenol) injections to treat specific muscles and muscle groups. This is commonly used for isolated issues such as an equinus pattern of spasticity at an ankle or a flexion synergy at a child's arm. The time course and the natural history of the underlying diagnosis are important considerations here due to the irreversible nature of these injections. While the lasting effects of these injections are limited, they should not be thought of in the same vein as a trial of an oral medication. Adjustments of the treatment regimen will be required as the child recovers and their tone evolves.

3. The more *generalized treatments* can either be systemic or act directly at the spinal cord level. These would include oral medications and intrathecal baclofen therapy. Oral medications often used include diazepam, baclofen, tizanidine, and dantrolene. When taken enterally, these medications are appropriate for tone issues that are diffuse or if involvement is widespread. However, as such, they also have potential to exhibit their known toxicities in competition with the desired effect. This includes potential sedation for the first three medications and possible liver toxicity for dantrolene. These adverse side effects may limit their efficacy. Intrathecal baclofen requires a surgical intervention to deliver baclofen directly to the intrathecal space via a catheter. The effect at the spinal cord is achieved at much lower quantities of baclofen than would be needed enterally. Intrathecal baclofen is rarely appropriate in the neurocritical care setting; however, some work has been done with intrathecal infusion initiated early in a brain injury for both tone management and reduction in some or all of the effects of dysautonomia (15).

■ PROGRESSION, TIME COURSE, AND TRANSITION TO INPATIENT REHABILITATION

Much like the progression of the care in a critical care unit, the intensity of rehabilitation is weaned over time. For a patient with a new neurologic injury, rehabilitation is initiated in the ICU, but is intensified when there is a transition to an appropriate inpatient rehabilitation unit. A patient usually remains there for weeks to months. They are discharged when there is a safe discharge plan and when it is deemed that they do not need several hours of therapy daily. This is not to say that their rehabilitation is complete. These patients will transition back into the community (often referred to as community reentry or school reentry) and continue outpatient therapies. These outpatient services often consist of regular (weekly or more frequent) therapies and evaluations by the rehabilitation team for the next several months. This care will be discontinued when it is noted that the patient has reached a plateau in function, however, that point is difficult to define. Thereafter, if there are further needs or functional deficits that may improve, then these therapies should continue in the school setting for these children.

■ INDICATIONS FOR TRANSFER TO AN INPATIENT REHABILITATION UNIT

For a patient to qualify for acute inpatient rehabilitation, they must have goals that would be reasonably attainable in a setting where they would benefit from daily therapy. Therefore, they must have significant and persistent neurologic deficits affecting the realms of mobility, self-care, communication, bowel or bladder control, swallowing, or cognition. They must be neurologically and medically stable. Current guidelines for most insurance companies indicate that there must be need for at least two therapies (PT or OT or speech therapy) daily, and that the patient must be able to tolerate a minimum of 3 hours of therapy daily. If the child cannot tolerate that much therapy, a more appropriate setting would be a subacute rehabilitation unit.

For adults to be candidates for inpatient rehabilitation, they must also be cognitively able to learn and be capable of interacting with their therapists. In our experience, we have sometimes been able to gain payer approval for a trial of rehabilitation for some pediatric patients who were not communicative or who had questionable ability to learn. These special circumstances have pertained to "lower level" patients who were either not communicative prior to their acute care course or who have had a very significant brain injury and their current communication or learning status is not clear. This has only been possible with clear, consistent documentation of their function and progress from the treating therapists and the physiatrist working with these patients in the ICU. This serves as a "trial" of therapy. Evidence of progress on standardized, cognitively based assessments done in the acute setting has proved very helpful in making a case for transferring such patients to an acute rehabilitation setting.

There are many reasons why appropriate patients are either delayed or never make it to inpatient rehabilitation at all. Many of them are specific to the resources of the patient or the patient's family, some are due to the wishes of the patient or the family, and yet still others have to do with the resources in their geographic area. One recent study surmised that common causes for delay to rehabilitation fall into two basic categories related to (1) bed availability and (2) financial support. This reflects the fact that there are not enough rehabilitation facilities qualified to treat children, as well as the fact that the facilities that are able to address these patients' rehabilitation needs are often full. There is also the challenge of long-distance transport for these fragile patients once a bed is actually available (3).

There are two other potential rehabilitation destinations for neurocritical care patients. One is to refer them directly to outpatient services. This is feasible only if they are medically stable and safe. This may be appropriate if the patient needs only one therapy, just PT or only OT, for example. This may be appropriate if their needs do not require daily therapy. This obviously implies a lesser severity of disability. The other setting would be a "day program" or "day hospital" setting. These settings are not offered at many hospitals and often have varying admission criteria, but they are essentially rehabilitation settings that are of intensity between inpatient rehabilitation and outpatient rehabilitation. In these programs, patients may get any of the therapies that an inpatient could receive, with regular oversight from a physician. The therapies are usually daily, and multiple therapies are attended daily. Once again, these patients must be medically stable and safe, but they must also have a means of getting to the therapies daily. Day programs fulfill the needs of this specific patient group extremely well, but are often difficult to utilize due to transportation issues, regional availability, or due to lack of payer coverage for this specific insurance benefit.

■ ISSUES AND CONTROVERSIES REGARDING REHABILITATION IN THE ICU

While there is no known effective "coma stimulation" program which has been found to improve recovery time or outcome of any age patient with a traumatic brain injury, there are stimulant medications which are often used, such as amantadine. There is a clear profile for adverse side effects, most of which are manageable or tolerable. There appear to be beneficial effects on alertness and arousal; however, it is difficult to prove conclusively (16,17). There are some promising innovative medical approaches to arousal problems that are being trialed currently. However, the concerns with these medications are their possible long-term effects on neural plasticity.

In terms of complementary and alternative therapies, there is very little support in the research literature for the use of hyperbaric oxygen therapy (18), craniosacral therapy to improve neurologic function, or chiropractic therapy to improve function (19).

Terminally ill patients present another aspect of rehabilitation. A common misperception about rehabilitation is that hospice care and rehabilitation are mutually exclusive. This is not always the case, and while the goals may be very different for this group of patients, they may be very important and reasonable. Goals directed at a shorter life expectancy often focus on mobility or activities of daily living. In a neurocritical care unit, these scenarios may occur with oncology patients, patients with inborn errors of metabolism, or patients with neurodegenerative disorders who have recently decompensated. The goals for these patients must be tailored to what is reasonably feasible in the projected time frame, and must obviously be desired by the patient and family. These are almost always hard choices for the family, because pursuing these goals requires some hard work during a period when time is the most precious. Yet it may be simpler to pose these limited goals if they are specific and have clear relevance for these patients in their

last days. Such goals might include things like better transfers, better toileting, increased independence with certain activities of daily living, reduced burden of care for a period, or even better positioning. Once again, goals must be discrete and clearly defined in order to have financial support from third party payers. With appropriate goal setting, the practical gains for these patients may be very dignifying for them and their families.

■ SUMMARY

Optimal outcomes for children admitted to a neurocritical care unit often require the collaboration of the rehabilitation team. Knowing who to consult is essential, and ideally, rehabilitation should begin as early as is reasonably feasible. A physiatrist has expertise in many of the sequelae of neurologic injuries. Finally, having clear decisions regarding possible transfers to inpatient rehabilitation allows caregivers to plan for the future.

■ REFERENCES

1. DeLisa JA. *Rehabilitation Medicine: Principles and Practice.* 3rd ed. Philadelphia, PA: Lippincott-Raven; 1998.
2. Macciocchi S et al. Spinal cord injury and co-occurring traumatic brain injury: assessment and incidence. *Arch Phys Med Rehabil.* 2008;89:1350–1357.
3. Tepas JJ III et al. The effect of delay in rehabilitation on outcome of severe traumatic brain injury. *J Pediatr Surg.* 2009;44:368–372.
4. Mackay LE et al. Early intervention in severe head injury: long-term benefits of a formalized program. *Arch Phys Med Rehabil.* 1992;73:635–641.
5. Cope DN, Hall K. Head injury rehabilitation: benefit of early intervention. *Arch Phys Med Rehabil.* 1982;63:433–437.
6. Hu MH et al. Early and intensive rehabilitation predicts good functional outcomes in patients admitted to the stroke intensive care unit. *Disabil Rehabil.* 2010;32:1251–1259.
7. Cremer R et al. Children with chronic conditions in pediatric intensive care units located in predominantly French-speaking regions: prevalence and implications on rehabilitation care need and utilization. *Crit Care Med.* 2009;37:1456–1462.
8. Bell MJ et al. Development of a pediatric neurocritical care service. *Neurocrit Care.* 2009;10:4–10.
9. Wrigley JM et al. Social and physical factors in the referral of people with traumatic brain injuries to rehabilitation. *Arch Phys Med Rehabil.* 1994;75:149–155.

10. Baguley IJ et al. A critical review of the pathophysiology of dysautonomia following traumatic brain injury. *Neurocrit Care*. 2008;8:293–300.

11. Citta-Pietrolungo TJ, Alexander MA, Steg NL. Early detection of heterotopic ossification in young patients with traumatic brain injury. *Arch Phys Med Rehabil*. 1992;73:258–262.

12. Radecki RT, Gaebler-Spira D. Deep vein thrombosis in the disabled pediatric population. *Arch Phys Med Rehabil*. 1994;75:248–250.

13. Castriotta RJ et al. Prevalence and consequences of sleep disorders in traumatic brain injury. *J Clin Sleep Med*. 2007;3: 349–356.

14. Whyte J et al. Effects of methylphenidate on attention deficits after traumatic brain injury: a multidimensional, randomized, controlled trial. *Am J Phys Med Rehabil*. 2004;83:401–420.

15. Turner MS. Early use of intrathecal baclofen in brain injury in pediatric patients. *Acta Neurochir Suppl*. 2003;87:81–83.

16. Williams SE. Amantadine treatment following traumatic brain injury in children. *Brain Inj*. 2007;21:885–889.

17. Green LB, Hornyak JE, Hurvitz EA. Amantadine in pediatric patients with traumatic brain injury: a retrospective, case-controlled study. *Am J Phys Med Rehabil*. 2004;83:893–897.

18. McDonagh M et al. Hyperbaric oxygen therapy for traumatic brain injury: a systematic review of the evidence. *Arch Phys Med Rehabil*. 2004;85:1198–1204.

19. Ylvisaker M et al. Rehabilitation and ongoing support after pediatric TBI: twenty years of progress. *J Head Trauma Rehabil*. 2005;20:95–109.

25 Psychological Reactions to Critical Care Events

PAUL M. ROBINS and MARY ROURKE

The experience of pediatric critical care is quite likely to be a traumatic one for children and families. It has been well documented that serious childhood illness—including cancer, burns, serious injury, and many other life-threatening pediatric conditions or experiences—is commonly associated with significant psychological trauma reactions for both the affected child and for his or her parents (1–4). The implied urgency of high-level intensive medical care, including the pervasiveness of significant life threat and the experience of pain and/or risky medical procedures, is clearly likely to intensify feelings of intense fear, horror, and helplessness—all of which are precursors to psychological trauma. Indeed, research indicates that high percentages of children in critical care environments and their parents report very high anxiety (5–6) as well as significant levels of trauma symptoms, with nearly a third of parents meeting diagnostic criteria for acute stress disorder while the child is being treated in a critical care unit (7). These symptoms usually include reexperiencing scary or horrifying aspects of the illness or care, experiencing very high levels of arousal and panic, and, when possible, avoiding events or people that are associated with the trauma (3).

Understanding trauma reactions in pediatric critical care is important for several reasons. It is well documented that early trauma reactions predict longer-term trauma reactions, which ultimately derail both long-term medical care as well as normal development and quality of life (2–3,8–10). Further, decision-making during the delivery of critical care is impacted when the parental decision-makers are

traumatized. Evidence supports the negative effect of trauma on decision-making, suggesting that trauma interferes with adult coping in two ways: it compromises individual coping and problem-solving skills and it impedes the ability of adults to come together and work collaboratively on coping with their intimate partners (11).

Despite the indications that trauma is an understandable and common experience when children are critically injured or sick, it may not be routinely or adequately recognized or addressed by physicians or nurses (12). Citing these concerns, the federally funded National Child Traumatic Stress Network has called for health care providers and others working with traumatized children and their families to develop models of care that are trauma-informed and that address coordination across the multiple systems in which children live and grow (9).

Following these guidelines, the purpose of this chapter is to present a trauma-informed and systems-based framework that might guide care provided to children and families in pediatric critical care environments. We first present an overview of pediatric medical traumatic stress (PMTS) and how it manifests in children and parents during intensive medical crises. Next, we discuss a systems-informed framework to understand psychological reactions related to acute trauma in pediatric health care settings. Using a case example, we then illustrate how those trauma-related systemic concerns might appear, and provide guidelines for how to use a systemic understanding of PMTS to work effectively at the bedside.

■ UNDERSTANDING PMTS

PMTS is a normative reaction of parents and children to the trauma of serious childhood illness and injury. While PMTS is derived from the construct of posttraumatic stress disorder (PTSD) (13), there are essential differences between the two constructs. Both are reactions to trauma, which is defined as "…experiencing, witnessing, or being confronted with an event or events that involve actual or threatened death or serious injury or a threat to the physical integrity of oneself or others" (13), and both occur after one experiences fear, horror, or helplessness as an initial reaction to the trauma. In the case of PMTS, the trauma may be the diagnosis or some aspect(s) of the illness or treatment. PTSD is a psychiatric diagnosis, and its symptoms cause global and clinically significant distress and/or impairment in social, occupational, or other important areas of functioning. In contrast, PMTS is defined as a normative set of psychological and physiologic responses of children and their families to pain, injury, serious illness, medical procedures, and invasive or frightening treatment experiences, and it occurs at some level in nearly all parents and many children who are faced with a serious medical illness (14). Though PMTS reactions are normative reactions to the nonnormative stressors of serious childhood illness, they lead to, and are intensified by, the challenges faced by parents of children experiencing medical trauma or illness. These challenges include role changes, parental stress, marital dissatisfaction, discontinuity of care, compromised condition management, communication barriers, anxiety surrounding decision making, conflict with the medical team and school system, lack of community and peer support, and lack of economic resources (15–21).

PMTS responses can vary in intensity, may be disruptive to functioning, and can be experienced simultaneously, but in different ways, by multiple members of the same family (8,22). As outlined by the National Child Traumatic Stress Network (NCTSN) (www.nctsn.org), PMTS symptoms include:

1. *Reexperiencing of the traumatic event.* Reexperiencing is a broad term that refers to the unintended and/or uncontrollable repeated experience of upsetting thoughts or feelings associated with the trauma. Reexperiencing can be unprovoked, or can be triggered by exposure to reminders in the environment. Examples of reexperiencing include intrusive and obsessive thoughts about aspects of the medical trauma (e.g., replaying the trip to the emergency department, or the moment at which a child was injured), periods of calm that are shattered by unwanted recollections of the traumatic event, recurrent distressing dreams, unpleasant visceral reactions when encountering triggers (e.g., smelling reminders of the trauma causes nausea or dizziness), and intense distress when reminded of prior scary events (e.g., panic when waiting for test results that previously had scary results).

2. *Avoidance and cognitive/emotional numbing related to the traumatic event(s).* This broad category refers to two kinds of symptoms. Parents and children may actively or passively avoid thinking about or dealing with issues related to the trauma or with people or places that remind them of the trauma. For example, parents may avoid a certain physician or nurse, or may, in extreme cases, be unable to come to the bedside. Passive avoidance can include a very limited or nonexistent memory for portions of the trauma experience. Parents or children may not remember important elements of the diagnosis or treatment, or the events that caused an injury; they may forget important parts of a treatment conversation. The second aspect of this cluster of symptoms involves a sense of emotional numbing. People experiencing this symptom may look unable to experience emotion of any kind, and may seem frozen, disoriented, or like they are not processing important parts of what is happening.

3. *Emotional arousal.* A high level of arousal is a common symptom during and after a medical trauma. While this arousal may look like a traditional panic response (e.g., palpitations, shortness of breath, dizziness), it may also include difficulties with organization and concentration, difficulty remembering medical responsibilities or organizing oneself for the next level of medical care, as well as angry, irritable, and inappropriate outbursts with medical staff.

There can be significant adaptive functions of PMTS. For example, reexperiencing events helps parents and children process and resolve trauma memories, while avoidance and distraction can help parents tolerate distress and get through the hospitalization and medical procedures (3). However, these thoughts, feelings, and behaviors can also substantially complicate an already complex care system. Making accurate medical assessments and delivering urgent interventions with a child experiencing traumatic distress can be a serious challenge. While the presence of parents at the bedside, a hallmark of family-centered pediatric care, allows parents to comfort children, it also introduces the possibility of parental trauma reactions interfering with care. It becomes increasingly difficult to work consistently with parents as medical decision-makers if parents are experiencing unpredictable periods of intense anxiety, mood lability, or moments of paniclike symptoms. Similarly, at the other extreme, parents who seem numb or frozen, as though they are not processing important information, may avoid seeing or talking to the care team or may not be able to partner effectively with team. Neither parent will be able to calm a scared or hurting child, or actively and effectively partner with the critical care team.

As the preceding paragraph suggests, demands on a child and family in a critical care unit are quite often inconsistent with good peritrauma care. People experiencing trauma require safe, predictable environments in which they have thorough information and experience support and control over what is happening (3,14). Paradoxically, critical care environments often are unpredictable, require quick decisions with no time to ponder information, and present multiple unplanned exposures to things that may trigger trauma responses. Multiple members of a family—all of whom may be present in the care environment—may be having simultaneous, but very different trauma reactions (8,22).

Additionally, there is an increasing awareness that pediatric health care providers may also have their own trauma reactions to children that they are treating or as a result of their chronic and cumulative exposure to and participation in multiple pediatric tragedies (23–25). Members of the medical care team may be aiming to deliver urgent medical care in a calming manner, while attempting to manage their own reactions.

A systems context for understanding the impact of medical trauma on children, families, and the health care team can help frame an understanding of how pediatric medical trauma can complicate care. In particular, family systems models can assist in understanding how family development can be disrupted by the experience of medical trauma. Effective clinical responses that can accommodate the effects of the trauma on the child, family, and health care team can be developed.

■ A SYSTEMIC UNDERSTANDING OF FAMILIES IN CRISIS

Pediatric medical trauma, like any major crisis, prompts a family to move unexpectedly and abruptly into a period of acute crisis. How the family responds to this turmoil and navigates their own traumatic reactions is based in part on two factors. First, understanding how the family was organized before the medical crisis can inform a team about a family's preexisting strengths/resources and vulnerabilities. While a solid family organization prior to a trauma may lead to a stronger response to trauma, processes that worked for a family in a time of health may be ineffective during a time of crisis. Therefore, the second important factor to consider is how the family's organization changes in response to and during the period of critical care. At the moment of a trauma, the medical well-being of the child becomes paramount, forcing all family members to abandon old patterns and urgently implement new patterns of behavior necessary to navigate the crisis. Understanding how families accomplish this transition provides an important window into their adaptive functioning.

Drawing from the family systems literature, it is helpful to examine the family's organization along the following six dimensions as described in Alderfer and Rourke (26):

1. *Structure and organization*
   Like any group, a family has a structure, with roles and leadership positions developing within and between family members. Some family structures are hierarchical and organized with clear leadership roles for parents. Others are flat organizations with relative equality and shared decision-making among all members. Still others have reversed hierarchies in which children are essentially in charge and do a great deal of parental caretaking. Most families have a structure that, if not entirely adaptive, is still stable enough to allow them to meet the demands that they need to meet, given the individual challenges of each member. When critical illness strikes, however, roles and leadership structures may no longer work, or may change by necessity. For example, when parents spend multiple days at the hospital, partners and other family members function in new roles in order to maintain stability. Such new organization can result in role strain (27–28).

2. *Adaptability, or flexibility in leadership, roles, and relationship rules*
   Family adaptability can range from extremely flexible (chaotic) to extremely inflexible (rigid). Examples of more chaotic family functioning may be characterized by multiple physical moves with inconsistent caretaking, or nonexistent schedules or routines in

the home; examples of more rigid functioning include one parent making all decisions despite input from the other parent, or families being tightly organized around only one way of doing things. In the face of illness, a good balance of adaptability is necessary; families must be able to organize and implement consistent care routines and to structure their own participation in their child's care (and to care for other family needs outside of the hospital), while also being flexible enough to adapt to changes in care that can occur with the often unpredictable changes in a child's status, or the changes in medical teams that occur daily.

3. *Cohesion, or the emotional bonds between family members*
Cohesion can be represented along a continuum, from enmeshed to disengaged. Enmeshed families have weak boundaries between individuals; people speak for each other, and have difficulty separating their own needs or roles from those of other family members. In disengaged families, at the other end of the spectrum, individual family members may be more isolated and cut off from each other. In the face of medical trauma, family members may retain their way of functioning, or may be pushed more in one direction or another. A challenge in decision-making can easily emerge in enmeshed families, as individuals may "lose their voice," and one person may (inaccurately) speak for another. In disengaged families, individuals may resist stepping in to make necessary decisions, or may seem less invested in or able to engage in the intimate nature of the care that is often necessary during the critical care experience.

4. *Communication, or the clarity of expression*
Communication patterns are a significant contributor to the sense of community in a family, and communication rules often dictate what can be spoken about in a family, how directly or indirectly family members can address an emotional situation, and how nonverbal messages, like care, comfort/nurturance, anger, and fear get expressed. Clearly, a family's patterns in this area will affect how they manage an event like medical crisis, and individuals' own trauma reactions will affect how communication patterns after the trauma get established. Awareness of a family's level of comfort with a particular communication style can inform how the critical care

team presents information to the family and conducts ongoing interactions.

5. *Affective environment, or the emotional tone of the family*
A family's affective environment is often intricately tied to communication. How a family expresses and navigates strong emotion results in an overriding emotional tenor, which in turn continues to shape patterns of communication and care. When a life-threatening event intervenes in a family's life, often the affective environment is shattered, and strong bursts of negative emotion (often fear) predominate. This can interact with a family's communication style to shape adaptation in both positive and negative ways (26).

6. *Problem-solving ability*
A family's problem-solving ability is defined as their goal-directed negotiation and task accomplishment—or the ability to come together as a group and get things done (26). For most families, most of the time, problem-solving is related to the normative tasks of mastering developmental milestones. For example, families must get their children through school, help them navigate social challenges, and provide food, shelter, and clothing. Clearly, families vary in their ability to come together and meet these tasks. Serious pediatric illness or injury, however, requires a more intense form of problem-solving, as families must make potentially life-altering medical decisions, while also managing to care for their family's needs more generally.

In addition to these structural/organizational constructs, the child's and the family's current developmental phase (i.e, early childhood, adolescence, young adulthood) affects the family response to the illness or medical crises. In addition, medical crises can require a family to operate in a way that is inconsistent with a new or different level of development. For example, medical crisis can force families to pull together in order to respond to the needs of the ill child, much like families organize around a baby or toddler. Traumatic illness may, in fact, accentuate or greatly prolong the normal period of pulling together. Over time, this pattern of pulling together can become problematic, and can affect family members' ability to become more independent and competent (e.g., a first grader may not have the experiences that support independence and may then be very frightened to go to school). Similarly, the traumatic illness of a teenager entering college often causes the postponement of this normative developmental shift. These out of sequence forces often derail normative developmental growth and can, over time, lead to significant role strain within and between family members.

Thus, it is essential to consider both the family life cycle as well as family structure when understanding psychological reactions to pediatric neurocritical care events, and to consider both how a family was functioning before the trauma, as well as how they have changed in response to the trauma. It must be emphasized, however, that changes in a family's organization after a trauma, in and of themselves, are not problematic. If changes in a family's structure or developmental level support the child and the parent's ability to effectively manage the medical crisis, if medical decisions are being made appropriately and caretaking is adequate, and if the pattern results in no distress, there is no reason for concern or intervention. If, however, the child, parent, or team finds that important medical decision-making or caretaking is compromised, or that the child or family experiences distress or negative developmental progress, then intervention is appropriate.

We now consider more explicitly how family reactions interact with symptoms of PMTS by presenting a case study. We discuss family level constructs, consider signs of disruption faced by the family, and outline possible responses by health care professionals to optimally manage responses to the medical trauma.

■ CASE OVERVIEW

Jesse was a 15-year-old boy who lived at home with his mother, who was a single parent. He had an older brother who was living independently, and had never known his father. His mother's extended family lived several hours from the family; neighbors and friends largely comprised the family's local support network.

Jesse had been battling a slowly growing tumor in his chest for 2 years. After a long period of treatment resulting in stable disease, Jesse's tumor grew quickly, spread to his spinal column, and had begun impeding his ability to breathe. He was intubated and placed on a ventilator emergently, and with great difficulty. Because of his fragile respiratory status, sudden and significant mental status changes, and changes in his

ability to control his arms and legs, Jesse was admitted to the pediatric intensive care unit. Jesse's mother was his sole caretaker, and was the only adult involved in Jesse's care. Jesse remained in intensive care for more than 60 days, until his condition stabilized and he could be extubated and moved to a rehabilitation floor. Over the next several months, Jesse remained in the hospital, and was periodically admitted to the Pediatric Intensive Care Unit (PICU) for various issues, until he died, as expected, in the PICU.

We will present a discussion of various issues that occurred over the course of Jesse's last several months of life and repeat PICU visits by reviewing the constructs outlined above.

■ DEVELOPMENT

Jesse was diagnosed with cancer as a young adolescent, which is normally a developmental time during which children become more independent and autonomous, and parents become less involved in caretaking. The demands of Jesse's illness, however, required the family to organize more like the family of a younger child. Jesse's mother had to remain involved in the high-stakes medical care and in Jesse's caretaking, and because of his illness, Jesse could not participate in usual young adolescent social activities. His respiratory crisis and periodic mental status changes, requiring PICU care and resulting in hospitalization for the rest of his life, cemented this pattern; Jesse could not attend school, for example, and could not ride his bike or skateboard with his friends. Because of his medical status and his fear, Jesse had the normative emotional reaction of regressing; he often whined and cried in his bed, and began acting like a much younger child, refusing to complete self-care tasks that were well within his ability. His mother had to pay attention to intimate details of his personal care, including how much he urinated and what he ate, in ways that are not typical of a family at adolescence. As a result of all these factors, Jesse's mother reacted by treating Jesse like a much younger child. She protected him from information, spoke for him, and overindulged him. Her own trauma was triggered when she heard Jesse's cries and complaints, and this dramatically amplified her fear and helplessness, which in turn exacerbated her attempts to "make this better." She therefore continued to "baby" Jesse, which allowed him to continue behaving more like a preschooler and less like an adolescent. He would beg nurses to do for him as his mother did, and throw a tantrum when people would not do for him what he wanted them to do.

Intervention: The following are some general guidelines for care when a family's developmental level appears to be causing difficulties for them or for the medical team:

- Normalize confusion and ambivalence about a child's developmental needs, and the ways in which the demands of critical care illness are often inconsistent with what a child needs developmentally.
- Partner with family (including child, when appropriate) to identify the roles a child and parent can take, and make those roles as developmentally appropriate as possible.
- Develop new routines gradually, with attention to soothing worry, supporting growth, and avoiding judgment and punishment.
- Coach children and parents through normative fears in developmentally appropriate ways ("I know this is hard/scary, but you can do it, and there is a team to support you"), rather than overindulging, overprotecting, or overfunctioning for them.

These guidelines shaped the team's response to the patterns in which Jesse and his mother found themselves stuck. Once extubated, Jesse wanted to eat anything and everything he could get his hands on, and was not able to respect the team's rules about what foods were safe given his limited swallowing abilities. Like a much younger child, he would demand a food, insist that his mother get it immediately, tantrum if she did not, and then, when the food arrived, insist that she be instrumentally involved in feeding him. Mom complied and, several times a day, was demanding that Jesse's requested food be delivered immediately to his room. She would then sit on the side of the bed and feed him with a spoon. The team's first step in addressing this behavior was to work with Mom to identify what Jesse could and could not do, reasonably. He could eat a limited list of foods, he could choose from those foods, and he could feed himself. Mom agreed with these abilities, and she worked with a team member to develop a food plan that gave Jesse more adolescentlike control and involvement. The team and Mom developed a menu of permissible foods, and Jesse could chose from items on this menu. Once foods were delivered, they were set up in a way that allowed Jesse to feed himself. At the same time, the plan had a role for Mom that allowed her to continue

to feel that she was actively parenting Jesse through this time. While it took a few days of Mom and the team partnering together to coach Jesse through a few tantrums of protest, within a few days, Jesse was sticking to the menu, feeding himself, and approaching his feeding team to have discussions about new foods he wanted to add to the menu.

■ ORGANIZATION/STRUCTURE

In many single-parent families, especially during adolescence, the hierarchy of the family may become less pronounced, with a child and parent looking somewhat like peers, and less like a rule-making parent caring for a rule-following child. During serious medical illness, this hierarchy may become even less apparent, with parents and children often sharing a hospital room and adopting a level of intimacy that minimizes the hierarchy that may have been more typical of a family. In two-parent families, the hierarchy between one parent and the sick child may be erased, while the second parent becomes marginalized. In some families, a reverse pattern happens, and a hierarchy becomes more pronounced and extreme. In cases like this, parents may become the central decision-makers, marginalizing the child to be the obedient patient.

Common signs that the hierarchy has been disrupted in a way that is not adaptive for the family include:

- Child trying to take care of the parent or protect the parent from news or information that may be upsetting.
- Child trying to make decisions without appropriate parental input.
- Parents abdicate decisions and are literally or figuratively absent from the bedside; child has to make decisions by default.
- Parent appears flustered and unable to manage the medical demands.
- Child appears very fearful.
- Parent becomes hyper-in-charge, and excludes both medical staff and the child from decision-making or important discussions.
- One parent, alone or with the child, becomes the decision-maker, while the second parent is marginalized and does not actively participate in the medical care or decision-making.

Jesse and his mother began the illness journey with a minimal level of hierarchy. Prior to his illness, Jesse was already known as "the man of the house," and typically took care of several adultlike concerns at home for his mother. As he became ill (prior to the emergent PICU admission), his mother's anxiety heightened, and Jesse, who looked older than his age, took on a primary role in managing his medical care. He made many of his own medical decisions, often attended medical appointments without his mother, and kept much of his suffering silent. Once in the PICU and newly intubated, Jesse clearly did not have the capacity to make decisions, but did everything in his power to communicate to his mother that he was in charge, and to protect his mother from "scary" information. This was confusing to the team, as Jesse also behaved in a regressed way, as described above. This kind of fragmented and seemingly incompatible set of behaviors is not atypical in families managing trauma. Though Jesse's mother was initially by his bedside, responding to Jesse's basic needs, she became increasingly overwhelmed by the medical events that triggered her own trauma, and began to avoid exposure to these triggers by pulling away. She found it increasingly difficult to make medical decisions and, over a few weeks, began to anticipate when the physicians would enter the room, and would be absent during those periods. When present, she began to "absent" herself by becoming very disorganized and overly emotional, prompting Jesse to increase his protective concern for her.

Intervention: The easiest ways in which to intervene to establish appropriate hierarchy in families managing medical crises involve respectfully and calmly assigning family members roles and responsibilities consistent with an appropriate place in the hierarchy. Often, this kind of intervention will require a team member designated to be a partner for the parent and/or for the child, to provide him or her with resources that will support the newly assigned responsibilities. In addition, simply treating the parent and child as competent and conveying your expectation that they will be able to execute their roles can help the parent and the child to see each other as competent, and can support a shift in hierarchy. Exposing families to groups of other families managing similar conditions (e.g., parent support group; teen group) can give family members role models and peers to help them take steps toward a more helpful family organization.

For Jesse, the first intervention was to give his mother a specific job at the bedside. She was given two daily responsibilities: to help Jesse complete his menus, and to make a list each morning of the issues that Jesse

wanted to discuss with the medical team. This "job" gave the family the task of discussing medical information, left Jesse with age-appropriate autonomy, but also included his mother in the conversation in a manageable and less scary way. It was not required that she be present for the conversation with the medical team, only that she help Jesse make his list of concerns each day. As she experienced some relief in knowing the concerns, and some confidence and competence in being able to tolerate the worry of knowing the concerns, she did begin participating in the care more effectively. As Jesse experienced his mother being able to handle information, he began being less protective and more inclusive of her in his overall care and decision-making. Jesse's mother would still sometimes become emotionally overwhelmed. However, with some very gentle coaching, she learned to communicate this to the team and to step out, allowing the team to work more directly with Jesse at these times so that he did not have to "cover" for her.

■ ADAPTABILITY

During a medical crisis, families must adapt in many ways. They must adapt to the emotional volatility of having a critically ill child, to the hospital realities of changing medical team members and rapidly changing medical needs and treatments, and to the practical realities of managing their child's medical care while also attending to the regular issues of life (e.g., managing work obligations, caring for other children, paying bills, getting themselves fed and housed, etc.). Clearly, families will manage most successfully when they balance consistency with flexibility. This kind of balance, however, requires solid problem-solving, good support, and emotional stability, all of which can be in short supply when one's child is in need of critical care. Being too consistent, or becoming anchored or fixed around rigid patterns of response, is one way in which adaptability challenges can emerge during the critical care experience. Rigid adherence to family and treatment routines can help parents, and even the child patient, feel a sense of control. When clinical needs demand quick changes, however, these families may become flooded with anxiety; changing up the routine may evoke intense fear, which can lead to opposition from both parents and children.

Being anchored at the other end of the adaptability continuum can be equally unhelpful. When families are traumatized by an illness or injury, they may be flooded with high anxiety and no sense of organization. They may abandon their routines and sense of order, and be unable to construct new routines to meet the needs. The result can appear to be chaos. Parents may have difficulty executing (or even understanding) care plans, they may have no predictable routines for being at the bedside, attending to their own needs, or communicating with the team. They may not show up at the bedside, or may appear too emotionally overwhelmed to participate in care when they do show up.

Some families, including Jesse and his mother, experience challenges at both ends of the continuum. Early in Jesse's care, and each time there was a major change in his condition, plan of care, or primary care team, his mother became completely chaotic and disorganized. Her attendance at the bedside was unpredictable, making it difficult for the team to execute care and make decisions, and when she was there, she was unable to organize herself to be a good support to Jesse. At other times, Mom became fully and rigidly organized around Jesse's routines. At times, this was helpful, and appeared to ground both her and Jesse. At other times, this was problematic. Jesse had to be changed in exactly the same way, always by the same nurse; he had to have his medications at exactly the same time, down to the minute. Slight changes in those routines were very difficult for Mom to tolerate. Changing the time or dose of a medication often precipitated an emotional crisis for Mom, and required several hours of team discussion to resolve.

Intervention: A few basic principles can help a team guide families to the middle of the adaptability continuum, promoting the ability of families to execute care and personal routines, while also maintaining the ability to change up those routines when necessary. Integrating good peritrauma care into family interactions can help. Specifically, helping families to feel a sense of safety, control, and information can help to reduce trauma-related anxiety that may exacerbate challenging family reactions (14). If families feel that they have access to clear information and feel that they have reasonable control over even some small aspects of care, they are more likely to be able to tolerate changes. Teams can help to maximize a sense of safety, control, and information by:

- Preparing families at the outset of a critical care experience to expect multiple changes, and letting families know that team members will help them develop routines to manage the changes.
- Providing clear, crisp information to parents each time there is a change in care, and taking a few moments to be sure they have understood it.
- Providing as much predictability as possible by helping families and children understand the general routines of a day in the PICU (e.g., giving information about times at which the doctors usually round, the meals are delivered, the nursing staff changes).
- Helping families to develop simple routines to manage their involvement in a child's care ("Here is how you can help us change your son"), as well as taking care of their own needs (e.g., prompting parents to set up schedules for being at the hospital, getting their own meals, communicating with others in their family).

Jesse's mother was strongly encouraged to set up a schedule for when she could be at the hospital, and was given a way to communicate with the nursing team when she had to change that schedule. Once Jesse was stabilized initially, a daily schedule of therapies was posted on his wall so that he and Mom could have a sense of predictability to their days. Changes were communicated by the same team member, as much as was possible, in a clear way and with as much notice as possible to Mom and Jesse. Over time, a sense of routine developed, and the rigidity and chaos extremes became less common.

■ COHESION

As described above, a family's patterns of involvement and closeness can support or undermine development. Preexisting patterns of cohesion that may have been functional for a family prior to an illness or injury may become less helpful during a critical care experience. Most often, issues related to family closeness emerge when patterns of connection between family members are not concordant with the developmental stage of the children or the family, and/or when parents have difficulty understanding that their own reactions to the events are separate and distinct from the reactions of their child, and vice versa. Mothers of babies, for example, may be traumatized considering that their babies are being emotionally scarred for life by the medical experience of critical care. While the experience is no doubt emotionally traumatizing for the mothers, it is likely to be less so for the youngest children.

For Jesse, the demands of his illness, as well as his family's preexisting patterns, resulted in an organization typical of a family with a much younger child. In many ways, Mom appeared to be overinvolved with Jesse, and violated his own autonomy by speaking for him, responding for him, and assuming that her emotional reactions were the same as his emotional reactions. Mom was reluctant to allow Jesse to take an age-appropriate role in learning about and managing his own medical issues. Jesse, a partner in this relational process, did the same with Mom; he assumed that he knew what her emotional reactions would be, and therefore made decisions to try to protect or shield her from information as a result.

For example, Jesse's mother, understandably devastated by Jesse's prognosis of having life-limiting disease, had insisted that he be protected from this information. After a surgery confirmed the prognosis, she and the medical team negotiated for nearly 2 weeks over whether or not he should be told. Mom could not understand that Jesse might not only be able to tolerate this information, but that open and honest discussion might relieve him of a burden and result in better care. Once it became clear that a discussion had to happen, Mom attempted to prepare for this discussion by calling the care team, including a psychologist and a social worker, to the bedside, and then, while crying, crawling into bed with her son as the physician began to speak.

Intervention: All of the intervention ideas listed above will also help in managing appropriate emotional connections between family members, while also promoting appropriate differentiation between family members. Three guiding principles may help:

- Prepare children and parents for the idea that while each will have a strong reaction to critical care, their reactions are likely to be different. Different things will scare them, different things will be hard for them, and each will surprise the other during the process. Simply providing this information can attune parents and children to look for differences, rather than to assume they are all having the same experience.
- Develop age-appropriate tasks and roles for parents and for patients, and support families in the execution of these routines.

- Help parents and children stay connected to roles and important others outside of the critical care experience. Parents can be encouraged to take brief breaks from the bedside, to attend to their other children or to each other, or to go to a hospital-sponsored group or support room. Children can be encouraged, as they are able, to communicate with siblings or friends, or to engage in developmentally appropriate activities or interests, even if they are only watching television or playing video games.

For Jesse, all of the team's work around establishing routines and engaging Jesse and Mom in ways that allowed Jesse to be a teenager helped to balance the level of Mom's involvement. Often this process required nuanced work. For example, when preparing Mom to be part of the conversation in which Jesse would be told of his prognosis, the team was careful to craft roles for Mom and others on the team that would allow Mom to take a parental role while allowing Jesse age-appropriate information. When Mom climbed tearfully into bed with her son to prepare him for the conversation, a team member privately, gently, and respectfully reminded Mom that Jesse would have his own reaction, and that she was demonstrating her reaction by climbing into bed. When encouraged to be his mother, she quickly acknowledged this, and stepped out of the bed, assuming her role by the bedside, more calmly. During the conversation, Jesse indicated that (as the team suspected) he already knew his prognosis ("I'm not stupid, you know"), but that he had not felt free to discuss it, or his very strong, and developmentally appropriate, reactions to it. The conversation showed both Jesse and Mom that they had separate experiences, with quite a bit of overlap, and this understanding opened up a new way for them to talk about the medical situation.

■ COMMUNICATION AND PROBLEM-SOLVING PROCESSES

Both communication and problem-solving processes are mechanisms that contribute to how a family is organized, and how they maintain that organization. In Jesse's family, communication was less than effective, largely because the overwhelming cohesion in the family left little room for real discussion about issues. Both Mom and Jesse believed they knew how the other felt, and spent most of their energy protecting each other from these imagined responses. Likewise, problem-solving was limited by the way in which the family bounced from rigidity to chaos.

Intervention: As was illustrated above, most interventions to address the issues of family organization involve using communication and problem-solving as tools. By helping families to communicate differently with each other and with the team, and by helping to develop new, consistent, and flexible problem-solving processes, teams can help families minimize the effects of trauma on their organization during the critical care experience (1,2).

■ AFFECTIVE ENVIRONMENT

The affective environment or emotional climate of a family can be an indicator of how families are adapting, and can help teams decide when intervention is necessary. While no one would expect the emotional climate of a family with a child in critical care to be rosy, there are clearly times when the climate is more strained than is typical, or when levels of emotion, most often trauma/anxiety, interfere with care. For Jesse's family, the emotional climate of this family was unpleasant, and despite their intense connection to each other, Mom and Jesse were both feeling terrible, but quite privately. Their rigid protection of each other did not allow either of them to process or express their own sadness and worry. They were often resentful of each other and unable to count on each other's support, leading them to feel alone and isolated. In short, the affective environment was strained, and in addition to feeling worried, sad, and being tearful, they were each often irritable and short-tempered with each other and with the medical team. No one's needs were being met.

Intervention: A family's affective environment is both a result of their organization, communication, and problem-solving processes, and a contributor to those same processes. As such, interventions that support appropriate organization, cohesion, and adaptability, as listed above, are likely to lead to a more adaptive affective environment. While in critical care, an affective environment may never feel casual, light, or sunny. However, honest communication patterns, the freedom to adapt to changes and respond to scary situations without constraint, will contribute to a more honest and

open environment that will foster each individual's and the family's mastery of the situation.

■ CONCLUSION

There is never a good time for a child to experience a neurocritical trauma. The child, family, and often health care team are inevitably challenged in multiple aspects of functioning when a child ends up on a critical care unit. A systems-informed framework for understanding the impact of the illness and resultant trauma on the child, family, and health care team helps to provide a care framework that is consistent, assuring, developmentally appropriate, and, as a result, medically optimized. Understanding a child's neurocritical status in the context of a family's structure and organization, adaptability, cohesion, developmental status/trajectory, problem solving, and affective environment are believed to enhance care in the short term and optimize psychosocial adjustment in the long term. It promotes a framework that depathologizes traumatic reactions and helps the patient, family, and health care team better understand their thoughts, feelings, and behaviors. A trauma-centered, systems-informed framework also provides concrete and accessible interventions to assist with optimal adjustment throughout the cycle of the trauma and illness. As a result, families are better able to adapt to the ever changing realities inherent in the critical care environment, teams and families are better able to participate in mutually informed medical care, and there is a pathway toward developmentally informed adjustment as the crisis resolves.

While nurses, physicians, and other critical care team members can occasionally attend to the constructs and processes outlined in this chapter, these issues can fall by the wayside when emergent high-stakes medical issues are present. Consistent attention to these issues, though hard to implement, will, however, reduce the barriers to providing medical care by developing more resources within the family and less conflict between the family and the team. One solution to this dilemma is to have a behavioral health provider colocated in a critical care unit. This provider can assist patients, families, and care team members in adopting a trauma-centered, systems-informed framework, develop and guide interventions, and assess outcomes. As an integrated member of the health care team, the behavioral health provider can assess the psychosocial status of new patients and families, monitor adjustment and adaptation throughout the hospital course, facilitate entry into a less intensive unit or the community, and maintain follow-up care as the patient or family members attempt to reestablish a new chapter in their lives. The behavioral health provider can also provide ongoing liaison to the medical team and thereby facilitate the incorporation of systems-based and trauma-informed care into their training. For example, over time, case specific consultation, psychosocial rounds, and well-planned didactics can help a critical unit care team develop greater sophistication in the medical and psychosocial care of children. The medical cost offset and value added of integrated behavioral health providers also contribute to overall patient quality and safety.

■ REFERENCES

1. Boyer BA et al. Prevalence and relationships of posttraumatic stress in families experiencing pediatric spinal cord injury. *Rehabil Psychol.* 2000;45(4):339–355. doi: 10.1037//0090-5550.45.4.339.

2. Kassam-Adarns N, Fleisher CL, Winston FK. Acute stress disorder and posttraumatic stress disorder in parents of injured children. *J Trauma Stress.* 2009;22(4):294–302. doi: 10.1002/jts.20424.

3. Kazak AE et al. An integrative model of pediatric medical traumatic stress. *J Pediatr Psychol.* 2006;31(4):343–355. doi: 10.1093/jpepsy/jsj054.

4. Saxe G et al. Relationship between acute morphine and the course of PTSD in children with burns. *J Am Acad Child Adolesc Psychiatry.* 2001;40(8):915–921. doi: 10.1097/00004583-200108000-00013.

5. Helfricht S et al. Posttraumatic stress disorder among parents of children on cancer treatment. *J Pediatr Psychol.* 2004;29(3):211–219.

6. Shudy M et al. Impact of pediatric critical illness and injury on families: a systematic literature review. *Pediatrics.* 2006;118:S203–S218. doi: 10.1542/peds.2006-0951B.

7. Balluffi A et al. Traumatic stress in parents of children admitted to the pediatric intensive care unit. *Pediatr Crit Care Med.* 2004;5(6):547–553. doi: 10.1097/01.pcc.0000137354.19807.44.

8. Kassam-Adams N, et al. Parent-child agreement regarding children's acute stress: the role of parent acute stress reactions. *J Am Acad Child Adolesc Psychiatry.* 2006;45(12):1485–1493. doi: 10.1097/01.chi.0000237703.97518.12.

9. Ko SJ, et al. Creating trauma-informed systems: child welfare, education, first responders, health care, juvenile justice. *Prof Psychol Res Pr.* 2008; 39(4), 396–404. doi: 10.1037/0735-7028.39.4.396.

10. Winthrop AL. Health-related quality of life after pediatric trauma. *Curr Opin Pediatr.* 2010;22(3):346–351. doi: 10.1097/MOP.0b013e3283394351.

11. Kramer U et al. Individual and dyadic coping strategies in the aftermath of a traumatic experience. *Swiss J Psychol.* 2005;64(4):241–248. doi: 10.1024/1421-0185.64.4.241.

12. Ziegler MF et al. Posttraumatic stress responses in children: awareness and practice among a sample of pediatric emergency care providers. *Pediatrics.* 2005;115(5):1261–1267. doi: 10.1542/peds.2004-1217.

13. American Psychiatric Association. *Diagnostic and Statistical Manual of Mental Disorders.* 4th ed. Washington, DC: American Psychiatric Association; 1994.

14. Child traumatic stress. The National Child Traumatic Stress Network Web site. http://www.nctsn.org/. Updated 2011. Retrieved June 30, 2011.

15. Ahl LE et al. Functional therapy for children with cerebral palsy: an ecological approach. *Deve Med Child Neurol.* 2005;47(9):613–619. doi: 10.1017/s0012162205001210.

16. Berge JM, Patterson JM, Reuter M. Marital satisfaction and mental health of couples with children with chronic health conditions. *Fam Syst Health.* 2006;24(4):267–285. doi: 10.1037/1091-7527.24.3.267.

17. Carpentier MY et al. The relationship of parent self-focused negative attributions to ratings of parental overprotection, perceived child vulnerability, and parenting stress. *Fam Syst Health.* 2008;26(2):147–163. doi: 10.1037/1091-7527.26.2.147.

18. Kratz L et al. Managing childhood chronic illness: parent perspectives and implications for parent provider relationships. *Fam Syst Health.* 2009;27(4):303–313. doi: 10.1037/a0018114.

19. Martland T, Cross HJ. Best clinical and research practice in pediatric neurology. *Epilepsy Behav.* 2009;15:51–54. doi: 10.1016/j.yebeh.2009.03.018.

20. Miller VA. Parent-child collaborative decision making for the management of chronic illness: a qualitative analysis. *Fam Syst Health.* 2009;27(3):249–266. doi: 10.1037/a0017308.

21. Power TJ. Collaborative practices for managing children's chronic health needs. In: Phelps L, ed. *Chronic Health-Related Disorders in Children: Collaborative Medical and Psychoeducational Interventions.* Washington, DC: American Psychological Association; 2006:7–23.

22. Kazak AE et al. Treatment of posttraumatic stress symptoms in adolescent survivors of childhood cancer and their families: a randomized clinical trial. *J Fam Psychol.* 2004;18(3):493–504. doi: 10.1037/0893-3200.18.3.493.

23. Mealer M et al. The prevalence and impact of post traumatic stress disorder and burnout syndrome in nurses. *Depress Anxiety.* 2009;26(12):1118–1126. doi: 10.1002/da.20631.

24. Robins PM, Meltzer L, Zelikovsky N. The experience of secondary traumatic stress upon care providers working within a children's hospital. *J Pediatr Nurs.* 2009;24(4):270–279. doi: 10.1016/j.pedn.2008.03.007.

25. Rourke MT. Compassion fatigue in pediatric palliative care providers. *Pediatr Clin North Am.* 2007;54(5):631–644. doi: 10.1016/j.pcl.2007.07.004.

26. Alderfer MA, Rourke MT. Family psychology in the context of pediatric medical conditions. In Bray JH, ed. *Wiley-Blackwell Handbook of Family Psychology.* New York, NY: John Wiley & Sons; 2009.

27. Mohlman Berg J, Patterson JM. Cystic fibrosis and the family: a review and critique of the literature. *Fam Syst Health.* 2004;22(1):74–100.

28. Quittner AL et al. Role strain in couples with and without a child with a chronic illness: associations with marital satisfaction, intimacy, and daily mood. *Health Psychol.* 1998;17(2):112-124. doi: 10.1037//0278-6133.17.2.112.

26 *End of Life Care*

VANESSA MADRIGAL and WYNNE MORRISON

Although mortality rates for children in developed countries have been decreasing over the past few decades, over 50,000 children still die yearly in the United States, with most of these deaths occurring in the hospital (1–4). From age 1 until young adulthood, unintentional injury is the leading cause of death. Compared to adults with life-threatening multisystem trauma, trauma in children is more likely to include a component of neurologic injury, which is a leading contributor to both morbidity and mortality in pediatric intensive care units (ICUs) (5–7).

In addition to patients with traumatic brain injury, clinicians in multidisciplinary pediatric ICUs (PICUs) may care for children with other life-threatening neurologic problems such as central nervous system infections, intractable seizures, brain tumors, hypoxic-ischemic brain injury, or congenital problems such as hydrocephalus or progressive neuromuscular weakness from many causes. In one large, multicenter study, 12% of children who died in PICUs were initially admitted for neurologic diagnoses (8). Children hospitalized with central nervous system disorders are more likely to be in the ICU than other children, and also are more likely to die, with as many as 46% of children who die in ICUs having a neurologic diagnosis as one component of their illness (9). To care for these children and their families, it is necessary to become comfortable providing effective, compassionate end of life care when lifesaving or life-prolonging therapies are either no longer possible or no longer in the child's best interests. Skillful care at the end of life requires an ability to help a family and health care team navigate the ethical and emotional concerns that may arise when a child is dying. It also requires a focus on pain and symptom management with special attention to how pharmacologic therapies differ when the goals of care shift to providing comfort rather than extending life. All pediatric intensivists and neurointensivists will care for dying children, and knowing how to guide children and families through this stage of life is an important complement to knowing how to save a life when doing so is possible.

■ HOW DEATHS OCCUR IN THE PICU

There are many different ways that children can die in an ICU. Some will be declared dead by neurologic criteria and others by traditional cardiopulmonary criteria. Some will die despite continued resuscitative efforts and escalation of therapies, and for others the family and medical team will decide to discontinue or not initiate potentially life-sustaining interventions such as mechanical ventilation.

Several single center studies in the United States have suggested that as many as one-third to half of deaths in PICUs are preceded by decisions to limit or discontinue life-sustaining interventions (10–14). The frequency with which support is withdrawn varies greatly from country to country, and individual practitioners likely have varying thresholds for when they would consider withdrawal of therapies (15). Withdrawal of technological support may be more frequent in children with prolonged ICU stays (16).

A recent study using a large, multi-institutional database in the United States suggested that it is becoming more common for children to die with some limitations on medical therapies in place. Although there was a wide variability between institutions, out of 1,263 deaths, 23% of children were declared dead by neurologic criteria, 16% had do not attempt resuscitation (DNAR) orders, 49% had medical therapies limited or withdrawn (and presumably also had DNAR orders by the time of death), and only 12% died despite ongoing medical interventions (8).

Declaration of Death by Neurologic Criteria

Children with brain injuries or other processes that lead to severely elevated intracranial pressure will often, over the course of hours or days, suffer an irreversible loss of all function of the brain, a state described as *total brain failure* or *brain death* (17). In recent years, the term *death diagnosed by neurologic criteria* has been suggested as being preferable to *brain death* in order to emphasize that it is the criteria used for diagnosing death that differ (either cardiopulmonary or neurologic), not the fact that the patient is dead. Brain death is discussed in Chapter 27.

The declaration of death by neurologic criteria can be confusing for many families, as they are told that their child is dead while the body is still warm, the heart is still beating, and the chest moving in respiration due to the mechanical and pharmacologic cardiopulmonary support in place in the ICU. Careful attention and patience is necessary to help families understand that the patient is truly dead. Many clinicians misspeak and make statements like "he will die" when the ventilator is discontinued, when in fact death has already occurred. Clarity in language used can help avoid confusion.

Although the death of a child is almost always a tragedy, being able to definitively determine when brain injury is complete and irreversible can be helpful to both the family and medical team. Once death has been declared, there is no need for the family to struggle with difficult decisions about whether to discontinue therapies like mechanical ventilation. The team is able to tell the family that the outcome is certain and the next steps are clear. Once a patient has been declared dead, a family should not be asked *whether* they want to discontinue a ventilator, only the timing of stopping needs to be discussed.

Another question that needs to be resolved once death has been declared is whether the family wishes to take the opportunity to donate the child's organs before the mechanical supports are discontinued. It is standard practice to separate the discussion of organ donation from the conversation in which the family is told that their child is dead, in order to give them time to process the news before being asked about donation (18). It is also important for organ donation to be discussed in conjunction with a representative from an organ procurement organization (OPO), who is the expert in the processes involved in donation. Effective collaboration with the OPO can be facilitated by an early referral of a severely brain injured and ventilator dependent patient for evaluation of eligibility as an organ donor. Although the family should not be approached about donation if death has not yet been declared, the OPO representative can review the case and talk with the team about whether donation would even be possible. Plans for when and how to approach the family can also be made.

Failed Resuscitation

Many children die in the ICU despite ongoing support with the full array of available life-sustaining measures and resuscitative attempts. Children with neurologic injury or diseases may die because of failure of other organ systems that are compromised by the same process that has affected the brain. In addition, severe neurologic dysfunction can also lead to cardiopulmonary failure, with arrhythmias, hemodynamic instability, or acute respiratory distress syndrome as reported sequelae.

When a child has died despite ongoing resuscitation, attention should turn to support of the family and the medical team. Many centers have begun to allow families to be present while cardiopulmonary resuscitative attempts are underway (19). Allowing a family to be present can reassure them that everything possible was done to try to save their child, and can sometimes help a family feel that they were able to say goodbye before the moment of death. Although staff may fear that family presence could interfere with their ability to provide appropriate care, there are reports in the literature that suggest that this is rarely a problem (20,21). It is important to have a staff member available to explain what is going on to family members and provide support, and no family member should be required to remain present for a resuscitation if it becomes overwhelming.

Withdrawal of Life-Sustaining Therapies

In many cases, a family and medical team will make a joint decision that the burdens of continuing medical therapies outweigh the benefits for a particular child. This decision is often made in cases where the medical team feels that death is highly likely to occur even if on-going aggressive measures continue. Sometimes survival may be possible, but the quality of life of the surviving child is expected to be so poor that the decision is made not to prolong suffering. In the minds of many, neurologic status and cognitive function are key determinants of quality of life, and therefore baseline cognitive function and expected deteriorations in neurologic status from baseline may both be important factors in helping a family and team decide whether ongoing medical therapies are overly burdensome. For other families, however, there may be inherent value in supporting life no matter how impaired the child is or is expected to be. Such decisions are therefore inherently value-laden and an individual patient's and family's opinions should be considered.

Ethically, there is little difference between withholding and withdrawing a medical treatment, and having begun a treatment does not impose an obligation to continue it if circumstances change and the intervention no longer offers a long-term benefit for the child (22–24). For many families, however, there is a tremendous emotional difference between deciding not to start what is felt to be a nonbeneficial therapy and discontinuing a therapy that is already in place. Some families may decide that they are comfortable limiting the further escalation of mechanical or pharmacologic supports, but want to continue support which is currently in place until the trajectory of a child's illness becomes absolutely clear. Flexibility on the part of the team is necessary to find a solution that is both emotionally acceptable to the family and medically appropriate for the child.

DNAR Orders

DNAR orders are orders that specify therapies that will not be applied if a patient's status deteriorates (25). A wide range of treatments could be limited by such orders, examples being intubation and mechanical ventilation, chest compressions, defibrillation, pharmacologic interventions like vasoactive infusions or cardiac arrest medications, transfusion of blood products or antibiotics. The goal of DNAR orders is to avoid medical treatments that are felt to be unlikely to be beneficial or

treatments which may merely prolong dying or a very poor quality of life. "Do not attempt resuscitation" is touted as a preferable phrase to "Do not resuscitate" due to concerns that the latter suggests that resuscitation would always be possible, when it is frequently not so. Some centers have also begun to use the term *allow natural death* instead of DNAR, as this may be a more acceptable term to patients and families (26,27).

In discussing DNAR orders with patients or families, it is usually best to clarify their overall goals of care, rather than presenting them with a list of possible interventions and proceeding to check off which they would or would not want. Such "goals" could include wanting to have their child suffer as little as possible, wanting to be home if possible, wanting to preserve life as long as possible in the hopes that things improve, or wanting to honor a particular wish expressed by the patient. The patient or family will usually need some guidance as to which therapies or limitations of therapies make sense in light of their overall goals of care (28–30).

It can be important to emphasize that placing a DNAR order is not equivalent to "doing nothing." Both the team and family should be aware that there are still many things to be done—assuring patient comfort, treating other difficult symptoms, and just being present with a family to assure them that the dying child is being well cared for and that they, as parents, are making loving, appropriate decisions.

Discontinuing Mechanical Ventilation

When a decision has been made to extubate and to discontinue mechanical ventilation for a patient who is expected to die, it is important to ensure that the process facilitates patient comfort rather than increasing suffering (31). Patient comfort may be improved by removing an endotracheal tube that has been a significant cause of distress, but there is also a risk that discontinuing the ventilator leads to dyspnea and respiratory distress. Treating anticipated distress pharmacologically is important, usually both with narcotics and sedative agents. Administering medications or increasing the rate of infusions already in place prior to the extubation can prevent suffering and having to "catch up" with symptoms afterward.

There are two approaches to discontinuing mechanical ventilation, each of which may be appropriate depending on the situation. One method is described in some literature as "terminal extubation," in which the endotracheal tube is removed and ventilation discontinued without weaning ventilation (22). Another approach, "terminal weaning," involves gradually decreasing the amount of ventilator support before extubating (32). One advantage of decreasing ventilator support prior to extubating is that it allows the clinician to better assess whether the patient will develop respiratory distress when ventilator support is removed and titrate medications accordingly. If this method is used, it should be possible to decrease the level of support fairly rapidly, over minutes, rather than prolonging "weaning" procedures. For patients who are on advanced modes of ventilation such as high frequency ventilation, switching to a conventional mode of ventilation prior to extubation may help the family be able to hold a child before death. If a patient is already obtunded or heavily sedated, decreasing ventilatory support prior to extubation is probably unnecessary. Regardless of which method is used, a medication plan should be in place for treating distress after extubation with doses readily available prior to removing the endotracheal tube.

It is important for the team and family to understand that discontinuing a ventilator, or any other therapy, does not mean that a child will absolutely die or that death will immediately occur. The family should understand how long the clinician anticipates the child will breathe independently but that there is uncertainty in any such prediction. Most intensivists can remember a handful of cases in their experience where a child did not die after treatments were discontinued. This uncertainty can sometimes be framed in such a way that it helps a family deal with a decision to withdraw—the disease process leads to the child's death, not the family's decisions, and therefore, we do not ultimately control the time of death.

The family should also be prepared for what the child may look like after the ventilator is discontinued. Discussion of color changes, work of breathing or irregular breathing, and possible noisy breathing like stridor is important. The clinician should also distinguish between symptoms that cause the patient discomfort and other symptoms, such as irregular or noisy breathing, that cause more distress for the observers than the child. The prior requires medical interventions and the latter reassurance. Checking in frequently after the withdrawal to reassure the family that the child looks comfortable, or to treat discomfort if it is present is essential.

Other measures which can improve the environment for the family include moving to a private room if possible, turning off monitors (or monitoring from outside the room), and helping a family to hold a child both before and after removal of the endotracheal tube. Temporarily relaxing restrictions on the number of family members that can be in the room can be helpful, although it is good practice to first ascertain whether the parents want extended family members present. A family may appreciate having a small child moved from a crib to a larger bed so that the parent can lie in bed holding the child.

Location of Death

Many factors determine the optimal location for medical care at the end of life. How long is the patient expected to survive? How intensive are the interventions required to keep the patient comfortable? At which location in the hospital does the staff know the child and family best? How stable is the home setting and can the child be kept comfortable there? The "best" location may change over time as circumstances or the child's status changes. Sometimes, the ICU is the best place for a child to be if careful attention and a low patient to nurse ratio is necessary to assure the patient's comfort. Sometimes it is also advantageous to have a child remain in the ICU if the family has not met staff elsewhere. Other families who are followed long-term on different floors in the hospital may prefer to have their child transferred out to their "primary" team. Many families also want to have their children home at the time of death. Hospice agencies can be invaluable partners in facilitating this desire, as nursing and other support services can then be available in the home. Over time as more of these services become available, more parents of children with complex chronic conditions are choosing to bring their children home to die (33).

Fluids and Nutrition

Although most argue that medically provided nutrition and hydration are medical interventions which can be withdrawn like any other, there are some important differences from other modalities often withheld or withdrawn, such as mechanical ventilation or cardiopulmonary resuscitation (34). For many families, continuing nourishment of their child is of great emotional importance, and discontinuing it may feel like "starvation." Guidelines have suggested that medically provided nutrition and hydration be withheld only from children with a permanent lack of consciousness, or from children who are actively dying for whom providing it may increase suffering (35). It is also important to consider whether the child is capable of experiencing hunger, and to take steps to ensure that suffering is not thereby increased by withholding medically provided nutrition.

Organ Donation After a Circulatory Determination of Death

Organ donation after a circulatory determination of death (DCDD), also known as donation after cardiac death or nonheart beating organ donation, may be an option for families who have made a decision to discontinue ongoing aggressive support in the care of their child. The process involves the discontinuation of mechanical ventilation and/or other therapies in or near the operating room, with plans in place for a relatively rapid procurement of organs after a brief waiting period following the declaration of death by traditional means (36). There are many controversies surrounding the process, including what constitutes an adequate waiting period and whether the patients can be considered "unresuscitatable" at the time of organ procurement (37). Institutions should have policies in place that guide clinicians in this process. DCDD is touted as a means of increasing the organ supply to prevent deaths on the transplant waiting list, and can also be a help to families who want to be able to find something meaningful in a tragic situation (38). It is important that decisions about withdrawing therapies be made independently from decisions about organ donation, and also important that the team providing the end of life care for the child at the time of ventilator withdrawal be different from the team that will procure organs if the child dies. Standard end of life care, with medications used as needed to relieve suffering, should be provided by clinicians who are accustomed to providing such care, and a location should be identified for ongoing care of the child if death does not occur soon enough after withdrawal to allow the procurement of organs.

■ PAIN AND SYMPTOM MANAGEMENT

An in-depth discussion of pain and symptom management at the end of life is beyond the scope of this chapter, and palliative medicine texts should be consulted for more guidance on this topic (39,40). A few guiding principles and some of the most common medications

used are discussed next. Although most patients in the ICU will have reliable intravenous access, it is important to remember that there are many routes of medication administration available other than intravenous—such as oral, sublingual, inhaled, transdermal patches, rectal, nasal, or subcutaneous. Use of other routes should be strongly considered, particularly for patients who may be transitioning to care at home.

Principle of Double Effect

Clinicians at the bedside may be hesitant to use large doses of narcotic or sedative agents at the end of life because of fear that the respiratory depressant side effects of such medications could lead to death. As long as such medications are used in reasonable doses for treating pain, dyspnea, or other symptoms, then it is ethically appropriate to accept that they may cause respiratory depression. This idea is known as the "Principle of Double Effect." The benefits of the intended effect (relief of suffering) outweigh and justify the harms of the anticipated but unintended effect (respiratory depression) (41). In reality, it is rarely necessary to invoke this principle, as medications which are titrated to effect do not usually cause a significant degree of respiratory depression. It is also important to realize that there is no "ceiling" on the doses of medications that may be needed to treat pain and dyspnea at the end of life. Patients who have become tolerant to narcotics or benzodiazepines may be on doses far higher than the typical starting doses listed in formularies or reference texts, and it is appropriate to continue to escalate doses when needed. Increasing a dose or infusion rate by 20% for mild symptoms or 50% for severe symptoms is perfectly reasonable, with frequent further increases possible for continuing symptoms (42).

Inappropriate Medications at the End of Life

It is inappropriate to give medications at the end of life that have the sole intent of hastening death, without providing symptomatic relief (22,24,43). Examples of such inappropriate medications would be neuromuscular blocking agents or potassium chloride. Neuromuscular blocking agents have the additional disadvantage of making it nearly impossible to assess whether the dying child is in distress and in need of more medication for pain. In rare instances where clearance of neuromuscular blocking agents will be prolonged and delay withdrawal of unwanted therapies, there are some who argue that withdrawal should not be delayed as long as the death of the patient is almost certain given the circumstances and sufficient analgesics and sedatives are administered to guarantee no conscious awareness. Withdrawing under these circumstances is controversial, however, and it is usually better to wait some period of time until reversal of neuromuscular blockade is possible. Most families will understand the need to wait if it is presented as the best way to guarantee that the child is not suffering.

Opioids

Opioid or narcotic agents are usually the primary means of treatment of pain and dyspnea at the end of life, with several options available for use (39). All work via μ-opioid receptors in the central nervous system leading to euphoria and analgesia, and may also cause side effects such as respiratory depression, constipation, nausea, itching, and urinary retention. It is important to anticipate and manage side effects to avoid suffering. Morphine is the longest-used of these agents, and is available in a variety of forms for administration as well as both short-acting and long-acting preparations. Morphine leads to a release of histamine which can sometimes worsen itching, and accumulation can lead to hyperalgesia or myoclonus (42). Switching to another agent can be beneficial if these or other severe side effects occur. Codeine is an agent which works after being metabolized to morphine, but more than 10% of the population are slow metabolizers, decreasing its usefulness. Codeine also tends to cause marked nausea, making it a less useful drug at the end of life. Hydromorphone is a more useful agent as a substitute when side effects of morphine have become difficult to manage. Oxycodone is an oral agent which may be another reasonable alternative for mild to moderate pain. Fentanyl is a short-acting, lipophilic agent available in intravenous and patch formulations. It is often used as an infusion, but tolerance may develop fairly rapidly requiring dose escalation. Meperidine should be avoided because a metabolite, normeperidine, can accumulate and lead to seizures. Methadone is unique among the narcotics in that it also has effects at the N-methyl-D-aspartate (NMDA) receptor. This benefit can sometimes help control pain when patients have become tolerant to other opioids and can also offer some benefit for neuropathic pain. Care should be taken because of its very long half-life. Frequent dosing may be needed to control pain initially, but the drug will then accumulate over days potentially leading to oversedation and respiratory depression.

Sedatives

Sedative agents are often a useful adjunct in treating suffering at the end of life, and can be useful for alleviating anxiety or for decreasing an awareness of pain when it is difficult to treat by other means. Benzodiazepines are a mainstay when sedation is required, and can be delivered orally, rectally, intramuscularly, or intravenously by either intermittent dosing or an infusion (44). Other agents may occasionally be necessary for sedation, such as barbiturates, but clinicians should be aware that barbiturates can increase the perception of pain so should only be used if the goal is depression of mental status. Neuroleptic agents may also be helpful, particularly when there is a component of delirium, but can have worrisome side effects (45). "Terminal sedation" is a phrase sometimes used to refer to the use of sedation to the level of unconsciousness at the end of life to treat symptoms that cannot be managed by any other means. Any sedative or anesthetic, such as propofol, could be used for this purpose, but such a degree of sedation is rarely necessary and should only be considered for intractable suffering not otherwise manageable. Ketamine is an NMDA receptor antagonist which functions as a dissociative anesthetic with excellent sedative and analgesic properties, but has the disadvantage of potentially leading to disturbing hallucinations, particularly in older children and at higher doses.

Other Agents and Adjuncts

Other medications such as tricyclic antidepressants or agents with anticonvulsant activity such as gabapentin and pregabalin can sometimes be useful in the treatment of neuropathic pain. Local techniques such as lidocaine patches or regional anesthetic blocks are also sometimes useful to control pain and enable a decrease in the total systemic dose of medications required. Nonpharmacologic interventions such as distraction, a calming environment, swaddling, and massage can also help with symptom management (39).

Treatment of Dyspnea

Nebulized analgesic agents such as morphine have been evaluated in several trials as a treatment of dyspnea, with mixed results (46). In the ICU, it is generally advantageous to use systemically delivered opioids for treating dyspnea, although nebulized agents can be tried if a patient or family wants a child to be able to remain as alert as possible. Physical measures such as blowing cool air in the face have also been touted as a treatment for dyspnea. Oxygen supplementation and noninvasive positive pressure ventilation are also potential options for treating breathlessness, but the burden-benefit balance should always be weighed of whether using such therapies leads to a greater or lesser degree of comfort.

Neurologic Symptoms

Many patients with neurologic injury or disease processes are at a high risk of disturbing events like seizures or myoclonus at the end of life. Benzodiazepines are often useful for intermittent seizures and the associated sedation may also be beneficial. For some children, such as those with brain tumors, in whom seizures may be possible, less sedating preventive agents like valproate or levetiracetam may be more appropriate (44). Myoclonus can be extraordinarily difficult to treat at the end of life, and the mainstay of therapy is to make sure that the child is adequately sedated, enough to prevent suffering and to reassure the family that the child is not aware of the movements.

Support of the Family

Family Needs

Each family with a child facing the end of life is unique with their own set of values and a wide variety of complex, changing needs. However, some common practices are discussed below.

Communication and Honesty

Communication is the cornerstone of providing good care at the end of a child's life. Parents consistently report a desire for ample information in nontechnical language (47–49). Even in the face of uncertainty, or bad news, parents prefer honesty (49,50). Providers should carefully consider the language that they use in the delivery of information, and express empathy and compassion. Studies have demonstrated that single events like insensitive delivery of bad news, feeling dismissed or patronized, perceived disregard for parents' judgment regarding the care of their child, and poor communication of important information can cause parents profound distress which can haunt and complicate grief long after their child has died (50).

Another aspect of communication is choosing the circumstances under which to deliver information—for example, choosing the setting, coordinating which members of the multidisciplinary team should be present, and which of the family members to include. The medical team must identify and respect the wishes of the parents or child regarding who should be present during discussions and in the patient's room. Alerting the parents to the possible topics to be discussed can be helpful. Particularly with the delivery of bad news, parents report wanting preparation that bad news is coming (49).

Unfortunately, although the importance of good communication is universally recognized, patient information is frequently not communicated well in the ICU (51). Institutions have a responsibility to develop robust systems and training programs to provide strong foundations in communication strategies.

Patient and family meetings may help foster communication. Discussions with families are an important place to identify goals, values, expectations, and the medical status of the child. Family members should be asked open-ended questions about what they understand about their loved one's condition, what they fear (52), and what they hope for (28). Then care providers should repeat what they have heard, which fosters trust and helps correct any misunderstandings. These meetings are also an important setting for identifying conflicts, whether they be between the medical team and family, between family members, and even between the family and the patient. Once identified, the family meetings can even serve as an appropriate environment to move toward resolving those conflicts. The American College of Critical Care Task Force calls for early and repeated care conferencing to reduce family stress and improve consistency in communication (49). In some adult studies, family meetings have actually affected patient outcomes. For example, in one study, the implementation of family meetings within the first 72 hours for patients at higher risk achieved significant reductions in ICU length of stay (53).

Including family members on rounds is a useful way to update parents and include them in daily decision making. Recommended as a standard of care (49,54), parents report preferring bedside rounds and feel better informed when they were present (55).

Partnership in Decision Making

Parents need to feel that they are active partners in the multiprofessional decision-making process. "Shared decision-making" is a process by which both the family and team share responsibility for making a good choice for a patient. The medical team may present a variety of acceptable medical options to a family, the family may share their perspective on the advantages of or problems with each option, and the team should then help guide the family to a reasonable decision (56). It can be problematic if the team insists on a certain course of action without considering a family's opinions, but it is also a problem if the team dispassionately offers a family a menu of choices and awaits a decision without providing guidance based on accumulated medical experience. Making recommendations in light of an understanding of the values of the patient and family is an important responsibility of the physician. Often a series of meetings is required for the family and team to reach a consensus about the best course of action. When possible, having some consistency in the members of the medical team that attend family meetings is helpful in allowing the medical team to understand how the family's views change over time. Innumerable authors and organizations now support some degree of shared decision-making (49,50,57). Recent studies in adult patients also suggest that incorporating the viewpoints of patients and families improves the quality of end of life care (58–62).

When a child is healthy, parents typically see their role as one of protector and provider for the child. This role is threatened by a critical illness and the ensuing loss of control. Helping parents to retain some sense of control can contribute to a higher quality of end of life care (60,63). Clinicians can help by supporting families in making whatever choices they are willing and able to make. Yet families must bear the burden of decisions long after the child has died. Partnering with the medical team should lessen the personal weight and be tailored to patients' preferences and beliefs (57).

Hope

High on the list of family needs is to maintain hope (49,50). The need to maintain hope is often pivotal in understanding family dynamics and in eliciting trust and achieving consensus at family meetings. The diversity of hopes can range from the miraculous to the mundane and can adapt and change (28). Even as some hopes die, others emerge as seen with a hope for freedom from pain, a dignified death, or more quality time together. Families' most bitter complaints have often been about physicians who dismiss their hopes (50).

Maintaining a Connection With Their Child

Parents express a variety of ways they wish to maintain a connection with their child both at the time of death and afterward. Creating memories with the child and family is extremely important. Helping the family be physically present around the time of a child's death is a powerful way to maintain that connection. Also, family members may wish to collect a locket of hair or make handprints and footprints with paints on paper. Kits can be provided that allow a family to make a hand impression on clay or casting material. Mementos and pictures provide a tangible connection long after the child has died. Some parents and families maintain a connection to their child by building memorials and performing altruistic acts such as organ donation, volunteer work, charitable fundraising, and support group development (48).

Religious and Cultural Needs

Families often have significant spiritual needs when a child is near the end of life (19,47,64). A child's death can shatter even the most well-grounded person's sense of purpose and meaning. Needs could include prayer, particular rituals, reading of sacred texts, and traditions for connecting with others, bereavement support, gratitude, and compassion (48).

Clinicians may understand the importance of spirituality and religious beliefs when a patient is near the end of life, but may feel unskilled and uncomfortable discussing these concerns (65,66). Studies recommend that physicians make an assessment of spiritual needs, identifying values, priorities, and help screen for spiritual crisis (48,67). Clinicians should listen empathetically without offering premature reassurance, or trying to alleviate the patient's spiritual suffering (66). Physicians should be aware of services available, such as the chaplain service for referrals if desired by the family (68). Many religious traditions call for ceremonies and rituals at the end of life (69–75). Asking patients and families to share their spiritual needs also helps in working out the logistics for such preferences. Some patients have reported not wanting to share their beliefs with clinicians (76). An alternative is to ask in such a way that gives families the option, rather than feeling like a requirement, of sharing their needs and concerns (77).

Many families will have specific cultural needs. Culture, as opposed to race or ethnicity, refers to a pattern of learned beliefs, shared values, and behaviors, including styles of communication and relationships roles within the family (78). Many cultures including some Asian, Mexican, Middle Eastern, and African American cultures view the individual not as an autonomous entity, but as part of a network of family and social relationships (79). These beliefs are in sharp contrast with mainstream American and European culture where the individual and his/her beliefs are of highest importance (80).

Language difference can be a major barrier to families receiving optimal communication and care. The use of a professional interpreter is essential for important conversations. Children and family members should not be placed in the difficult and embarrassing situation of interpreting (81). Without a common language, the parents' ability to understand and acquire complete information about their child's condition is compromised. Language-discordant parents have reported feeling isolated, confused, and distrustful of the hospital system (50). Clinicians should make reasonable efforts to round with or be available to families when an interpreter is present. When having a sequence of family meetings, particularly surrounding difficult decisions, having the same interpreter helps foster consistent communication. Finally, a preconference meeting with the interpreter might be helpful to clarify what topics will be discussed, terminology that will be used, and whether the role of the interpreter will be one of strict linguistic translation or that of a "cultural broker" (82).

Support for Siblings

Families often worry about when to allow children to visit their dying sibling. Hospitals should support visiting protocols that allow siblings to visit even when typical visitation rules may exempt young family members. Child life specialists have valuable skills to prepare a sibling for what they are about to see, and provide creative outlets to express their emotions through various forms of play and artwork. These activities can sometimes be done in conjunction with family meetings, and provide a form of distraction for the young family members as the parents are making difficult decisions. Studies have reported that siblings benefit from access to playrooms during hospital visits, support groups, and respectful attention from staff (50,83).

Visiting Hours

The ability to visit the patient at any time is extremely important to families toward the end of life (49). Many hospitals have restrictions in place on the number of visitors allowed in a room at a time in order to allow staff to focus on safe and effective care for all patients. If a patient is dying, it may be possible to ease restrictions or perhaps rotate two family members into the room at a time. Creative ways of managing large families are important.

The Multidisciplinary Team Approach

Modern medicine can become extremely fragmented and requires extraordinary coordination of care involving interdisciplinary communication. This collaborative approach is crucial when working with a child and family near the end of life (84). Family meetings should include members of the multidisciplinary team, including the specialists involved so as to foster consensus on information delivered to the family. A team meeting a few minutes prior to bringing the family into the conversation is often helpful to achieve consensus. It may be important to include nurses, respiratory therapists, child life specialists, social workers, chaplains, and trainees. For some families, however, avoiding too large a group is also important as having the family be overwhelmed if substantially outnumbered by medical professionals.

Patient-Family Discussions, Controversies, and Resolving Disagreements

Difficulties in Prognosis

One of the most difficult questions, and one upon which so much hinges for both clinician and family is prognosis. Accurate predictions are elusive to even the most experienced clinicians and can be distorted by bias and previous experience. Validated, objective prognostic models have been viewed as a mechanism for improving clinical decision making in ICU, such as APACHE I-III (Acute Physiology and Chronic Health Evaluation), and MPM-II (Mortality Probability Models) (62) for adults, and the PRISM III (Pediatric Risk of Mortality) score (85) for children. Most such scores, however, are more appropriate for benchmarking populations or ICU performance and were not designed to be predictors of outcome for individual patients. Accurate prognostic information can be viewed as a tool to help save the lives of the salvageable and offer the dying a peaceful and dignified death (86), but such accuracy is often difficult to achieve in practice. A family undertaking a difficult decision deserves best estimates determined by validated tools and clinician experience, but clinicians should avoid being overly confident in their predictions in the timing of death, particularly when there is uncertainty. Family trust can be lost when such predictions turn out to be incorrect.

Resolving Conflict With Families

As discussed earlier, families need honest, complete information with good communication. A breakdown in these needs can quickly unravel into a relationship of distrust. In addition to planning structured family meetings, when conflict arises it can be important to take a step back and focus on building an alliance with the family, stressing common goals such as providing the best possible care for the child. Continuing to argue the same point of disagreement again and again is rarely productive.

Primary Attendings

A primary ICU attending can be helpful in resolving conflicts with families. Particularly at larger institutions, prolonged ICU hospitalizations expose the family to a myriad of differing management and communication styles. Some families may appreciate the differing opinions that this rotation offers. However, evidence in the adult literature shows that family dissatisfaction increases if more than two ICU physicians care for the patient (87,88). Contradictory information or conflicting recommendations regarding their child's treatment can cause confusion and emotional turmoil adding an additional layer of stress (50). Having the family choose a primary ICU attending can offer consistency in style of communication and help build a trusting relationship. Although a primary attending will not be able to make every day-to-day management decision for the child, he or she can be a consistent person to attend sequential family meetings and provide a longer-term perspective to the team than can be extraordinarily valuable when having to make difficult decisions at the end of life.

Including Bedside Nursing Staff in Conversations

Of all the members of the multidisciplinary team, the bedside nurse spends the most time with the patient and family, and has a unique and important perspective. Including the bedside nurse on rounds, in conversations with the family, and in particular in family meetings can be of great importance in resolving conflict and ensuring a consistent message is delivered. Nurses often serve as a voice for families and through their advocacy role, help inform doctors about parents' wishes (89,90), and

make family meetings more productive and pertinent. After formal meetings are over, the bedside nurse is the staff member who most often helps the family summarize, clarify, and formulate new questions.

The role of the nurse at the end of life goes far beyond the benefit of helping to reduce conflict. Once the decision to discontinue life support has been made, for example, the burden of comfort care often rests with nursing staff (91,92). Some parents report the nurse being more involved during the dying process than other family members or friends (92). The bedside nurse can help parents anticipate color and temperature changes as well as assist with bathing and other activities. Nurses, however, should take caution to avoid imposing their value systems at the end of life. Some parents have been reported to act against their own cultural values, for example by being made to feel they had to hold their child after death, simply to please the nurse (93).

Education for nurses in end of life care has increasingly become recognized as a fundamental part of the nursing curriculum. In 1998, the American Association of Colleges of Nursing developed the document "Peaceful Death: Recommended Competencies and Curricular Guidelines for End-of-Life Nursing Care" that focused on core competencies now considered requisite for each graduate (94). The End-of-Life Nursing Education Consortium (ELNEC) is a national education initiative that gives nursing leaders training in palliative care skills for dissemination to nursing students and practicing nurses (94). Evidence is showing that the ELNEC project has increased effectiveness of new graduates and faculty expertise in end of life care (95). In addition to the initial training, ongoing end of life education has also been shown to be essential to meet the needs of all staff working in the PICU (96).

Other Support Personnel

Other members of the multidisciplinary team can often help provide support to the family and are often the source of conflict resolution when it exists between members of the staff and patients or families.

Social workers often develop relationships with the family and can explore social aspects affecting care. At the end of life, they can often assist in helping families find financial assistance with funerals and other expenses in addition to connecting with bereavement groups.

A chaplain can be a comfort to the child's family, in the absence of or in addition to a family's outside spiritual advisor. Chaplains are familiar with a variety of religious practices and can serve as intermediaries when understanding a particular ritual or practice that may be unfamiliar or even uncomfortable to the medical members of the team. They are trained to support families of varying beliefs nonjudgmentally. Even families with no expressed religious preference may suffer from spiritual distress when faced with a child's death.

The primary care provider or primary specialist often have a long-standing relationship with the family, and can help illuminate sources of conflict or concern. Community pediatricians have been reported to fill unique roles of medical interpreter, advisor, and emotional support to families (92). Additionally, there may be other children in the family that the pediatrician follows, and whereas there may be little interaction with the rest of the medical team after a child's death, the pediatrician may have a continuing relationship with the family and can be mindful of extended grief, depression, and the possible need for intervention.

Role of Palliative Care Physicians

Palliative care, which can be provided by the primary medical team or a dedicated service, is medical care focused on the relief of suffering and support for the best possible quality of life for patients and families facing life-threatening illness (97). Families sometimes experience a feeling of abandonment when the primary team that has an emphasis on a cure does not appear as active in the daily comfort care (98). Having a team that can focus on the transition from cure to comfort, and has the ability to work across the inpatient and outpatient setting can significantly reduce those feelings of abandonment. Palliative care teams are usually multidisciplinary, incorporating many of the disciplines described above including advanced practice nurses, social workers, child life specialists, and chaplains in addition to physicians who specialize in end of life care for children. Some hospices are often underprepared to care for children, particularly with regard to pain management (50), and will benefit from working closely with a pediatric team.

Ethics Committees

The responsibility for medical care and resolution of ethical issues lies primarily with the physician, the health care team, and the patient and his/her family. Additional techniques and personnel, as described above, are often

sufficient for addressing challenging questions. When the medical team's efforts have been exhausted, an ethics committee should be available for conflict consultation or advice about ethical dilemmas. Additionally, members of these committees may be particularly adept in facilitating physician and family/patient communication. Bringing in an "outside" perspective in this way can often help a family and team find creative solutions to entrenched conflicts. As a broader role, the ethics committee also serves to develop and implement care policies that support the decision-making process and promote care coordination (84).

Courts

Rare circumstances exist, where despite the best efforts of all the services involved, the family, patient, and medical team cannot come to a consensus. The escalation conflict can arrive to a point where resolution is impossible without legal intervention. The movement of decision making from the bedside to the courtroom, however, virtually eliminates those other roles described above that are skilled in conflict resolution. Additionally, the involvement of the courts necessarily makes adversaries of those involved by declaring a winning and losing side (99). The courts should therefore be used as a last resort when it comes to conflict resolution.

■ SUPPORT OF STAFF AND SELF-CARE

All members of the multidisciplinary team who work closely with patients at the end of life are subject to a wide variety of profound emotions. Identifying and acknowledging distress in staff members must be a goal. Fallibility, anger, sense of loss, frustration at lack of control, and grief are only some of the complex emotional issues described. Some team members also report moral distress and loss of professional integrity (100,101). These emotions can create future interdisciplinary conflicts and can substantially impact personal and professional life. Inadequate resolutions are not sustainable, and can eventually burnout. Proactive attention to preventing staff burnout is therefore essential (100).

Debriefings

Debriefing provides a structured setting for staff to manage and respond to their grief. Discussions should help staff realize that the physical, emotional, social, and spiritual responses they experience are normal, natural responses (100). Open-ended questions like "what was it like taking care of this patient?" can help different members of the team acknowledge the importance of communication, feel less isolated, and connect with colleagues. Ideally, the facilitator should be trained in the group processes, and in recognizing potential complications of grief. The session should also provide education on identifying important coping and self-care strategies, healthy expressions of grief, and the use of support systems (102).

Finding Meaning

When the team cannot save the patient, one important aspect of supporting the staff is by shifting the focus. Instead of finding purpose and meaning in saving the patient, focus must be transitioned to relieving patient suffering and helping the family. These goals are often attainable, and can provide an enormous amount of satisfaction even in the setting of tragic loss. Staff should be encouraged to make meaningful memories, and during debriefings discuss how they will remember the patient and family (100).

■ CONCLUSION

End of life care in pediatrics presents unique challenges for all families and clinicians. Ultimately, goals focus on managing pain and other distressing symptoms, communicating honest and accurate information, making decisions consistent with a family's value system, and minimizing suffering whenever possible. Intensivists have the knowledge and experience gained from years of caring for children and their families at the end of life to be able to maximize comfort and be a guide through incredibly difficult circumstances. Skillful management of this transition is an essential final act in our care for our patients.

■ REFERENCES

1. Mathews TJ et al. Annual summary of vital statistics: 2008. *Pediatrics.* 2011;127(1):146–157.
2. Centers for Disease Control. WISQARS Leading Causes of Death Reports, National and Regional, 1999–2010. Centers for Disease Control Website. http://webappa.cdc.gov/sasweb/ncipc/leadcaus10.html.
3. Feudtner C, Connor SR. Epidemiology and health services research. In: Carter BS, Levetown M, eds. *Palliative Care for Infants, Children, and Adolescents: A Practical Handbook.* Baltimore, MD: Johns Hopkins University Press; 2004:xvi, 399 p.
4. Feudtner C et al. Characteristics of deaths occurring in children's hospitals: implications for supportive care services. *Pediatrics.* 2002;109(5):887–893.
5. Thakker JC et al. Survival and functional outcome of children requiring endotracheal intubation during therapy for severe traumatic brain injury. *Crit Care Med.* 1997;25(8):1396–1401.
6. Kochanek PM et al. Severe traumatic brain injury in infants and children. In: Fuhrman BP, Zimmerman JJ, eds. *Pediatric Critical Care.* (3rd ed.) Philadelphia, PA: Mosby-Elsevier; 2006:1595–1617.
7. Morrison WE et al. Gender and age effects on outcome after pediatric traumatic brain injury. *Pediatr Crit Care Med.* 2004;5(2):145–151.
8. Lee KJ, Tieves K, Scanlon MC. Alterations in end-of-life support in the pediatric intensive care unit. *Pediatrics.* 2010; 126(4):e859–e864.
9. Moreau J et al. ICU use and mortality are higher among children with acute CNS disorders than children with other acute disorders. *Crit Care Med.* 2010;38(12)(suppl):A22.
10. Lantos JD, Berger AC, Zucker AR, Do-not-resuscitate orders in a children's hospital. *Crit Care Med.* 1993;21(1):52–55.
11. Mink RB, Pollack MM. Resuscitation and withdrawal of therapy in pediatric intensive care. *Pediatrics.* 1992;89(5): 961–963.
12. Vernon DD et al. Modes of death in the pediatric intensive care unit: withdrawal and limitation of supportive care. *Crit Care Med.* 1993;21(11):1798–1802.
13. Levetown M et al. Limitations and withdrawals of medical intervention in pediatric critical care. *JAMA.* 1994;272(16): 1271–1275.
14. Keenan HT et al. Attitudes toward limitation of support in a pediatric intensive care unit. *Crit Care Med.* 2000;28(5): 1590–1594.
15. Randolph AG et al. Variability in physician opinion on limiting pediatric life support. *Pediatrics.* 1999;103(4):e46.
16. Naghib S et al. Mortality in very long-stay pediatric intensive care unit patients and incidence of withdrawal of treatment. *Intensive Care Med.* 2010;36(1):131–136.
17. The President's Council on Bioethics. *Controversies in the Determination of Death: A White Paper by the President's Council on Bioethics.* Washington, DC: 2008. www.bioethics.gov or http://bioethics.georgetown.edu/pcbe/.
18. Gortmaker SL et al. Improving the request process to increase family consent for organ donation. *J Transpl Coord.* 1998;8(4):210–217.
19. Davidson JE et al. Clinical practice guidelines for support of the family in the patient-centered intensive care unit: American College of Critical Care Medicine Task Force 2004–2005. *Crit Care Med.* 2007;35(2):605–622.
20. Robinson SM et al. Psychological effect of witnessed resuscitation on bereaved relatives. *Lancet.* 1998;352(9128): 614–617.
21. Hanson C, Strawser D. Family presence during cardiopulmonary resuscitation: Foote Hospital emergency department's nine-year perspective. *J Emerg Nurs.* 1992;18(2):104–106.

22. Truog RD et al. Recommendations for end-of-life care in the intensive care unit: the Ethics Committee of the Society of Critical Care Medicine. *Crit Care Med.* 2001;29(12):2332–2348.

23. Solomon MZ et al. New and lingering controversies in pediatric end-of-life care. *Pediatrics.* 2005;116(4):872–883.

24. American Academy of Pediatrics Committee on Bioethics: Guidelines on foregoing life-sustaining medical treatment. *Pediatrics.* 1994;93(3):532–536.

25. Morrison W, Berkowitz I. Do not attempt resuscitation orders in pediatrics. *Pediatr Clin North Am.* 2007;54(5):757–771, xi–xii.

26. Knox C, Vereb JA. Allow natural death: a more humane approach to discussing end-of-life directives. *J Emerg Nurs.* 2005;31(6):560–561.

27. Cohen RW. A tale of two conversations. *Hastings Cent Rep.* 2004;34(3):49.

28. Feudtner C. The breadth of hopes. *N Engl J Med.* 2009; 361(24):2306–2307.

29. Tulsky JA. Beyond advance directives: importance of communication skills at the end of life. *JAMA.* 2005;294(3):359–365.

30. Sulmasy DP, Snyder L. Substituted interests and best judgments: an integrated model of surrogate decision making. *JAMA.* 2010;304(17):1946–1947.

31. Munson D. Withdrawal of mechanical ventilation in pediatric and neonatal intensive care units. *Pediatr Clin North Am.* 2007;54(5):773–785, xii.

32. Gianakos D. Terminal weaning. *Chest.* 1995;108(5):1405–1406.

33. Feudtner C, Silveira MJ, Christakis DA. Where do children with complex chronic conditions die? Patterns in Washington State, 1980–1998. *Pediatrics.* 2002;109(4):656–660.

34. Casarett D, Kapo J, Caplan A. Appropriate use of artificial nutrition and hydration—fundamental principles and recommendations. *N Engl J Med.* 2005;353(24):2607–2612.

35. Diekema DS, Botkin JR. Clinical report—forgoing medically provided nutrition and hydration in children. *Pediatrics.* 2009;124(2):813–822.

36. Herdman R, Beauchamp TL, Potts JT. The Institute of Medicine's report on non-heart-beating organ transplantation. *Kennedy Inst Ethics J.* 1998;8(1):83–90.

37. Carcillo JA et al. A call for full public disclosure and moratorium on donation after cardiac death in children. *Pediatr Crit Care Med.* 2010;11(5):641–643; author reply 643–645.

38. Koogler T, Costarino Jr AT. The potential benefits of the pediatric nonheartbeating organ donor. *Pediatrics.* 1998; 101(6):1049–1052.

39. Friedrichsdorf SJ, Kang TI. The management of pain in children with life-limiting illnesses. *Pediatr Clin North Am.* 2007;54(5):645–672, x.

40. Ferrell B, Coyle N. *Oxford Textbook of Palliative Nursing.* 3rd ed. New York, NY: Oxford University Press; 2010.

41. Beauchamp TL, Childress JF. *Principles of Biomedical Ethics.* New York, NY: Oxford University Press; 2009.

42. Zernikow B et al. Pediatric palliative care: use of opioids for the management of pain. *Paediatr Drugs.* 2009;11(2):129–151.

43. Truog RD et al. Pharmacologic paralysis and withdrawal of mechanical ventilation at the end of life. *N Engl J Med.* 2000;342(7):508–511.

44. Wusthoff CJ, Shellhaas RA, Licht DJ. Management of common neurologic symptoms in pediatric palliative care: seizures, agitation, and spasticity. *Pediatr Clin North Am.* 2007;54(5):709–733, xi.

45. Mysiw WJ, Sandel ME. The agitated brain injured patient. Part 2: pathophysiology and treatment. *Arch Phys Med Rehabil.* 1997;78(2):213–220.

46. Ullrich CK, Mayer OH. Assessment and management of fatigue and dyspnea in pediatric palliative care. *Pediatr Clin North Am.* 2007;54(5):735–756, xi.

47. Meyer EC et al. Improving the quality of end-of-life care in the pediatric intensive care unit: parents' priorities and recommendations. *Pediatrics.* 2006;117(3):649–657.

48. Meert KL, Thurston CS, Briller SH. The spiritual needs of parents at the time of their child's death in the pediatric intensive care unit and during bereavement: a qualitative study. *Pediatr Crit Care Med.* 2005;6(4):420–427.

49. Davidson JE et al. Clinical practice guidelines for support of the family in the patient-centered intensive care unit: American College of Critical Care Medicine Task Force 2004-2005. *Crit Care Med.* 2007;35(2):605–622.

50. Contro N et al. Family perspectives on the quality of pediatric palliative care. *Arch Pediatr Adolesc Med.* 2002;156(1):14–19.

51. Azoulay E et al. Half the families of intensive care unit patients experience inadequate communication with physicians. *Crit Care Med.* 2000;28(8):3044–3049.

52. Lo B. *Resolving Ethical Dilemmas: A Guide for Clinicians.* 2nd ed. Philadelphia, PA: Lippincott Williams & Wilkins; 2000.

53. Lilly CM et al. An intensive communication intervention for the critically ill. *Am. J. Med.* 2000;109:469–475.

54. Pediatrics, Committee on Hospital Care American Academy of Pediatrics. Family-centered care and the pediatrician's role. *Pediatrics.* 2003:691–697.

55. Landry MA et al. A randomized, controlled trial of bedside versus conference-room case presentation in a pediatric intensive care unit. *Pediatrics.* 2007;120:275–280.

56. Kon AA. The shared decision-making continuum. *JAMA.* 2010;304(8):903–904.

57. Institute of Medicine, Commitee on Quality of Health Care in America. *Crossing the Quality Chasm: A New Health System for the 21st Century.* 2001. National Academies Press; 1 edition (July 18, 2001) Washington, DC.

58. Curtis JR et al. Studying communication about end-of-life care during the ICU family conference: development of a framework. *J Crit Care.* 2002;17(3):147–160.

59. Mcdonagh JR et al. Family satisfaction with family conferences about end-of-life care in the intensive care unit: increased proportion of family speech is associated with increased satisfaction. *Crit Care Med.* 2004;32(7):1484–1488.

60. Steinhauser KE et al. Factors considered important at the end of life by patients, family, physicians, and other care providers. *JAMA.* 2000;284(19):2476–2482.

61. Steinhauser KE et al. In search of a good death: observations of patients, families, and providers. *Ann Intern Med.* 2000;132(10):825–832.

62. Ohno-Machado L, Resnic FS, Matheny ME. Prognosis in critical care. *Annu Rev Biomed Eng.* 2006;8:567–599.

63. Lo B. Improving care near the end of life. Why is it so hard? *JAMA.* 1995;274(20):1634–1636.

64. Garros D, Rosychuk RJ, Cox PN. Circumstances surrounding end of life in a pediatric intensive care unit. *Pediatrics.* 2003;112(5):e371.

65. Grossoehme DH et al. Pediatrician characteristics associated with attention to spirituality and religion in clinical practice. *Pediatrics.* 2007;119(1):e117–e123.

66. Lo B et al. Discussing religious and spiritual issues at the end of life: a practical guide for physicians. *JAMA.* 2002;287:749–754.

67. Puchalski C et al. Improving the quality of spiritual care as a dimension of palliative care: the report of the Consensus Conference. *J Palliat Med.* 2009;12(10):885–904.

68. Wall RJ et al. Spiritual care of families in the intensive care unit. *Crit Care Med.* 2007;35:1084–1090.

69. Baggini J, Pym M. End of life: the humanist view. *Lancet.* 2005;366:1235–1237.

70. Dorff EN. End-of-life: Jewish perspectives. *Lancet.* 2005; 366:862–865.

71. Engelhardt HT, Iltis AS. End-of-life: the traditional Christian view. *Lancet.* 2005;366:1045–1049.

72. Firth S. End-of-life: a Hindu view. *Lancet.* 2005;366:682–686.

73. Keown D. End of life: the Buddhist view. *Lancet.* 2005; 366:952–955.

74. Markwell H. End-of-life: a Catholic view. *Lancet.* 2005; 366:1132–1135.

75. Sachedina A. End-of-life: the Islamic view. *Lancet.* 2005; 366:774–779.

76. Daaleman TP, Nease DE Jr. Patient attitudes regarding physician inquiry into spiritual and religious issues. *J Fam Pract.* 1994;40(4):330, 406.

77. Morrison W, Nelson RM. Should we talk to patients (and their families) about God? *Crit. Care Med.* 2007;35(4):1208–1209.

78. Betancourt J. Cultral competence—marginal or mainstream movement?. *JAMA.* 2004;351(10):953–954.

79. Kagawa-Singer M, Blackhall LJ. Negotiating cross-cultural issues at the end of life: "You got to go where he lives." *JAMA.* 2001;286(23):2993–3001.

80. Robinson A, Thomson R. Variability in patient preferences for participating in medical decision making: implication for the use of decision support tools. *Qual Health Care.* 2001;10(suppl 1):i34–i38.

81. Norris WM et al. Communication about end-of-life care between language-discordant patients and clinicians: insights from medical interpreters. *J Palliat Med.* 2005;8(5):1016–1024.

82. Pham K et al. Alterations during medical interpretation of ICU family conferences that interfere with or enhance communication. *Chest.* 2008;134(1):109–116.

83. Children and the death of a sibling. In: Charles A. Corr and Donna M. Corr, eds. *Handbook of Childhood Death and Bereavement.* New York, NY: Springer Publishing Co Inc; 1996:149–164.

84. Baker JN et al. Integration of palliative care practices into the ongoing care of children with cancer: individualized care planning and coordination. *Pediatr Clin North Am.* 2008;55(1):223–250, xii.

85. Pollack MM. PRISM III: an updated Pediatric Risk of Mortality Score. *Crit Care Med.* 1996;24(5):743–752.

86. Kollef MH. Outcome prediction in the ICU. In: Rubenfeld CA, ed. *Managing Death in the ICU.* New York, NY: Oxford University Press, Inc.; 2001:39–59.

87. Azoulay E et al. Meeting the needs of intensive care unit patient families: a multicenter study. *Am J Respir Crit Care Med.* 2001:163(1):135–139.

88. Johnson D, Wilson M, Cavanaugh B. Measuring the ability to meet family needs in an intensive care unit. *Crit Care Med.* 1998;26:266–271.

89. Brien IO. Medical futility in children's nursing: making end-of-life decisions. *Br J Nurs.* 2010;19(6):352–356.

90. Copnell B. Death in the pediatric ICU: caring for children and families at the end of life. *Crit Care Nurs Clin North Am.* 2005;17(4):349–360, x.

91. Curley MA, Meyer EC. The impact of the critical care experience on the family. In: M-H PA, ed. *Critical Care Nursing of Infants and Children.* Philadelphlia, PA: WB Saunders; 2001:47–67.

92. Meyer EC et al. Parental perspectives on end-of-life care in the pediatric intensive care unit. *Crit Care Med.* 2002;30(1):226–231.

93. McKinley D, Blackford J. Nurses' experiences of caring for culturally and linguistically diverse families when their child dies. *Int J Nurs Pract.* 2001;7(4):251–256.

94. American Association of Colleges of Nursing. *End-of-Life Nursing Education Consortium (ELNEC)* [cited 2011 August 8].

95. Ferrell BR et al. Evaluation of the End-of-Life Nursing Education Consortium undergraduate faculty training program. *J Palliat Med.* 2005;8(1):107–114.

96. Roberts KE, Boyle LA. End-of-life education in the pediatric intensive care unit. *Crit Care Nurse.* 2005;25:51–57.

97. Teno JM et al. Family perspectives on end-of-life care at the last place of care. *JAMA.* 2004;291(1):88–93.

98. Hinds PS et al. Key factors affecting dying children and their families. *J Palliat Med.* 2005;8(suppl 1):S70–S78.

99. Roscoe LA, Osman H, Haley WE. Implications of the Schiavo case for understanding family caregiving issues at the end of life. *Death Stud.* 2006;30(2):149–161.

100. Rushton CH et al. Interdisciplinary interventions to improve pediatric palliative care and reduce health care professional suffering. *J Palliat Med.* 2006;9(4):922–933.

101. Jellinek MS et al. Pediatric intensive care training: confronting the dark side. *Crit Care Med.* 1993;21(5):775–779.

102. Keene EA et al. Bereavement debriefing sessions: an intervention to support health care professionals in managing their grief after the death of a patient. *Pediatr Nurs.* 2010; 36(4):185–189; quiz 190.

27 *Brain Death*

MUDIT MATHUR and STEPHEN ASHWAL

Brain death is a clinical state characterized by coma and apnea with continued absence of all cortical function as well as brainstem reflexes after exclusion of confounding diagnoses, and a period of observation that establishes irreversibility. By general consensus among the medical community and legislation in the United States, brain death is death.

■ HISTORICAL PERSPECTIVE

Technological advances in the 1950s made it possible to continue to support patients who had lost all brain function by assisting their breathing and circulation. Previously, these unconscious patients lacking brainstem control of their spontaneous respirations would have been pronounced dead using the traditional cardiopulmonary criteria of cardiac asystole and apnea. This clinical state was described in 1959 as "a state beyond coma"—le coma depassé—by Mollaret and Goulon (1). They recognized that patients who had lost cortical and brainstem function could be maintained for a period of time, though deterioration in cardiopulmonary function would occur eventually despite continued mechanical support.

The recognition that cardiorespiratory functions could be supported artificially despite the lack of brain function led to efforts in the United States to redefine death. In 1968, the Harvard criteria were established based on the concept of whole brain death (2). These criteria (unreceptivity and unresponsivity, no movements or breathing off the respirator for 3 minutes, no brainstem and deep tendon reflexes, and isoelectric electroencephalogram [EEG]) formed the basis for determining brain death in older children and adults. The validity of these criteria depended on excluding temperature below 90°F (32.2°C) and central nervous system depressants (such as barbiturates). Persistence of the Harvard criteria after 24 hours of observation would confirm brain death. A prospective observational study involving 503 comatose and apneic patients at nine centers geographically distributed throughout the United States confirmed the general validity of these criteria (3). A confirmatory test demonstrating the absence of cerebral blood flow was suggested "when an early diagnosis of brain death is desired, in patients with small amounts of sedative drugs in the blood, in patients undergoing therapeutic procedures making the examination of 1 or more cranial nerves impossible, and in patients with small pupils." Clinical "Guidelines for the Determination of Death" were developed by an expert group of medical consultants using these principles to clarify accepted medical standards and provide specific guidance for physicians using neurological tests to determine death (4). The clinical guidelines for determining brain death in adults have undergone updates in 1995 and 2009, although the underlying principles of establishing coma, absent brainstem reflexes, and apnea off ventilator support endure (5,6).

■ EVOLUTION OF BRAIN DEATH GUIDELINES FOR INFANTS AND CHILDREN

Brain death guidelines were generally applied to children older than 5 years initially as "the brains of infants and young children have increased resistance to damage and may recover substantial functions even after exhibiting unresponsiveness for longer periods compared with adults" (4). A special taskforce was convened by the American Academy of Pediatrics and American Academy of Neurology to develop guidelines for determining brain death in infants and children of all ages. These guidelines were published simultaneously in several journals and widely disseminated in 1987 (7,8). Two neurologic examinations and confirmatory testing separated by varying intervals from 12 to 48 hours based on the patient's age were recommended. Confirmatory testing by an EEG to document electrocerebral silence (ECS) was recommended for all children younger than 1 year. Neonates under 7 days of age were excluded from the guidelines due to the limited clinical experience and lack of sufficient data in this population. The validity of applying these specific guidelines in newborns greater than 34 weeks of conceptual life was confirmed later (9).

A joint taskforce convened by the Society of Critical Care Medicine, American Academy of Pediatrics and Child Neurology Society reviewed and revised these guidelines in 2011 (10). There are several key changes from the 1987 guidelines. The initial waiting period before conducting the first neurologic examination, who should conduct the examination, number of examinations, interexamination interval, number of apnea tests, P_{CO_2} thresholds during apnea testing, and when an ancillary test may be conducted to reduce the interexamination observation interval or assist with the diagnosis of brain death are all clearly defined. A sample checklist is also now provided to assist clinicians with consistent performance and documentation of examination elements and ancillary testing (10).

■ DEFINITION OF BRAIN DEATH: MEDICAL AND LEGAL CONSIDERATIONS

The Uniform Determination of Death Act (UDDA; 1981) has been adopted as the legal basis of defining death throughout the United States (11). The UDDA states:

"An individual who has sustained either (1) irreversible cessation of circulatory and respiratory functions, or (2) irreversible cessation of all functions of the entire brain, including the brainstem, is dead. A determination of death must be made in accordance with accepted medical standards." Some states (New York, New Jersey) have stipulated religious exemptions to brain death, specified the number of examinations (a second physician must confirm findings in California, Alabama, Iowa, Florida, Kentucky, Louisiana, and Virginia), and physician qualification to conduct them (one of the examiners must be a specialist in the field of neurology, neurosurgery, or EEG in Virginia) (12,13).

As originally conceived by the National Conference of Commissioners of Uniform State Laws, the medical profession remains free to formulate acceptable medical practices and to utilize new biomedical knowledge, diagnostic tests, and equipment to diagnose brain death (11). Achieving uniformity in determining death was one of the goals of the U.S. President's Commission for the Study of Ethical Problems in Medicine and Biomedical and Behavioral Research as described in their analysis "Defining Death" (14). Coma and apnea with continued absence of all cortical function and brainstem reflexes after exclusion of conditions that may confound the clinical assessment, and an adequate period of observation following the initial insult to the brain to establish irreversibility are widely accepted medical principles for brain death determination in the United States.

■ INCIDENCE AND ETIOLOGY

The precise population-based incidence of brain death in infants and children is not known. There may have been approximately 1,500 infants and children who suffered brain death in the United States in 2009, based on the United Network for Organ Sharing report of 919 deceased pediatric solid organ donors, and a consent rate of 60% (percentage of eligible patients becoming donors). The incidence of brain death was reported to be 0.9% of all admissions to two pediatric intensive care units (PICUs) in one retrospective study (15). In this study, the most common cause for brain death was trauma, followed by drowning and meningitis. In another tertiary care PICU, brain death was the mechanism of death in 23% of 300 deaths, and occurred in about 1.1% of all admissions over a 54-month period (16). Cases occur throughout the pediatric age group. A list of conditions that may lead to brain death is listed in Table 27.1.

■ PATHOGENESIS

The absence of intracranial circulation precluding oxygen and nutrient delivery to brain tissue is the underlying common pathophysiology irrespective of the proximate cause of brain death. Hypoxia and ischemia result in brain injury and edema that continues to evolve during the intensive care unit (ICU) stay, and may ultimately progress to brain death after rostrocaudal brainstem herniation. Irreversible and total brain injury may also be present upon admission to the PICU, but can only be diagnosed as brain death after a period of observation and serial neurological examinations.

Neuropathologic findings in brain death are not diagnostic (17). Various findings described include the gross dusky, featureless pathological appearance described as "respirator brain," brain edema, congestion, and evidence of cerebellar tonsillar herniation. These changes appear to manifest about 12 hours after ECS is observed on EEG and are unaffected by the time interval between withdrawal of ventilator support and autopsy (18). Histologically, neuronal cytoplasm may be pale and ghostlike. White matter myelin staining appears pale, and glial cell nuclei are shrunken and pyknotic. Autolysis of the cerebellar granular layer and the pituitary gland was seen in all 60 cases in one series (19). In a recent study, moderate to severe ischemic changes were observed throughout the brain. These changes occurred in the cerebral cortex and basal ganglia in 53% to 68%, thalamus in 34%, midbrain 37%, pons 37%, medulla 40%, and cerebellum in 52% of the cases (17). The lack of uniformity in brain pathology illustrates that the whole brain death definition used in the United States follows a functional rather than a structural paradigm.

■ CLINICAL COURSE AND INTENSIVE CARE UNIT MANAGEMENT

Patients who eventually progress to meet brain death criteria are often in a deep coma upon admission to the PICU or develop a comatose state while in the ICU. Close collaboration between neurologists, neurosurgeons, and pediatric intensivists is essential in providing optimal care to these critically ill infants or children. Meticulous attention to maintenance of airway, breathing, and circulation is fundamental in avoiding secondary brain injury. A detailed history of the events leading to the patient's present condition, serial physical examination to monitor changes, and essential laboratory investigations to exclude plausible alternative diagnoses must be undertaken while stabilizing the patient in the ICU. Investigation for the cause of coma may include a blood chemistry profile with glucose, sodium, potassium, blood urea nitrogen, calcium, magnesium, and ammonia, metabolic studies, plasma and urine toxicology screens, drug levels, EEG, and neuroimaging with computed tomographic (CT) scan or magnetic resonance imaging. For a detailed approach to the initial workup and stabilization of the comatose infant or child, please refer to the Chapter "Approach to Acute Encephalopathy and Coma."

Correction of severe electrolyte and metabolic disturbances, maintaining normothermia, assurance of absence of neuromuscular blocking agents or intoxicating substances, a normal blood pressure, and optimal oxygenation and ventilation should be undertaken by the critical care team even as potential causes of coma are being investigated. This is essential to identify and treat potentially reversible causes of coma, and also sets the stage for performing a brain death examination if the patient does not improve.

■ Table 27.1 Causes of Brain Death

1. Hypoxic-ischemic brain injury: cardiopulmonary arrest, submersion injury, carbon monoxide poisoning, cyanide poisoning, strangulation, sudden infant death syndrome
2. Infectious: meningitis-bacterial or viral, viral encephalitis
3. Traumatic: (caused by closed or penetrating head trauma): cerebral contusion, epidural hematoma, intracerebral hematoma, diffuse axonal injury, shaken-baby syndrome
4. Space occupying intracranial lesions/elevated intracranial pressure: brain tumor, cyst, abscess, obstructive hydrocephalus
5. Vascular events: massive cerebral infarction, intracranial bleeding from vascular malformations, venous sinus thrombosis, embolism
6. Poisoning: lead, alcohols, drugs of abuse, insecticides, pharmacological agents, snake bite
7. Metabolic disorders: Reye syndrome, diabetic ketoacidosis, hepatic encephalopathy, uremia, urea cycle disorders, disorders of fatty acid metabolism, mitochondrial disorders

Despite optimization of physiologic parameters to maximize neuroprotection, some patients remain in or evolve to a deep unresponsive coma. These patients require a detailed neurologic examination to establish whether they meet criteria for brain death. In some cases progression to brain death may be heralded by development of a brief period of hypertension and bradycardia, signifying brainstem herniation. In other patients, some combination of pupillary changes, extreme elevation of intracranial pressure, sustained elevation of intracranial pressure above the mean arterial blood pressure precluding cerebral perfusion, development of diabetes insipidus, loss of temperature regulation, and recurrence or progression of hemodynamic instability may indicate progression to brain death. In a recent study involving adult patients, acute hypotension and polyuria signified brain death (20). Diabetes insipidus has been reported in only 38% to 41% of children with confirmed brain death and cannot be relied upon as the sole indicator of brain death (15,21). Newer modalities such as brain tissue oxygenation monitoring can also reveal the clinical progression toward brain death (22). However, the exact time-point that brain death occurs may not be clear. Indeed, the guidelines for the determination of brain death were formulated with a view to safeguard against making this diagnosis prematurely. Therefore, only after exclusion of other causes, stabilization of the patient's hemodynamic and respiratory status, and an appropriate observation period should brain death examination and testing be undertaken.

■ DIAGNOSING BRAIN DEATH

A flow chart illustrating the process for diagnosing brain death in infants and children under the current clinical guidelines is shown in Figure 27.1 (10).

Number of Examinations and Examiners

The 2011 pediatric guidelines recommend that separate attending physicians conduct the initial and confirmatory brain death examination. Apnea testing must be conducted in conjunction with each examination, but may be performed by any of the examining physicians as it is considered an objective test (10). In contrast, only one neurologic examination and apnea test is recommended according to the 2010 American Academy of Neurology guidelines to pronounce brain death in adults (6). Most brain death statutes do not specify the

qualifications of the physicians performing the examination, and local hospital policies are variable (23,24). At a minimum, the physician performing brain death examination and apnea testing should have experience in performing all the components of the neurologic examination and apnea testing. The physician should also be familiar with state law and local hospital policy and procedures before conducting this examination. There is a general consensus, and in many states specific legislation (California, Louisiana, Alabama, New Jersey) that transplant surgeons not be involved in the clinical diagnosis of brain death due to an inherent conflict of interest. It is also advisable that there be agreement among the physicians caring for a particular child in the ICU setting, that the child meets criteria for brain death.

Prerequisites

Some key prerequisites must be met before conducting brain death examination and testing in a comatose infant or child. The etiology of coma must be known, its irreversibility established, and any variables that may confound the physical examination corrected. This may require a period of observation of 24 hours or more after some inciting events such as cardiopulmonary arrest or acute traumatic brain injury in children (10). Before initiating the brain death examination, variables that can influence the clinical examination by generating an appearance of coma must be corrected to a physiologic range. These include achieving normal body temperature (using external warming if necessary) and a blood pressure that is in the normal range for age (using fluid resuscitation and/or inotropic and vasopressor support as needed). Severe electrolyte and acid-base disturbance should be corrected to physiologic values. Drug or metabolic intoxication should be excluded. Anticonvulsants, sedative medications, and neuromuscular blocking agents should be discontinued for a time period based on the half-life of the medication to ensure clearance. Elimination half-life for some medications commonly used in critical care units is provided in Table 27.2. Waiting for several half-lives in order to achieve adequate clearance of medications that may confound the clinical examination is recommended. Clinicians should keep in mind that clearance of drugs and their metabolites may be affected by factors such as the age of the child, organ dysfunction or failure, and spontaneous or induced hypothermia. Serum levels of medications with sedative properties such as barbiturates should be checked to ensure clearance to a low therapeutic range before conducting the brain death examination. Clearance of neuromuscular blocking agents can be established at the bedside by using a nerve stimulator to confirm a nondecremental "train of four" muscle twitch response (10).

Physical Examination Components

A detailed neurologic examination must be conducted to document the persistence of coma, absence of brainstem reflexes, and apnea in order to establish

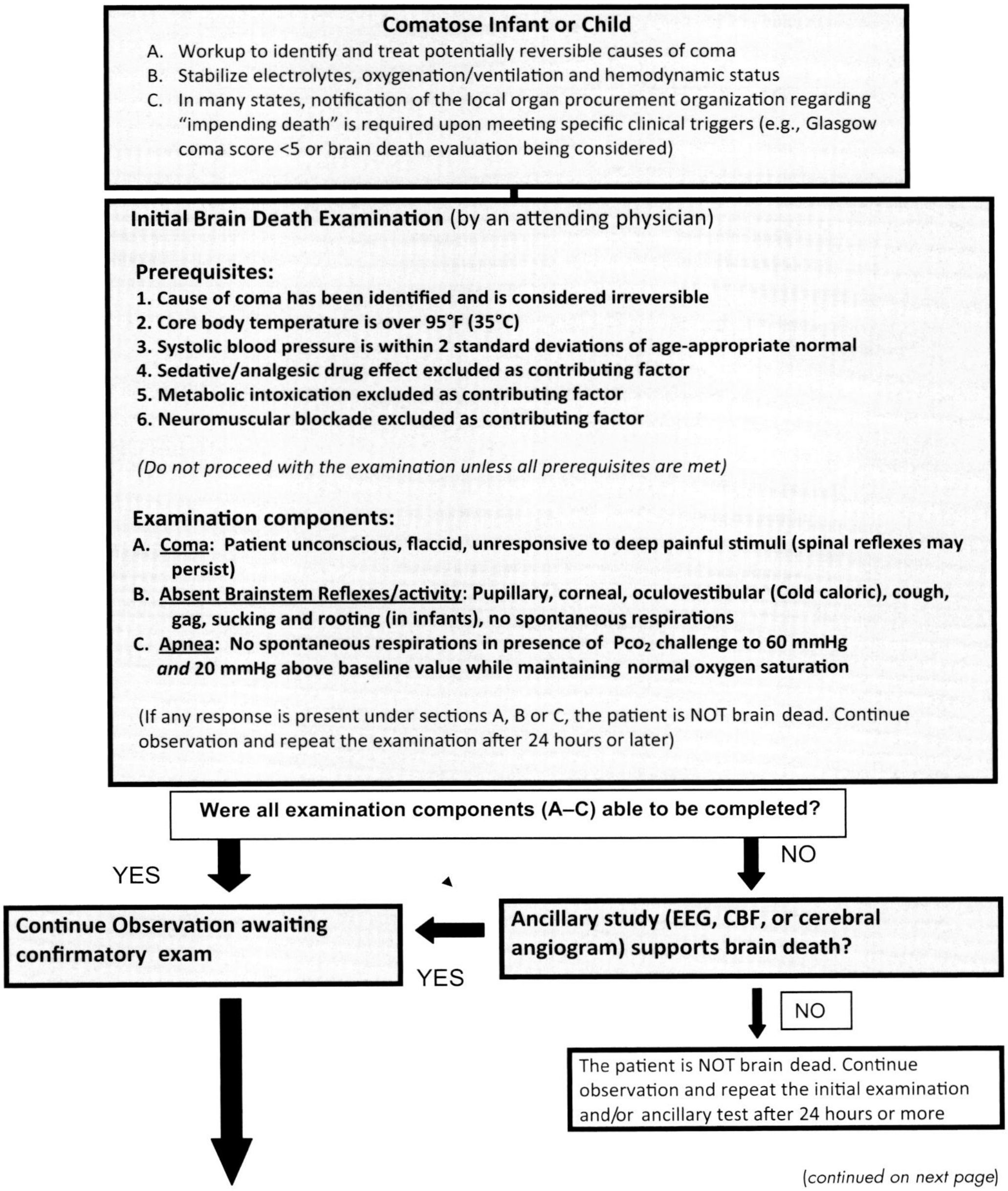

FIGURE 27.1 Evaluation for brain death in a comatose infant or child.
Based on Nakagawa TA, Ashwal S, Mathur M. et al, Guidelines for the determination of brain death in infants and children: an update of the 1987 task force recommendations. *Crit Care Med* 2011.

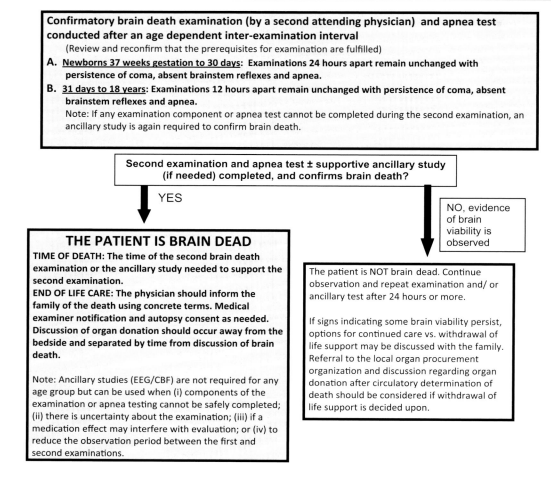

Confirmatory brain death examination (by a second attending physician) and apnea test conducted after an age dependent inter-examination interval
(Review and reconfirm that the prerequisites for examination are fulfilled)

A. <u>Newborns 37 weeks gestation to 30 days</u>: Examinations 24 hours apart remain unchanged with persistence of coma, absent brainstem reflexes and apnea.

B. <u>31 days to 18 years</u>: Examinations 12 hours apart remain unchanged with persistence of coma, absent brainstem reflexes and apnea.
Note: If any examination component or apnea test cannot be completed during the second examination, an ancillary study is again required to confirm brain death.

Second examination and apnea test ± supportive ancillary study (if needed) completed, and confirms brain death?

YES

NO, evidence of brain viability is observed

THE PATIENT IS BRAIN DEAD

TIME OF DEATH: The time of the second brain death examination or the ancillary study needed to support the second examination.
END OF LIFE CARE: The physician should inform the family of the death using concrete terms. Medical examiner notification and autopsy consent as needed. Discussion of organ donation should occur away from the bedside and separated by time from discussion of brain death.

Note: Ancillary studies (EEG/CBF) are not required for any age group but can be used when (i) components of the examination or apnea testing cannot be safely completed; (ii) there is uncertainty about the examination; (iii) if a medication effect may interfere with evaluation; or (iv) to reduce the observation period between the first and second examinations.

The patient is NOT brain dead. Continue observation and repeat examination and/ or ancillary test after 24 hours or more.

If signs indicating some brain viability persist, options for continued care vs. withdrawal of life support may be discussed with the family. Referral to the local organ procurement organization and discussion regarding organ donation after circulatory determination of death should be considered if withdrawal of life support is decided upon.

FIGURE 27.1 *(continued)*

the diagnosis of brain death. The patients should have a flaccid tone and no spontaneous or induced movements. Response to painful stimuli, pupillary light reflex, cough, gag, corneal, oculovestibular, sucking, and rooting reflexes must all be tested systematically (10). The parts of the brain and brainstem evaluated by each component of the neurologic examination are listed in Table 27.3 and the Loma Linda Brain Death Examination form is provided in Figure 27.2. According to the current guidelines, testing the oculocephalic response is no longer required (10). The examination must remain consistent throughout the period of observation and testing. It should be noted that spinal reflexes or myoclonus may occur despite brain death, although these movements are brief, slow, and rarely persistent.

Apnea Testing

Current brain death guidelines specify that arterial $Paco_2$ should rise at least 20 mmHg above the baseline and the final value should be $\geq$ 60 mmHg with no respiratory effort during the testing period to establish apnea consistent with brain death (10).

There are several considerations that clinicians must keep in mind in preparation for conducting an apnea test. Prior to initiating apnea testing, it is important that the critical care team assess the extent of preexisting lung injury, the ventilator settings, and hemodynamics and decide whether the patient will tolerate a prolonged period of apnea. Apnea testing should be deferred if there are conditions that would invalidate the apnea test (such as high cervical spine injury) or raise safety

■ **Table 27.2** Elimination Half-Life of Some Commonly Used Medications		
Medication	Half-Life in Newborns	Half-Life in Infants and Children
Phenobarbital	45–500 hours	Infants: 20–133 hours
		Children: 37–73 hours
Pentobarbital		25 hours
Midazolam	6.5–12 hours	0.78–3.3 hours
Lorazepam	40 hours	Infants: 40.2 hours (range 18–73 hours)
		Children: 10.5 hours (range 6–17 hours)
Morphine	7.6 hours (range 4.5–13.3 hours)	Infants 1–3 months: 6.2 hours (5–10 hours)
		6 months–2.5 years: 2.9 hours (1.4–7.8 hours)
		Children: 1–2 hours
Fentanyl	1–15 hours	0.5–14 years: 21 hours (range 11–36 hours for long-term infusions)

concerns for the patient (e.g., high oxygen requirement, high ventilator settings, high frequency oscillatory ventilation, potential for cardiovascular instability due to the respiratory acidosis inherent in apnea testing). If apnea testing is contraindicated or cannot be completed safely, an ancillary test (EEG or cerebral blood flow determination) may be used to assist with the determination of brain death. In general, the apnea test should be conducted by a physician who can not only make the assessment of pretest stability, but is also prepared to intervene if the patient has a clinical deterioration during the test. In a retrospective single center review of 228 adults with brain death, an apnea test could not be performed in 7% due to poor baseline hemodynamics or oxygenation and had to be aborted in 3% of patients due to hypoxemia or hypotension (25). In another case series, hypotension occurred in 24% and arrhythmias in 2.7% of 145 apnea tests (26). Greater alveolar-arterial oxygen gradient and acidosis preceding apnea test initiation have been associated with test completion failure in adult patients (27).

To create the safest possible environment for conducting an apnea test, the patient should be preoxygenated well. The simplest way to achieve this is to raise the Fio_2 on the ventilator to 1.0 for several minutes. A baseline blood gas should be obtained and recorded. Previous studies and mathematical modeling suggest that Pco_2 rises about 4 mmHg for every minute of apnea during the first 5 minutes, and 2 to 3 mmHg per minute thereafter (assuming that the patient is at a basal metabolic rate). Thus, reaching the Pco_2 threshold of 60 mmHg necessary to corroborate brain death requires at least 5 minutes of apnea in initially normocapnic infants and children (28–30). To minimize the period of apnea, a baseline blood gas should be obtained, and ventilator settings adjusted so the baseline Pco_2 is as

close to 40 mmHg as possible. Monitoring transcutaneous Pco_2 during apnea testing may help determine when the threshold of 60 mmHg has been reached, thereby limiting the occurrence of complications related to prolonged apnea (31).

The patient's upper body and abdominal area should be exposed completely to observe for any spontaneous respiratory effort throughout the apnea test. The patient can then be disconnected from the ventilator completely, connected to a T-piece attached to the endotracheal tube (ETT) or a self-inflating bag valve system such as a Mapleson circuit connected to the ETT; or maintained on continuous positive airway pressure (CPAP) mode. CPAP may provide better maintenance of oxygenation during apnea than using a T-piece (32). Tracheal insufflation of oxygen at 6 L/min using a catheter inserted through the ETT to provide apneic oxygenation has also been described, however, if this catheter obstructs the ETT significantly, barotrauma may result (33,34). Bedside monitor tracings or ventilator triggering should not be relied upon to identify respiratory effort as transmitted cardiac pulsations or a large air leak around the ETT can sometimes create a false impression of spontaneous breathing. Caution should also be observed if the CPAP mode is used during apnea testing as some ventilators may have default settings that provide an assisted breath following a preset period of apnea or a sensitive flow-by trigger mechanism giving the false appearance of a patient-initiated respiratory effort (35,36).

A follow-up blood gas should be obtained again after about 5 minutes of apnea. If the rise in Pco_2 does not meet the threshold described and the patient is clinically stable, the apnea test should be continued and blood gases repeated every few minutes until an appropriate rise in Pco_2 has occurred. The baseline and final

■ **Table 27.3** Required Elements of the Brain Death Examination

	Manner of Application	**Cranial Nerves and Brain Area Tested**	**Findings Consistent With Brain Death**
Response to painful stimulus	Pressure on supraorbital nerve, tympanomandibular joint, or nail bed	Afferent V and efferent VII (supraorbital pressure); ascending sensory fibers, reticular activating system, sensory and motor cortex (nail bed stimulation)	Absence of purposeful motor response, no decorticate or decerebrate posturing confirms unresponsive coma consistent with brain death
Pupillary response	Bright light shone on both pupils to assess direct and consensual pupillary light reflex	Cranial nerves II and III (midbrain)	Midposition pupils 4–6 mm in diameter with no response to light
Cold caloric stimulation (oculovestibular reflex)	After confirming tympanic membranes are intact, irrigation of bilateral tympanic membranes with at least 20 mL of ice water with the head of the bed at 30° elevation	Cranial nerves III, IV, VI, and VIII (medial longitudinal fasciculus, pons, and midbrain)	No eye deviation toward the cold stimulus
Corneal reflex	Touching the edge of the cornea with a swab	Cranial nerves III, V, and VII (pons)	Bilateral absence of corneal reflex (blinking)
Cough reflex	Introduction of a suction catheter through the endotracheal tube into the bronchi	Cranial nerves IX and X	No cough observed
Gag reflex	Stimulation of posterior pharynx with a tongue blade	Cranial nerves IX and X	No gag observed
Sucking reflex (in infants)	Stimulating the tongue and inside of the mouth using a finger or pacifier	Cranial nerves V, VII, XII	No sucking movements of tongue
Rooting reflex (in infants)	Stroking the cheeks toward the lips	Cranial nerves V, VII, XI	No turning toward the stimulus
Apnea test	Suspension of ventilator support while maintaining oxygenation (see text for further details)	Respiratory centers in medulla oblongata	No spontaneous respirations despite rise in P_{CO_2} 20 mmHg above baseline and final $P_{CO_2} \geq$ 60 mmHg

blood gas P_{CO_2} and the period of apnea should be recorded. Oxygen saturation should be monitored closely throughout the apnea testing. If the patient develops significant arterial desaturation or cardiovascular instability at any point, apnea testing should be stopped. The patient should be provided manually assisted ventilation immediately and placed back on the ventilator. In such cases where apnea testing cannot be completed safely, ancillary testing may be pursued to assist with diagnosing brain death (10).

Interexamination Interval, Second Brain Death Examination, and Time of Death

The current guidelines recommend that a second brain death examination and apnea test be conducted to confirm brain death after a 24 hour interval in term newborns (> 37 weeks gestation) up to the age of 30 days (recommendations for preterm neonates < 36 weeks gestation were not made because of insufficient data). Twelve hours of observation are indicated for patients

31 days or older up to the age of 18 years (10). Longer intervals are recommended for younger infants, reflecting a more cautious approach to the diagnosis of brain death in this population. The recommended intervals could be shortened if an ancillary test is conducted. The physician performing the second examination should again carefully review the patient's clinical records to ensure that there have not been any interval changes in the neurologic status. Prerequisites for brain death examination and testing as outlined previously must be reconfirmed. All elements of the neurologic examination and apnea testing should be repeated. The continued absence of all cortical and brainstem function confirms brain death. An ancillary study should be pursued in situations where a specific part of the clinical assessment cannot be performed or is unreliable. The time of the

Two attending physicians (At least one must be Neurosurgeon or Neurologist) must perform independent examinations & apnea tests separated by prescribed intervals

Age of Patient	Timing of first exam (to be documented by first examiner)	Inter-exam. Interval (to be documented by second examiner)
Term newborn 37 weeks gestational age and up to 30 days old	☐ First exam may be performed ≥ 24 hours after birth OR ≥ 24 hours following cardiopulmonary resuscitation or other severe brain injury	☐ At least 24 hours ☐ Interval shortened to ≥12 hours because ancillary study (section 4) is consistent with brain death
31 days to 18 years old	☐ First exam may be performed ≥ 24hours following cardiopulmonary resuscitation or other severe brain injury	☐ At least 12 hours OR ☐ Interval shortened to ≥ 6 hours because ancillary study (section 4) is consistent with brain death

Section 1. PREREQUISITES for brain death examination and apnea test

A. IRREVERSIBLE AND IDENTIFIABLE Cause of Coma (Please check)

☐ Traumatic brain injury ☐ Anoxic brain injury ☐ Known metabolic disorder ☐ Other (Specify) _____

B. Correction of contributing factors that can interfere with the neurologic examination		Examination One		Examination Two	
a.	Core Body Temp is over 95° F (35° C)	☐ Yes	☐ No	☐ Yes	☐ No
b.	Systolic blood pressure or MAP in acceptable range (Systolic BP not less than 2 standard deviations below age appropriate norm)based on age	☐ Yes	☐ No	☐ Yes	☐ No
c.	Sedative/analgesic drug effect excluded as a contributing factor	☐ Yes	☐ No	☐ Yes	☐ No
d.	Metabolic disturbance/intoxication excluded as a contributing factor	☐ Yes	☐ No	☐ Yes	☐ No
e.	Neuromuscular blockade excluded as a contributing factor	☐ Yes	☐ No	☐ Yes	☐ No

If ALL prerequisites are marked YES, then proceed to section 2, OR if any prerequisite is marked NO during either Exam 1 or Exam 2, a confounding variable exists. Correct confounding variable before proceeding further, OR list below and perform an ancillary study to establish brain death and document in Section 4.
☐ Exam 1: _____ confounding variable was present. Ancillary study EEG/ CBF (select one) was therefore performed
☐ Exam 2: _____ confounding variable was present. Ancillary study EEG/ CBF (select one) was therefore performed

Section 2. PHYSICAL EXAMINATION (Please check) NOTE: SPINAL CORD REFLEXES ARE ACCEPTABLE		Examination One Date/ time:		Examination Two Date/ Time:	
a.	Flaccid tone, patient unresponsive to deep painful stimuli	☐ Yes	☐ No	☐ Yes	☐ No
b.	Pupils are midposition or fully dilated and light reflexes are absent	☐ Yes	☐ No	☐ Yes	☐ No
c.	Corneal, cough, gag reflexes are absent	☐ Yes	☐ No	☐ Yes	☐ No
	Sucking and rooting reflexes are absent (in neonates and infants)	☐ Yes	☐ No	☐ Yes	☐ No
d.	Oculovestibular and/or oculocephalic reflexes are absent	☐ Yes	☐ No	☐ Yes	☐ No
e.	Spontaneous respiratory effort while on mechanical ventilation is absent	☐ Yes	☐ No	☐ Yes	☐ No

If ALL examination elements are marked YES, then proceed to section 3. If any examination element is absent due to a preexisting condition or cannot be completed due to current pathology, an ancillary study MUST be performed with each examination. List the specific examination element below, perform an ancillary study to establish brain death and document in Section 4.
☐ Exam 1: The _____ (specify) element of the exam was absent due to preexisting condition/could not be performed because:_____ Ancillary study EEG/ CBF (select one) was therefore performed to document brain death. (Section 4).
☐ Exam 2: The _____ (specify) element of the exam was absent due to preexisting condition/could not be performed because:_____ Ancillary study EEG/ CBF (select one) was therefore performed to document brain death. (Section 4).

Section 3. APNEA Test	Examination One Date/ Time_____	Examination Two Date/ Time_____
☐ No spontaneous respiratory efforts were observed despite final $PaCO_2$ ≥ 60 mmHg and a ≥ 20 mmHg increase above baseline. (Examination One) ☐ No spontaneous respiratory efforts were observed despite final $PaCO_2$ ≥ 60 mmHg and a ≥ 20 mmHg increase above baseline. (Examination Two)	Pretest $PaCO_2$: _____ Apnea duration: _____min Posttest $PaCO_2$: _____	Pretest $PaCO_2$: _____ Apnea duration: _____min Posttest $PaCO_2$: _____

(continued on next page)

FIGURE 27.2 Brain death examination for infants and children checklist.

☐ Exam 1: Apnea test is contraindicated or could not be performed to completion		
because_____. Ancillary study <u>EEG/ CBF</u> (select one) was therefore performed		
☐ Exam 2: Apnea test is contraindicated or could not be performed to completion		
because_____. Ancillary study <u>EEG/ CBF</u> (select one) was therefore performed to document brain death. (Section 4).		

Section 4. ANCILLARY STUDY

An ancillary study is only required when (1) any components of the examination or apnea testing cannot be completed; (2) if there is uncertainty about the results of the neurologic examination; or (3) if a medication effect may be present.

Ancillary studies may also be used to shorten the observation period: If an ancillary study, used in conjunction with the first neurologic examination, supports the diagnosis of brain death, the inter-examination observation interval can be shortened and the second neurologic examination and apnea test (or all components that can be completed safely) can be performed at least 6 or 12 hours later depending on the patient's age. (A second ancillary study is not necessary in this situation)

Date/Time: _____	☐ Final Electroencephalogram (EEG) report documents electrocerebral silence OR	☐ Yes ☐ No
	☐ Final Cerebral Blood Flow(CBF) study report documents no cerebral perfusion	☐ Yes ☐ No
Date/Time: _____	☐ Final Electroencephalogram (EEG) report documents electrocerebral silence OR	☐ Yes ☐ No
	☐ Final Cerebral Blood Flow(CBF) study report documents no cerebral perfusion	☐ Yes ☐ No

Section 5. Signatures

Examiner One

I certify that my examination is consistent with cessation of function of the brain and brainstem. Confirmatory exam to follow.

_____   _____
(Printed Name)   (Signature)

_____   _____ _____ _____
(Specialty)   (Pager #/License #) (Date mm/dd/yyyy)   (Time)

Examiner Two

I certify that my ☐examination (☐ and/or ancillary test report) confirms unchanged and irreversible cessation of function of the brain and brainstem. The patient is declared brain dead at this time. Date/Time of death: _____

_____   _____
(Printed Name)   (Signature)

_____   _____ _____ _____
(Specialty)   (Pager #/License #) (Date mm/dd/yyyy)   (Time)

FIGURE 27.2 (continued)

second examination confirming brain death (or of the supportive ancillary study if needed) is the legal time of death (10).

Ancillary Studies

Ancillary tests are not required for determination of brain death in infants and children under the 2011 guidelines. An ancillary study is required only if (1) any components of the examination or apnea testing cannot be completed; (2) there is uncertainty about the results of the neurologic examination; or (3) a medication effect may be present. Ancillary studies may also be used to shorten the interexamination interval to accelerate the determination of death. If the first neurologic examination and an ancillary study both support the diagnosis of brain death, the second neurologic examination and apnea test (or components that can be completed safely) can be performed at any time thereafter (10).

Ancillary studies used to support a diagnosis of brain death can be divided broadly into tests assessing cerebral blood flow (Table 27.4) and those assessing brain activity: EEG, brainstem auditory evoked potentials (BAERs), and somatosensory evoked potentials (SSEPs) (6,10). The choice of the test performed depends on clinician preference, institutional availability, as well as the advantages and disadvantages associated with each ancillary test in the context of a specific patient. Some of the commonly used tests are discussed further.

Electroencephalography

There are several advantages of using EEG as an ancillary test for brain death determination. It is portable, noninvasive, available at most hospitals, and relatively inexpensive. However, there are several problems which complicate the use of EEG. First, EEG tracings can be affected by electrical interference from bedside monitors and equipment at the highly sensitive thresholds set for brain death recordings (37,38). Second, an isoelectric EEG may occur soon after a cardiac arrest if sedative or anesthetic agents (e.g., barbiturates, benzodiazepines, narcotics, thiopental, ketamine, halothane, and isoflurane) are still impacting the brain (39). The American Electroencephalographic Society Guidelines have recommended criteria for brain death recordings (40). The EEG recording should be isoelectric for a minimum of 30 minutes and show no electrical activity beyond 2 µV at a sensitivity of 2 µV/mm, with filter settings at 0.1 or 0.3 second at 70 Hz.

■ Table 27.4 Ancillary Studies That Assess Cerebral Blood Flow

Method	Measurement	Absent Cerebral Circulation Indicated by
Cerebral angiography	High pressure and rapid, intraarterial injection of contrast agent	Absence of intracranial filling of large cerebral arteries and their major branches
Nuclear medicine scan (cerebral blood flow scan)	Intravenous rapid bolus injection of radionuclide isotope such as Tc99m diethylene-triamine-penta-acetic acid or HMPAO Tc99m hexa-methyl-propylene-amine oxide, Tc99m pertechnate	Absence of radionuclide detection in blood pools in the distribution of large vessels and brain parenchyma
Tc99m HMPAO SPECT	Similar to radionuclide imaging but with high resolution, 3 dimensional imaging system; lateral static images can assess the brainstem and cerebellum	Absence of activity on dynamic scintigraphy and absent brain isotope uptake on static images
CT angiography	Use of conventional CT scanning combined with use of rapid infusion of contrast agent to visualize intracranial vessels	Relatively new method with data from adult studies that show lack of filling of intracranial arteries
MRI and MRA	Use of conventional MRI to detect red blood cells within intracranial arteris as an indicator of blood vessel structure	MRI demonstrates edema; MRA demonstrates lack of filling of intracranial blood vessels
Transcranial Doppler	Measures blood velocity from large intracranial vessels during diastole and systole	Serial changes with loss of diastolic flow, flow reversal, and loss of systolic flow
Digital subtraction angiography	Imaging that provides visualization of cerebral vessels	Absence of contrast material within large cerebral vessels
Spiral CT	Sequential scans in 10 mm sections 20 and 60 seconds after injection of contrast	Absence of bilateral cortical middle cerbral artery and internal cerbral vein opacification
Xenon CT	Provides quantitative measure of cerebral blood flow by inhalation of xenon gas detected with cranial CT	Cerebral blood flow values < 5–10 mL/min/100 g indicate absence of cerebral circulation

Abbreviations: CT, computed tomography; HMPAO, Hexamethylpropyleneamine oxime; MRA, magnetic resonance angiography; MRI, magnetic resonance imaging; SPECT, Single Photon Emission Computed Tomography; Tc99m, Technetium99m.

Measuring Cerebral Blood Flow: Angiography and Radionuclide Cerebral Imaging

The technique of assessing cerebral blood flow (CBF) using radionuclide cerebral imaging has been evaluated against 4-vessel dye contrast arteriography (cerebral angiogram) in children and shows complete agreement (41,42). Although cerebral angiogram has been considered the gold standard for ancillary testing as it directly evaluates the intracranial circulation, it is rarely performed in clinical practice (10). It is expensive, invasive, time consuming, and requires the patient to be moved to the angiography suite. There are risks associated with contrast material itself such as allergic reaction or potential renal damage. These drawbacks have led clinicians to increasingly use CBF as the ancillary test for direct evaluation of cerebral blood flow. The advantages of CBF include that it is noninvasive, portable to the patient's bedside, and has lower costs. CBF has an important added benefit similar to cerebral angiography in that it is unaffected by the presence of sedative medications that obscure the clinical and EEG examination (43–45).

EEG vs CBF

Although EEG continues to be a reliable modality, contemporary practice appears to be shifting toward the use of CBF as the preferred ancillary test in infants and children (46,47). It should be noted that though CBF may be more commonly utilized, the diagnostic yield when both EEG and CBF are initially performed is about 70% for either study in infants and children older than 1 month of age (10). For newborns, CBF should be the preferred modality as EEG with ECS is less sensitive (40%) than absence of CBF (63%) when confirming the diagnosis of brain death (10).

Other Ancillary Tests

Bispectral (BIS) monitoring: BIS is an EEG-derived method of assessing brain activity and may be useful in assessing progression to brain death (48,49). However, being EEG derived, it shares all its disadvantages. Also, BIS readings may decrease to zero prior to brain death (50). Thus, its utility as a definitive ancillary test appears to be limited at this time.

Brainstem auditory and somatosensory evoked potentials: The role of BAERs and SSEPs in brain death determination have been studied in children (51,52) but are not among the recommended ancillary tests in the current guidelines (10).

CT angiography: CT angiogram is a rapid, less invasive test with wider availability than conventional angiography, though it still requires patient transport. It has been compared directly against a nuclear medicine perfusion scan in adult subjects for brain death confirmation. CT angiogram appeared to be an efficient test with no demonstrated false negatives; and an increased sensitivity to detecting minimal cerebral blood flow in patients with open skull defects (53). In another analysis, its sensitivity was 85.7% and specificity 100% in confirming brain death (54). However, some other studies have described poor sensitivity and concordance with 4-vessel cerebral angiography (55,56).

Transcranial Doppler: The observation of reverberant flow and short systolic spikes on transcranial Doppler are indicative of absence of cerebral blood flow. This technique is easier to perform in pediatric and neonatal patients due to thin temporal bone windows; however, the presence of nonossified fontanelles in infants may alter the observed flow pattern and affect interpretation (57,58).

Brain tissue oxygenation: This technique uses invasive monitors that monitor brain tissue oxygenation directly. These monitors have been used to optimize neurocritical care therapy in patients with elevated intracranial pressure. Incidentally, it was observed that brain tissue oxygenation decreased to zero in five children who progressed to brain death, and remained above this threshold in 80 others who did not (59). Comparative data against established modalities is needed to evaluate the utility of this ancillary test.

■ END-OF-LIFE CONSIDERATIONS

Communication With the Family

The role of the critical care and neuroscience physicians is not complete after the confirmatory brain death examination. Lay persons have a poor understanding of brain death, and families may question the diagnosis of death. Their child continues to feel warm to touch, has a heartbeat, and is breathing though all these functions are maintained only as a result of technological ICU support. In one study, only half the families surveyed reported receiving an explanation regarding brain death and in others only one-third of families understood that death had occurred (60–62). It is important for the physician to use concrete terms in conveying the diagnosis of death to the family. Allowing the family to be present during the examination and apnea testing, allowing time for them to understand the diagnosis, and enlisting the assistance of organ procurement organization family care support personnel may help in this process.

In some situations, the critical care team may have to balance the added time needed for the family to come to terms with the diagnosis of brain death against scarce ICU resources needed to assist other critically ill children. For example, California law requires hospitals to consider the needs of other patients and prospective patients in urgent need of care while providing a "reasonably brief" period of accommodation for family or next of kin to gather at the patient's bedside. No new medical intervention is required during this period, though previous cardiopulmonary support is continued (63).

Consideration of Organ Donation

The family must be given time to understand that their loved one has died before any discussions regarding organ donation. "Uncoupling" the request for donation from the pronouncement of death and a trained requestor making the request in a private setting improve consent rates for donation (64). Early referral to the designated organ procurement organization and the presence of an in-house organ procurement organization representative to coordinate the request for donation may be helpful in improving donation rates (65, 66). Approval from the coroner/medical examiner's office should be obtained in cases of suspected child abuse before organ donation can proceed. If the family declines organ donation, ventilator support can be discontinued at any time thereafter.

Organ Donor Management

Hypotension, hypothermia, diabetes insipidus, hypernatremia, hyperglycemia, pulmonary edema, pneumonia, and coagulopathy may all occur in brain dead children and require ongoing management when organ donation is being considered (67). Such management may include the initiation of hormonal replacement therapy with thyroxine, vasopressin, and corticosteroids as well as precise hemodynamic titration and ventilator adjustments that optimize organ function (68–71). A detailed discussion of organ donor management is beyond the scope of this chapter. Ideally, the critical care team should continue to provide consultation to the personnel managing the potential donor. Aggressive and protocol-driven donor management has been shown to improve donor stability and increase organ yield (72–74). Ultimately, optimal donor management has the potential to help the thousands of potential recipients waitlisted for solid organ transplantation in the United States.

Patients Who Do Not Fulfill Brain Death Criteria

Some children who undergo brain death examination may have remnants of brain function, with clinical examination findings or ancillary test results that do not support the diagnosis of brain death. The clinicians must discuss these findings and probable long-term prognosis with the family. Magnetic resonance spectroscopy may provide additional information and assist with prognostication (75–76). Options for long-term placement in a chronic care facility after surgical placement of tracheostomy and feeding tubes versus withdrawal of life support should be discussed. If the family elects to withdraw life support, the local organ procurement organization should be consulted again as organ donation after circulatory determination of death may be a consideration.

■ SPECIAL SITUATIONS AND FUTURE DIRECTIONS

Lazarus Sign

Unusual spontaneous movements described in brain dead patients typically occurring during terminal apnea after disconnection from the ventilator are sometimes referred to as the "Lazarus sign." These may include finger jerks, triple flexion response, arching of the back, neck turning, stiffening of the legs, and upper extremity flexion. These spinal movements can be categorized into monosegmental muscle stretch reflexes, oligosegmental cutaneomuscular reflexes, and polysegmental spinal automatism patterns (77). They may produce distress among health care personnel or family members, but these nonpurposeful stereotypical movements are spinal cord induced and in no way inconsistent with the diagnosis of brain death (78–81).

Pitfalls in the Diagnosis of Brain Death

Cases of drug intoxication, delayed clearance of medications (such as barbiturates, tricyclic antidepressants, baclofen, lidocaine, neuromuscular blockers), severe hypothermia, locked-in syndrome, Guillain-Barré syndrome or other acute neuromuscular disorders involving central and peripheral nerves, brainstem encephalitis, organophosphate poisoning, and high spinal cord injury can all appear clinically similar to brain death (82–88). In most of the reported cases of apparent "brain death," at least one discrepancy from established brain death examination findings can be identified. Appropriate laboratory tests such as plasma drug screening to characterize the unknown agent and neuroimaging including the cervical spinal cord should be conducted if there are inconsistencies in the patient's clinical history or neurologic examination. It is imperative that the patient be observed for a longer period, the clinical examination repeated, and ancillary studies obtained if the proximate cause of coma is unclear. The advent of new treatment modalities such as therapeutic hypothermia after cardiac arrest may also change the severity of brain injury, or the time course in which it manifests (89–90). Clinicians should extend the observation period as necessary, or obtain an ancillary test to diagnose brain death under such circumstances (10). By carefully following these principles, an inaccurate diagnosis of brain death can be avoided.

Improving Consistency in the Implementation of Brain Death Guidelines

Physician documentation of clinical examination and ancillary tests used for determining brain death is inconsistent, and frequently incomplete in both adults and children (47,91). The Presidential Commission's goals were to develop guidelines that are clear, consistent, uniform, and reliable for diagnosis, declaration, documentation, and reporting of brain death. Previous pediatric guidelines were also intended to fit these needs, but in practice have not proven to do so as individual providers variably translated them into clinical practice (46,47,92). Codifying brainstem death guidelines into the simpler format of a checklist has proved useful in improving documentation of this crucial determination in the United Kingdom in two of three reported studies (93–95). A checklist is also provided in the Canadian forum's recommendations for neurologic determination of death, although there are no published data describing its utilization and effectiveness (96). There is emerging data suggesting that a computerized template or checklist may be useful in improving the consistency of brain death documentation in infants and children at the hospital level in the United States (97,98). Using the checklist included with the 2011 update of the pediatric brain death guidelines could standardize their implementation across variable state laws, hospital policies, and individual preferences, making the documentation of this crucial determination more uniform nationally. A sample checklist based on the 2011 guidelines is shown in Figure 27.2. Accuracy in the determination and documentation of brain death is important to retain the confidence of our communities in the medical profession and the process of organ donation and transplantation.

■ CONCLUSIONS

Brain death is a clinical diagnosis made in a patient with coma and apnea after a period of observation and systematic evaluation and exclusion of confounding factors. The clinical examination must demonstrate complete cessation of functions of the entire brain including the brainstem. Two complete neurologic examinations and apnea tests separated by age-dependent intervals must be performed to establish brain death. Using a checklist based on the current brain death guidelines may help to standardize their implementation and documentation

across variable state laws, hospital policies, and individual preferences. Neurocritical care specialists must provide a supportive environment while communicating the diagnosis of brain death to the family using unambiguous terms. End of life options such as autopsy and organ donation should be discussed at a later time once the family has understood that their child has died. Further care decisions regarding patients who do not fulfill brain death criteria should be made considering the family's wishes, and may include withdrawal of life support or ongoing chronic care in a specialized long-term care facility.

■ REFERENCES

1. Mollaret P, Goulon M. Le coma depasse. *Rev Neurol.* 1959;101:3–15.
2. A definition of irreversible coma; report of Ad Hoc Committee of the Harvard Medical School to Examine the Definition of Brain Death. *JAMA.* 1968;205:337–340.
3. Collaborative study on brain death: an appraisal of the criteria of cerebral death: A summary statement. *JAMA.* 1977;237:982–986.
4. Guidelines for the determination of death. Report of the Medical Consultants on the Diagnosis of Death to the President's Commission for the Study of Ethical Problems in Biomedical and Behavioral Research. *JAMA.* 1981;246(19):2184–2186.
5. The Quality Standards Subcommittee of the American Academy of Neurology. Practice parameters for determining brain death in adults (summary statement). *Neurology.* 1995;45:1012–1014.
6. Wijdicks EFM, Varelas PN, Greer DM. Determining brain death in adults: 2009 guideline update. *Neurology.* 2010;74:1911–1918.
7. Report of Special Task Force: Guidelines for determination of brain death in children. *Pediatrics.* 1987;80:298–300.
8. Guidelines for determination of brain death in children. *Pediatr Neurol.* 1987;3(4):242–243.
9. Ashwal S, Schneider S. Brain death in the newborn: clinical, EEG and blood flow determinations. *Pediatrics.* 1989;84:429.
10. Nakagawa TA et al. Guidelines for the determination of brain death in infants and children: an update of the 1987 task force recommendations. *Crit Care Med.* 2011;39:2139–2155.
11. Uniform Brain Death Act. Uniform Laws annot 12:63 (west 1993; west suppl. 1997). Paper presented at: National Conference of Commissioners of Uniform State Laws Meeting; 1980; Kauai, HI; p2.
12. Determination of death. 10 N.Y.C.R.R. § 400.16, e(3).
13. New Jersey Declaration of Death Act. Death not declared in violation of individual's religious beliefs. L1991. ch 90; NJSA 26:6A–5.
14. President's Commission for the Study of Ethical Problems in Medicine and Biomedical and Behavioral Research. *Defining Death: Medical, Legal and Ethical Issues in the*

Determination of Death. Washington, DC: US Government Printing Office, 1981.

15. Staworn D et al. Brain death in pediatric intensive care unit patients: incidence, primary diagnosis, and the clinical occurrence of Turner's triad. *Crit Care Med*. 1994;22(8):1301–1305.
16. Vernon DD et al. Modes of death in the pediatric intensive care unit: withdrawal and limitation of supportive care. *Crit Care Med*. 1993;21:1798–1802.
17. Wijdicks EFM, Pfeifer EA. Neuropathology of brain death in the modern transplant era. *Neurology*. 2008;70:1234–1237.
18. Leestma JE, Hughes JR, Diamond ER. Temporal correlates in brain death. EEG and Clinical relationships to the respirator brain. *Arch Neurol*. 1984;41:147–152.
19. Ujihara N, Hasizume Y, Takahasi A. A clinico-neuropathological study on brain death. *Nagoya J Med Sci*. 1993;56(1-4):89–99.
20. Wijdicks EFM et al. Pronouncing brain death. Contemporary practice and safety of the apnea test. *Neurology*. 2008;71:1240–1244.
21. Fiser DH et al. Diabetes insipidus in children with brain death. *Crit Care Med*. 1987;15(6):551–553.
22. Palmer S, Bader MK. Brain tissue oxygenation in brain death. *Neurocrit Care*. 2005;2:17–22.
23. Greer DM et al. Variability of brain death determination guidelines in leading neurologic institutions. *Neurology*. 2008;70:284–289.
24. Powner DJ, Hernandez M, Rives TE. Variability among hospital policies for determining brain death in adults. *Crit Care Med*. 2004;32:1284–1288.
25. Wijdicks EFM et al. Pronouncing brain death. Contemporary practice and safety of the apnea test. *Neurology*. 2008;71:240–1244.
26. Goudreau JL, Wijdicks EFM, Emery SF. Complications during apnea testing in brain death-predisposing factors. *Neurology*. 2000;55(7)1045–1048.
27. Lee AH et al. Predictors of apnea test failure during brain death determination. *Neurocrit Care*. 2010;12:352–355.
28. Rowland TW, Donnelly JH, Jackson AH. Apnea documentation for determination of brain death in children. *Pediatrics*. 1984;74:505–508.
29. Paret G, Barzilay Z. Apnea testing in suspected brain dead children—physiological and mathematical modeling. *Intensive Care Med*. 1995;21:247–252.
30. Outwater KM, Rockoff MA. Apnea testing to confirm brain death in children. *Crit Care Med*. 1984;12:357–358.
31. Vivien B et al. An evaluation of transcutaneous carbon dioxide partial pressure monitoring during apnea testing in brain-dead patients. *Anesthesiology*. 2006;104(4):701–707.
32. Levesque S et al. Efficacy of a T-piece system and a continuous positive airway pressure system for apnea testing in the diagnosis of brain death. *Crit Care Med*. 2006;34(8):2213–2216.
33. Bar-Joseph G, Bar-Levie Y, Zonis Z. Tension pneumothorax during apnea testing for the determination of brain death. *Anesthesiology*. 1998;89:1250–1251.
34. Monterrubio-Villar J, Cordoba-Lopez A. Barotrauma during apnoea testing for brain death determination in a five-year-old boy. *Anaesth Intens Care*. 2008;36(3):462–463.
35. Wijdicks EFM, Manno EM, Holets SR. Ventilator self-cycling may falsely suggest patient effort during brain death determination. *Neurology*. 2005;65(5):774.

36. Willatts SM, Drummond G. Brain death and ventilator trigger settings. *Anaesthesia*. 2000;55:676–684.
37. Moshe SL. Usefulness of EEG in the evaluation of brain death in children: the pros. *Electroencephalogr Clin Neurophysiol*. 1989;73:272–274.
38. Schneider S. Usefulness of EEG in the evaluation of brain death in children: the cons. *Electroencephalogr Clin Neurophysiol*. 1989;73:276–278.
39. Schmitt B et al. Resuscitation after severe hypoxia in a young child: temporary isoelectric EEG and loss of BAEP components. *Intensive Care Med*. 1993;19:420–422.
40. American Electroencephalographic Society. Guideline three: minimum technical standards for EEG recording in suspected cerebral death. *J Clin Neurophysiol*. 2006;23(2):97–104.
41. Schwartz JA, Baxter J, Brill DA. Diagnosis of brain death in children by radionuclide cerebral imaging. *Pediatrics*. 1984;73(1):14–18.
42. Singh NC et al. Usefulness of (Tc99m) HM-PAO scan in supporting clinical brain death in children: uncoupling flow and function. *Clin Intensive Care*. 1994;5(2):71–74.
43. Conrad G, Sinha P. Scintigraphy as a confirmatory test of brain death. *Semin Nucl Med*. 2003;33(4):312–323.
44. Goodman JM, Heck LL, Moore BD. Confirmation of brain death with portable isotope angiography: a review of 204 consecutive cases. *Neurosurgery*. 1985;16(4):492–497.
45. Holzman BH et al. Radionuclide cerebral perfusion scintigraphy in determination of brain death in children. *Neurology*. 1983;33(8):1027–1031.
46. Mejia RE, Pollack MM. Variability in brain death determination practices in children. *JAMA*. 1995;274(7):550–553.
47. Mathur M et al. Variability in pediatric brain death determination and documentation in southern California. *Pediatrics*. 2008;121(5):988–993.
48. Misis M et al. Bispectral EEG monitoring for early detection of brain death. *Transpl Proc*. 2008;40(5):1279–1281.
49. Okuyaz C et al. Bispectral index monitoring in confirmation of brain death in children. *J Child Neurol*. 2006;21:799–801.
50. Vivien B et al. Detection of brain death onset using the bispectral index in severely comatose patients. *Intensive Care Med*. 2002;28:419–425.
51. Ruiz-Garcia M et al. Brain death in children: clinical, neurophysiological and radioisotopic angiography findings in 125 patients. *Childs Nerv Syst*. 2000;16:40–45.
52. Ruiz-Lopez MJ et al. Brain death and evoked potentials in pediatric patients. *Crit Care Med*. 1999;27:412–416.
53. Berengeur CM, Davis FE, Howington JU. Brain death confirmation: comparison of computed tomographic angiography with nuclear medicine perfusion scan. *J Trauma*. 2010;68:553–559.
54. Frampas E et al. CT angiography for brain death diagnosis. *Am J Neuroradiol*. 2009;30:1566–1570.
55. Quesnel C et al. Limitations of computerized tomographic angiography in the diagnosis of brain death. *Intensive Care Med*. 2007;33:2129–2135.
56. Combes JC et al. Reliability of computed tomographic angiography in the diagnosis of brain death. *Transpl Proc*. 2007;39:16–20.
57. de Freitas GR, Andre C. Sensitivity of transcranial Doppler for confirming brain death: a prospective study of 270 cases. *Acta Neurol Scand*. 2006;113:426–432.

58. Vincenzini E et al. Transcranial Doppler for brain death in infants: the role of the fontanelles. *Eur Neurol*. 2010;63: 164–169.

59. Figaji AA, Kent SJ. Brain tissue oxygenation in children diagnosed with brain death. *Neurocrit Care*. 2010;12:56–61.

60. Franz HG et al. Explaining brain death: a critical feature of the donation process. *J Transpl Coord*. 1997;7(1): 14–21.

61. Pearson IY et al. A survey of families of brain dead patients: their experiences, attitudes to organ donation and transplantation. *Anaesth Intensive Care*. 1995;23(1):88–95.

62. Siminoff LA, Mercer MB, Arnold R. Families' understanding of brain death. *Prog Transplant*. 2003;13(3):218–224.

63. CA health and safety code, section 1254.4.

64. Gortmaker SL et al. Improving the request process to increase family consent for organ donation. *J Transpl Coord*. 1998;8(4):210–217.

65. Siminoff LA et al. Factors influencing families' consent for donation of solid organs for transplantation. *JAMA*. 2001;286(1):71–77.

66. Shafer TJ et al. Location of in-house organ procurement organization staff in level I trauma centers increases conversion of potential donors to actual donors. *Transplantation*. 2003;75:1330–1335.

67. Lutz-Dettinger N, de Jaeger A, Kerremans I. Care of the potential pediatric organ donor. *Pediatr Clin North Am*. 2001; 48:715–749.

68. Katz K et al. Vasopressin pressor effects in critically ill children during evaluation for brain death and organ recovery. *Resuscitation*. 2000;47:33–40.

69. Zuppa AF et al. The effect of a thyroid hormone infusion on vasopressor support in critically ill children with cessation of neurologic function. *Crit Care Med*. 2004;32: 2318–2322.

70. Schnuelle P et al. Effects of catecholamine application to brain-dead donors on graft survival in solid organ transplantation. *Transplantation*. 2001;72(3):455–463.

71. Nakagawa TA. Updated pediatric donor management and dosing guidelines. NATCO, the Organization for Transplant Professionals Web site. www.natco1.org/prof_development/index.htm#guidelines. Updated 2008. Accessed Nov 1, 2010.

72. Rosendale JD et al. Increased transplanted organs from the use of a standardized donor management protocol. *Am J Transplant*. 2002;2:761–768.

73. Finfer S et al. Intensive care management of paediatric organ donors and its effect on post-transplant organ function. *Intensive Care Med*. 1996;22:1424.

74. Rosendale JD et al. Aggressive pharmacologic donor management results in more transplanted organs. *Transplantation*. 2003;75:482–487.

75. Babikian T et al. MR spectroscopy: predicting long-term neuropsychological outcome following pediatric TBI. *J Magn Reson Imaging*. 2006;24(4):801–811.

76. Shutter L, Tong KA, Holshouser BA. Proton MRS in acute traumatic brain injury: role for glutamate/glutamine and choline for outcome prediction. *J Neurotrauma*. 2004;21(12): 1693–1705.

77. Spittler JF et al. Phenomenological diversity of spinal reflexes in brain death. *Eur J Neurol*. 2000;7:315–321.

78. Marti-Fabregas J et al. Decerebrate-like posturing with mechanical ventilation in brain death. *Neurology*. 2000;54: 224–227.

79. Ropper A. Unusual spontaneous movements in brain-death patients. *Neurology*. 1984;34:1089.

80. Saposnik G et al. Spontaneous and reflex movement in brain death. *Neurology*. 2000;54:221.

81. Christie JM, O'Lenie TD, Cane RD. Head turning in brain death. *J Clin Anaesth*. 1996;8:141–143.

82. Wijdicks EFM. The diagnosis of brain death. *N Engl J Med*. 2001;344(16):1215–1221.

83. Joffe AR, Anton N, Blackwood J. Brain death and the cervical spinal cord: a confounding factor for the clinical examination. *Spinal Cord*. 2010;48:2–9.

84. Freidman Y et al. Simulation of brain death from fulminant de-afferentation. *Can J Neurol Sci*. 2003;30:397–404.

85. Ostermann ME et al. Coma mimicking brain death following baclofen overdose. *Intensive Care Med*. 2001;27(5):945–947.

86. Kainuma M, Miyake T, Kanno T. Extremely prolonged vecuronium clearance in a brain death case. *Anesthesiology*. 2001;95:1023–1024.

87. Peter JV, Prabhakar AT, Pichamuthu K. In-laws, insecticide and a mimic of brain death. *Lancet*. 2008;371(9612):622.

88. Richard IH et al. Non-barbiturate, drug induced reversible loss of brainstem reflexes. *Neurology*. 1998;51(2)639–640.

89. Joffe AR et al. A 10 month old with reversible findings of brain death. *Pediatr Neurol*. 2009;41(5):378–382.

90. Shemie SD, Langevin S, Farrell C. Therapeutic hypothermia after cardiac arrest: another confounding factor in brain-death testing. *Pediatr Neurol*. 2010;42(4):304.

91. Wang MY, Wallace P, Gruen JP. Brain death documentation: analysis and issues. *Neurosurgery*. 2002;51:731–736.

92. Harrison AM, Botkin JR. Can Pediatricians define and apply the concept of brain death? *Pediatrics*. 1999;103(6):e82.

93. Keogh AT, Akhtar TM. Diagnosing brain death: the importance of documenting clinical test results. *Anesthesiology*. 1999;54:81–83.

94. Kafrawy U, Stewart D. An evaluation of brainstem death documentation: the importance of full documentation. *Pediatr Anesth*. 2004;14:584–588.

95. Goh AYT, Mok Q. Clinical course and determination of brainstem death in a children's hospital. *Acta Paediatr*. 2004; 93:47–52.

96. Shemie SD et al. Severe brain injury to neurological determination of death: Canadian forum recommendations. *Can Med Assoc J*. 2006;174:S1–S12.

97. Stockwell JA, Pham N, Fortenberry JD. Impact of a computerized note template/checklist on documented adherence to institutional criteria for determination of neurologic death in a pediatric intensive care unit. *Pediatr Crit Care Med*. 2011;12(3):271–276.

98. Mathur M, Syed A, Ashwal S. Using a checklist improves pediatric brain death documentation. *Crit Care Med*. 2010;12(suppl):A720.

28 *Ethical Issues*

MATTHEW P. KIRSCHEN and CHRIS FEUDTNER

■ INTRODUCTION

What are the ethical issues that clinicians should anticipate and consider when caring for children with critical
neurologic illnesses and their families in the intensive
care unit (ICU)? The first step in addressing clinical ethical dilemmas is recognizing them when they arise, from
the time of hospital admission through to discharge.
After recognizing and defining an ethical conflict—
important steps that can be quite challenging—an appropriate resolution may be simple or intricate, and may
require input from third parties like ethics committees.
This chapter aims to help pediatric neurocritical care clinicians to be better able to anticipate, recognize, examine, and manage ethically problematic situations in the
care of these critically ill patients.

■ FRAMEWORK OF ANTICIPATORY GUIDANCE FOR ADDRESSING ETHICAL ISSUES

Anticipate is a key word in the paragraph above. During
ICU hospitalizations, conflicts emerge between the medical team and family frequently enough that they should
be anticipated. In one prospective study of pediatric
critical care physicians and nurses, conflicts arose in
managing nearly half of the children admitted for more
than 8 days (1). Drawing on guidelines developed for
the ethical treatment of critically ill infants and children
(2), we have organized this chapter so as to provide the

reader with a framework for anticipating and either
preventing or managing ethical problems when treating
children with brain injury in the ICU.

Identifying an Authorized Decision-Maker

A prerequisite for ethical decision-making is to identify a person who has the authority to speak on behalf
of the patient. Parents or guardians typically serve as
authorized decision makers for children with neurologic injuries and determine goals of care and consent
to (grant permission for) medical care. The standards
that an authorized decision maker must meet to consent
to medical treatment include: (1) they appreciate that
they have a choice; (2) they appreciate the situation and
prognosis as well as risks, benefits, and consequences
of treatments; (3) their decisions are stable over time
and not impulsive; and (4) their decisions are consistent
with their personal values and goals of care (3,4). If a
member of the medical team feels that the authorized
decision-maker lacks competence to make treatment
decisions, that medical provider is ethically required to
request a capacity evaluation.

In rare circumstances, children can make medical
decisions for themselves if they have been emancipated
or deemed a mature minor for medical decision-making
purposes (5). Common reasons for emancipation include
marriage, pregnancy or having a child, military service,
financial independence, and living apart from parents.
State courts determine mature minor status by weigh-
ing age, ability, experience, education, training, degree
of maturity or judgment, and capacity to appreciate the

nature, risks, and consequences of procedures (6–8). Most often, a child must be at least 14 years old to be considered, as some studies have shown that children this age have the same ability to make health care decisions as adults (9).

The American Academy of Pediatrics (AAP) has defined the concept of assent for older children and adolescents who are not their own medical decisions makers. The four components of assent are: (1) an appropriate awareness of the nature of their condition; (2) knowledge of what they can expect with tests and treatments; (3) a positive clinical assessment of their understanding of the situation and the factors influencing their response; and (4) an expression of the patient's willingness to accept care (5). The AAP argues that all children are entitled to understandable medical information and the opportunity to assent or dissent, and emphasizes that a child's views, once solicited, should be given serious weight. The AAP also advises that if a child is forced to undergo care despite objection, the reasons for doing so should be made clear to them. Dissent in other contexts should be used as an opportunity to explore the child's discomfort with a test, therapy, or the trajectory of the care plan, and to find an amicable solution with mutual understanding between the patient, parents, and physician (5,10).

Children or young adults who have sustained damage to specific language networks in their brains either by a stroke or other focal injury can have difficulty providing assent or consent. Assessing competence in aphasic patients can be very challenging (11,12). A patient might be able to understand their medical situation, but unable to express their preferences. Likewise, they may be able to speak fluently and express their thoughts, but unable to appreciate the scope and potential consequences of their medical situation and treatment options. It is important to involve specialists like speech and occupational therapists to try to understand the viewpoints and wishes of these children.

In certain circumstances in the ICU, the process of consent may be bypassed. This usually occurs during emergency treatment where an authorized decision-maker is not identified or available. In these scenarios, treatment may be provided with implied consent according to the standard of care with the understanding that the child and surrogate would have provided consent were they able (4,13,14). Importantly, this provision only applies during the acute emergency and does not extend beyond that point. For example, emergency

placement of a central venous catheter or endotracheal tube during resuscitation does not allow elective future placement of a more permanent venous access port or a tracheostomy.

Some children are at greater risk for progression of their disease necessitating urgent interventions, and are at greater risk for poor outcomes. Frequent discussions with a child's family about goals of care are crucial for these medically fragile children so that emergency interventions can be carried out in an ethical manner with as much informed consent as possible. These discussions can be of great benefit to the patient and family even if they are less structured than standard "advanced directives" which are authored by competent adult patients and describe the care they would wish to receive in various potentially end-of-life situations, clarifying preferences for interventions such as cardiopulmonary resuscitation or tracheal intubation. These can be in the form of a typed and signed letter, or better, on the official "out of hospital resuscitation status" forms that exist for most states in the United States (accessible at www.ohsu.edu/polst/programs/state+programs.htm). During the time that the patient is hospitalized, these preferences can be set forth in code status orders with an accompanying note in the medical record documenting the discussion on which the orders were based.

Providing Emotional, Social, and Spiritual Support

Having a gravely ill child in an ICU is an extraordinarily stressful and distressing experience for families. Parents of children with life-threatening diseases report that they turn for support to the medical team as well as their support network outside of the hospital, often (but not always) including a faith or religious community (15). Family members, including parents, siblings, and even grandparents, require ongoing emotional, social, and spiritual support during a childhood critical illness, particularly in the acute phases (16). These forms of support—which can range from helping a parent find a quite room to sleep to providing meal vouchers to the timely visit of a hospital chaplain—can demonstrate the caring feelings that the intensive care team extends to the family and the patient, help families to better cope with the situation, and in a variety of ways facilitate better communication and collaboration between the family and the medical team, and avert some potential conflicts.

Establishing a Pre-Illness Neurologic Baseline

Before prognosticating for a child with a neurologic injury, one must know the child's prior baseline. Brain injuries from strokes, hypoxia-ischemia, or trauma can have very different implications depending on baseline capabilities. Many children have normal baselines, meaning that they met their developmental milestones on time, performed appropriately in school, and had normal motor and cognitive functions. Children with chronic neurologic and developmental conditions may have had a wide range of abilities and limitations, ranging from mild learning disabilities or motor impairments to being nonverbal, noncommunicative, and totally dependent. Other children have progressive disorders like Duchenne muscular dystrophy, spinal muscular atrophy, or mitochondrial, metabolic, or genetic disorders; for these patients one must inquire about the patient's level of function or impairments before the injury.

When a child with a chronic static encephalopathy develops an infection, seizure, or dehydration, and is admitted to the ICU, the medical staff often passes judgment on the child's pre-illness neurologic impairment and poor quality of life. It is far better to pause, forestall judgment, and gather information. The medical team's assessment should incorporate both the medical (e.g., neurologic/developmental evaluations, therapist reports, neuroimaging and electroencephalographic [EEG]) data, and familial assessments (e.g., the parents' interpretation of the child's function) when determining the child's pre-illness neurologic baseline, covering domains like mental and respiratory status, motor function, communication (including language and cognition), feeding, and sensory function (e.g., hearing and vision) (17). Pictures and videos can be helpful in providing information about a child's prior behavior and neurologic condition. Acknowledging and agreeing upon a child's baseline can help minimize conflict and facilitate discussions about prognosis and outcomes. Focusing on capabilities and strengths instead of disabilities and weaknesses is particularly helpful.

Defining Quality of Life

The prognosis for a child's post-illness "quality of life"—typically focusing on pain and suffering, requirements for ongoing treatment, and levels of cognitive and motor function (17,18)—can be a great source of conflict between health care providers and families. Quality of life assessments are even more challenging after brain injury since the prediction of functional outcome is difficult and accuracy can vary by training and experience of the predictor (19–21).

Physicians and hospital staff must be careful about imposing their personal views and beliefs about quality of life when discussing treatment options and expectations of therapy with families. Several studies have demonstrated differences in attitude between physicians, nurses, and parents about the optimal treatment plan for children with severe impairment. One study found discrepancy between what neonatologists, cardiologists, and cardiac surgeons would recommend for children born with hypoplastic left heart syndrome and what they would want for their own children (22). Physicians were more likely to choose nonsurgical approaches for their own children than recommend them to families. Another study comparing neonatologists and neonatal nurses with adolescents and their parents found that a greater percentage of health care professionals thought a childhood of profound neurologic impairment was worse than death (23). Ultimately—and perhaps inevitably—basing treatment decisions on projected neurologic capabilities and quality of life is difficult, uncertain, and often painful for both parents and physicians.

Establishing the Goals of Care

Discrepancies between family goals of care and the medical team's assessment of likely outcomes are common sources of conflict and are usually best mediated proactively once detected, at the onset of a change in a child's condition, or when a prognostic milestone occurs, rather than allowing the discrepancy to linger into a protracted ICU course. While it is becoming more common for outpatient neurologists to discuss issues like life-sustaining therapies with families of children with chronic neurologic conditions, the responsibility to initiate conversations about acute treatment options, and their rationale often falls on the intensivist.

A common mistake made by intensivists is to ask families which specific therapies they want for their child without first clarifying the goals of care (24). Goals of care are usually articulated as pursuits, such as curing disease, alleviating pain and suffering, and improving or maintaining quality of life. Once goals of care have been established with the family, the intensivist can recommend interventions or treatments. Some therapies aim to cure disease or radically extend life, while others focus on enhancing physical or emotional comfort. Establishing goals of care serves to reinforce the therapeutic alliance between care team and family. If the family's goals of care are in the view of the intensive care team implausible, then this is a point for discussion.

Considering Palliative Care

Palliative care is often an option that warrants consideration for the care of children with grave neurologic injury or diseases. Palliative care focuses on improving a patient's quality of life, often by treating pain or other distressing systems, and also by attending to emotional, social, and spiritual needs. Compared to other modes of care, palliative care may place less emphasis on duration of life, yet most children who receive palliative care at the same time also receive a variety of life-prolonging treatments; to introduce palliative care into the mix of the child's overall treatment plan does not require foregoing other aspects of care. Starting palliative care does not require a limitation of resuscitation status, such as a do not attempt resuscitation order; one can get palliative care (or enroll in hospice) and still be a "full code." Starting palliative care also is not tantamount to the end of life; in a recent prospective cohort study of children receiving hospital-based palliative care services—a cohort in which many of the patients had underlying neurologic conditions—three-quarters of the patients were still alive after a year (25). Many children's hospitals have over the past decade established dedicated pediatric palliative care teams. Members of these teams are often adept at discussing a child's medical condition, goals of care, and treatment options with family members, and can help explain what palliative care is and can do for a child with a life-threatening condition.

Contemplating "Futility"

"Futility" is often mentioned during discussions about treatment options for the sickest patients in ICUs. Determining futility has important treatment implications because if an intervention is deemed futile, physicians do not have an ethical duty to prescribe it (13). The practical difficulty with using futility as an ethical argument for withholding or withdrawing therapy is that physicians are not uniform in their understandings of futility (26) or criteria for limiting life-sustaining

therapies (27), and often conflate futility with vague expressions like "uncommon," "rare," "hopeless," or "useless" (28). If futility has a useful meaning, it is built upon goals of treatment and the likelihood of therapeutic success with regard to those goals.

The concept and application of futility is hotly debated. Some scholars view futility disputes as a power struggle between physicians and children and their families (29). Others see these disputes as the consequence of the breakdown of the physician-patient relationship. If futility determinations are serving as a facade for quality of life assessments, they should be identified as such and dealt with accordingly (30). These concerns notwithstanding, medical futility, while debated in academic circles and hospital committees, has a lower incidence in ICUs than one may expect given the severity of the illnesses managed there. One study conducted in pediatric ICUs found that only 2.7% of patient-days met at least one definition of futility (31). In clinical situations with potential for futile care, the issues should be identified and addressed prospectively.

Preventing Miscommunication

Miscommunication can occur on many levels during a child's ICU stay, and commonly results from inconsistent or incomplete sharing of clinical data, assessment, prognosis, or treatment recommendations. Miscommunication can occur between the medical team and family or between the primary medical team and consultants. In one prospective study, physicians and nurses were asked about conflict sources for children whose ICU stay exceeded 8 days, and reported that 60% of all conflicts were between the medical team and families (1). Poor communication (48%), unavailability of parents (39%), and disagreements over the care plan (39%) were most commonly cited.

Avoiding miscommunication can be challenging, especially when children have complex, multisystem involvement to their illness, unclear prognosis, and no standard treatment. The keys to prevention are open discussion regarding the unfolding clinical course, consensus on the treatment plan, and complete transparency in discussions with families. Many institutions now have a family centered care approach and allow parents to participate in daily rounds (32). This model intimately includes parents in their child's care and provides a forum to speak about their child's condition and treatment plan. Meetings with the family can also facilitate better communication. Approaches to family conferences vary widely and often depend on the personality and experience of the primary attending physician and the availability of other staff including social workers, chaplains, and nurses. Several guides are available for how to structure and lead effective family conferences (24,33), as well as offering more general communication strategies and suggestions for discussing distressing information with children and families (34,35).

Managing Framing

Framing refers to the portrayal of facts when explaining potential care options, and can include changes in inflection, facial expressions, and gestures. Framing can influence a parent's informed decision (13,24,36). Framing also plays a key role when phrasing questions to assess preferences or presenting outcome statistics. For example, when discussing a child's resuscitation status, Murphy and colleagues (37,38) got different responses asking "Would you want us to do everything possible to save your life if your heart stopped beating?" versus explaining CPR mechanics and showing outcomes. Studies have also found that absolute risk reduction is less misleading than relative risk reduction when talking about therapeutic options, and that the order of information and time frame of outcomes can bias understanding (39). Some experts recommend double framing to minimize bias, wherein parents are presented the chances of benefit and no benefit (24). For example, instead of saying, "There is an 80% to 90% chance that treatment will not help," the statement could be double framed by saying, "There is an 80% to 90% chance that treatment will not help, which also means there is a 10% to 20% chance that it will help." Because framing can profoundly influence treatment decisions, physicians should be as mindful to frame treatment options and recommendations appropriately.

Handling Prognostic Uncertainty and Timeliness

Neurologic prognostication has evolved from simply estimating the probability of survival to predicting recovery of function. Extensive research has assessed prognosis after events like cardiac arrest and traumatic brain injury (40–42). Most studies have focused on mortality statistics, but some more recent studies have evaluated functional outcomes (17,43). Attempts have also been made to use information like exam findings, secondary systemic injuries, neuroimaging findings, biochemical markers, and electrophysiologic markers to help clarify the severity of injury and chance of recovery (41,44–46). Unfortunately, the data in these studies are too coarse to guide individual patient care, especially in pediatric patients where injuries vary greatly and data are more limited. Several functional outcome measures have been developed to minimize dependence on subjective assessments and apply to the broadest possible age range (17,47,48). Further complicating neuroprognostication is the influence of individual physicians making the prognosis, as one study found that prognostication profiles exist among intensivists and vary according to age and clinical experience (21). It is essential to involve consultants, particularly neurologists, developmental pediatricians, and physical medicine and rehabilitation specialists as these clinicians are usually the ones to provide long-term care for these children and may offer valuable advice in predicting whether goals of care are attainable.

The timeliness of prognostication is another great challenge if the prognosis is to be of use in guiding treatment toward either a radical life-extending path or a palliative care path. After brain injury, the extent of injury is often not evident until swelling and inflammation have subsided. If the child is technologically supported through the acute phase of their brain injury and has time to recover from secondary injuries, and only then the prognosis clearly becomes one of a permanent vegetative state—which may be contrary to the goals of care—then there are no intensive life-sustaining therapies to withdraw. The withholding or cessation of artificially routed nutrition and hydration, which in adults can be justified if the adult patient had previously expressed a preference to not be sustained in an highly impaired state through the use of artificially routed nutrition and hydration, is viewed by many to be different in children who never have had the cognitive capacity to hold or express such a preference. If the provision of artificially routed nutrition and hydration is a cause of ongoing suffering to the child, then it can be stopped (as can any therapy when the benefits are outweighed by the harms), but because "feeding" is such a fundamental aspect of what adults do for children, and stopping feeding and providing hydration has such a certain fatal outcome, the process of doing so requires much deliberation, communication, and collaboration with the family and the medical staff.

Deciding on the Extent of Testing

Questions often arise as to how much information is necessary prior to confidence in a prognosis. Are clinical exams after the injury sufficient, or do advanced tests like EEG and magnetic resonance imaging (MRI) provide essential information? One study found that abnormal exam signs (pupil reactivity and motor response), absent N20 waves bilaterally on sensory evoked potentials, electrocerebral silence or burst suppression patterns on EEG, and abnormal MRI with diffusion restriction in the cortex and basal ganglia are each highly predictive of poor outcome when performed 24 hours after injury (41). If these diagnostic tools do provide crucial information, it is unclear exactly when these tests should be performed to reveal the nature and severity of injury.

Physicians should also be prepared to address the potentially added value of primarily research-based functional neuroimaging studies as another window into the current and potential functionality of the brain. It is still unclear whether noninvasive advanced neuroimaging like functional MRI, positron emission tomography, arterial spin labeled perfusion MRI, or neuromodulatory technology like transcranial magnetic stimulation or transcranial direct current stimulation contribute vital data to neurologic prognosis. Several neuroimaging studies have examined patients in vegetative and minimally conscious states and shown that some speech perception, emotional processing, command following, language comprehension, and even conscious awareness might be retained in some behaviorally vegetative patients (49–51). While these results raise the possibility of misdiagnosis or misclassification, they show an opportunity for imaging technology to be helpful in diagnosing, classifying, and prognosticating. Functional imaging may be able to identify children who will benefit from rehabilitation services or those whose conditions are irreversible. In the near future, families may request or demand these scans as confirmatory tests prior to decisions about life-sustaining therapies. The ultimate goal of this type of imaging is not to replace clinical assessments, but to aid in improving diagnosis and prognostication. This evolving technology may become key in characterizing brain function after injury, but for now one must be transparent when discussing the capabilities and limitations of this technology with families who seek functional imaging.

Determining Whether Brain Death Has Occurred

Physicians, ethicists, and lawmakers have worked to define brain death, particularly in children, and especially with modern life-sustaining technologies and the potential for organ donation after death (4,52–56). Conflicts can arise over the meaning of brain death and the cessation of support after brain death as there is widespread misunderstanding about brain death in the public, media, and among physicians and nurses (57–59).

Brain death can be difficult for parents and families to comprehend, especially when life signs such as heartbeat, warmth, and breathing are present (60). Because these visible signs exist, families may disagree with the diagnosis of death and insist that mechanical support continue. Although most major western religions have accepted the concept of brain death, some families, particularly from some conservative Roman Catholic or Orthodox Jewish communities, believe that cessation of the heart is the only sign of death (4). In situations where families do not accept the diagnosis, physicians must effectively communicate the concept, criteria, and legality of brain death. Since a child who has been declared brain dead is medically and legally dead, physicians should be careful to avoid delivering contradictory messages. For example, referring to ventilation as "life-support" is inaccurate since the child is dead. Similarly, phrases like "allowing the child to die" when extubating convey mixed messages since the child has already died. Taken to the extreme, some argue that family permission should not be required to turn off the ventilator after brain death since permission would not be requested after circulatory failure. Despite physicians' best efforts to explain the finality of brain death, there have been reports of brain-dead people being mechanically ventilated for months or years (61).

Most families understand the diagnosis of brain death and agree to stop intensive interventions. Families who do not accept the diagnosis or finality of brain death must be handled compassionately and diplomatically. While withdrawal is legal, doing so may create anxiety and guilt among family members and medical staff. Physicians have an ethical responsibility in these situations to balance legal obligations, avoidance of futile therapies, respect for family wishes, compassionate care, and limited medical resources (4,62).

Discharging from the ICU

Disposition from the ICU can present ethical dilemmas or disputes. While most parents want to take their children home, this might not be the best or safest option, and caring for these children at home is often a logistical and financial struggle. Every situation is unique. Social workers, discharge planners, therapists, and physical medicine and rehabilitation specialists can be valuable when deciding the optimal location after discharge. Factors such as insurance coverage, county services, and geographic proximity of facilities affect the family's options. There is an ethical obligation to advocate appropriately for home nursing care, which is often essential for children with neurologic injury, especially if the child is technology dependent. If the medical team's collective judgment is that home is not the best location for ongoing care for the child and conflict arises with the family, consultation of an ethics consultant may be helpful.

Seeking Ethics Consultation

Ethical dilemmas are inevitable when dealing with sick children, particularly critically ill children with neurologic problems. Physicians and medical teams often need ethical advice on decisions or conflicts within or between the team and the family. An interdisciplinary ethics consultation service or ethics advisory committee can help identify and analyze ethical problems and find a resolution (63,64). While their recommendations can and often do steer clinical decisions, the attending physician is ultimately responsible for a child's care (65). Ethics committees and consultation procedures vary by institution, but any member of the care team, including physicians, nurses, therapists, residents, fellows, social workers, and family, should be able to seek consultation. Neurologists or neurosurgeons must participate in cases dealing with neurologic injury, as they can provide an experienced and specialized neurologic exam, offer guidance on prognosis, and clarify criteria for brain death and vegetative states. Ethicists have devised several methods for approaching medical-ethical dilemmas in current practice (4,66,67,68), including one adopted by the American Academy of Neurology Ethics, Law and Humanities Committee as a tool to analyze ethics teaching cases (69).

While barriers exist to ethics consultation (70,71), several studies have shown that physicians and care providers find consultation advice valuable in resolving conflict (72,73). In one multicenter randomized controlled trial of ethics consultations in the adult ICU, 87% of physicians, nurses, and patients or surrogates found that ethics consultation was helpful in addressing treatment conflict, and more than 90% of physicians and nurses would seek consultation again (74). Proactive ethics consultation is one way to maintain communication between care teams and families and has been shown to reduce length of stay in the ICU for dying patients (75).

The boundaries of "standard" and appropriate medical practice are clarified not only by ethical considerations but also by laws. When irreconcilable differences in goals of care or specific treatment plans persist, despite the best efforts of the primary care intensivist team and the ethics consultants, hospital legal counsel can help clarify what is permitted by law in these situations and may provide guidance regarding how to proceed.

■ CONCLUSION

The care of children with acute neurologic injuries, which is inherently complex and demanding, can benefit by proactively anticipating some of the potential sources of ethical conflict that commonly arise when devising and implementing treatment plans for these children. This chapter provides a framework that aims to allow neurointensivists and the patients and families that they serve to feel more secure in their decisions and collaborate more effectively in the care of their patients and children.

■ REFERENCES

1. Studdert DM et al. Nature of conflict in the care of pediatric intensive care patients with prolonged stay. *Pediatrics*. 2003;112:553–558.
2. Benitz WE. A paradigm for making difficult choices in the intensive care nursery. *Camb Q Healthc Ethics*. 1993;2:281–294.
3. Lo B. Assessing decision-making capacity. *Law Med Health Care*. 1990;18:193–201.
4. Bernat JL. *Ethical Issues in Neurology*. 3rd ed. Philadelphia, PA: Wolters Kluwer/Lippincott Williams & Wilkins; 2008.

5. Informed consent, parental permission, and assent in pediatric practice. Committee on Bioethics, American Academy of Pediatrics. *Pediatrics*. 1995;95:314–317.
6. Hickey K. Minors' rights in medical decision making. *JONAS Healthc Law Ethics Regul*. 2007;9:100–104; quiz 105–106.
7. Sigman GS, O'Connor C. Exploration for physicians of the mature minor doctrine. *J Pediatr*. 1991;119:520–525.
8. Diaz A et al. Legal and ethical issues facing adolescent health care professionals. *Mt Sinai J Med*. 2004;71:181–185.
9. Weithorn LA, Campbell SB. The competency of children and adolescents to make informed treatment decisions. *Child Dev*. 1982;53:1589–1598.
10. Shield JP, Baum JD. Children's consent to treatment. *BMJ*. 1994;308:1182–1183.
11. Braunack-Mayer A, Hersh D. An ethical voice in the silence of aphasia: judging understanding and consent in people with aphasia. *J Clin Ethics*. 2001;12:388–396.
12. Stein J, Brady Wagner LC. Is informed consent a "yes or no" response? Enhancing the shared decision-making process for persons with aphasia. *Top Stroke Rehabil*. 2006;13:42–46.
13. Beauchamp TL, Childress JF. *Principles of Biomedical Ethics*. 6th ed. New York, NY: Oxford University Press; 2009.
14. Rosoff AJ. Treatment undertaken without express consent. *Med Staff Couns*. 1989;3:7–14.
15. Hexem KR et al. How parents of children receiving pediatric palliative care use religion, spirituality, or life philosophy in tough times. *J Palliat Med*. 2011;14:39–44.
16. Shudy M et al. Impact of pediatric critical illness and injury on families: a systematic literature review. *Pediatrics*. 2006;118(suppl 3):S203–S218.
17. Pollack MM et al. Functional Status Scale: new pediatric outcome measure. *Pediatrics*. 2009;124:e18–e28.
18. Vazquez Mata G et al. Analysis of quality of life in polytraumatized patients two years after discharge from an intensive care unit. *J Trauma*. 1996;41:326–332.
19. Marcin JP et al. Prognostication and certainty in the pediatric intensive care unit. *Pediatrics*. 1999;104:868–873.
20. Marcin JP et al. Certainty and mortality prediction in critically ill children. *J Med Ethics*. 2004;30:304–307.
21. Racine E et al. Profiles of neurological outcome prediction among intensivists. *Neurocrit Care*. 2009.
22. Kon AA, Ackerson L, Lo B. Choices physicians would make if they were the parents of a child with hypoplastic left heart syndrome. *Am J Cardiol*. 2003;91:1506–1509, A1509.
23. Saigal S et al. Differences in preferences for neonatal outcomes among health care professionals, parents, and adolescents. *JAMA*. 1999;281:1991–1997.
24. Larriviere D, Williams, MA. Neurocritical care. In: Torbey MT, ed. *Neurocritical Care*. Cambridge, MA: Cambridge University Press; 2010:308–318.
25. Feudtner C et al. Pediatric palliative care patients: a prospective multicenter cohort study. *Pediatrics*. 2011;127:1094–1101.
26. Solomon MZ. How physicians talk about futility: making words mean too many things. *J Law Med Ethics*. 1993;21:231–237.
27. Randolph AG et al. Variability in physician opinion on limiting pediatric life support. *Pediatrics*. 1999;103:e46.
28. Schneiderman LJ, Jecker NS, Jonsen AR. Medical futility: its meaning and ethical implications. *Ann Intern Med*. 1990;112:949–954.
29. Morreim EH. Profoundly diminished life. The casualties of coercion. *Hastings Cent Rep*. 1994;24:33–42.
30. Lantos J. When parents request seemingly futile treatment for their children. *Mt Sinai J Med*. 2006;73:587–589.
31. Sachdeva RC et al. Resource consumption and the extent of futile care among patients in a pediatric intensive care unit setting. *J Pediatr*. 1996;128:742–747.
32. Muething SE et al. Family-centered bedside rounds: a new approach to patient care and teaching. *Pediatrics*. 2007;119:829–832.
33. Hardart G, Devictor, DJ, Truog, RD. Ethics. In: Nichols DG, ed. *Rogers' Textbook of Pediatric Intensive Care*. 4th ed. Philadelphia, PA: Wolters Kluwer/Lippincott Williams & Wilkins; 2008:xxxi, 1839 p.
34. Levetown M. Communicating with children and families: from everyday interactions to skill in conveying distressing information. *Pediatrics*. 2008;121:e1441–e1460.
35. Feudtner C. Collaborative communication in pediatric palliative care: a foundation for problem-solving and decision-making. *Pediatr Clin North Am*. 2007;54:583–607, ix.
36. Tversky A, Kahneman D. The framing of decisions and the psychology of choice. *Science (NY)*. 1981;211:453–458.
37. Murphy DJ. Do-not-resuscitate orders. Time for reappraisal in long-term-care institutions. *JAMA*. 1988;260:2098–2101.
38. Murphy DJ et al. The influence of the probability of survival on patients' preferences regarding cardiopulmonary resuscitation. *N Engl J Med*. 1994;330:545–549.
39. Epstein RM, Alper BS, Quill TE. Communicating evidence for participatory decision making. *JAMA*. 2004;291:2359–2366.
40. Jagannathan J et al. Long-term outcomes and prognostic factors in pediatric patients with severe traumatic brain injury and elevated intracranial pressure. *J Neurosurg*. 2008;2:240–249.
41. Abend NS, Licht DJ. Predicting outcome in children with hypoxic ischemic encephalopathy. *Pediatr Crit Care Med*. 2008;9:32–39.
42. Moler FW et al. In-hospital versus out-of-hospital pediatric cardiac arrest: a multicenter cohort study. *Crit Care Med*. 2009;37:2259–2267.
43. Johnson P et al. Long-term outcomes of pediatric acquired brain injury. *Brain Cogn*. 2006;60:205–206.
44. Moran LM et al. Apolipoprotein E4 as a predictor of outcomes in pediatric mild traumatic brain injury. *J Neurotrauma*. 2009;26:1489–1495.
45. Figaji AA et al. Pressure autoregulation, intracranial pressure, and brain tissue oxygenation in children with severe traumatic brain injury. *J Neurosurg*. 2009;4:420–428.
46. Lo TY, Jones PA, Minns RA. Pediatric brain trauma outcome prediction using paired serum levels of inflammatory mediators and brain-specific proteins. *J Neurotrauma*. 2009;26:1479–1487.
47. Fiser DH et al. Relationship of pediatric overall performance category and pediatric cerebral performance category scores at pediatric intensive care unit discharge with outcome measures collected at hospital discharge and 1- and 6-month follow-up assessments. *Crit Care Med*. 2000;28:2616–2620.
48. Fiser DH. Assessing the outcome of pediatric intensive care. *J Pediatr*. 1992;121:68–74.

49. Schiff ND et al. fMRI reveals large-scale network activation in minimally conscious patients. *Neurology*. 2005;64:514–523.

50. Owen AM, Coleman MR. Functional neuroimaging of the vegetative state. *Nat Rev Neurosci*. 2008;9:235–243.

51. Owen AM et al. Detecting awareness in the vegetative state. *Science (NY)*. 2006;313:1402.

52. Farrell MM, Levin DL. Brain death in the pediatric patient: historical, sociological, medical, religious, cultural, legal, and ethical considerations. *Crit Care Med*. 1993;21:1951–1965.

53. Shemie SD et al. Diagnosis of brain death in children. *Lancet Neurol*. 2007;6:87–92.

54. Veatch RM. *The Basics of Bioethics*. 2nd ed. Upper Saddle River, NJ: Prentice Hall; 2003.

55. Ashwal S, Serna-Fonseca T. Brain death in infants and children. *Crit Care Nurse*. 2006;26:117–124, 126–118.

56. Nakagawa TA et al. Guidelines for the determination of brain death in infants and children: an update of the 1987 Task Force recommendations. *Crit Care Med*. 2011;39:2139–2155.

57. Youngner SJ et al. 'Brain death' and organ retrieval. A cross-sectional survey of knowledge and concepts among health professionals. *JAMA*. 1989;261:2205–2210.

58. Siminoff LA, Burant C, Youngner SJ. Death and organ procurement: public beliefs and attitudes. *Kennedy Inst Ethics J*. 2004;14:217–234.

59. Harrison AM, Botkin JR. Can pediatricians define and apply the concept of brain death? *Pediatrics*. 1999;103:e82.

60. Hardwig J. Treating the brain dead for the benefit of the family. *TJ Clin Ethics*. 1991;2:53–56.

61. Shewmon DA. Chronic "brain death": meta-analysis and conceptual consequences. *Neurology*. 1998;51:1538–1545.

62. Cranford RE. Discontinuation of ventilation after brain death. Policy should be balanced with concern for the family. *BMJ*. 1999;318:1754–1755.

63. Fletcher JC, Siegler M. What are the goals of ethics consultation? A consensus statement. *J Clin Ethics*. 1996;7:122–126.

64. Schneiderman LJ. Ethics consultation in the intensive care unit. *Curr Opin Crit Care*. 2005;11:600–604.

65. American Medical Association. Council on Ethical and Judicial Affairs. *Code of Medical Ethics: Current Opinions with Annotations*. Chicago, IL: American Medical Association; 2010.

66. Snyder L, Leffler C. Ethics manual: fifth edition. *Ann Intern Med*. 2005;142:560–582.

67. Lo B. *Resolving Ethical Dilemmas: A Guide for Clinicians*. 4th ed. Philadelphia, PA: Wolters Kluwer Lippincott Williams & Wilkins; 2009.

68. Siegler M. Decision-making strategy for clinical-ethical problems in medicine. *Arch Intern Med*. 1982;142:2178–2179.

69. Fletcher JC et al. *Fletcher's Introduction to Clinical Ethics*. 3rd ed. Hagerstown, MD: University Pub. Group; 2005.

70. Davies L, Hudson LD. Why don't physicians use ethics consultation? *J Clin Ethics*. 1999;10:116–125.

71. DuVal G et al. A national survey of U.S. internists' experiences with ethical dilemmas and ethics consultation. *J Gen Intern Med*. 2004;19:251–258.

72. Schneiderman LJ. Effect of ethics consultations in the intensive care unit. *Crit Care Med*. 2006;34:S359–S363.

73. Schneiderman LJ, Gilmer T, Teetzel HD. Impact of ethics consultations in the intensive care setting: a randomized, controlled trial. *Crit Care Med*. 2000;28:3920–3924.

74. Schneiderman LJ et al. Effect of ethics consultations on nonbeneficial life-sustaining treatments in the intensive care setting: a randomized controlled trial. *JAMA*. 2003;290:1166–1172.

75. Dowdy MD, Robertson C, Bander JA. A study of proactive ethics consultation for critically and terminally ill patients with extended lengths of stay. *Crit Care Med*. 1998;26:252–259.

Index

Note: Locators followed by '*f*' and '*t*' refer to figures and tables respectively.